Essential Neurology Board Review Q & A

Tyler Ellis Smith • Vito Arena

Editors

Essential Neurology Board Review Q & A

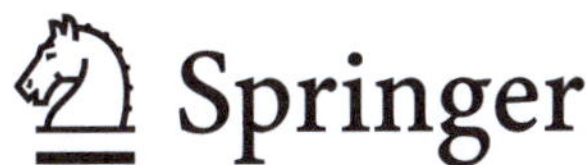 Springer

Editors
Tyler Ellis Smith
Neurology - Multiple Sclerosis
New York University Langone Medical Center
New York, NY, USA

Vito Arena
Neurology - Multiple Sclerosis
New York University Langone Medical Center
New York, NY, USA

ISBN 978-3-032-17212-9   ISBN 978-3-032-17213-6 (eBook)
https://doi.org/10.1007/978-3-032-17213-6

This Springer imprint is published by the registered company Springer Nature Switzerland AG
The registered company address is: Gewerbestrasse 11, 6330 Cham, Switzerland

If disposing of this product, please recycle the paper.

To students, residents, fellows, and all lifelong learners, remember why we learn and study. Remember the patient, the person coming to you for help.
To my daughter, Lily, I love you.
—Tyler Smith, MD.
To my daughter, Remi. You'll always be my baby girl, you pinky-promised. I love you.
—Vito Arena, MD.

Foreword

It is with honor and enthusiasm that I introduce *Essential Neurology Board Review Q&A*—a valuable tool designed to support students, residents, and all learners in mastering the complex and ever-evolving field of neurology. As a Program Director of an adult neurology residency for 9 plus years, I have seen firsthand the critical role that active learning plays in developing both foundational knowledge and clinical acumen. I appreciate learners' eagerness for "bite sized" information, repetition, and reinforcement. This book provides just that.

Now more than ever there is so much to learn and know about the field of neurology to take comprehensive and holistic care of our patients. What makes this book particularly effective is its balance between breadth and depth. It covers essential topics across the spectrum of neurological disease while emphasizing the clinical relevance of each question. The real-world application of neurologic knowledge is exactly the skill we educators aim to develop in our trainees.

The authors of this book bring a vast array and diversity of expertise. I applaud them for creating a resource that provides succinct overviews of each topic, practical frameworks for approach to neurologic symptoms, and practice questions with illustrative explanations and references for further reading. I am confident this book will contribute to the tools we need to build successful neurologists.

New York, NY, USA   Arielle Kurzweil

Introduction

Dear Colleague,

We hope this book finds you well—getting adequate sleep, eating healthy, and with only a modicum of stress.

We write this book to help you understand some of the key topics in neurology and prepare for the neurology board exam. We have recruited authors from across various subspecialties to write questions highlighting some of the most important and up-to-date topics in neurology. You may notice some overlap in question topics throughout these chapters, and this underscores the interconnected nature of neurology in this age.

We recommend approaching these questions as if you are taking the board exam, review the answers, and then pursue a deeper dive into the associated references for areas of interest or difficulty. The explanations are designed to both elaborate on the correct answer, but equally important, to provide background and understanding of the incorrect options to broaden your understanding.

Whether you are in the final stages of residency or fellowship and preparing for your board exam, or reading this at the start of your residency, we hope studying this book will prove to be an enlightening experience for you.

All the best, Tyler Smith, Vito Arena

New York, NY, USA

Tyler Smith
Vito Arena

Contents

Sleep Medicine

Michelle Goodman and Tejwant Bindra

1. A 35-year-old female corrections officer is requested to work a double shift which involves working overnight. She is found unintentionally napping at her station reporting inability to maintain wakefulness. Which brain structure is primarily involved in promoting her sleepiness?
   A. Ventrolateral preoptic nucleus (VLPO)
   B. Suprachiasmatic nucleus (SCN)
   C. Ascending reticular activation system (ARAS)
   D. Lateral pontine tegmentum
   Correct answer: A

Explanation

The VLPO plays a prominent role in promoting sleep by releasing inhibitory neurotransmitters. These neurotransmitters suppress the wake-promoting regions of our brain, primarily located within the ARAS. Given this patient's symptoms, the brain structure primarily involved in promoting sleep is the VLPO.

The SCN, considered the central circadian clock or pacemaker, is located within the anterior hypothalamus. It does not directly promote sleep, but instead uses sensory input such as light to create our daily rhythm. This patient's circadian rhythm is likely misaligned given her night shifts, but her SCN is not directly promoting sleepiness.

The ARAS is a wake-promoting network which arises in the brainstem and projects to the thalamus and cortex, promoting arousal. Pathological dysfunctions of the ARAS can result in sleepiness.

The lateral pontine tegmentum is also part of the sleep-wake circuitry. It has cholinergic neurons which are involved in the generation of REM sleep.

M. Goodman
NYU Langone, New York, NY, USA
e-mail: Michelle.Goodman@nyulangone.org

T. Bindra (✉)
Child Neurology/Epilepsy/Sleep Medicine, NYU Langone-Long Island, New York, NY, USA
e-mail: Tejwant.Bindra@nyulangone.org

Reference

Patel AK, Reddy V, Shumway KR, et al. Physiology, Sleep Stages. [Updated 2024 Jan 26]. In: StatPearls [Internet]. Treasure Island (FL): StatPearls Publishing; 2025 Jan-.

2. Neurotransmitters are involved in sleep promoting and wake promoting. Which of these neurotransmitters is incorrectly paired with the neural structure it is released from?
   A. Locus coeruleus—norepinephrine
   B. tuberomammillary nucleus—histamine
   C. lateral hypothalamus—orexin
   D. basal forebrain—serotonin
   Correct answer: D

Explanation

The locus coeruleus releases norepinephrine which plays a prominent role in promoting wakefulness and arousal.

The tuberomammillary nucleus of the hypothalamus is the only known location in the brain that produces histamine, which functions to promote wakefulness.

The lateral hypothalamus releases orexin (hypocretin), which is important in maintaining wakefulness and transitioning between sleep and awake states. Dysfunction here is central to the mechanism behind narcolepsy.

The basal forebrain releases acetylcholine, not serotonin. The release of acetylcholine from the basal forebrain increases cortical activation and subsequently promotes both wakefulness and REM sleep. Serotonin is produced in the raphe nuclei, which is located in the brainstem (Table 1.1).

Reference

Patel AK, Reddy V, Shumway KR, et al. Physiology, Sleep Stages. [Updated 2024 Jan 26]. In: StatPearls [Internet]. Treasure Island (FL): StatPearls Publishing; 2025 Jan-.

3. A 45-year-old female presents to the office with complaints that she has minimal to no sleep almost every night. She has a history of hypertension well managed

T. E. Smith, V. Arena (eds.), *Essential Neurology Board Review Q & A*, https://doi.org/10.1007/978-3-032-17213-6_1

Table 1.1 Main neurotransmitters/neuromodulators associated sleep/wake function and area of release

Neurotransmitter	Primary brain region of release	Function
Norepinephrine	Locus coeruleus	Promotes wakefulness, arousal
Histamine	Tuberomammillary nucleus (hypothalamus)	Promotes wakefulness
Orexin (Hypocretin)	Lateral hypothalamus	Promotes wakefulness
Serotonin	Raphe nuclei (brainstem)	Promotes wakefulness
Acetylcholine	Basal forebrain, laterodorsal/pedunculopontine tegmentum	Promotes wakefulness and REM sleep
Dopamin	Ventral tegmental area (VTA), substantia nigra	Promotes wakefulness and REM sleep
Glutamate	Presynaptic vesicles in nerve terminals	Promotes wakefulness and REM sleep
GABA	Ventrolateral preoptic nucleus (VLPO)	Promotes sleep, inhibits arousal systems
Galanin	Ventrolateral preoptic nucleus (VLPO)	Promotes sleep, inhibits arousal systems
Adenosine (neuromodulator)	Intracellularly throughout the CNS	Promotes sleep, inhibits arousal systems

with metoprolol and anxiety disorder well managed on Lexapro. She goes to bed at 10 pm every night but has trouble initiating sleep. Once asleep, she will have frequent arousals, tossing and turning throughout the night. She feels she gets her best sleep in the early morning when she has to wake at 7 am. This makes waking in the morning difficult. She feels excessive fatigue throughout the day. No unintentional napping reported. She attempted several behavioral modifications including decreasing screen time prior to bedtime without impact. She reports that her mind is often moving topic to topic although there is no acute stressor. She has tried melatonin and diphenhydramine with intermittent impact but not sustained. She feels the lack of sleep affects her daytime function and performance at work, which frustrates her. Which of the following is true regarding this condition?

A. Associated with agrypnia excitata
B. Cognitive behavioral therapy added to medications options does not provide additional benefit over medications alone
C. Can be comorbid with other medical and psychiatric conditions
D. Is considered chronic if occurs for >1 month

Correct answer: C

Explanation

This patient presents with hallmark features of chronic insomnia, demonstrating difficulty with sleep initiation and maintenance, non-restorative sleep, and worsening fatigue and daytime function. The chronic nature of her symptoms (occurring most nights for more than 3 months) and the absence of a clear, reversible cause are consistent with a diagnosis of chronic insomnia disorder.

Insomnia can be comorbid with other medical and psychiatric conditions. Chronic insomnia is often seen with other conditions such as substance abuse, depression, anxiety, chronic pain, cardiovascular disease, and neurological disorders, among others. Insomnia can be both a symptom and an independent risk factor for psychiatric disorders. While this patient's anxiety appears well controlled, it is common for cognitive arousal such as racing thoughts without overt anxiety, to contribute to insomnia.

Agrypnia excitata is an extremely rare and severe form of insomnia associated with conditions such as fatal familial insomnia and Morvan syndrome. These disorders are characterized with a progressive loss of sleep, autonomic dysfunction, and neuropsychiatric symptoms, which is fortunately not seen in this patient.

Cognitive behavioral therapy for insomnia (CBT-I) is the first-line treatment for chronic insomnia and has been shown to be more effective long-term than pharmacotherapy alone. Combining CBT-I with medications may offer short-term benefit, but medications alone are typically not curative and come with their own risks, such as dependence and tolerance.

Current diagnostic criteria define chronic insomnia as symptoms occurring at least 3 nights per week for at least 3 months. Insomnia occurring for less than 3 months is considered short-term insomnia.

Reference

Schutte-Rodin S; Broch L; Buysse D; Dorsey C; Sateia M. Clinical guideline for the evaluation and management of chronic insomnia in adults. *J Clin Sleep Med 2008*;4(5):487–504.

4. Which of the following sleep promoting agents is incorrectly paired with the target receptor?
   A. Zolpidem is a GABA-A receptor agonist
   B. Ramelteon is melatonin receptor agonist
   C. Diphenhydramine is a histamine receptor antagonist
   D. Suvorexant is an orexin receptor agonist

Correct answer: D

Explanation

Medications that facilitate sleep often do so by enhancement of gamma-aminobutyric acid (GABA) but there are also other mechanisms of action to promote sleep.

Zolpidem is a "non benzodiazepine" benzodiazepine receptor agonist that binds selectively to the benzodiazepine-1 subunit of the GABA-A receptor, enhancing inhibitory neurotransmission and promoting sleep onset.

Ramelteon acts as a melatonin receptor agonist, specifically targeting melatonin receptor-1 (MT1) and melatonin receptor-2 (MT2) in the suprachiasmatic nucleus of the hypothalamus. These receptors help regulate sleep initiation and phase shifting effects of melatonin on circadian rhythms, making ramelteon useful for sleep-onset insomnia.

Diphenhydramine, an over-the-counter antihistamine, promotes sleep through histamine H1 receptor antagonism. Histamine plays a key role in maintaining wakefulness, and blocking its action can lead to sedation.

Suvorexant is actually an orexin receptor antagonist, not an agonist. It blocks the orexin-1 and orexin-2 receptors, which are involved in promoting wakefulness. By inhibiting the orexin system, suvorexant reduces arousal and facilitates sleep onset and maintenance.

Reference

Sateia MJ, Buysse DJ, Krystal AD, Neubauer DN, Heald JL. Clinical practice guideline for the pharmacologic treatment of chronic insomnia in adults: an American Academy of Sleep Medicine clinical practice guideline. *J Clin Sleep Med.* 2017;13(2):307–349.

5. A 17-year-old female presents with complaints of trouble initiating sleep and excessive daytime somnolence. She will usually have an unintentional nap on the sofa for around 30 min before eating dinner. She will then sit on her bed to complete her homework followed by watching TV until her planned 10 pm bedtime. She is unable to sleep until 12–1 am during which time she will watch something on her phone which she feels relaxes her. Once asleep, she does not usually wake until morning. Her parents report difficulty waking her in the morning at 6 am. She usually falls asleep on the ride to school, and her teachers have been noticing unintentional napping during classes throughout the day. Which of the following is the most likely cause of her complaints?
   A. Inadequate sleep hygiene
   B. Psychophysiologic insomnia
   C. Paradoxical insomnia
   D. Behavioral insomnia of childhood
   Correct answer: A

Explanation

The features that this teenager is presenting with are most consistent with inadequate sleep hygiene, which involve behaviors and environmental factors which impede her ability to fall asleep. Some examples as portrayed in this case include the use of her bed/bedroom for activities other than sleep, evening naps, and prolonged screen time before bedtime.

Psychophysiologic insomnia is a condition in which patients become anxious while trying to fall asleep, leading to a learned association of the bed with an inability to sleep. There is no report of excessive focus or worry about sleep in this patient. These patients will usually find it easier to sleep in a setting away from their typical sleep environment such as when on vacation.

Paradoxical insomnia, previously known as sleep state misperception, consists of an individual underestimating the amount of sleep they are attaining as can be proven by polysomnography or actigraphy data.

Behavioral insomnia of childhood refers to issues with sleep usually in younger children due to learned patterns or behaviors which impede the ability to fall asleep independently. The two common subtypes are sleep onset association and limit setting. In sleep onset association type, the child has a specific setting or object required to initiate or return to sleep. In limit setting type, there is often stalling or bedtime refusal due to inadequate limits set by the parent or caregiver.

Reference

American Academy of Sleep Medicine. International classification of sleep disorders, 3rd ed. Darien, IL: American Academy of Sleep Medicine, 2014; 19–46.

6. A 38-year-old male with history of a Chiari I malformation presents with progressively increasing night-time awakenings and worsening unrefreshed sleep. He has more lately reported gasping arousals at times feeling like he was not breathing. This will often scare him and prevent him from returning to sleep. He has never been told he snores. He reports when idle for longer periods during the day like watching TV he will have unintentional napping. He has a BMI of 24 and Mallampati class 2 airway. Polysomnography obtained in further evaluation revealed multiple episodes throughout the night of cessation of airflow with absent signs of respiratory effort. Which of the following is correct regarding this condition?
   A. Surgical intervention is unlikely to improve these events
   B. This condition may also be associated with congestive heart failure and high-altitude situations
   C. Is not associated with an increased risk for adverse cardiovascular outcomes
   D. Low chemoreceptor sensitivity to changes in carbon dioxide (CO_2) will result in worsening of these events
   Correct answer: B

Explanation

This patient is presenting with signs consistent of central sleep apnea (CSA), defined by repetitive episodes of cessation of airflow in the setting of absent or severely reduced respiratory effort (Fig. 1.1). The fact that he has a history of a Chiari I malformation which indicates caudal displacement of the cerebellar tonsils can disrupt cerebrospinal fluid (CSF) flow and lead to compression of his brainstem respiratory centers. This can result in failure to initiate ventilatory effort which is consistent with CSA.

The only correct option above is that CSA may also be associated with congestive heart failure and high-altitude situations. The instability of the respiratory control system is worse in these conditions, which exacerbates symptoms of CSA. Other conditions which have been associated with CSA include arrhythmias, cheyne-stokes breathing, cerebrovascular accident, opiate, and other medications among others.

If CSA is secondary to Chiari I malformation, then a Chiari decompression surgery can improve, if not resolve, the CSA events.

CSA as well as OSA are both correlated with increased risks of adverse cardiovascular outcomes.

It is the high chemoreceptor sensitivity, not the low chemoreceptor sensitivity, that leads to over-responsiveness to CO_2 changes which results in the instability of breathing patterns in CSA.

References

American Academy of Sleep Medicine. International classification of sleep disorders, 3rd ed. Darien, IL: American Academy of Sleep Medicine, 2014; 19–46.

Le T, Kawanjit. Medical image of the week: Cheyne Stokes breathing on polysomnography. Southwest J Pulm Crit Care. 2016 Apr;12(4):163–4.

7. A 61-year-old obese male with history of myasthenia gravis well managed for years now presents accompanied by his wife with reports of progressively worsening issues with recall and concentration. On further questioning, his wife reports loud nightly snoring with witnessed apneas for many years. He has had snorting and gasping arousals which at times result in difficulty returning to sleep. He wakes unrefreshed with daytime somnolence. He had taken a planned nap for many years while working but now has frequent episodes of unintentional napping as he is more idle since retirement. In-lab diagnostic polysomnography revealed an apnea-hypopnea index (AHI) of 20 events/hr (normal <5 events/hr) with intermittent desaturations and no hypercapnea. This patient is most likely to be diagnosed with which sleep disorder?

A. Obstructive sleep apnea
B. Central sleep apnea
C. Sleep-related hypoventilation
D. Insufficient sleep syndrome

Correct answer: A

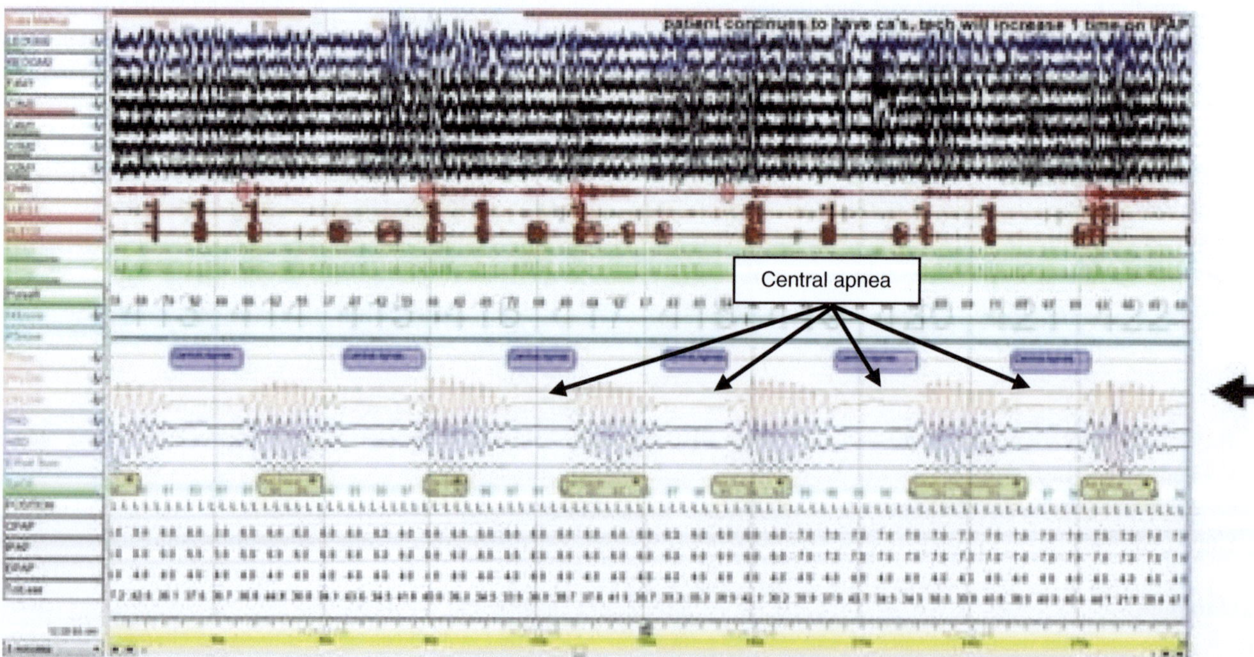

Fig. 1.1 Polysomnography—this figure demonstrates a lack of air flow combined with a lack of chest and abdomen effort consistent with a central apnea. (Source: Le T, Kawanjit S. CC BY-SA 4.0 (https://creativecommons.org/licenses/by-sa/4.0/deed.en) via *Southwest J Pulm Crit Care*. Image has not been modified. Please see full attribution with citation above in references section for this question.)

Explanation

This patient is presenting with the classic features of obstructive sleep apnea (OSA) including loud snoring, gasping followed by arousal, daytime sleepiness, cognitive decline, and apnea witnessed by his wife. OSA is characterized by collapse of the upper airway during sleep, which occurs repeatedly throughout the night, leading to breathing pauses, oxygen desaturation, sleep fragmentation, and consequently, excessive daytime sleepiness (Fig. 1.2). While his obesity is a risk factor, his history of myasthenia gravis has also been shown to be associated with OSA. Neuromuscular weakness can predispose to airway collapse during sleep. Even patients with mild neuromuscular disease can develop symptoms of OSA.

Apnea-hypopnea index (AHI) from an overnight polysomnogram can help determine presence and severity of OSA. In adults, an AHI of 5–15 events/hr is indicative of mild elevation, 15–30 events/hr is indicative of moderate OSA and >30 events/hr is consistent with severe OSA.

Central sleep apnea is defined as a sleep-disordered breathing with repetitive episodes of absent or severely reduced respiratory effort during sleep. Notably, there is no airway obstruction in this disorder. In OSA, respiratory effort continues despite the block to airflow, whereas in central sleep apnea no respiratory effort is made.

Sleep-related hypoventilation is defined by elevated carbon dioxide (hypercapnia) during sleep. This is most often seen in patients with obesity hypoventilation syndrome or neuromuscular disorders. This patient's PSG had no report of hypercapnia, making hypoventilation less likely.

Insufficient sleep syndrome is seen in patients who chronically restrict their sleep duration. This ultimately results in sleep deprivation symptoms such as daytime sleepiness and cognitive decline. It is unlikely in this patient with no evidence of chronic sleep restriction.

References

American Academy of Sleep Medicine. International classification of sleep disorders, 3rd ed. Darien, IL: American Academy of Sleep Medicine, 2014; 19–46.

Arikawa, Takuo & Nakajima, Toshiaki & Yazawa, Hiroko & Kaneda, Hiroyuki & Haruyama, Akiko & Obi, Syotaro & Amano, Hirohisa & Sakuma, Masashi & Toyoda, Shigeru & Abe, Shichiro & Tsutsumi, Takeshi & Matsui, Taishi & Nakata, Akio & Shinozaki, Ryo & Miyamoto, Masayuki & Inoue, TeruoClinical Usefulness of New R-R Interval Analysis Using the Wearable Heart Rate Sensor WHS-1 to Identify Obstructive Sleep Apnea: OSA and RRI Analysis Using a Wearable Heartbeat Sensor. Journal of Clinical Medicine. 9. 3359. https://doi.org/10.3390/jcm9103359

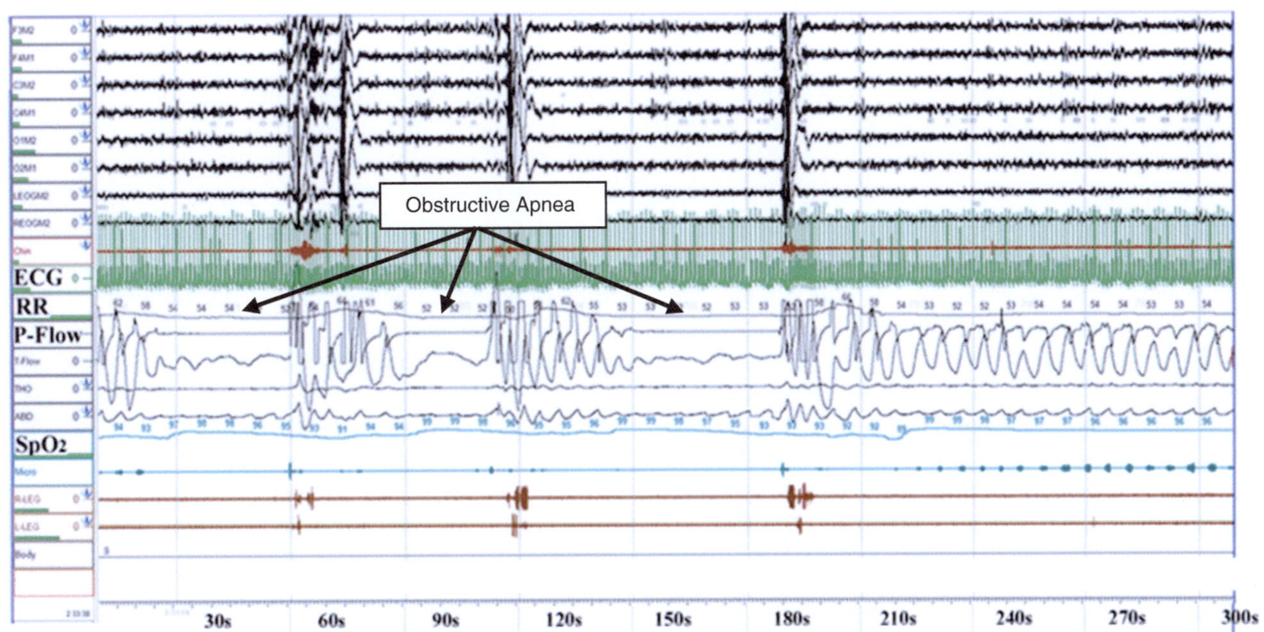

Fig. 1.2 Polysomnography—This figure demonstrates lack of air flow (pflow/tflo) with sustained chest (tho) and abdomen (abo) effort consistent with an obstructive apnea (OA). (Source: Arikawa, et al. (2020). CC BY 4.0 (https://creativecommons.org/licenses/by/4.0/) via *Journal of Clinical Medicine*. Modification of original image to include arrows pointing to obstructive sleep apnea. Please see full attribution with citation above in references section for this question.)

Linked questions: 8–9

8. A 14-year-old male with a history of frequent night-time awakenings presents with complaints of excessive daytime sleepiness despite stable sleep schedule. His parents report no issues with sleep onset but he has had trouble staying asleep for many years. They have tried melatonin and diphenhydramine in the past without much change. Teachers have reported he is falling asleep in classes, and this is starting to affect his previously excellent grades. At times of increased stress or anxiety, he will feel sudden weakness and have near falls. There have been occasional episodes of him waking during the night seeing a cloaked dark figure hovering over him at which time he feels like he cannot move for a few minutes. The most appropriate diagnostic test to confirm his diagnosis is:
   A. Polysomnography (PSG) with multiple sleep latency tests (MSLT)
   B. Serum hypocretin (orexin) level measurement
   C. Overnight pulse oximetry
   D. Brain MRI to rule out structural lesions
   Correct answer: A

Explanation

This patient is presenting with the classic features of narcolepsy, and in particular, narcolepsy type 1 (narcolepsy with cataplexy). Narcolepsy is defined by symptoms similar to those seen in this patient including cataplexy, sleep paralysis, sleep-related hallucinations, and excessive daytime sleepiness. The episodes of sudden weakness and near falls without loss of consciousness as in this case is an example of cataplexy. Hallucinations can be hypnagogic (at sleep onset) or hypnopompic (on waking). Polysomnography (PSG) is the first step to analyzing sleep architecture and ruling out other diagnoses, followed by a multiple sleep latency test (MSLT), which assesses for mean sleep latency and presence of REM sleep during 20-min naps. In narcolepsy, this test will demonstrate a mean SOL of <8 min with 2 or more sleep onset REM periods over 5 naps.

While reduced CSF hypocretin (orexin) levels (<100 pg/mL) is highly specific and sensitive for the diagnosis of narcolepsy type 1, serum hypocretin level has unclear clinical utility. Narcolepsy type 2 (narcolepsy without cataplexy) will generally not have reduced CSF hypocretin level.

Overnight pulse oximetry would help identify patients with various sleep breathing disorders but has no role in the diagnosis of narcolepsy.

Brain MRI is usually indicated if there is concern for hypersomnia in the setting of an underlying brain lesion, which is not suggested in this patient's clinical history.

Of note, genetic abnormality in the human leukocyte antigen (HLA) subtypes DR2/DRB1*1501 and DQB1*0602 are closely associated with narcolepsy with cataplexy.

Reference

Slowik JM, Collen JF, Yow AG. Narcolepsy. [Updated 2023 Jun 12]. In: StatPearls [Internet]. Treasure Island (FL): StatPearls Publishing; 2025 Jan-.

Linked question

9. Which of the following would be the ***least*** likely to improve his symptoms?
   A. sodium oxybate
   B. pitolisant
   C. modafinil
   D. melatonin or diphenhydramine
   Correct answer: D

Explanation

Treatment of narcolepsy primarily focuses on improving daytime wakefulness as well as managing the REM phenomena including cataplexy, sleep paralysis, sleep-related hallucinations that might be present.

Sodium oxybate improves both cataplexy and excessive daytime sleepiness. The exact mechanism is not fully understood, however, it is hypothesized to bind both gamma-aminobutyric acid B (GABA-B) receptors as well as gamma-hydroxybutyrate (GHB) receptors in the brain, subsequently resulting in consolidated slow wave sleep.

Pitolisant is a histamine receptor inverse agonist specifically targeting the H-3 receptor in the brain. It is an approved therapy for cataplexy and excessive daytime somnolence seen in narcolepsy.

Modafinil and armodafinil are considered one of the first-line agents used in the treatment of excessive daytime sleepiness. It is not exclusively used in narcolepsy and has been used to treat daytime sleepiness in OSA and in patients with shift work sleep disorder as well. The mechanism of action of modafinil involves several neurotransmitters including inhibiting the reuptake of dopamine and norepinephrine as well as potential indirect effects on glutamate, GABA, orexin, and histamine.

Melatonin and diphenhydramine would likely worsen this patient's daytime sleepiness. Melatonin can be used in patients with circadian rhythm disorders and REM behavioral disorder. It would not decrease daytime somnolence or increase alertness in this patient. Diphenhydramine is an antihistamine with sedative effects. Neither of these medications would address the patient's daytime functioning.

Reference

Maski K, Trotti LM, Kotagal S, et al. Treatment of central disorders of hypersomnolence: an American Academy of Sleep Medicine clinical practice guideline. *J Clin Sleep Med.* 2021;17(9):1881–1893.

10. A 19-year-old male presents to your clinic with his third episode in the past year of excessive somnolence lasting up to a week at a time associated with hyperphagia, irritability, and disinhibition. Which of the following is a proposed pathophysiology of this syndrome?
    A. Abnormal hypothalamic regulation of the sleep-wake cycle
    B. Dysfunction of the REM sleep center in the brainstem
    C. Impaired orexin secretion due to an autoimmune process
    D. Genetic dysfunction of the paternally inherited chromosome 15

    Correct answer: A

Explanation

This patient presents with classic symptoms of Kleine-Levin Syndrome (KLS), a rare sleep disorder characterized by at least 2 recurrent episodes of hypersomnia with at least 1 of the following: cognitive dysfunction, altered perception, eating disorder (anorexia or hyperphagia), or disinhibited behavior (such as hypersexuality). Episodes typically last 2 days to 5 weeks and are separated by periods of normal behavior and sleep at least once every 18 months. This disorder is more prevalent among adolescent males. While the precise pathophysiology of KLS is not fully understood, dysfunction in the hypothalamus, which plays a key role in regulating the sleep-wake cycle, appetite, and behavior, is considered central to the disorder.

Dysfunction of the REM sleep center in the brainstem is more relevant to disorders of REM sleep regulation, such as REM sleep behavior disorder or narcolepsy, but it is not the primary mechanism in KLS, which affects global sleep-wake homeostasis rather than REM-specific control.

Impaired orexin secretion due to an autoimmune process describes a proposed pathophysiology of narcolepsy type 1, not KLS. Narcolepsy type 1 manifests with excessive daytime sleepiness, cataplexy (which is the sudden loss of muscle tone triggered by strong emotions like laughter or anxiety), sleep paralysis, hypnagogic or hypnopompic hallucinations, and disrupted nocturnal sleep. It does not feature the recurrent hypersomnolence episodes with behavioral changes and hyperphagia typical of KLS.

Genetic dysfunction of the paternally inherited chromosome 15 refers to Prader-Willi syndrome (PWS), a genetic disorder resulting from the absence of paternally expressed genes in the 15q11.2-q13 region. PWS presents in early infancy with hypotonia, feeding difficulties, and poor growth, which subsequently evolve into hyperphagia, obesity, intellectual disability, short stature, hypogonadism, and often behavioral problems as the child grows. Though hypersomnia and sleep-disordered breathing (obstructive sleep apnea or central sleep apnea) may occur in PWS, the sleep disturbances are chronic, not episodic as in KLS. Importantly, while hyperphagia is common to both conditions, PWS is again not characterized by acute, intermittent episodes of hypersomnia or behavior change, distinguishing it clinically from KLS.

Reference

Prabhoo Dayal, Virendra Vikram Singh, Ravikant Kumar. A 5-year follow-up of a female patient with Kleine-Levin syndrome: Diagnosis,disease course and management. Rare, Volume 1, 2023, 100003.

11. A 24-year-old male presents with complaints of trouble waking in the morning. He keeps a set bedtime of 10 pm with stable bedtime routine. Regardless of bedtime routine, he will take 3–4 h for sleep onset which is usually around 2 am. Once asleep, he will not wake until around 10 am. He has missed attending morning meetings due to this. He recalls in college he performed poorly in all morning classes. He feels well-rested when able to sleep on this schedule from 2 am to 10 am. These symptoms and sleep schedule have been present since childhood. He denies any mood symptoms, substance use, or other medical conditions. What is the most likely diagnosis?
    A. Advanced sleep-wake phase disorder
    B. Delayed sleep-wake phase disorder
    C. Non-24-h sleep-wake rhythm disorder
    D. Irregular sleep-wake rhythm disorder

    Correct answer: B

Explanation

Circadian rhythm sleep-wake disorders are characterized by a substantial misalignment between the internal circadian rhythm and the sleep-wake schedule required by the environment (school, work, or social activities) (Fig. 1.3). These disorders are characterized by symptoms of insomnia, excessive daytime sleepiness or both.

This patient has a delayed sleep-wake phase disorder (DSWPD) which is characterized by a significant delay in the timing of sleep compared to societal norms. This is more common in adolescents and young adults. Individuals with DSWPD have difficulty falling asleep at conventional times and often struggle to wake up in the morning, even when they need to adhere to an early schedule. In this case, the patient consistently stays awake until 2 am and experiences difficulty waking up before noon, which is a hallmark of DSWPD. It is often a chronic condition that can impair social, educational, and occupational functioning but is not typically associated with underlying psychiatric or medical conditions.

Advanced sleep-wake phase disorder (ASWPD) involves a shift in the sleep-wake cycle toward earlier times. Advanced

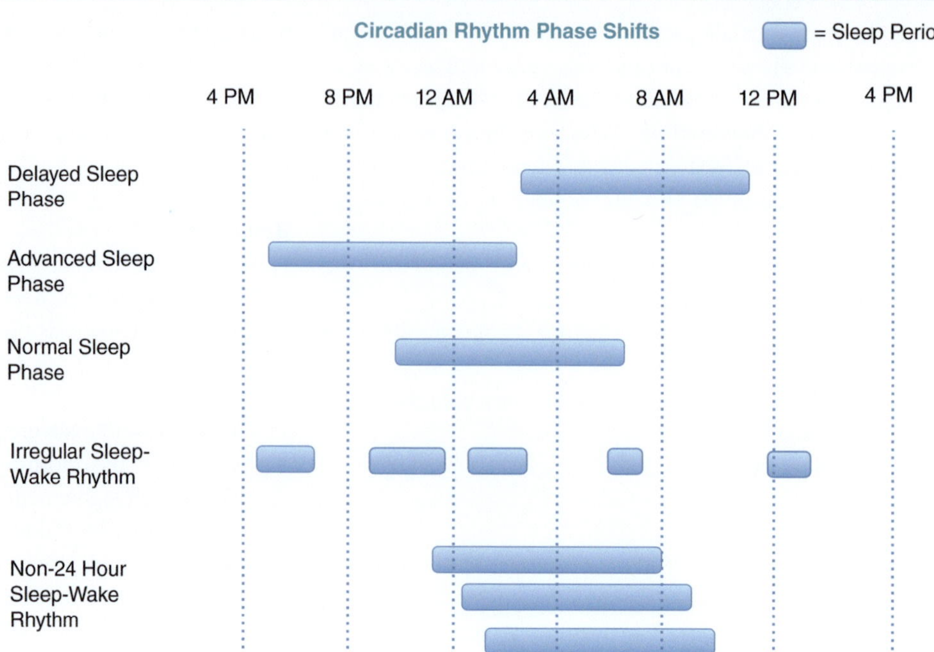

Fig. 1.3 Circadian rhythm phase shifts associated with medically recognized circadian rhythm sleep disorders. (Source: Wells, Mary Ellen and Overton, Auburne. CC BY 4.0 (https://creativecommons.org/licenses/by/4.0/deed.en) via *Primary Health Care*. Image has not been modified. Mary Ellen Wells and Auburne Overton (2014) Circadian Rhythm Sleep Disorders. Primary Health Care 4:158. F3)

age tends to be a risk factor. Individuals with ASWPD tend to fall asleep and wake up much earlier than societal norms, such as falling asleep around 7 pm and waking up at 3 am.

Non-24-hour sleep-wake rhythm disorder is most commonly seen in blind individuals who lack the ability to perceive light cues that help regulate their circadian rhythms. These individuals experience a sleep-wake cycle that progressively delays daily resulting in a misaligned sleep schedule. The patient in this case does not report a progressive shift in their sleep-wake times, making non-24-hour sleep-wake rhythm disorder less likely.

Irregular sleep-wake rhythm disorder is characterized by a fragmented sleep-wake cycle with multiple sleep periods throughout the 24-h day, rather than a single consolidated sleep episode. Individuals with this disorder often have no regular sleep-wake timing and may sleep at different times throughout the day and night. This is more commonly observed in several neurologic disorders, such as dementia or developmental disorders in children.

Reference

Mary Ellen Wells and Auburne Overton (2014) Circadian Rhythm Sleep Disorders. Primary Health Care 4:158

12. A 4-year-old female presents with nocturnal disturbances occurring multiple times a week. She falls asleep at 8 pm within a few minutes and wakes between 11 pm and 12 am with episodes characterized by screaming, crying, appearing scared with heart racing, heavy breathing, and sweating lasting for 15 min. Her mother reports difficulty waking her or consoling her. She will eventu-

ally return to sleep without any recollection of the events the next morning. What is the most likely diagnosis?
A. Confusional arousal
B. Nightmare disorder
C. Exploding head syndrome
D. Sleep terrors
Correct answer: D

Explanation

Sleep terrors are a type of non-REM parasomnia typically seen in children aged 4–12. They occur during slow-wave sleep, usually in the first third of the night, consistent with this patient's symptoms occurring between 11 pm. and midnight after falling asleep at 8 pm. Sleep terrors are characterized by sudden arousals from sleep accompanied by screaming, crying, intense fear, autonomic nervous system activation, and confusion. Children often appear inconsolable and are difficult to awaken. Subsequently, they do not recall the episode the next morning.

Nightmare disorder, in contrast, occurs during REM sleep, usually in the second half of the night, and the child typically wakes fully from the dream with clear recall of the disturbing content. Unlike sleep terrors, nightmares do not involve confusion or autonomic signs and the child can often be consoled.

Confusional arousals are another non-REM parasomnia that also occurs in the first part of the night. They may include disorientation, mumbling, or sitting up in bed, but they are not as pronounced as with sleep terrors and usually lack the symptoms of intense fear or autonomic symptoms.

Exploding head syndrome is characterized by a sudden loud noise or sensation of explosion in the head without pain either at sleep onset or upon awakening during the night. There is recollection of the event with associated fear. On occasion, the episode may be accompanied by a flash of light or myoclonic jerks. This is more commonly seen in females and adults.

Reference

Singh S, Kaur H, Singh S, Khawaja I. Parasomnias: A Comprehensive Review. Cureus. 2018 Dec 31;10(12):e3807

13. A 36-year-old female presents with a history of sleep onset and maintenance insomnia. She started taking zolpidem CR 12.5 mg at bedtime with improvement noted. Shortly after, she started to notice recurrence of her daytime somnolence. In the morning, she would find multiple items in her kitchen eaten without recollection. At times she would find crumbs in her bed. This has led to significant weight gain. Which of the following is the most likely diagnosis?
    A. Sleepwalking
    B. Night eating syndrome
    C. Sleep-related eating disorder
    D. Kleine-Levin syndrome
    Correct answer: C

Explanation

Sleep-related eating disorder (SRED) is a parasomnia characterized by recurrent episodes of involuntary eating during partial arousals from sleep, typically with little or no memory of the events. Individuals often consume unusual or high-calorie foods, and sometimes even inedible or hazardous substances. Injuries can occur in pursuit of food or while cooking food. These episodes occur during non-REM sleep, particularly during the first half of the night. The key features in this case including recurrent nocturnal eating, amnesia for the events, and resultant weight gain are classic for SRED. This may be precipitated by non-benzodiazepine benzodiazepine receptor agonist medications as in this case. This disorder is more common in women and young adults.

Sleepwalking (somnambulism) involves complex motor behaviors during partial arousals from slow-wave sleep but typically does not involve eating. It is a non-REM parasomnia that occurs during slow-wave sleep, typically in the first third of the night. While both conditions are non-REM parasomnias and may coexist, sleepwalking alone would not explain the focused, repeated nocturnal eating or the weight gain described here.

Night eating syndrome (NES) is an eating disorder, not a parasomnia. In NES, patients are aware of their nocturnal eating episodes, and it often includes evening hyperphagia and/or insomnia. The key distinction is that individuals with NES retain full awareness of their behaviors and often eat to fall back asleep, unlike the amnestic behaviors in SRED.

Kleine-Levin syndrome (KLS) is characterized by episodic hypersomnia associated with cognitive dysfunction, altered perception, eating disorder with anorexia or hyperphagia, and disinhibited behavior. KLS can present with inappropriate nocturnal eating but its predominance in adolescent males and its complex periodic nature distinguish it from SRED.

Reference

Singh S, Kaur H, Singh S, Khawaja I. Parasomnias: A Comprehensive Review. Cureus. 2018 Dec 31;10(12):e3807

Linked questions: 14–15

14. A 76-year-old male with Parkinson's disease (PD) presents with reports that he often acts out his dreams during sleep, including kicking and shouting, noted by his wife. This is particularly problematic at night and has at times led to minor injuries. He is fully coherent after his wife wakes him from these events. An overnight diagnostic polysomnogram is ordered (Fig. 1.4) which revealed a lack of atonia during REM sleep. What is the most likely diagnosis?
    A. Sleepwalking
    B. Confusional arousals
    C. REM sleep behavior disorder
    D. Periodic limb movement disorder
    Correct answer: C

Explanation

REM sleep behavior disorder (RBD) is characterized by the loss of normal muscle atonia during REM sleep with dream enactment behavior including vocalizations and complex motor behaviors that are often violent in nature. As these episodes occur in REM, they are more common in the second half of sleep. Upon awakening from the episode, the person is alert and coherent as opposed to most non-REM parasomnias. They are more common in males and prevalence increases with advancing age. This disorder has a strong association with synucleinopathies like Parkinson's disease, Multisystem Atrophy and Lewy Body Dementia, making it especially relevant in this patient.

Sleepwalking (somnambulism) is a non-REM parasomnia that occurs during slow-wave sleep, typically in the first third of the night. It involves ambulation and other complex motor behaviors with limited awareness and is more common in children than in older adults. Importantly, it does not involve dream enactment, and the person is usually confused if awakened.

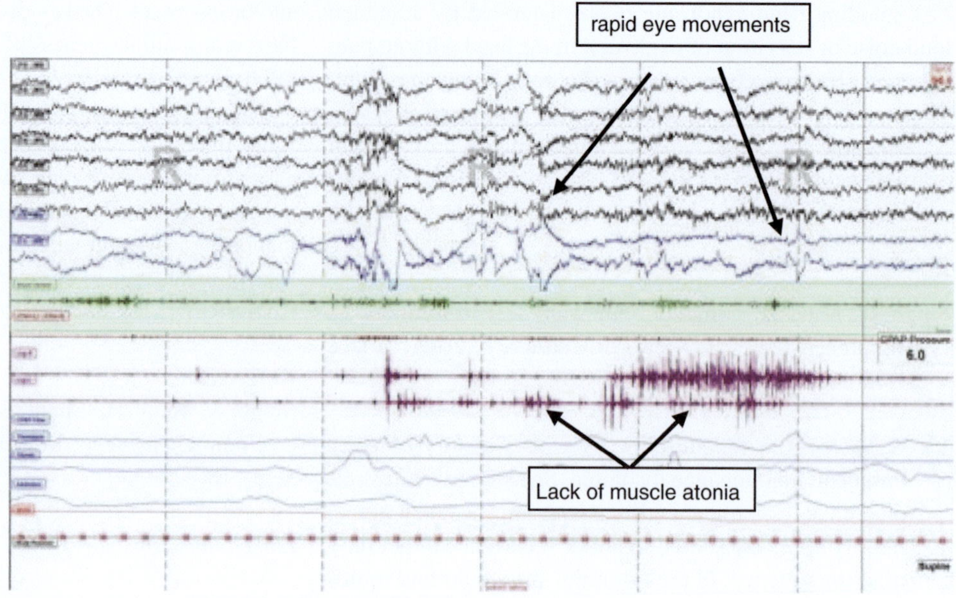

Fig. 1.4 Polysomnography showing rapid eye movements and lack of muscle atonia. (Source: Bartell J, Shetty S and Knox KS. CC BY-SA 4.0 (https://creativecommons.org/licenses/by-sa/4.0/deed.en) via *Southwest J Pulm Crit Care*. Image has been modified with arrows pointing to rapid eye movement and lack of muscle atonia. Please see full attribution with citation below in references section for this question.)

Confusional arousal is another non-REM parasomnia, in which individuals may sit up, mumble, or appear disoriented during the arousal but do not ambulate. Like sleepwalking, it typically occurs in the first part of the night and is not associated with complex dream enactment behavior.

Periodic limb movement disorder consists of periodic limb movements of sleep (PLMS). These involve repetitive, stereotyped limb jerks (usually in the lower extremities) that occur during sleep. These movements are not typically associated with dream enactment or abnormal behaviors, and patients are usually unaware of them unless they are awakened or their bed partner observes them.

References

Bartell J, Shetty S, Knox KS. Medical image of the week: REM without atonia. Southwest J Pulm Crit Care. 2015;10(3):147–8

Howell M, Avidan AY, Foldvary-Schaefer N, et al. Management of REM sleep behavior disorder: an American Academy of Sleep Medicine clinical practice guideline. *J Clin Sleep Med.* 2023;19(4):759–768.

Linked question

15. What is the most appropriate treatment for the sleep disorder in this patient?
    A. Selective serotonin reuptake inhibitors (SSRIs)
    B. Dopaminergic therapy
    C. Melatonin
    D. Clonazepam
    Correct answer: C

Explanation

American Academy of Sleep Medicine management of RBD guidelines recommends immediate- release melatonin or clonazepam as a conditional recommendation.

Melatonin is the best treatment for RBD in this patient. It has been shown to reduce dream enactment behaviors and improve sleep quality, with minimal side effects. Unlike other sleep medications, melatonin is less sedating, does not impair cognition, and carries fewer risk of falls or respiratory depression, making it especially appropriate in an elderly population.

Clonazepam, a benzodiazepine, is effective in treating RBD as well. However, it is not as preferred in older adults due to concerns of daytime sedation, cognitive impairment, falls, and potential worsening of comorbid sleep apnea.

Selective serotonin reuptake inhibitors (SSRIs) are not a treatment for RBD. SSRIs and other antidepressants such as tricyclic antidepressants and serotonin norepinephrine reuptake inhibitors (SNRIs) can worsen RBD symptoms or even precipitate the disorder by disrupting REM sleep regulation.

Dopaminergic therapy is vital to managing motor symptoms of Parkinson's disease but has not been found to have a direct benefit in treating RBD.

Reference

Howell M, Avidan AY, Foldvary-Schaefer N, et al. Management of REM sleep behavior disorder: an American Academy of Sleep Medicine clinical practice guideline. *J Clin Sleep Med.* 2023;19(4):759–768.

16. A 56-year-old male reports occasional awakenings and daytime somnolence. His primary medical doctor ordered a home sleep study which did not reveal sleep disordered breathing. On further questioning, his wife notes that he has frequent jerking limb movements during the night. He tried over- the-counter diphenhydramine which worsened nocturnal awakenings and leg movements. What is the most likely diagnosis?
    A. Restless legs syndrome
    B. Periodic limb movement disorder
    C. Sleep-related leg cramps
    D. Propriospinal myoclonus
    Correct answer: B

Explanation

Periodic limb movement disorder is a sleep-related movement disorder characterized by repetitive, involuntary limb movements (typically in the legs) (Fig. 1.5). The movements often consist of rhythmic extension of the big toe often in combination with dorsiflexion of the ankle, the knee, and sometimes the hip typically with lack of awareness. When the periodic limb movements of sleep lead to sleep fragmentation, frequent awakenings, daytime fatigue or impact on social functioning, it is termed periodic limb movement disorder. Criterion is met with PLMS index more than >5/hr in children and >15/hr adults on polysomnography.

Restless leg syndrome (RLS) is a related but distinct condition. It involves an urge to move the legs, usually accompanied by uncomfortable sensations that worsen at rest and improve with movement. Importantly, RLS symptoms occur while the person is awake or drowsy, particularly in the evening or at night prior to sleep. They must result in some level of distress, concern, and impairment in important areas of daytime functioning. In contrast, PLMS/PLMD occurs during sleep, and the individual is unaware of them except through disrupted sleep or bed partner observations.

Sleep-related leg cramps are characterized by a painful sensation usually occurring in the calf or foot associated with sudden, involuntary muscle contraction. These contractions occur while in bed although they can arise from wakefulness or sleep. They are relieved by forceful stretching which releases the contraction but can also remit spontaneously. Predisposing factors can include prior vigorous exercise, diabetes mellitus, amyotrophic lateral sclerosis, peripheral vascular disease among other metabolic disorders.

Propriospinal myoclonus is a rare movement disorder characterized by sudden axial jerks involving the abdomen and trunk then propagated to proximal muscles of the limbs and neck, usually occurring at sleep onset. It is distinct from PLMS in both phenomenology and distribution of movements and would not typically cause repeated awakenings throughout the night.

Reference

Anguizola E SS, Botta P LM, Castro-Villacañas A, Garcia-Borreguero D. The Clinical Evaluation of Sleep-Related Movement Disorders. Sleep Med Clin. 2021 Jun;16(2):223–231.

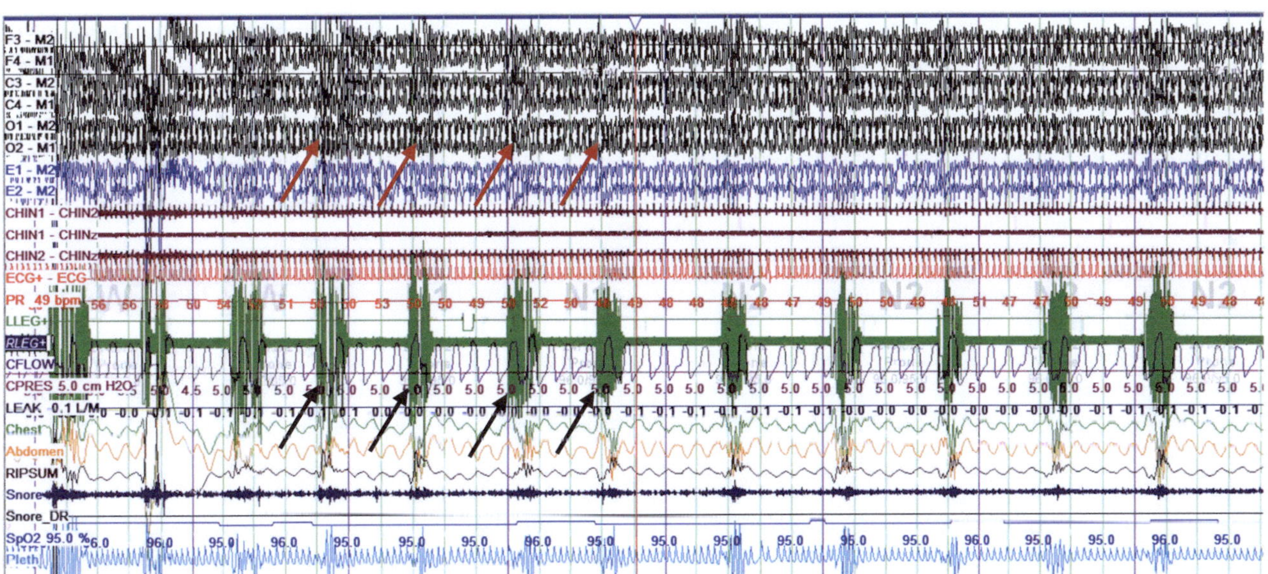

Fig. 1.5 This figure demonstrates periodic limb movements of sleep as shown by the black arrows. The red arrows are associated arousals. (Permission obtained from patient to reproduce image)

17. A 64-year-old female comes to your office with complaints of leg discomfort in the evening which often prevent sleep onset. She will usually walk around the house and stretch after which she feels improvement. Her husband reports noticing frequent leg movements and kicking throughout the night which limits his sleep. She finds it difficult to wake in the morning and feels fatigued throughout the day regardless of hours slept. She reports when she lays down for bed, she will have sensations of something crawling on her legs with an intense need to move them. This will resolve her symptoms for short period of time before it recurs. Which of the following is false regarding this condition?
    A. Diagnosis requires an in-lab monitored polysomnogram
    B. Overnight polysomnography can reveal periodic limb movements of sleep
    C. Augmentation can occur on treatment with dopamine agonists
    D. Worsens during pregnancy or from selective serotonin reuptake inhibitors

Correct answer: A

Explanation

This patient presents with classic symptoms of Restless Leg Syndrome (RLS) which is characterized by an uncomfortable sensation in the legs accompanied by an urge to move the limbs that is worse at rest, particularly in the evening or night, and temporarily relieved by movement. These symptoms often delay sleep onset and contribute to daytime fatigue. Her husband's report of frequent leg kicking during the night suggests coexisting periodic limb movements of sleep (PLMS), which are often seen in individuals with RLS and can further disrupt sleep quality. RLS is a clinical diagnosis based on patient history. Polysomnography (PSG) is not required for diagnosis of RLS. Increased risk for the development of RLS include a positive family history, female sex, and genetic variants. Precipitating factors include iron deficiency, certain medications such as antihistamines, antidepressants and dopamine receptor antagonists, pregnancy, chronic renal failure, and prolonged immobility.

A state of dopaminergic dysfunction is suspected to cause RLS potentially mediated through deficiencies in central nervous system iron. Therefore, one of the initial goals of therapy is iron replacement with monitoring of ferritin level even in the absence of anemia. Iron supplementation is recommended if ferritin is <75 ng/mL in adults and <50 ng/mL in children. Iron stores should be monitored regularly as part of initial and ongoing treatment.

Although not necessary for the diagnosis, PSG in RLS patients can reveal repetitive, stereotyped limb movements defined as periodic limb movements of sleep. Periodic limb movements of sleep index >5/hr in children or >15/hr in adults are considered elevated.

While dopamine agonists like pramipexole and ropinirole are often effective initially, chronic use can lead to augmentation, a paradoxical worsening of symptoms with earlier onset, increased severity, and/or spread to other body parts.

RLS is common in pregnancy, especially in the third trimester, and symptoms often resolve postpartum. Several medications, including SSRIs, SNRIs, and certain antihistamines, are known to worsen or uncover RLS symptoms.

Reference

American Academy of Sleep Medicine. International classification of sleep disorders, 3rd ed. Darien, IL: American Academy of Sleep Medicine, 2014; 281–299.

18. A 2-month-old female presents to your clinic with her parents reporting rhythmic movements that occur during sleep. The movements are only seen during sleep and have been consistently occurring since 3 weeks of age without significant change or worsening over time. The movements are described as very brief twitches of the arms, legs, or the whole body. An EEG was performed which captured the events and was normal. Which of the following is the most likely condition?
    A. Benign sleep myoclonus of infancy
    B. Sleep-related rhythmic movement disorder
    C. Sleep-related leg cramps
    D. Benign myoclonic epilepsy of infancy

Correct answer: A

Explanation

In this infant, the movements are occurring only during sleep and are characterized by brief jerks and twitches of her body. Given this description, the most likely answer is benign sleep myoclonus of infancy which is considered a non-epileptic disorder characterized by repetitive, rhythmic myoclonic jerks that occur only during sleep. Most commonly, this is seen in full-term infants in the early months of life. The jerks are described as symmetric, synchronous, and bilateral, with cessation upon awakening.

Sleep-related rhythmic movement disorder is defined by repetitive, rhythmic, and stereotyped large muscle movements during drowsiness or sleep. Examples include body rocking and head banging and is most often seen in infants and young children. Though typically benign and stops in early childhood, it can continue into adolescence, and in very rare cases, adulthood. These behaviors result in sleep fragmentation, possible injury, or impairment in daytime function.

Sleep-related leg cramps are characterized by a painful sensation usually occurring in the calf or foot associated with sudden, involuntary muscle contraction. Predisposing factors can include prior vigorous exercise, diabetes mellitus, amyotrophic lateral sclerosis, peripheral vascular disease among other metabolic disorders. These can occur from wakefulness or sleep and are more common in adults. They would not result in the twitching movements seen in this patient.

Benign myoclonic epilepsy of infancy (BMEI) is a rare idiopathic generalized epilepsy syndrome that is characterized by myoclonic seizures that are brief, generalized, and easy to treat. They present in neurotypical infants in the first 3 years of life and generally have a favorable prognosis with resolution. EEG will typically show generalized spike-wave or polyspike-wave discharges during the jerking episodes.

Reference

Hillary Eichelberger, Aaron L.A. Nelson. Nocturnal events in children: When and how to evaluate. Current Problems in Pediatric and Adolescent Health Care, Volume 50, Issue 12, 2020, 100893.

19. A 74-year-old woman with Alzheimer disease (AD) presents with fragmented sleep, excessive daytime sleepiness, and confusion. She often wanders around the house during the night and has trouble distinguishing between day and night. Sleep disturbances are a commonly seen in AD.

     What is not typical of AD?
    A. Circadian rhythm disruption
    B. Decreased risk of sleep disordered breathing (SDB)
    C. Decrease in REM sleep
    D. Sundowning
    Correct answer: B

Explanation

AD is the most common dementia and is characterized by neuronal loss and deposition of amyloid beta, neurofibrillary tangles, and tau in the hippocampus and cerebral cortex. Sleep disturbances frequently occur in patients with AD. There is a reciprocal relationship between AD and sleep which can further worsen cognitive function. Circadian rhythm disruption is very common in Alzheimer's disease. Atrophy of the suprachiasmatic nucleus results in disruption of the day/night cycle.

Decrease in REM sleep due to possible degeneration of cholinergic neurons is also commonly seen in this patient population which is not a feature of healthy aging.

Sundowning is characterized by increased confusion, agitation, and anxiety into the early evening seen in elderly patients with dementia and is particularly common in AD. This is also due to circadian rhythm misalignment.

There is an increased risk of sleep-disordered breathing (SDB) seen with AD. This is proposed to be due to degeneration of the brainstem respiratory neurons and supramedullary respiratory pathways. The e4 allele of the apolipoprotein (APOE4) gene is a genetic risk factor for AD and also has been linked to obstructive sleep apnea.

Reference

Avidan Alon Y. Review of Sleep Medicine. 4th ed., 2018; 288–292.

20. A 58-year-old male with a history of a cerebrovascular accident (CVA) 2 years ago presents with palpitations and shortness of breath. On evaluation in the emergency department, he is found with new onset atrial fibrillation. He and his wife also report a long history of snoring with witnessed apneas, gasping arousals, and worsening daytime somnolence. These symptoms have worsened since prior CVA along with mild dysarthria and dysphagia requiring a modified diet. What is the most likely explanation for the development of atrial fibrillation?
    A. Intermittent hypoxia and autonomic dysfunction from OSA
    B. Hyperthyroidism
    C. Acute myocardial infarction
    D. Sleep-related hypoventilation
    Correct answer: A

Explanation

OSA has been found to be a prominent risk factor for atrial fibrillation, in part due to the recurrent episodes of intermittent hypoxia which result in sympathetic nervous system activation. These stressors start a cascade of oxidative stress, systemic inflammation, and changes in arterial structure, all of which increases risk of atrial fibrillation. OSA and AF are independent risk factors for CVAs. Given this patient's snoring, witnessed apneas, gasping arousals, and daytime somnolence suggesting a diagnosis of untreated OSA, this is the most likely underlying cause of his new onset atrial fibrillation (AF).

While hyperthyroidism is a classic cause of AF, it is unlikely in this patient without evidence of weight loss, tremors, hyperhidrosis, heat intolerance, mood swings, and other clinical features that appear in hyperthyroidism.

Acute myocardial infarction can also precipitate AF in the setting of atrial ischemia or increase atrial pressure, however, the question does not give any evidence of an acute coronary event, making this an unlikely cause.

Sleep-related hypoventilation can occur in syndromes such as obesity hypoventilation or neuromuscular diseases, which can result in persistent hypercapnia rather than the intermittent hypoxia that occurs in OSA. Though chronic hypoventilation can contribute to cardiopulmonary complications, it is less associated with AF than the increased sympathetic nervous system activation seen in OSA.

Reference

Marulanda-Londoño E, Chaturvedi S. The Interplay between Obstructive Sleep Apnea and Atrial Fibrillation. Front Neurol. 2017 Dec 11;8:668.

2

Sydney Chatfield, Kristen Yang, and Devorah Segal

Linked questions: 1–2

1. A 1-month-old infant boy is brought into the pediatrician's office for a routine wellness check-up. During the interview, the patient's father reports his son has been vomiting multiple times daily and unable to keep formula down. He also noticed when changing wet diapers that his urine has a very pungent smell. The infant was born at home, and this is his first doctor's visit. On examination, the infant is noted to have a lower weight than at birth and poor head control. A blood test is most likely to reveal which of the following?
   A. Elevated serum tyrosine levels
   B. Elevated serum homocysteine levels
   C. Decreased serum tyrosine levels
   D. Elevated serum branched-chain amino acids
   Correct answer: C

Explanation

The infant's presentation of vomiting, restricted growth, musty ("pungent") odor to the urine and signs of developmental delay all are suggestive of a diagnosis of Phenylketonuria (PKU). This autosomal recessive genetic disorder is due to a deficiency in the enzyme phenylalanine hydroxylase, which normally converts phenylalanine into tyrosine. Absence of this enzyme results in elevated phenylalanine and low tyrosine levels, which can be directly measured with serum testing. When phenylalanine accumulates, it can result in neurological impairment. PKU can be detected on newborn screening but can be missed in patients born outside a hospital setting. Elevated tyrosine levels can be seen with tyrosinemia or liver failure. These can present with poor weight gain and vomiting but would also demonstrate signs of liver failure such as hepatomegaly, elevated LFTs, and abnormal PT/INR. Elevated serum branched-chain amino

S. Chatfield · K. Yang · D. Segal (✉)
Department of Neurology, NYU Langone Health,
New York, NY, USA
e-mail: Sydney.Chatfield@nyulangone.org;
Kristen.yang@nyulangone.org; Devorah.Segal@nyulangone.org

acids would be found in maple syrup urine disease (MSUD), in which the enzyme that breaks down branched chain amino acids such as leucine, isoleucine, or valine is absent or diminished. MSUD characteristically presents in the first week of life with encephalopathy, dystonia, and sweet-smelling urine. Elevated homocysteine is usually secondary to cystathionine β-synthase deficiency. This disorder can cause developmental delay, hypotonia, and poor feeding but one would also expect to see marfanoid body habitus, ectopia lentis, thromboembolic complications, and no change in urine smell.

References

Louis, E. D., Mayer, S. A., & Noble, J. M. (Eds.). (2021). Merritt's neurology (14th ed.). Wolters Kluwer Health.
Vernon, H. (2016). Phenylketonuria. In M. V. Johnston (Ed.), Neurobiology of disease (2nd ed., pp. 447–450). Oxford University Press.

Linked question

2. After making the diagnosis above, you advise the family that the next best initial step in management of the infant is which of the following options?
   A. Low phenylalanine diet
   B. Supplement with high protein diet
   C. Enzyme replacement
   D. Removal of phenylalanine through dialysis
   Correct answer: A

Explanation

Phenylketonuria (PKU) is a result of a deficiency in the enzyme phenylalanine hydroxylase. This enzyme works to convert phenylalanine into tyrosine, so when this enzyme is absent, there is an accumulation of phenylalanine. To prevent neurological damage, it is imperative to prevent the buildup of phenylalanine. This is achieved by a life-long strict low phenylalanine diet. Toward this end, patients are advised to pursue a low protein diet, as phenylalanine is often found in high levels in sources of protein such as meat, eggs, dairy, and

T. E. Smith, V. Arena (eds.), *Essential Neurology Board Review Q & A*, https://doi.org/10.1007/978-3-032-17213-6_2

nuts. Most patients are responsive to dietary changes and do well after initiation. However, if phenylalanine levels remain elevated despite dietary changes, patients may require supplementation with tetrahydrobiopterin (BH4) or pegvaliase, an injectable enzyme that helps to metabolize phenylalanine. Dialysis is rarely used and only in severe cases of neurological damage and need for immediate phenylalanine removal.

Reference

van *Spronsen FJ, Blau N, Harding C, Burlina A, Longo N, Bosch AM. Phenylketonuria. Nat Rev Dis Primers. 2021;7(1):36. https://doi.org/10.1038/s41572-021-00267-0*

Linked questions: 3–4

3. While rounding on consults, the team discusses a 3-day old infant boy in the neonatal intensive care unit. He is currently on a ventilator after he was found to be severely tachypneic and hypotonic this morning. At birth, he had APGAR scores of 8 and 9 and initially did well with formula feeding. On examination, he has low weight, reduced tone and intermittent, rhythmic shaking of his arms that lasts less than 1 min. Initial labs show elevated ammonia, normal LFTs, normal glucose, and normal electrolytes. His mother believes that her brother had similar symptoms when he was born but died at 1 week of age. Additional serum testing shows elevated orthotic acid and low arginine levels. Which enzyme is the infant most likely to be deficient in?
   A. Argininosuccinate synthetase
   B. Carbamyl phosphate synthetase
   C. Argininosuccinase
   D. Ornithine transcarbamylase
   E. Arginase

   Correct answer: D

Explanation

An infant who was initially healthy at birth with quick development of lethargy, poor feeding, and vomiting, increasing difficulty breathing, and seizures displays symptoms highly concerning for hyperammonemia. Hyperammonemia shortly after birth can be the result of multiple etiologies including transient hyperammonemia of birth, liver dysfunction, or an inborn error of metabolism that directly or indirectly affects the urea cycle. Urea cycle disorders usually present a few days after birth when the infant has received increasing amounts of protein in their diet. All urea cycle disorders present similarly with the exception of arginase deficiency, which causes a much milder hyperammonemia and typically presents later in life with developmental delay, seizures, and spasticity. This is due to arginase's place in one of the last steps of the urea cycle, when ammonia has already been partially detoxified and incorporated into arginine, which can be excreted. To help differentiate from the remaining urea cycle disorders, genetic testing as well as measuring plasma amino acids and orotic acids is essential. OTC deficiency is the only X-linked urea cycle disorder (and not autosomal recessive) and should be considered in a male infant, particularly with a family history of similar symptoms in other male infants. OTC converts ornithine to citrulline, so citrulline will be low, orotic acid high, and arginine low in this disorder. Carbamoyl phosphate synthetase 1 (CPS1) converts carbon dioxide and ammonia into carbamoyl phosphate, which is used by OTC in the process of making citrulline. Therefore, deficiencies in this enzyme will have low orotic acid compared to OTC deficiency. Argininosuccinate synthetase (ASS) is next in the cycle converting citrulline to argininosuccinate, so citrulline will be high when this enzyme is deficient. Finally, argininosuccinase (arginosuccinate lyase (ASL)) converts argininosuccinate into arginine, so a deficiency in this enzyme will result in decreased arginine, increased citrulline, and normal orotic acid levels.

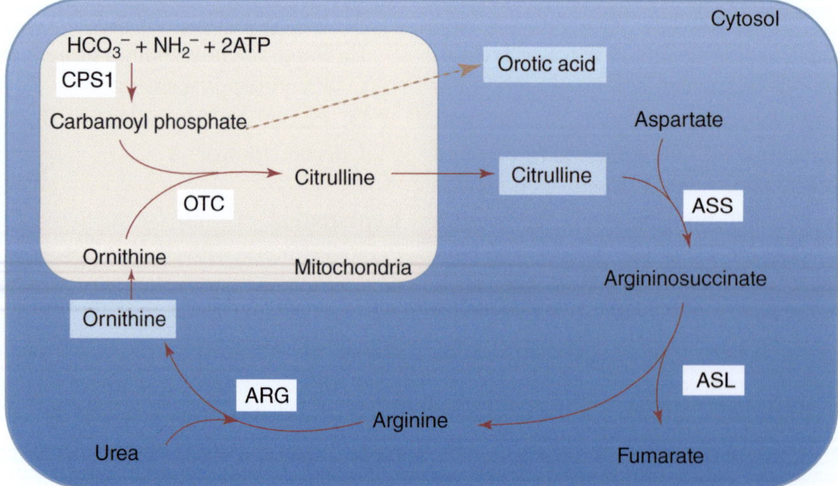

Urea Cycle (Source: Acharya, G., Mehra, S., Patel, R., Frunza-Stefan, S., Kaur, H. CC-BY 4.0 (https://creativecommons.org/licenses/by/4.0/) via *Case Reports in Critical Care*. Image has not been modified from source. Acharya G, Mehra S, Patel R, Frunza-Stefan S, Kaur H. Fatal Nonhepatic Hyperammonemia in ICU Setting: A Rare but Serious Complication following Bariatric Surgery. Case Rep Crit Care. 2016;2016:8531591. https://doi.org/10.1155/2016/8531591)

References

Acharya G, Mehra S, Patel R, Frunza-Stefan S, Kaur H. Fatal Nonhepatic Hyperammonemia in ICU Setting: A Rare but Serious Complication following Bariatric Surgery. Case Rep Crit Care. 2016;2016:8531591. https://doi.org/10.1155/2016/8531591

Louis, E. D., Mayer, S. A., & Noble, J. M. (Eds.). (2021). Merritt's neurology (14th ed.). Wolters Kluwer Health.

Maestri NE, Clissold D, Brusilow SW. Neonatal onset ornithine transcarbamylase deficiency: A retrospective analysis. J Pediatr. 1999;134(3):268–72. https://doi.org/10.1016/s0022-3476(99)70448-8.

Linked question

4. Genetic testing confirms the diagnosis above. The infant remains stable on a ventilator while weaning sedation and has no further episodes concerning for seizures. Neurological exam demonstrates pupils are 3 mm, equal, and reactive to light with withdrawal to noxious stimuli in all extremities. When placing the infant back in the bed, you notice symmetric arm extension with subsequent flexion. Repeat ammonia level is 175 µmol/L (normal range is 20–80 µmol/L). Given the infant's current medical status, which of the below treatment options is most appropriate to initiate at this time?
   A. Start IV sodium benzoate and glucose therapy
   B. Initiate high protein enteral feeds to restore nitrogen balance
   C. Administer oral arginine and citrulline supplementation
   D. Start lactulose to help lower ammonia levels
   E. Immediate initiation of hemodialysis to remove excess ammonia in the blood
   Correct answer: A

Explanation

Prolonged high levels of ammonia can cause significant neurological damage, so it is essential to rapidly reduce serum ammonia concentration. Initial treatments include IV glucose to help prevent muscle breakdown and the potential increase in nitrogen, which can further be converted to ammonia. Additionally, limiting protein intake in diet is important to help further reduce ammonia build up. Sodium benzoate is helpful to reduce ammonia as it utilizes a different pathway to help excrete nitrogen into the urine, therefore lowering the ammonia level. This infant is overall clinically stable and improving but continues to have elevated serum ammonia levels. He has no signs of cerebral edema or increased pressure at this time such as papilledema, pupillary abnormalities, or posturing and displays a normal Moro reflex. He should receive treatment to reduce his serum ammonia concentration but does not require urgent invasive therapy. If he was minimally responsive to initial measures, showed signs of worsening neurological function, or had ammonia levels that were significantly high (>500 µmol/L), he would require immediate hemodialysis to prevent cerebral edema, which can result in increased intracranial pressure, brain herniation and compression, cerebral hypoxia, and potential brain death. Due to the inability to convert ornithine to citrulline and produce further downstream products, it will be helpful to supplement arginine and citrulline in the future, but this will not affect his current ammonia concentration or prevent neurological decline. Lastly, lactulose is helpful for liver dysfunction and reducing ammonia in liver failure but not in OTC deficiency.

References

Stone WL, Basit H, Jaishankar GB. Urea Cycle Disorders. StatPearls. Treasure Island (FL): StatPearls Publishing Copyright © 2025, StatPearls Publishing LLC.; 2025.

Uta Lichter-Konecki LC, Hiroki Morizono, Kara Simpson, Nicholas Ah Mew, Erin MacLeod. Ornithine Transcarbamylase Deficiency. GeneReviews. Seattle: University of Washington; 2022.

5. Which of the following is a common long-term neurological complication of galactosemia even with dietary galactose restriction?
   A. Epilepsy
   B. Sensorineural hearing loss
   C. Cerebral infarct
   D. Progressive spasticity
   E. Dystonia
   Correct answer: B

Explanation

Galactosemia is due to a deficiency in the Galactose-1-phosphate uridyltransferase (GALT) enzyme responsible for the breakdown of galactose. When galactose cannot be broken down, toxic metabolites build up and cause multi-organ damage, including the nervous system. Galactosemia characteristically presents at birth with hypotonia, jaundice and hyperbilirubinemia, cataracts, and hypoglycemia. Treatment includes early initiation of a galactose-free and lactose-free diet with nutritional supplementation and therapy for cognitive and motor delays as needed. Patients generally respond well to dietary treatment, but a common long-term complication is the development of sensorineural hearing loss. This is thought to be due to toxic metabolite build-up, metabolic stress, and impaired glycosylation in the cochlea leading to damage over time. Patients with galactosemia should have regular audiology screening. Seizures and cerebral infarcts are not common symptoms directly related to galactosemia. Spasticity can develop as a result of damage to motor pathways, but hypotonia is more commonly seen, and dystonia is a rare finding. Children can have tremors or ataxia that progress with age, but extrapyramidal symptoms are rare.

References

Raynor E, Robison WG, Garrett CG, McGuirt WT, Pillsbury HC, Prazma J. Consumption of a high-galactose diet induces diabetic-like changes in the inner ear. Otolaryngol Head Neck Surg. 1995;113(6):748–54. https://doi.org/10.1016/s0194-59989570015-3

Rubio-Gozalbo ME, Haskovic M, Bosch AM, Burnyte B, Coelho AI, Cassiman D, et al. The natural history of classic galactosemia: lessons from the GalNet registry. Orphanet J Rare Dis. 2019;14(1):86. https://doi.org/10.1186/s13023-019-1047-z

6. Which MRI findings are most characteristic for Alexander Disease?
    A. Symmetric periventricular white matter abnormalities with sparing of the subcortical U-fibers
    B. Frontal predominant white matter abnormalities with contrast enhancement of periventricular regions
    C. Posterior predominant leukodystrophy with involvement of subcortical U-fibers
    D. Diffuse white matter abnormalities with cerebellar atrophy

Correct answer: B

Explanation

Alexander disease is a one of the classic leukodystrophy disorders characterized by progressive neurodegeneration secondary to myelin destruction. This disorder is specifically caused by a mutation in the glial fibrillary acidic protein (GFAP) gene, which results in accumulation of proteins forming Rosenthal fiber aggregates in astrocytes. The disease-causing mutation is often de novo but can be inherited in an autosomal-dominant fashion in rare cases. Build-up of protein aggregates leads to disruption of myelin maintenance and ultimately progressive loss of the myelin sheath. Alexander Disease can present as infantile, juvenile, or adult-onset forms with more severe features seen in forms presenting at a younger age. Genetic testing ultimately confirms the diagnosis, but MRI brain has several key characteristics that distinguish Alexander Disease from other leukodystrophies and can guide targeted genetic testing. The demyelination and white matter abnormalities seen in Alexander disease have a frontal predominance and often demonstrate contrast enhancement in the periventricular regions and sometimes the basal ganglia, thalami, or brainstem structures. The subcortical U-fibers are typically involved, although they may be spared in the early stages of the disease. Symmetric periventricular involvement with sparing of the U-fibers can be seen in metachromatic leukodystrophy. Leukoencephalopathy with vanishing white matter can cause posterior-predominant white matter changes with

U-fiber involvement in the mid to later stages. Diffuse white matter abnormalities with cerebellar atrophy is seen in alpha-mannosidosis, a type of lysosomal storage disease that causes hearing loss, skeletal abnormalities, and cognitive delay.

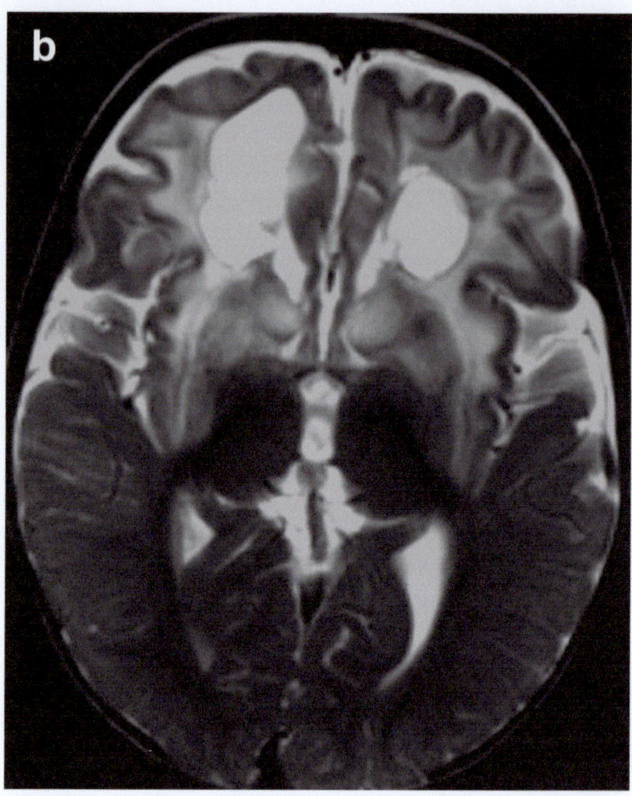

MRI brain of Alexander disease at 12 months of age. (Source: Nishibayashi, F., Kawashima, M., Katada, Y., Murakami, N., Nozaki, M. CC-BY 2.0 (https://creativecommons.org/licenses/by/2.0/) via *Journal of Medical Case Reports.* Image has been cropped from source. Nishibayashi F, Kawashima M, Katada Y, Murakami N, Nozaki M. Infantile-onset Alexander disease in a child with long-term follow-up by serial magnetic resonance imaging: a case report. J Med Case Rep. 2013;7:194. https://doi.org/10.1186/1752-1947-7-194)

References

Nishibayashi F, Kawashima M, Katada Y, Murakami N, Nozaki M. Infantile-onset Alexander disease in a child with long-term follow-up by serial magnetic resonance imaging: a case report. J Med Case Rep. 2013;7:194. https://doi.org/10.1186/1752-1947-7-194

Sabetrasekh, P., Alper, G., & Vanderver, A. (2017). Alexander disease type II. In E. Waubant & T. E. Lotze (Eds.), Pediatric demyelinating diseases of the central nervous system and their mimics (pp. 129–135). Springer.

Thakkar RN, Patel D, Kioutchoukova IP, Al-Bahou R, Reddy P, Foster DT, et al. Leukodystrophy Imaging: Insights for Diagnostic Dilemmas. Med Sci (Basel). 2024;12(1). https://doi.org/10.3390/medsci12010007

7. A 5-month-old child is referred for evaluation of hypotonia with high suspicion for Tay-Sachs disease. Which of the following findings would most strongly argue against this diagnosis?
   A. Development of hyperacusis
   B. Normal serum Arylsulfatase A activity
   C. Exaggerated startle response
   D. No organomegaly on ultrasound
   E. Normal serum hexosaminidase A activity
   Correct answer: E

Explanation

Tay-Sachs disease is a lysosomal storage disorder caused by a mutation in the HEXA gene. This mutation results in decreased or absent activity of hexosaminidase A, an enzyme which normally converts GM2 ganglioside into GM3 ganglioside as part of the breakdown pathway. Normal serum levels of hexosaminidase A activity are therefore not typically seen in children who have symptomatic Tay-Sachs Disease. Classic findings of this disorder present a few months after birth and include cherry red spot on the macula, hypotonia, exaggerated startle response, developmental delay, and hyperacusis. A cherry-red spot on the macula can also be seen in Niemann-Pick Types A and B, but those patients have hepatosplenomegaly, which is not seen in Tay-Sachs disease. Arylsulfatase A activity is reduced or absent in metachromatic leukodystrophy and not in Tay-Sachs disease.

References

Doe, J. A., & Smith, R. B. (2022). Lysosomal storage diseases: Pathogenesis and clinical features. In M. K. Johnson & L. P. Martinez (Eds.), Advances in neurogenetics (pp. 145–178). Academic Press.

McGinnis, S. (2023). Tay-Sachs disease: Pathophysiology, clinical features, and management. In R. Smith (Ed.), Neurogenetic disorders: Advances and treatments (2nd ed., pp. 145–170). Elsevier.

8. An 11-year-old girl presents to her pediatrician's office for an increasing rash this summer after coming back from summer camp. On further interview, development thus far has been notable for a mild delay in developmental milestones and intermittent mood swings. Examination demonstrates a wide-based gait, difficulty with performing rapid alternating hand movements, and rash as shown below. Laboratory tests demonstrate an elevated level of neutral amino acids in the urine. What is the best treatment for this condition?

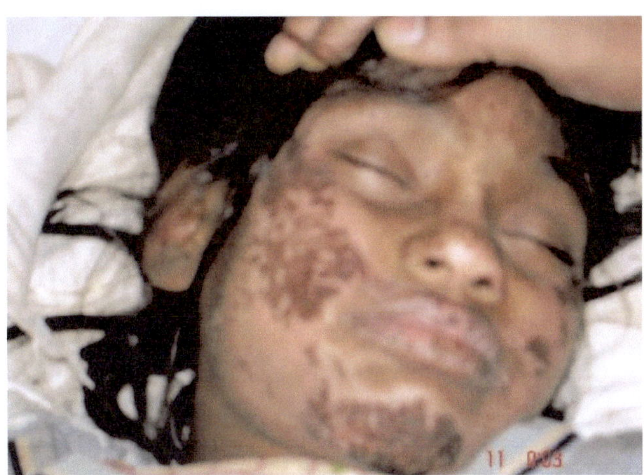

Skins lesions. (Source: Patel, A. B., Prabhu, A. S. CC-BY 2.0 (https://creativecommons.org/licenses/by/2.0/) via *Indian Journal of Dermatology*. Image has not been modified from source. Please see full attribution with citation below in references section for this question.)

A. Vitamin B3 (niacin) supplementation
B. Initiate chelation therapy
C. Vitamin E supplementation
D. Start a low protein diet
Correct answer: A

Explanation

This patient presents with developmental delays, photosensitivity (as evidenced by the red, scaly rash on areas of skin exposed to sun), psychiatric symptoms, and difficulty with coordinated movements and ataxia. These symptoms are all characteristic and key features of Hartnup disease. This is due to a mutation in the *SLC6A19* gene encoding the B0AT1 protein, which is responsible for reabsorbing neutral amino acids in the kidney such as tryptophan and phenylalanine. Thus, a urine test can reveal elevated levels of these amino acids that are being excreted at higher rates than normal. Tryptophan is a precursor to synthesis of niacin (Vitamin B3). Niacin deficiency can result in pellagra, which is characterized by multiple symptoms including dermatitis, diarrhea, and dementia. Additionally, tryptophan is the precursor to serotonin, which is important for motor control and mood. Supplementing with niacin and a high protein diet is the standard treatment for Hartnup Disease with good response in patients. Additionally, antidepressants can be utilized to help with mood-related symptoms. A high protein diet is usually initiated to help supplement the lost amino acids in the urine. Vitamin E deficiency can cause similar neurological symptoms of ataxia and neuropathy but is unlikely to have the skin manifestations and psychiatric comorbidities described here. Chelation therapy is the treatment of choice for iron or other heavy metal toxicity. Iron toxicity presents more chronically with multi-organ damage such as diabetes, skin pigmentation, joint pain, and heart failure or arrhythmia.

References

Patel AB, Prabhu AS. Hartnup disease. Indian J Dermatol. 2008;53(1):31–2. https://doi.org/10.4103/0019-5154.39740.

Smith, L. J., & Nguyen, T. M. (2021). Hartnup disease: Clinical presentation and management. In R. P. Thompson & A. K. Lee (Eds.), Inherited metabolic disorders in neurology (pp. 220–235). Springer.

9. In the pediatric neurology clinic, you see a follow-up for a 10-year-old boy initially presenting for recent onset of seizures and difficulty walking. At the prior visit, a physical exam described a tall boy with a depressed sternum and eye exam as below. Initial work-up demonstrated elevated urine homocysteine levels. Which of the following is an important primary neurological complication to advise the patient and family about?

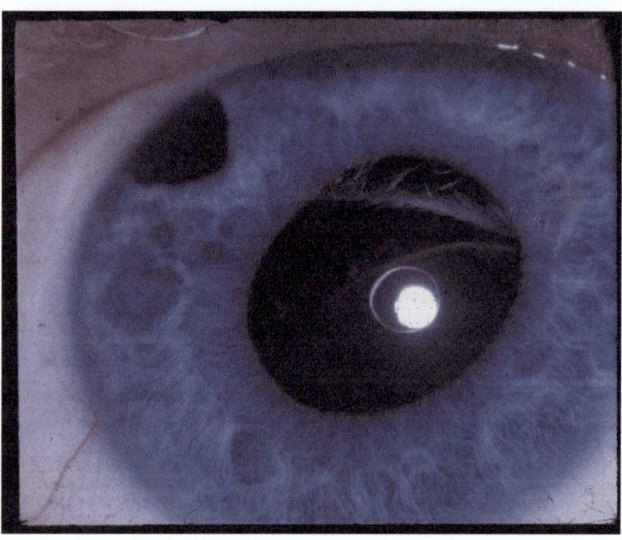

Eye. (Source: National Eye Institute, Public domain, via Wikimedia Commons)

A. Spontaneous subarachnoid hemorrhage
B. Cerebral infarction
C. Noncommunicating hydrocephalus
D. Parkinson's disease
E. Epidural hematoma
Correct answer: B

Explanation

This patient has symptoms of ataxia, seizures, a marfanoid habitus, and elevated urine homocysteine concentration, all of which are consistent with a diagnosis of homocystinuria.

The picture demonstrates downward subluxation of the lens in the eye. The downward displacement is a key feature seen in homocystinuria as opposed to Marfan Syndrome, which is associated with upward lens displacement. Homocystinuria is usually a result of cystathionine beta-synthase deficiency, which works to convert homocysteine to cystathionine. When the enzyme is deficient, it results in buildup of homocysteine and multiple neurological complications, including cognitive impairment, irritability and aggression, and seizures and induces a prothrombotic state. The prothrombotic state affects both venous and arterial systems, putting patients at high risk for ischemic cerebral infarction. Families and patients should be educated about signs of a stroke in order to seek immediate medical help. Due to the associated prothrombotic state, homocystinuria is more likely to cause ischemic infarcts than hemorrhagic infarcts. Hydrocephalus is not a common complication seen with this disease, but could be a secondary effect due to insults such as ischemic infarct. While homocystinuria can cause abnormal movements, such as dystonias and Parkinson-like symptoms, it is usually as a result of cerebral infarctions to the basal ganglia and not a primary effect of the disease itself. Lastly, epidural hematomas are secondary to trauma or iatrogenic interventions and not commonly seen with homocystinuria.

References

Garcia, L. F., & Thompson, H. J. (2018). Homocystinuria: Diagnosis and therapeutic strategies. In S. K. Miller & R. D. Carter (Eds.), Metabolic disorders of the nervous system (pp. 198–215).

Jones, M. R., & Patel, S. K. (2020). Homocystinuria: Biochemical basis and clinical management. In D. L. Harrison & P. R. Williams (Eds.), Inherited metabolic diseases: Clinical and molecular aspects (pp. 312–330). Elsevier.

National Eye Institute, Public domain, via Wikimedia Commons

10. A 1-year-old boy presents to the pediatric clinic for follow-up of worsening vision. His mother states he is no longer tracking objects and is not reaching for toys in front of him over the past few months. On physical examination, the patient is noted to have bilateral decreased red reflex, hypotonia, and prominent forehead with sunken cheeks. Initial labs show low serum phosphate and bicarbonate with normal anion gap and glycosuria. Which of the following is the most likely diagnosis?
A. Hurler syndrome
B. Zellweger spectrum disorder
C. Congenital CMV infection
D. Cystinosis
E. Lowe syndrome
Correct answer: E

Explanation

The child described has overall worsening vision over a sub-acute period. His exam is concerning for bilateral cataracts and low tone with facial dysmorphism. His lab results demonstrate a metabolic acidosis with low bicarbonate. This, in combination with low phosphate and elevated glucose in the urine, are suggestive of renal tubular disease, particularly Fanconi syndrome. This triad of cataracts (eye), hypotonia/intellectual disability (brain), and Fanconi syndrome (kidney) are classic for Lowe syndrome. Lowe syndrome is caused by a genetic mutation in the *OCRL* gene responsible for the OCRL-1 enzyme and is X-linked. This enzyme is essential for membrane trafficking and cytoskeletal structure with high expression in the kidneys, eye, and brain. While there is no cure, early treatment revolves around electrolyte and amino acid replacement, cataract removal, and physical and developmental therapies. Hurler syndrome is a mitochondrial disorder that can cause intellectual disability and has coarse facies, hepatosplenomegaly, and corneal clouding but not cataracts. Zellweger spectrum is a group of disorders affecting peroxisomes that can cause hypotonia and facial dysmorphisms but typically has a severe clinical presentation with rapid neurological decline due to lack of myelination; it is often lethal within the first 1–2 years of life. While congenital cytomegalovirus (CMV) infection can cause developmental delay and hypotonia, one would not expect to see cataracts or electrolyte abnormalities. Characteristic brain imaging in congenital CMV infection would also show periventricular calcifications. Cystinosis is a result of impaired cysteine removal by lysosomes. It is also a known cause of Fanconi syndrome but demonstrates cystine crystal in the cornea, not congenital cataracts.

References

Louis, E. D., Mayer, S. A., & Noble, J. M. (Eds.). (2021). Merritt's neurology (14th ed.). Wolters Kluwer Health.

Smith, J., & Brown, T. (2020). Lowe syndrome: Neurological manifestations and management. In K. F. Swaiman & S. Ashwal (Eds.), Pediatric Neurology: Principles and Practice (pp. 400–415). Elsevier.

11. In infants with Crigler-Najjar syndrome, what is the mechanism for neurological dysfunction such as poor feeding, lethargy, and low tone?
    A. Bilirubin-induced neurotoxicity
    B. Hyperammonemia secondary to liver failure
    C. Hypoxic-ischemic encephalopathy
    D. Cerebral infarction
    Correct answer: A

Explanation

Crigler-Najjar syndrome is due to a mutation in a gene causing deficiency of the enzyme uridine glucuronosyltransferase. This enzyme is key for conjugating bilirubin in the liver. Without this enzyme, unconjugated bilirubin increases and can lead to accumulation in the brain, resulting in bilirubin-induced neurotoxicity or kernicterus. This can lead to significant neurological dysfunction including low tone, decreased feeding, and seizures. Early intervention with phototherapy or exchange transfusion is essential. The liver in these patients otherwise functions normally, so would expect to see normal levels of AST, ALT, and ammonia and a normal appearing liver on imaging. Hypoxic-ischemic encephalopathy is secondary to lack of blood flow to the brain and can cause similar neurological symptoms but would have normal bilirubin and characteristic birth history and MRI findings. Crigler-Najjar syndrome does not place individuals at increased risk of ischemic or hemorrhage stroke.

Reference

Labrune, P., Myara, A., Hadchouel, M., & Sinaasappel, M. (2016). Neonatal jaundice and disorders of bilirubin metabolism. In Liver Disease in Children (pp. 157–174). Cambridge University Press.

12. A 2-month-old infant is referred to the neurology clinic after she was noted to have low tone and an abnormal cry. Her mother had an uncomplicated pregnancy and delivery. Since birth though, her mother has noted a high-pitched and sharp cry that sounds different from her siblings. On exam, she is unable to hold her head up and has head circumference in the 3rd percentile. It is suspected she has a genetic syndrome. Which of the following would be the next best test to confirm diagnosis?
    A. Chromosomal microarray
    B. Whole exome sequencing
    C. Brain MRI
    D. Karyotype analysis
    Correct answer: A

Explanation

Cri-du-chat syndrome, also known as 5p-syndrome, is a genetic condition resulting from deletion of the short arm of chromosome 5 that can be inherited or can occur spontaneously. Patients with this syndrome present with microcephaly, micrognathia, low birth weight, developmental delays in speech and motor skills, and intellectual disability. The most notable feature is a high-pitched, cat-like cry that occurs due to structural laryngeal abnormalities. Chromosomal microarray is the best test for detecting small chromosomal deletions as seen in cri-du-chat syndrome. Whole exome sequencing can miss small deletions and is best for single gene disorders. Brain MRI can show nonspecific changes such as atrophy but will not confirm the specific diagnosis. Karyotype analysis looks at chromosome banding patterns and can pick up large chromosome deletions but can miss the small microdeletions seen in disorders such as cri-du-chat syndrome.

References

Chen, H. (2016). Cri-Du-Chat Syndrome. In Atlas of Genetic Diagnosis and Counseling (pp. 675–683). Springer.

Su J, Fu H, Xie B, Lu W, Li W, Wei Y, et al. Prenatal diagnosis of cri-du-chat syndrome by SNP array: report of twelve cases and review of the literature. Mol Cytogenet. 2019;12:49. https://doi.org/10.1186/s13039-019-0462-0.

Linked questions: 13–14

13. A 13-year-old boy is seen as a new patient in the neurology clinic for increasing difficulty writing at school and clumsiness. The patient reports that his hand will twist at times, making it hard to hold onto his pencil. Additionally, he has had increasing difficulty walking in gym class and often finding himself tripping over his own feet. His mother reports similar symptoms in the patient's father, who died in a car crash when he was in his 20 s. Neurological exam shows mask-like facial expression, dysarthria, abnormal head tilt to the right, and generalized hyperreflexia. MRI of the brain is obtained and is shown below. Which of the following is the most likely diagnosis?

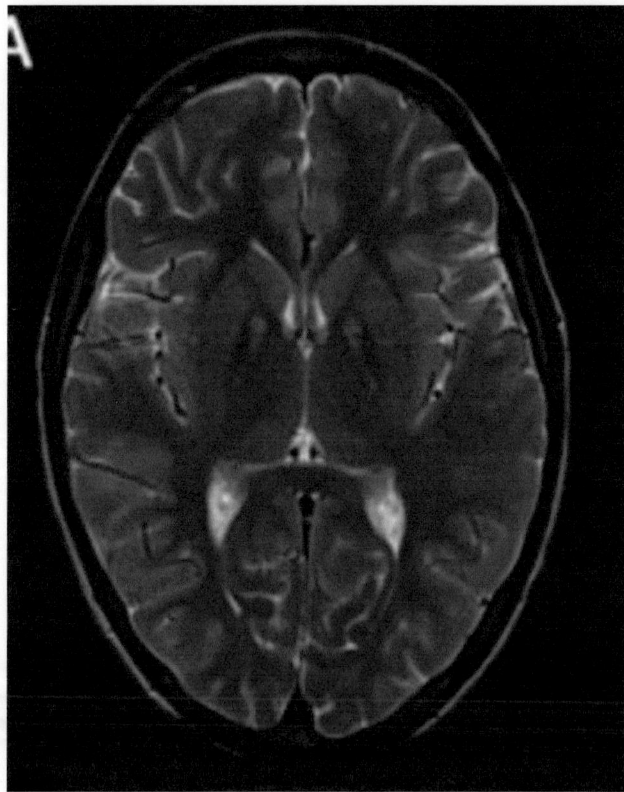

Axial MRI brain. (Source: Horache, K., Messaoud, O., Elkettani, N., Fikri, M., Jiddane, M., Touarsa, F. CC-BY 4.0 (https://creativecommons.org/licenses/by/4.0/) via *International Journal of Case Reports and Images*. Image has been cropped from source. Please see full attribution with citation below in references section for this question.)

A. Fredrich's ataxia
B. Huntington's disease
C. Pantothenate kinase-associated neurodegeneration
D. Wilson disease
E. Tay-Sachs disease

Correct answer: C

Explanation

Pantothenate kinase-associated neurodegeneration or PKAN is a neurodegenerative disorder due to a mutation in the PANK2 gene. Typical onset of symptoms occurs in pre-teen to teenage years with development of dystonias, rigidity, and spasticity, dysarthria, dysphagia, and later more cognitive decline. Life expectancy is usually 10–15 years after onset of symptoms with death occurring due to complications such as malnutrition, aspiration, or respiratory failure. In the atypical form of the disorder, symptoms are milder, start later in life, and generally are slower to progress with patients living to middle age. Only supportive therapy is available with no cure at the time of publication, but there is ongoing research into gene therapies.

The image above shows a *T2-weighted MRI showing the classic "eye-of-the-tiger" sign in the globus pallidus in a patient with PKAN.*

References

Hayflick, S. J., & Kurian, M. A. (2013). Pantothenate kinase (PANK2)-associated neurodegeneration. In C. Falup-Pecurariu, J. Ferreira, P. Martinez-Martin, & K. Ray Chaudhuri (Eds.), International Review of Neurobiology (Vol. 110, pp. 49–71). Academic Press.

Horache K., Messaoud, O., Elkettani, N., Fikri, M., Jiddane, M., Touarsa, F. Pantothenate kinase-associated neurodegeneration (PKAN) with a typical "eye of the tiger": A radiology case report. International Journal of Case Reports and Images. 2024;15(1):66–8. https://doi.org/10.5348/101447Z01KH2024CI.

Linked question

14. What is the mechanism of action by which the disorder above causes neurotoxicity?
    A. Protein misfolding and aggregation
    B. Copper accumulation in the brain
    C. Iron accumulation in the brain
    D. Impaired lysosomal storage within neurons

Correct answer: C

Explanation

PKAN is a result of a mutation in the PANK2 gene which encodes pantothenate kinase 2. This protein is a regulatory enzyme necessary for synthesis of Coenzyme A (CoA). CoA is essential for cellular energy and lipid synthesis. PANK2 is particularly highly concentrated in mitochondria in neurons. CoA is essential to multiple cell cycles that produce energy, including the citric acid cycle. Without functional CoA, cells are unable to produce enough energy and develop toxic accumulation of other downstream products such as cysteine. Cysteine in high concentrations can create a complex with iron in mitochondria. Over time, this iron accumulation leads to oxidative stress and neuronal cell death. It is unclear why, but these complexes particularly accumulate in the basal ganglia, causing the characteristic "eye of the tiger" sign as seen on MRI above. Huntington's disease is a result of trinucleotide repeat expansion of CAG creating a mutant protein that undergoes misfolding and aggregation. Wilson disease occurs due to copper accumulation in the brain. Tay-Sachs disease is caused by a gene mutation resulting in loss of the lysosomal enzyme β-hexosaminidase A.

Reference

Barton, J. C., Edwards, C. Q., Phatak, P. D., Britton, R. S., & Bacon, B. R. (2011). Pantothenate kinase (PANK2)-associated neurodegeneration. In Handbook of Iron Overload Disorders (pp. 437–448). Cambridge University Press.

15. A 5-year-old child presents with progressive ataxia, hepatosplenomegaly, and bone pain. Neurologic exam demonstrates oculomotor abnormalities and cognitive decline. Initial laboratory studies show decreased glucocerebrosidase activity. Based on the most likely diagnosis, what is the best initial treatment for this patient?
    A. Enzyme replacement therapy
    B. High-dose steroids
    C. Bone-marrow transplant
    D. Stem-cell gene therapy
    E. Dietary restriction of substrate
    Correct answer: A

Explanation

The child's presenting symptoms and decreased glucocerebrosidase activity are all suggestive of Gaucher disease. This is a lysosomal storage disorder that occurs as a result of decreased activity of the glucocerebrosidase enzyme, causing build-up of glucocerebroside in macrophages. The classic presenting symptoms of this disease include hepatosplenomegaly, bone pain/crises, pancytopenias, and neurological complications including ataxia, oculomotor apraxia, and cognitive decline. First-line treatment is enzyme replacement therapy with imiglucerase, but neurological symptoms are often refractory to treatment. High-dose steroids and dietary restrictions do not directly target the cause or effects of the disease. Bone marrow transplant is restricted

to patients who are refractory to first-line treatment. Stem-cell therapy is still in the experimental phase and not yet standard treatment at time of publication.

References

Aboobacker FN, Kulkarni UP, Korula A, Devasia AJ, Selvarajan S, Lionel S, et al. Hematopoietic Stem Cell Transplantation is a cost-effective alternative to enzyme replacement therapy in Gaucher Disease. Blood Cell Ther. 2022;5(3):69–74. https://doi.org/10.31547/bct-2021-020.

Patel, R. S., & Williams, D. L. (2022). Gaucher disease: Pathophysiology and clinical management. In M. K. Johnston & L. P. Harrison (Eds.), Handbook of inherited metabolic disorders (third ed., pp. 320–345).

Linked questions: 16–17

16. A 4-year-old boy is brought into the neurology clinic for abnormal movements. The boy's mother states that for the past few years, she has noted abnormal twisting movements of his arms that have become more frequent. When she asks him to stop, he is not able to. On chart review of his pediatrician's notes, the boy is behind in all developmental milestones and has had two hospital visits for chewing on his lips and fingers requiring stitches. Exam shows intermittent flailing and jerking of his arms as well as muscle stiffness with difficulty relaxing. Lab tests show elevated serum uric acid. Which of the following enzyme deficiencies is the cause of this patient's condition?
    A. Xanthine oxidase
    B. Guanidinoacetate methyltransferase
    C. Ornithine transcarbamylase
    D. Hypoxanthine-guanine phosphoribosyltransferase
    Correct answer: D

Explanation

This boy presents with classic symptoms of Lesch-Nyhan Syndrome. This disease is caused by a deficiency in hypoxanthine-guanine phosphoribosyl transferase, which is an essential enzyme involved in purine metabolism. Without this enzyme, uric acid accumulates in multiple organs and causes various symptoms. These include abnormal movements such as dystonia, chorea, or ballismus, as well as developmental delay, gout, kidney stones, and characteristic self-injurious behaviors such as biting lips and fingers or head-banging. Xanthine oxidase is the enzyme that converts xanthine to uric acid, so a deficiency in this enzyme would result in low, not high, uric acid levels. Guanidinoacetate methyltransferase is involved in creatine formation important for energy metabolism. While it can cause similar symptoms of developmental delay and movement disorders, the uric acid level would be normal and creatine would be low. Ornithine trancarbamylase deficiency is a classic urea cycle disorder that leads to elevated ammonia causing nausea, vomiting, and lethargy. It does not cause elevated uric acid or abnormal movements.

References

Burkitt, A. S. G. W. (Ed.). (2019). Neurogenetics: A guide to the molecular genetics of neurological disease. Elsevier.

Gahl, W. A., & Smith, M. A. L. (2020). Lesch-Nyhan syndrome. In A. R. Toth & R. P. Greenberg (Eds.), GeneReviews [Online]. University of Washington.

Linked question

17. After formal genetic testing, the suspected diagnosis above is confirmed. The boy is started on treatment with allopurinol and uric acid levels normalize. However, at the follow-up visit, his mother continues to report repeated episodes of tongue biting. What is the next best step in management?
    A. Start tetrabenazine with the allopurinol
    B. Increase the dose of allopurinol
    C. Add baclofen to the current regimen
    D. Initiate Febuxostat in addition to the allopurinol
    E. Begin behavioral therapy without additional medications
    Correct answer: C

Explanation

This boy with Lesch-Nyhan syndrome was appropriately treated with allopurinol to help decrease uric acid accumulation and prevent the associated hyperuricemia symptoms such as gout and kidney stones. However, allopurinol does not directly address the neurological manifestations of the disease, including self-injurious behavior. These behaviors can persist despite normalization of uric acid levels, therefore increasing the dose of allopurinol or adding an additional uric acid lowering agent such as febuxostat will not help manage these specific symptoms. The self-injurious behavior in Lesch-Nyhan is often a result of the abnormal movements, therefore targeting those movements directly has been shown to be effective. Thus, the next step would be starting a muscle relaxant like baclofen to help decrease dystonic and spastic manifestations and prevent further injury. Tetrabenazine is used for hyperkinetic movements and is not the first-line therapy for dystonia. Behavioral therapy can be effective in addressing ways to manage frustration and demonstrate safe behaviors, but should not be the sole therapy and can be used in conjunction with pharmacological interventions.

Reference

Jinnah, H. A., & DeGregorio, L. M. (2009). Neurologic and behavioral manifestations of Lesch-Nyhan disease and their treatment. Developmental Disabilities Research Reviews, 15(2), 146–155.

18. A 9-month-old full-term girl presents to the hospital for increasing difficulty breathing. The infant's parents have noticed increasing respiratory effort and often find her gasping for air. History is notable for being able to grasp with both hands, unable to sit independently, and able to roll from back to front. On exam, she is hypoxemic, hypotonic, with macroglossia, and hepatosplenomegaly. EKG shows a shortened PR interval. A muscle biopsy demonstrates vacuolated fibers with periodic acid–Schiff positive staining. Which of the following is the most likely diagnosis?
    A. Spinal Muscular Atrophy Type I
    B. Pompe Disease
    C. Cori Disease
    D. Leigh Syndrome
    E. Zellweger syndrome
    Correct answer: B

Explanation

This infant presents with respiratory distress and is noted to have low tone with motor developmental delay, large tongue, and hepatosplenomegaly. These are characteristic of a diagnosis of Pompe disease, an autosomal recessive disorder that causes reduced levels of the enzyme acid α-glucosidase (GAA). This enzyme is involved in breaking down glycogen. When glycogen accumulates in muscle, it can lead to muscle weakness and respiratory distress. EKG reveals a prolonged PR interval, likely secondary to build up of glycogen in the heart's conduction system. Muscle biopsy shows glycogen vacuoles within muscle fibers which are PAS-positive due to the glycogen accumulation. Diagnosis can be made with muscle biopsy, genetic testing, or enzyme activity measurement. Treatment involves early initiation of enzyme replacement therapy, but prognosis remains poor with death often occurring in the first decades of life. While the other answer choices can present with similar neurological features of muscle weakness and low tone, none of them would cause the PAS-positive vacuoles on muscle biopsy.

References

Polin, R. A., & Chung, W. K. (2011). Glycogen storage disease type II (Pompe's disease). In R. A. Polin & J. M. Lorenz (Eds.), Neonatology (pp. 165–167). Cambridge University Press.

Wokke, J. H. J., van Doorn, P. A., Hoogendijk, J. E., & de Visser, M. (2013). Glycogen storage disease type 2, Pompe disease. In Neuromuscular Disease (pp. 205–211). Cambridge University Press.

19. What is the pathophysiological mechanism of Krabbe disease?
    A. Increasing sphingomyelin accumulation
    B. Deficiency of arylsulfatase A enzyme
    C. Decreased hexosaminidase A levels
    D. Accumulation of galactocerebroside and psychosine
    Correct answer: D

Explanation

Krabbe disease is a lysosomal storage disorder caused by a deficiency in the enzyme galactosylceramidase. This is due to a mutation in the *GALC* gene and is autosomal recessive. The enzyme is central to the breakdown of galactolipids. When the enzyme is deficient, galactosylceramide and psychosine accumulate in neurons and are cytotoxic, ultimately leading to demyelination and formation of the characteristic globoid cells seen in Krabbe disease. Increased levels of sphingomyelin are seen in Niemann-Pick types A and B disease due to decreased sphingomyelinase activity. Metachromatic leukodystrophy is due to decreased arylsulfatase A enzyme activity causing build-up of sulfatides. Tay-Sachs disease is due to decreased hexosaminidase A enzyme activity leading to the build-up of GM2 gangliosides.

References

Mehta, A. B., & Winchester, B. (Eds.). (2012). Lysosomal storage disorders: A practical guide (2nd ed.). Wiley-Blackwell.

Schuchman, E. H., & Wasserstein, M. P. (2018). Lysosomal storage diseases: Perspectives and principles. In Hematology: Basic Principles and Practice (pp. 740–746). Elsevier Inc.

20. An 8-month-old presents with hypotonia and difficulty feeding. On a fundoscopic exam, the infant is noted to have a cherry-red spot. Enzyme testing reveals a lysosomal storage disorder. Which of the following clinical features would be more suggestive of Niemann-Pick disease rather than Tay-Sachs disease?
    A. Early onset cardiomyopathy
    B. Presence of startle reflex
    C. Coarse facial features
    D. Hepatosplenomegaly
    E. Developmental regression
    Correct answer: D

Explanation

Niemann-Pick and Tay-Sachs are both lysosomal storage disorders that present with neurodegeneration. However, they differ in mechanism, pathology, and a few key clinical characteristics. Both diseases cause developmental regression and a cherry red spot on the macula. One major distinction between the two is that Niemann-Pick has hepatosplenomegaly while Tay-Sachs does not. Exaggerated startle reflex is more characteristic of Tay-Sachs disease. Neither Niemann-Pick nor Tay-Sachs present with significant coarse and specific facial features. Coarse facial features can be seen with Hurler or Hunter syndrome.

Reference

Louis, E. D., Mayer, S. A., & Noble, J. M. (Eds.). (2021). Merritt's neurology (14th ed.). Wolters Kluwer Health.

21. Which of the following neurological features is most characteristic of Trisomy 13?
    A. Chiari malformation
    B. Holoprosencephaly
    C. Periventricular leukomalacia
    D. Cerebellar hypoplasia
    E. Corpus callosum agenesis
    Correct answer: B

Explanation

Trisomy 13, also known as Patau syndrome, classically presents with microcephaly, cleft palate, congenital heart defects, polydactyl, low set ears, and neurodevelopmental and growth delays. Neurological complications also include spinal cord malformations, scalp defects, and holoprosencephaly. Holoprosencephaly occurs when the brain does not divide into two hemispheres during development. This in turn can cause intellectual disabilities, developmental delays, seizures, pituitary disorders, cleft lip/palate, and close-spaced eyes. The other answer choices are not commonly seen in Trisomy 13.

References

Lechpammer, M., Del Bigio, M., & Folkerth, R. (2021). Patau syndrome (trisomy 13). In Perinatal Neuropathology (pp. 269–272). Cambridge University Press.

Louis, E. D., Mayer, S. A., & Noble, J. M. (Eds.). (2021). Merritt's neurology (14th ed.). Wolters Kluwer Health.

22. A teenage boy presents as a new patient for progressive muscle weakness. He has particular difficulty with standing from sitting and has worsening hearing loss. He has also noticed brief, involuntary jerking movements of his arms. Neurological exam demonstrates proximal muscle weakness, ophthalmoplegia, and ataxic gait. A muscle biopsy is performed and is shown below. Which of the following is the most likely diagnosis?

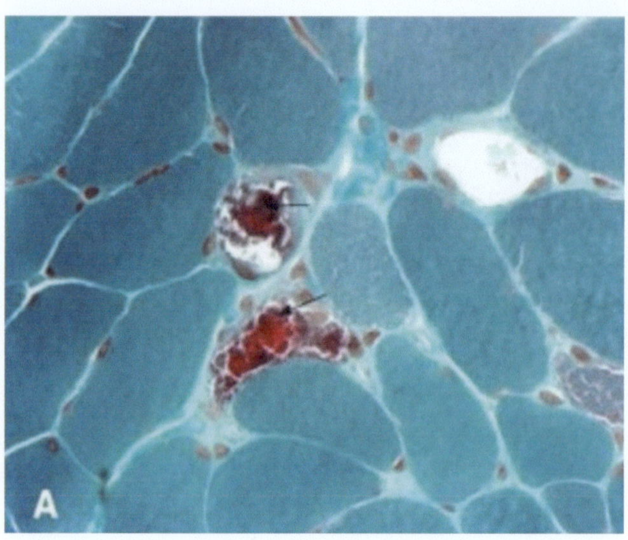

Micrograph. (Source: Abu-Amero, K. K., Al-Dhalaan, H., Bohlega, S., Hellani, A., Taylor, R. W. CC-BY 2.0 (https://creativecommons.org/licenses/by/2.0/) via *Journal of Medical Case Reports*. Image has been cropped from source. Please see full attribution with citation below in references section for this question.)

A. Myoclonic epilepsy with ragged red fibers (MERRF)
B. Duchenne muscular dystrophy
C. Spinal muscular atrophy type III
D. Charcot-Marie-Tooth disease
E. Becker muscular dystrophy

Correct answer: A

Explanation

The patient has proximal muscle weakness associated with hearing loss, ataxia, and ophthalmoplegia. Additionally, he has involuntary jerking movements that are likely myoclonus. These symptoms in combination with the muscle biopsy demonstrating red-ragged fibers are most consistent with myoclonic epilepsy with ragged red fibers (MERRF). MERRF is a mitochondrial disorder caused by a mutation leading to impaired mitochondrial protein synthesis. It is diagnosed via genetic testing and/or muscle biopsy. While there is no definitive treatment, patients with this condition should have regular hearing, vision, and cardiac function testing as well as physical therapy. Duchenne and Becker muscular dystrophy also cause proximal muscle weakness and elevated CK but would not cause red-ragged fibers on biopsy. Spinal muscular atrophy III also causes proximal muscle weakness but would not have myoclonus or ragged-red fibers. Lastly Charcot-Marie-Tooth disease presents with more distal weakness and sensory loss and would not cause myoclonus.

The micrograph above shows biopsy with Gömöri trichome staining demonstrating ragged red fibers.

References

Abu-Amero KK, Al-Dhalaan H, Bohlega S, Hellani A, Taylor RW. A patient with typical clinical features of mitochondrial encephalopathy, lactic acidosis and stroke-like episodes (MELAS) but without an obvious genetic cause: a case report. J Med Case Rep. 2009;3:77. https://doi.org/10.1186/1752-1947-3-77.

Engel, A. G. (n.d.). Mitochondrial encephalomyopathy with lactic acidosis and stroke-like episodes (MELAS). Washington University Neuromuscular Disease Center.

Nyhan, W. L., Hoffmann, G. F., Al-Aqeel, A. I., & Barshop, B. A. (2020). Myoclonic epilepsy with ragged-red fibers. In Mitochondrial diseases: Clinical and molecular aspects (pp. 123–145). Springer.

23. An 18-month-old girl is brought into the clinic for developmental regression. She had been meeting developmental milestones until around 14 months of age. She now has stereotyped hand-wringing movements and is no longer speaking. Her head circumference, which was at the 75th percentile in infancy, is now below the 3rd percentile. Which of the following genetic or molecular abnormalities is the most likely cause?
A. MECP2 de novo mutation
B. CGG expansion repeat in FMR1
C. TSC gene mutation
D. ARSA gene deficiency

Correct answer: A

Explanation

This child is presenting with features consistent with Rett syndrome. This is a neurodevelopmental disorder that primarily affects females with characteristic symptoms of developmental regression between 6 and 18 months, stereotypical midline hand-wringing movements, and secondary microcephaly after a period of normal head circumference. It is caused by a mutation in the methyl CpG binding protein 2 (MECP2) gene on the X chromosome, which encodes for a protein essential to normal brain development. These mutations are usually de novo, and treatment is supportive. CGG expansion repeat in the Fragile X Messenger Ribonucleoprotein 1 (FMR1) gene causes Fragile X syndrome, which is more commonly seen in boys with intellectual disability, hyperactivity, and impulsivity, and characteristic facial and body dysmorphic features. Tuberous sclerosis complex (TSC) gene mutations lead to tuberous sclerosis complex, which would present with multi-organ symptoms including characteristic skin findings, developmental delay, seizures, and cardiac and renal masses but does not have developmental regression or hand-wringing. Arylsulfatase A (ARSA) gene deficiency is seen in metachromatic leukodystrophy, which results in marked cognitive and motor regression but does not include stereotyped hand movements or secondary microcephaly.

References

Han ZA, Jeon HR, Kim SW, Park JY, Chung HJ. Clinical characteristics of children with rett syndrome. Ann Rehabil Med. 2012;36(3):334–9. https://doi.org/10.5535/arm.2012.36.3.334.

Louis, E. D., Mayer, S. A., & Noble, J. M. (Eds.). (2021). Merritt's neurology (14th ed.). Wolters Kluwer Health.

24. A 10-year-old boy with Down syndrome presents to the emergency room with 2 days of difficulty walking and clumsiness. He is also experiencing urinary incontinence. He has had no falls or trauma. Neurological exam reflexes diffuse hyperreflexia, up-going toes bilaterally, and spastic tone throughout extremities. MRI of the brain and C-spine are ordered. Which of the following is the most likely finding?
    A. Cervical myelopathy secondary to atlanto-axial instability
    B. Acute flaccid myelitis
    C. Cervical spondylotic myelopathy
    D. Segmental demyelinating lesion
    E. Cervical syringomyelia
    Correct answer: A

Explanation

This child's exam shows signs of loss of urinary control, ataxia, hyperreflexia with positive Babinski, and increased tone. These signs all point toward an upper motor neuron lesion at a high level given arm involvement. Children with Down syndrome are at risk for multiple neurological complications that should be considered. This includes atlanto-axial instability due to bony abnormalities and laxity in the corresponding ligaments in the upper neck. This can spontaneously cause compression of the spinal cord and the associated symptoms listed above. When suspected, the cervical spine should be immobilized and MR imaging obtained. If confirmed, early surgical intervention with fusion is the standard treatment of choice to prevent further long-term nerve damage. Without any clear signs of trauma, proceeding illness, or progressive nature, most other answer choices are less likely. Acute flaccid myelitis usually occurs after an illness and would cause more lower motor neuron signs on examination. Spondylotic myelopathy, while would cause similar symptoms, is uncommon in this age group, as it is a degenerative disease seen in older adults. Segmental demyelination can be seen in disorders such as multiple sclerosis (MS) and although MS relapses can occur in pediatric patients, this is relatively uncommon. With an existing history of Down's syndrome, the more likely answer is cervical myelopathy secondary to atlanto-axial instability. A cervical syringomy-

elia would also be slowly progressive and likely cause a cape-like distribution of sensory loss across the shoulders and upper extremities.

Reference

Staheli, L. T. (2019). Atlanto-axial instability. In R. M. Kliegman, J. W. St. Geme III, & N. F. Schor (Eds.), Nelson Textbook of Pediatrics (21st ed.). Elsevier.

25. A 9-month-old boy is referred to the neurology clinic as the infant is unable to sit independently and has poor head control. On neurological examination, the infant has rhythmic back and forth eye movements that persist in all directions and with fixation. Additionally, he has increased tone of the legs and truncal hypotonia. MRI findings are shown below. Genetic testing is still pending but is most likely to show a mutation in which of the following genes?

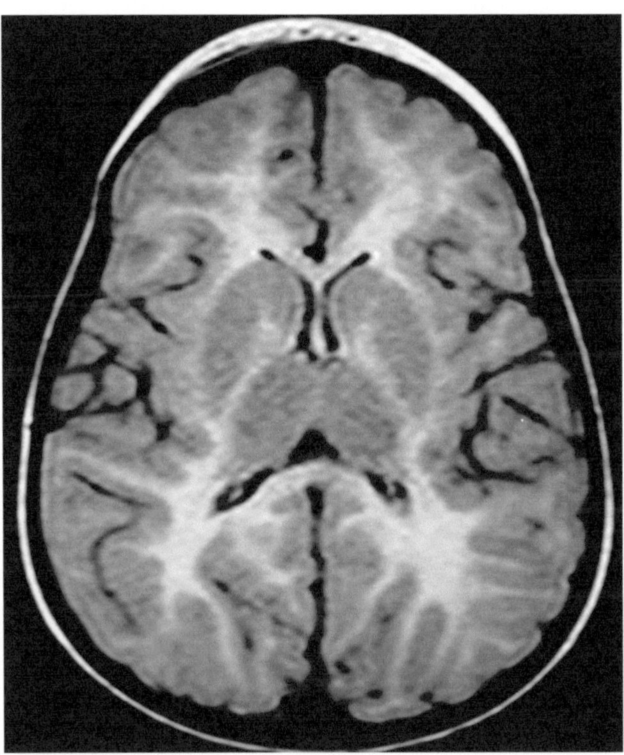

Axial MRI brain. (Source: Masliah-Planchon, J., Dupont, C., Vartzelis, G., Trimouille, A., Eymard-Pierre, E., Gay-Bellile, M., Renaldo, F., Dorboz, I., Pagan, C., Quentin, S., Elmaleh, M., Kotsogianni, C., Konstantelou, E., Drunat, S., Tabet, A-C., Boespflug-Tanguy, O. CC-BY 4.0 (https://creativecommons.org/licenses/by/4.0/) via *BMC Medical Genetics*. Image has been cropped from source. Please see full attribution with citation below in references section for this question.)

    A. ABCD1
    B. ARSA
    C. PLP1
    D. GALC
    Correct answer: C

Explanation

This infant presenting with motor developmental delay, pendular nystagmus, increased tone, and truncal hypotonia most likely has Pelizaeus-Merzbacher disease (PMD). This is caused by a mutation in the *PLP1* gene on the X chromosome leading to a duplication of the gene and overproduction of the proteolipid protein. When this protein is expressed in high quantities, it can disrupt normal myelination and cause the neurodevelopmental symptoms described. Specifically, pendular nystagmus with smooth, back and forth movements is characteristic for PMD. Diagnosis is confirmed via genetic testing, but MRI brain may demonstrate a "tigroid" appearance resulting from patchy myelination, with T2-hyperintense signal seen in areas of preserved myelin interspersed with T2-hypointense regions of hypomyelination. Alternatively, MRI brain may show diffuse increased T2-hyperintense signal (as shown in the image above). ABCD1 mutation causes adrenoleukodystrophy, a peroxisomal disorder. This also causes progressive demyelination but would be more diffuse due to the accumulation of very long-chain fatty acids. ARSA gene mutation causes arylsulfatase enzyme deficiency resulting in metachromatic leukodystrophy. This usually causes progressive severe motor and cognitive impairments and would not cause the MRI findings above. Krabbe disease is caused by a mutation in the GALC gene leading to demyelination in the central nervous system which would also result in more diffuse white matter changes rather than the patchy appearance seen on the MRI above. None of these other disorders typically present with pendular nystagmus.

References

Kohlschütter A, Eichler F. Childhood leukodystrophies: a clinical perspective. Expert Rev. Neurother. 2011;11(10):1485–96. https://doi.org/10.1586/ern.11.135.

Masliah-Planchon J, Dupont C, Vartzelis G, Trimouille A, Eymard-Pierre E, Gay-Bellile M, et al. Insertion of an extra copy of Xq22.2 into 1p36 results in functional duplication of the PLP1 gene in a girl with classical Pelizaeus-Merzbacher disease. BMC Med Genet. 2015;16:77. https://doi.org/10.1186/s12881-015-0226-6.

Pascual, J. M. (2017). Pelizaeus–Merzbacher disease. In Progressive Brain Disorders in Childhood (pp. 188–190). Cambridge University Press.

Ropper, A. H., Samuels, M. A., Klein, J. P., & Prasad, S. (2023). Adams and Victor's principles of neurology (12th ed.). McGraw-Hill Education.

26. What is the most common neurological complication of acute intermittent porphyria?
    A. Symmetric proximal motor neuropathy
    B. Generalized tonic-clonic seizures
    C. Distal symmetric length-dependent sensory neuropathy
    D. Cranial neuropathies
    E. Multifocal mononeuritis multiplex

Correct answer: A

Explanation

Acute intermittent porphyria (AIP) is a disease that occurs secondary to the accumulation of porphyrin resulting from a deficiency of the enzyme porphobilinogen deaminase. It most commonly causes symptoms of severe abdominal pain, constipation, nausea, vomiting, autonomic instability, and palpitations. Porphyrin itself is also highly neurotoxic, interfering with nerve function and maintenance. Common neurological symptoms include seizures, confusion, hallucinations, and most commonly acute neuropathy. The associated neuropathy primarily affects the motor nerves and often more proximal muscles first. The proximal muscles often rely more on larger motor neurons that are more subject to damage from accumulation of these neurotoxic substrates. Distal symmetric length-dependent sensory neuropathy is not classically seen in AIP but rather other metabolic conditions such as diabetes, vitamin deficiencies, chronic alcohol use, or hypothyroidism. Diagnosis is confirmed with elevated urinary porphyrin precursor markers, and treatment includes avoiding precipitating factors such as fasting or alcohol use and administration of heminin to reduce the level of the precursors that have built up. While AIP can cause seizures, it is an uncommon complication. AIP is not known to cause cranial neuropathies or multifocal mononeuritis multiplex, usually seen in vasculitis.

References

Bissell, D. M., & Korman, S. (2018). Acute intermittent porphyria: Diagnosis and management. Textbook of Medical Neurology, 4(2), 256–267.

Smith, J. A., & Johnson, R. B. (2023). The pathophysiology and clinical management of AIP motor neuropathy. Journal of Neurological Disorders, 15(2), 123–135.

Smith, J. D., & Thompson, A. P. (2020). Motor neuropathy in acute intermittent porphyria: A review of the neurological manifestations. Journal of Neurology and Clinical Neuroscience, 58(3), 202–210.

27. A teenage boy presents with episodes of burning pain in his hands and feet. He describes it as if his hands and feet were falling asleep and notices it most when he is in gym class or when he is playing soccer. He also has a history of small, dark red spots on his thighs. Neurologic examination shows decreased sensation to temperature and pain in his hands and feet. His mother describes similar symptoms in her brother. Which of the following is the most likely diagnosis?

A. Charcot-Marie-Tooth disease
B. Fabry disease
C. Diabetic neuropathy
D. Guillain-Barré syndrome
E. Chronic inflammatory demyelinating polyneuropathy (CIDP)

Correct answer: B

Explanation

This teenage boy is presenting with a painful peripheral neuropathy in a stocking-glove distribution triggered by exercise, which is characteristic of Fabry disease. Additionally, he has small, dark red spots which are likely angiokeratomas. The family history of similar symptoms in a maternal uncle is supportive of this diagnosis, as Fabry disease has an X-linked pattern of inheritance. Fabry disease is caused by a deficiency in the enzyme α-galactosidase A. This leads to build up of glycosphingolipids in nerves, leading to the neuropathic symptoms. It can also cause distal sensory neuropathy, cardiomyopathy, kidney damage, hearing loss, and stroke. Treatment involves enzyme replacement therapy to help improve symptoms and prevent organ damage but would also involve treatment of downstream end-organ complications such as arrhythmias or renal failure. Charcot-Marie-Tooth disease can also cause pain and burning sensations but is usually not episodic and more classically presents with progressive weakness as well as notable foot deformities. Diabetic neuropathy is usually a long term complication of uncontrolled diabetes and is not usually episodic or related to exercise and hot weather. Guillain-Barré syndrome presents after a recent infection with ascending motor and sensory polyneuropathy and would demonstrate weakness with areflexia on examination. Chronic inflammatory demyelinating polyneuropathy (CIDP) is a progressive or relapsing disease of weakness and loss of sensation. It is not usually episodically triggered by exercise or presenting with angiokeratomas.

References

Desnick, R. J., & Brady, R. O. (2021). Fabry disease: The molecular and clinical aspects. Elsevier.

Fitzpatrick, M. M., & Kieffer, E. T. (2019). Clinical management of Fabry disease: A review. Neurology Clinical Review, 29(3), 112–119.

Ropper, A. H., Samuels, M. A., Klein, J. P., & Prasad, S. (2023). Adams and Victor's principles of neurology (12th ed.). McGraw-Hill Education.

28. A 5-month-old infant is referred by the pediatrician for progressive hypotonia. On chart review, the infant was previously in the 25th percentile for head circumference and 50th percentile for length. Now 3 months later, the infant is in 90th percentile for head circumference and 60th percentile for length. MRI of the brain was obtained and shown below. On further work-up, MR spectroscopy showed an increased N-acetylaspartate peak. Which of the following is the most likely diagnosis?

A. Krabbe disease
B. Metachromatic leukodystrophy
C. Canavan disease
D. Hurler syndrome
E. Leigh syndrome

Correct answer: C

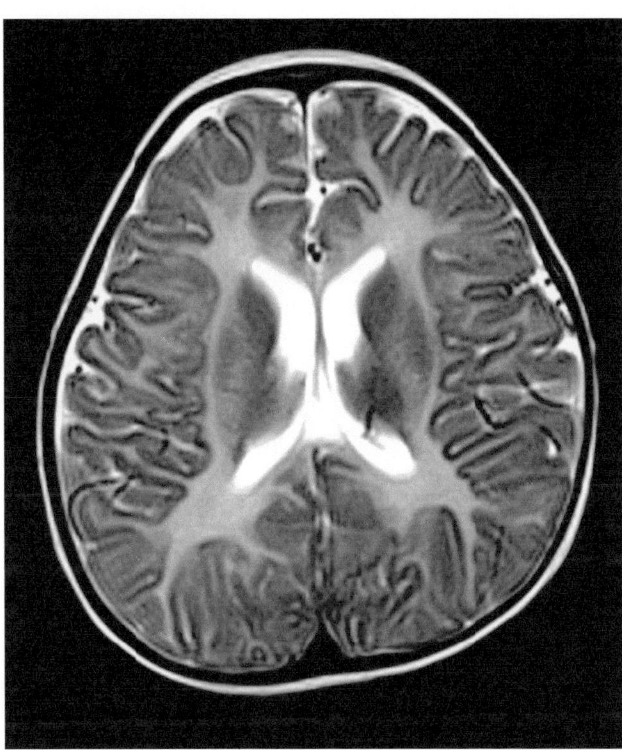

Axial T2 MRI image. (Source: Karimzadeh, P., Jafari, N., Nejad Biglari, H., Rahimian, E. Ahmadabadi, F., Nemati, H., Nasehi, M. M., Ghofrani, M., Mollamohammadi, M. CC-BY 3.0 (https://creativecommons.org/licenses/by/3.0/) via *Iranian Journal of Child Neurology*. Image has been cropped from source. Please see full attribution with citation below in references section for this question.)

Explanation

The most likely diagnosis for this patient is Canavan disease, a leukodystrophy caused by a mutation in the ASPA gene. This gene encodes aspartoacylase, an enzyme responsible for converting N-acetylaspartate into aspartate and acetate to use for protein synthesis. When N-acetylaspartate accumulates in the brain, it disrupts myelin synthesis and causes a spongiform degeneration in the white matter. This results in symptoms of macrocephaly, delayed motor and cognitive milestones, developmental regression, progressive hypotonia, and seizures. MR imaging demonstrates diffuse T2 hyperintensities in the white matter with involvement of the subcortical U-fibers, but often spares the basal ganglia and corpus callosum as shown in the image. MR spectroscopy can be helpful in the diagnosis as it will show elevations or peaks in N-acetylaspartate due to the accumulation in the brain. These patients have a poor prognosis and short life span with most dying by 5 years of age. Krabbe disease is also a leukodystrophy caused by galactocerebrosidase deficiency which can cause muscle weakness and visual changes but would have elevated lactate on MR spectroscopy. Metachromatic leukodystrophy is secondary to arylsulfatase A deficiency and presents with progressive motor and cognitive decline and an elevated sulfatide peak on MR spectroscopy. Hurler syndrome is a result of glycosaminoglycan accumulation in multiple organs and classically shows ventriculomegaly and cerebellar atrophy on MRI. Leigh syndrome is a mitochondrial disorder presenting with respiratory failure, milestone regression, and ataxia. MRI in Leigh syndrome can show bilateral basal ganglia lesions and MR spectroscopy may show elevated lactate.

References

Alshammari, M. (2017). Magnetic Resonance Spectroscopy in Leukoencephalopathies and Leukodystrophies: A Review. Brain and Development, 39(6), 467–477.

Gaillard, F., Campos, A., Knipe, H., & El Helou, S. (2024). Canavan disease. Radiopaedia.org. https://doi.org/10.53347/rID-1045.

Karimzadeh P, Jafari N, Nejad Biglari H, Rahimian E, Ahmadabadi F, Nemati H, et al. The Clinical Features and Diagnosis of Canavan's Disease: A Case Series of Iranian Patients. Iran J Child Neurol. 2014;8(4):66–71.

Louis, E. D., Mayer, S. A., & Noble, J. M. (Eds.). (2021). Merritt's neurology (14th ed.). Wolters Kluwer Health.

Matalon, R., Michals-Matalon, K., & Bley, A. E. (2025). Defects in metabolism of amino acids: N-acetylaspartic acid (Canavan disease). In R. M. Kliegman, J. W. St. Geme, N. J. Blum, & M. D. Shah (Eds.), Nelson Textbook of Pediatrics (22nd ed., Vol. 2, pp. 1234–1238). Elsevier.

29. A 6-year-old healthy child is brought to the clinic for evaluation of new-onset seizures. Over the course of the past year, the patient's mother noticed she has been falling more frequently. Additionally, she has had to attend multiple school conferences with the child's teacher about an inability to read and speak at the expected level and concern that she cannot see the board very clearly. On the initial exam, fundoscopic exam reveals bilateral retinal degeneration. Brain MRI shows diffuse cerebral and cerebellar atrophy. A routine EEG is obtained as part of the work-up and shown below. Which of the following is the most likely diagnosis?

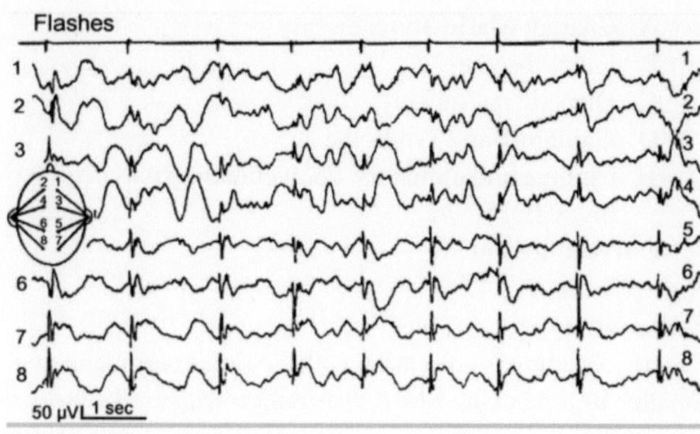

EEG. (Source: Schulz, A., Kohlschütter, A. CC-BY 3.0 (https://creativecommons.org/licenses/by/3.0/) via *Iranian Journal of Child Neurology*. Image has not been modified from source. Please see full attribution with citation below in references section for this question.)

A. Neuronal ceroid lipofuscinosis
B. Krabbe disease
C. Leigh syndrome
D. Tay-Sachs disease

Correct answer: A

Explanation

This child presents with features of vision loss, cognitive decline, multiple falls, and now seizures. Examination shows retinal degeneration likely causing progressive vision loss. Additionally, EEG is obtained and demonstrates that during photic stimulation, the child develops a bi-occipital spike-wave response. This is known as photoparoxysmal response, where flashes of light trigger abnormal electrical discharges in those who are prone to epilepsy or have specific neurological conditions. This, in combination with the MRI findings of diffuse cerebral and cerebellar atrophy, strongly suggests a diagnosis of neuronal ceroid lipofuscinosis (NCL) or Batten disease. NCL is an autosomal recessive neurodegenerative disorder caused by build-up of lipofuscin in the brain, as lysosomes are not able to properly break it down. There are multiple subtypes of the disease with varying ages of onset and prognosis, but more severe forms often include vision loss, regression with severe cognitive decline, seizures, and ataxia. Diagnosis involves assessing the clinical picture, EEG, MRI, and genetic testing. Treatment is mostly supportive, but new enzyme replacement therapies for some forms of NCL can help slow the progression of the more severe subtypes. Krabbe disease is a lysosomal storage disorder that can cause vision loss, seizures, and regression. However, it usually presents earlier in life and does not cause retinal degeneration or extensive atrophy within the brain as seen on MRI in this case shown below. Leigh syndrome is a mitochondrial disorder that can cause regression, seizures, ataxia and falls, and vision loss due to optic atrophy. It also presents early in life and has a more severe and rapid course. Tay-Sachs disease is a lysosomal storage disorder that can also cause neurological decline, seizures, and vision loss, but characteristically has a cherry-red spot on fundoscopy.

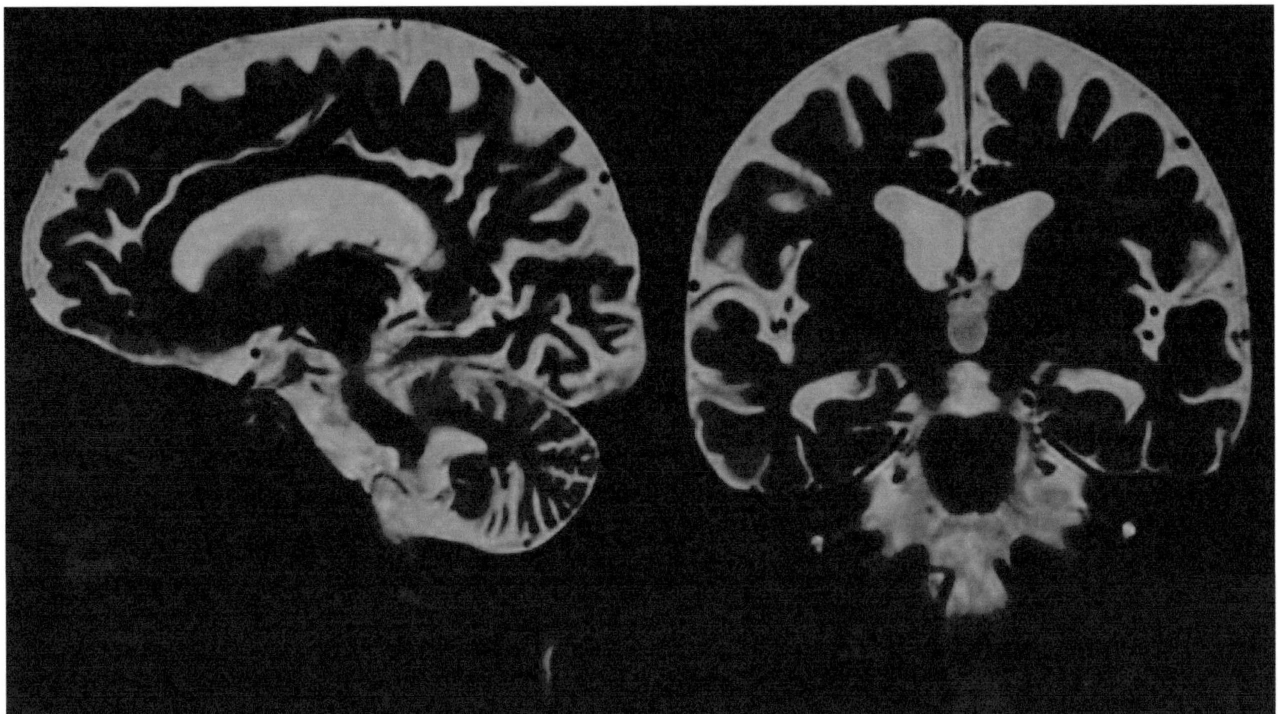

Axial and coronal MRI brain sections of neuronal ceroid lipofuscinosis. (Source: Schulz, A., Kohlschütter, A. CC-BY 3.0 (https://creativecommons.org/licenses/by/3.0/) via *Iranian Journal of Child Neurology.* Image has not been modified from source. Schulz A, Kohlschütter A. NCL Disorders: Frequent Causes of Childhood Dementia. Iran J Child Neurol. 2013;7(1):1–8)

References

Albert DV, Yin H, De Los Reyes EC, Vidaurre J. Unique Characteristics of the Photoparoxysmal Response in Patients With Neuronal Ceroid Lipofuscinosis Type 2: Can EEG Be a Biomarker? J Child Neurol. 2016;31(13):1475–82. https://doi.org/10.1177/0883073816658659.

Ropper, A. H., Samuels, M. A., Klein, J. P., & Prasad, S. (2023). Adams and Victor's principles of neurology (12th ed.). McGraw-Hill Education.

Schulz A, Kohlschütter A. NCL Disorders: Frequent Causes of Childhood Dementia. Iran J Child Neurol. 2013;7(1):1–8.

Simonati A, Williams RE. Neuronal Ceroid Lipofuscinosis: The Multifaceted Approach to the Clinical Issues, an Overview. Front Neurol. 2022;13:811686. https://doi.org/10.3389/fneur.2022.811686.

30. Which of the following serum laboratory findings is most suggestive of adrenoleukodystrophy?
    A. Decreased hexosaminidase A activity
    B. Increased lactate to pyruvate ratio
    C. Decreased arylsulfatase A activity
    D. Increased very long-chain fatty acids
    Correct answer: D

Explanation

Adrenoleukodystrophy is a peroxisomal disorder caused by a mutation in the ABCD1 gene. This is responsible for oxidation of very long-chain fatty acids. When absent, these very long-chain fatty acids accumulate especially in brain and adrenal tissue. Therefore, when considering adrenoleukodystrophy on the differential, very long-chain fatty acids should be directly measured. Diagnostic accuracy is high in males, but levels can be normal in some females, so genetic testing is often preferred for diagnosis. Decreased hexosaminidase A activity is seen in Tay-Sachs disease. Metachromatic leukodystrophy is due to mutation leading to decreased arylsulfatase A activity and build-up of sulfatides. Increased lactate to pyruvate ratio can be seen in some mitochondrial disorders.

References

Engelen, M., Kemp, S., & Eichler, F. (2024). Adrenoleukodystrophy. In Handbook of Clinical Neurology (Vol. 204, pp. 133 138). Elsevier.

Ropper, A. H., Samuels, M. A., Klein, J. P., & Prasad, S. (2023). Adams and Victor's principles of neurology (12th ed.). McGraw-Hill Education.

31. Anencephaly is the result of which of the following processes:
    A. Defective cleavage of the embryonic forebrain
    B. Defective neuroblast migration
    C. Defective closure of the anterior neuropore
    D. Defective closure of the posterior neuropore
    Correct answer: C

Explanation
Children with anencephaly are born with an absent scalp and open skull, resulting in exposure of the brain. This is the result of defective closure of the anterior neuropore. Holoprosencephaly describes the spectrum of abnormalities that result from the defective cleavage of the embryonic forebrain. Lissencephaly results from defective neuroblast migration. Myelomeningocele is a result of defective closure of the posterior neuropore.

Reference
Swaiman, K. F., Ashwal, S., Ferriero, D. M., Schor, N. F., Finkel, R. S., Gropman, A. L., & Pearl, P. L. (2017). *Swaiman's pediatric neurology e-book: Principles and practice*. Elsevier Health Sciences.

32. Where is the most common location of an encephalocele?
    A. Midline-frontal
    B. Midline-parietal
    C. Nasal cavity
    D. Midline-occipital
    Correct answer: D

Explanation
An encephalocele describes the protrusion of the brain and meninges covered by skin through a defect in the skull. The most common location is the midline-occipital; however, among the Asian population, the defects are generally midline-frontal.

Reference
Swaiman, K. F., Ashwal, S., Ferriero, D. M., Schor, N. F., Finkel, R. S., Gropman, A. L., & Pearl, P. L. (2017). *Swaiman's pediatric neurology e-book: Principles and practice*. Elsevier Health Sciences.

33. Which of the following is a late presentation of syringomyelia?
    A. Changes in temperature sensation
    B. Loss of pain sensation
    C. Headache
    D. Changes in vibratory sensation
    Correct answer: D

Explanation
Syringomyelia usually has a gradual progression. The initial symptoms consist of changes in pain and temperature sensation because the crossing spinothalamic fibers are usually first affected by the expanding fluid cavity. As the cavity slowly expands, the posterior columns are affected, causing changes in fine touch and vibratory sense.

Reference
Heiss JD, Snyder K, Peterson MM, Patronas NJ, Butman JA, Smith RK, et al. Pathophysiology of primary spinal syringomyelia. J Neurosurg Spine. 2012;17(5):367–80. https://doi.org/10.3171/2012.8.Spine111059.

34. Which of the following would likely not be found on MRI in a patient with tethered cord syndrome?
    A. Spinal infarction
    B. Diastematomyelia
    C. Lipoma
    D. Arteriovenous Fistula
    Correct answer: D

Explanation
The tethering of the cord can lead to stretching, causing the lumbosacral region to be at risk of ischemia. Diastematomyelia is a congenital anomaly that consists of the division of the lower spinal cord into two halves. This can result in tethered cord syndrome due to the abnormal ascent of the spinal cord. In more than 50% of patients with tethered cord syndrome, a spinal dysraphism is present such as a lipoma or tuft of hair.

Reference
Swaiman, K. F., Ashwal, S., Ferriero, D. M., Schor, N. F., Finkel, R. S., Gropman, A. L., & Pearl, P. L. (2017). *Swaiman's pediatric neurology e-book: Principles and practice*. Elsevier Health Sciences.

Linked questions: 35–36

35. A 12-year-old girl presents for follow-up in clinic. Her MRI brain is significant for progressive calcifications in the right hemisphere. Her exam demonstrates a large right facial angioma and mild weakness in the left upper and lower extremities. She also has a history of refractory seizures that begin clinically with left sided tonic-clonic movements. What condition does this child most likely have?
    A. Neurofibromatosis
    B. Tuberous sclerosis
    C. Sturge-Weber syndrome
    D. Incontinentia pigmenti
    Correct answer: C

Explanation

Sturge-Weber syndrome is a neurocutaneous condition characterized by a triad of abnormal brain vessels, eye conditions including glaucoma, and a port-wine stain birthmark. Patients may present with unilateral weakness and refractory seizures. The characteristic MRI finding is calcifications in the cortical area on the same side as the birthmark. Patients with conditions affecting one hemisphere, including Sturge-Weber syndrome and Rasmussen's encephalitis, are often good candidates for a potential hemispherectomy to assist with seizure management.

Reference

Thomas-Sohl KA, Vaslow DF, Maria BL. Sturge-Weber syndrome: a review. Pediatr Neurol. 2004;30(5):303–10. https://doi.org/10.1016/j.pediatrneurol.2003.12.015.

Linked question

36. Regarding the patient in the previous question, which medication should be started at diagnosis?
    A. ACTH
    B. Low-dose aspirin
    C. Vitamin K
    D. Prednisone
    Correct answer: B

Explanation

Low-dose aspirin is recommended in children with Sturge-Weber Syndrome, particularly those with unilateral calcifications on MRI brain. This may decrease the frequency of stroke-like episodes including transient and permanent episodes of hemiparesis.

Reference

Sánchez-Espino LF, Ivars M, Antoñanzas J, Baselga E. Sturge-Weber Syndrome: A Review of Pathophysiology, Genetics, Clinical Features, and Current Management Approache. Appl Clin Genet. 2023;16:63–81. https://doi.org/10.2147/tacg.S363685.

37. A 5-year-old girl presents to neurology clinic to establish care. He recently immigrated from Algeria and has medical records with him. Growing up, mom reports he had profound weakness and feeding problems. His surgical history is significant for an orchiopexy. His BMI tracks along the 98th percentile. On exam, he has noticeable almond-shaped eyes, small hands and feet, and enamel hypoplasia. Which of the following findings would NOT be supportive of this patient's suspected syndrome?
    A. Abnormal EMG
    B. Sleep apnea
    C. Hypopigmentation
    D. Speech delay
    Correct answer: A

Explanation

This patient has characteristic findings of Prader-Willi Syndrome. Early-onset hyperphagia and obesity is a hallmark finding, along with almond-shaped eyes and hypotonia. Additional minor criteria for Prader-Willi Syndrome includes sleep apnea and hypopigmentation. Developmental delay is a major criterion for diagnosis.

Reference

Cassidy SB, Schwartz S, Miller JL, Driscoll DJ. Prader-Willi syndrome. Genet Med. 2012;14(1):10–26. https://doi.org/10.1038/gim.0b013e31822bead0.

38. Which of the following is NOT a long-term sequela of incontinentia pigmenti?
    A. Retinal detachment
    B. Alopecia
    C. Cardiomyopathy
    D. Hemiparesis
    Correct answer: C

Explanation

Incontinentia pigmenti (also known as Bloch-Sulzberger Syndrome) is a rare neurocutaneous syndrome that primarily affects the eyes, skin, teeth, and central nervous system. Cardiac complications are rare and usually consist of pulmonary hypertension. There have been some case reports associating incontinentia pigmenti with congenital heart defects.

References

Onnis G, Diociaiuti A, Zangari P, D'Argenio P, Cancrini C, Iughetti L, et al. Cardiopulmonary anomalies in incontinentia pigmenti patients. Int J Dermatol. 2018;57(1):40–5. https://doi.org/10.1111/ijd.13835.

Swinney CC, Han DP, Karth PA. Incontinentia Pigmenti: A Comprehensive Review and Update. Ophthalmic Surg Lasers Imaging Retina. 2015;46(6):650–7. https://doi.org/10.3928/23258160-20150610-09.

Linked questions: 39–40

39. A 9-year-old girl presents to the emergency room for a respiratory illness. On chart review, she is observed to have several ED visits for sinopulmonary infections. Her exam is significant for head thrusting when asked to fixate on an object and unsteadiness when ambulating in a straight line. What underlying condition is most consistent with this child's presentation?
    A. Joubert's Syndrome
    B. Marinseco-Sjogern syndrome
    C. Miller-Fisher Syndrome
    D. Ataxia-telangiectasia
    Correct answer: D

Explanation

The patient's description of the inability to visually fixate on an object with compensatory head movements is consistent with oculomotor apraxia, which is present in ~90% patients with ataxia-telangiectasia (AT). Patients with AT are also more susceptible to recurrent sinopulmonary infections due to the disturbance of B and T cell functions. Oculomotor apraxia and ataxia can also be seen in Joubert Syndrome, but recurrent infections are not a common feature. Ataxia can also be seen in Marinesco-Sjogren syndrome; however, other expected hallmark features would include cataracts and myopathy. Although Miller-Fisher Syndrome is also associated with ataxia, recurrent infections are not associated with the diagnosis and the abnormal eye findings in Miller-Fisher syndrome are typically ophthalmoplegia rather than oculomotor apraxia.

References

Rothblum-Oviatt, C., Wright, J., Lefton-Greif, M. A., McGrath-Morrow, S. A., Crawford, T. O., & Lederman, H. M. (2016). Ataxia telangiectasia: a review. Orphanet journal of rare diseases, 11, 1–21.

Swaiman, K. F., Ashwal, S., Ferriero, D. M., Schor, N. F., Finkel, R. S., Gropman, A. L., & Pearl, P. L. (2017). Swaiman's pediatric neurology e-book: Principles and practice. Elsevier Health Sciences.

Linked question

40. Which of the following lab abnormalities would this child most likely have?
    A. Decreased IgM
    B. Elevated alpha-fetoprotein
    C. Elevated IgA
    D. Decreased vitamin A
    Correct answer: B

Explanation

Elevated alpha-fetoprotein level is a common marker for ataxia-telangiectasia. The underlying pathophysiology is unclear, however, it may be related to deficits in DNA repair resulting in liver cell damage and dysfunction. Other lab abnormalities seen in this condition include absent IgA which may result in a compensatory increase in IgM.

References

Rothblum-Oviatt C, Wright J, Lefton-Greif MA, McGrath-Morrow SA, Crawford TO, Lederman HM. Ataxia telangiectasia: a review. Orphanet J Rare Dis. 2016;11(1):159. https://doi.org/10.1186/s13023-016-0543-7.

Swaiman, K. F., Ashwal, S., Ferriero, D. M., Schor, N. F., Finkel, R. S., Gropman, A. L., & Pearl, P. L. (2017). Swaiman's pediatric neurology e-book: Principles and practice. Elsevier Health Sciences.

41. Which of the following statements regarding megalencephaly is incorrect?
    A. Megalencephaly in patients with achondroplasia rarely causes increases in intracranial pressure
    B. Most infants with metabolic megalencephaly have a normal head circumference at birth
    C. Metabolic disorders are not associated with the development of megalencephaly
    D. Hemimegalencephaly can be an indication of a neurocutaneous disorder
    Correct answer: C

Explanation

Megalencephaly describes the abnormal enlargement of the brain. The primary causes include anatomical and metabolic disorders. Achondroplasia and gigantism are examples of anatomical megalencephaly. With anatomical megalencephaly, children are found to have macrocephaly at birth with normal intracranial pressure. Meanwhile, children with metabolic disorders may have normal head circumferences at birth with subsequent rapid increase over time as metabolic products accumulate resulting in cerebral edema and subsequent enlargement of the brain.

Linked questions: 42–43

42. The following image is suggestive of which of the following conditions?

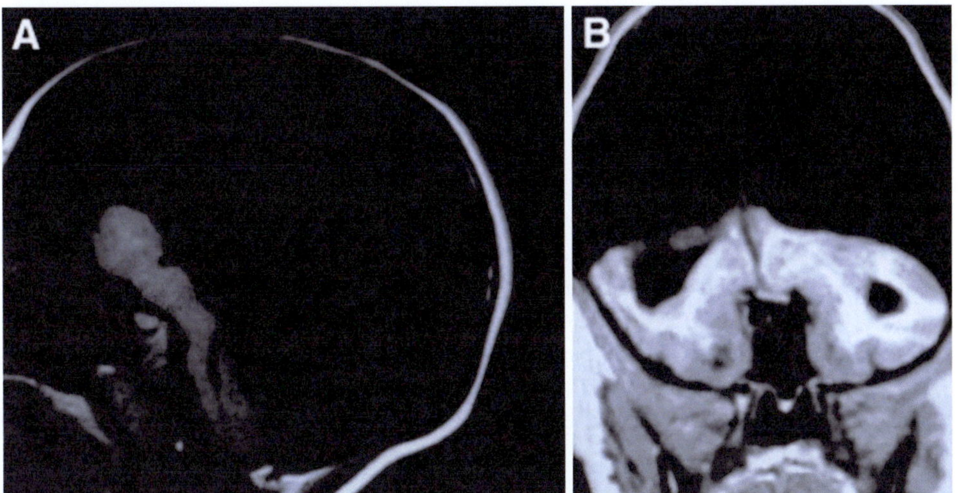

Sagittal and coronal MRI brain sections. (Source: Pavone, Piero, Praticò, A. D., Vitaliti, G., Ruggieri, M. Rizzo, R., Parano, E., Pavone, L., Pero, G., Falsaperla, R. CC-BY 4.0 (https://creativecommons.org/ licenses/by/4.0/) via *Italian Journal of Pediatrics*. Image has not been modified from source. Please see full attribution with citation below in references section for this question.)

A. Hydranencephaly
B. Schizencephaly
C. Porencephaly
D. Megalencephaly
Correct answer: A

Explanation

Hydranencephaly is a rare congenital post-neurulation disorder characterized by the replacement of the bilateral cerebral hemispheres with a sac filled with cerebrospinal fluid. Porencephaly also describes the presence of cystic cavities in the brain however rather than the complete absence of the hemispheres, there is residual brain tissue present. The MRI above shows T1-weighted images demonstrating hydranencephaly.

Reference

Pavone P, Praticò AD, Vitaliti G, Ruggieri M, Rizzo R, Parano E, et al. Hydranencephaly: cerebral spinal fluid instead of cerebral mantles. Ital J Pediatr. 2014;40:79. https://doi.org/10.1186/s13052-014-0079-1.

Linked question

43. Which of the following conditions is NOT associated with the MRI finding in Question 42?
    A. Blockage of the carotid artery
    B. Diffuse rhythmic slowing on EEG
    C. Cytomegalovirus
    D. Twin pregnancy
    Correct answer: B

Explanation

Given the absence of cerebral hemispheres, the EEG pattern would demonstrate flat or severely decreased electrical activity. Although the exact pathophysiology of hydranencephaly is unknown, the most commonly proposed mechanisms include vascular insults and intrauterine infections. Bilateral occlusion of the internal carotid arteries during fetal development results in brain tissue necrosis with subsequent replacement with CSF. In monochorionic pregnancies, the surviving twin is at risk of developing hydranencephaly due to the release of emboli or thromboplastin from the deceased twin. There have been reports involving viruses including toxoplasmosis, cytomegalovirus, enterovirus, and adenovirus related to the development of hydranencephaly.

Reference

Sandoval JI, De Jesus O. Hydranencephaly. StatPearls. Treasure Island (FL): StatPearls Publishing Copyright © 2025, StatPearls Publishing LLC.; 2025.

Linked questions: 44–45

44. A 15-year-old boy presents to neurology clinic for follow up. His head circumference tracks along the 97th percentile. Exam is significant for hypertelorism, hypoplastic maxilla, and bilateral hearing loss. His mother reports concern regarding increased bulging of his eyes bilaterally. What disorder is most consistent with this patient's presentation?
    A. Apert Syndrome
    B. Gigantism

C. Crouzon Syndrome
D. Aicardi Syndrome
Correct answer: C

Explanation

The patient's presentation is most consistent with Crouzon Syndrome (craniofacial dysostosis). Crouzon Syndrome is the premature closure of cranial sutures and maldevelopment of the facial bones. Apert Syndrome and Crouzon Syndrome both involve premature fusion of the skull bones; however, Apert Syndrome also involves syndactyly in the hands/feet while Crouzon Syndrome primarily affects the face and skull.

Reference

Bowling EL, Burstein FD. Crouzon syndrome. Optometry. 2006;77(5):217–22. https://doi.org/10.1016/j.optm.2006.03.005.

Linked question

45. Which of the following statements is correct regarding this patient's disorder?
    A. This disorder is autosomal recessive
    B. This disorder is associated with a mutation in the growth hormone gene
    C. Patients with this disorder have a poor life expectancy
    D. This disorder usually involves sleep apnea
    Correct answer: D

Explanation

Crouzon Syndrome is an autosomal-dominant disorder that involves a missense mutation in the fibroblast growth receptor gene. The life expectancy for these patients is favorable especially with early surgical correction of the cranial abnormalities. Due to midface hypoplasia, patients are at risk for upper and lower airway obstructions including sleep apnea.

Reference

Da Silva, D. L., Palheta Neto, F. X., Carneiro, S. G., Palheta, A. C. P., Monteiro, M., & Cunha, S. C. (2008). Crouzon's syndrome: literature review. *Intl Arch Otorhinolaryngol*, *12*(3), 436–441.

46. An 11-year-old girl is being evaluated for cardiac failure. Her exam is significant for cranial bruits and macrocephaly. MRI brain is significant for dilation of the lateral and third ventricles. Which of the following is most likely her diagnosis?
    A. Vein of Galen malformation
    B. Pompe's Disease

C. Hypertrophic cardiomyopathy (HCOM)
D. Leigh syndrome
Correct answer: A

Explanation

The condition depicted is most consistent with a Vein of Galen malformation (VGM) which involves the direct connection of the cerebral arteries to the veins. By bypassing the capillaries, this results in elevated blood flow and potentially high-output cardiac failure. MRI brain may demonstrate non-communicating hydrocephalus due to the compression of the cerebral aqueduct by the dilated vein of Galen. Pompe disease can result in cardiomyopathy due to weakening of the heart muscles, however, this would not be associated with hydrocephalus or cranial bruits. HCOM may result in cardiac failure and is usually not associated with intracranial findings. Leigh syndrome is a mitochondrial disorder which may result in HCOM and hydrocephalus but also often involves marked neurodevelopmental regression and seizures; death usually occurs at 2–3 years of age due to respiratory or cardiac failure.

References

Gupta AK, Varma DR. Vein of Galen malformations: review. Neurol India. 2004;52(1):43–53.

Swaiman, K. F., Ashwal, S., Ferriero, D. M., Schor, N. F., Finkel, R. S., Gropman, A. L., & Pearl, P. L. (2017). Swaiman's pediatric neurology e-book: Principles and practice. Elsevier Health Science

47. Which of the following is NOT a diagnostic criterion for Neurofibromatosis (NF) Type 1?
    A. Greater than 2 Lisch nodules
    B. Sphenoid dysplasia or other distinctive bone lesions
    C. Vestibular Schwannoma
    D. Optic glioma
    Correct answer: C

Explanation

Vestibular schwannomas are tumors characteristic of NF2-related schwannomatosis and not NF1. The other answer choices are all included in the diagnostic criteria for NF1.

References

Friedman JM. Neurofibromatosis 1. In: Adam MP, Feldman J, Mirzaa GM, Pagon RA, Wallace SE, Amemiya A, editors. GeneReviews(®). Seattle (WA): University of Washington, Seattle

Copyright © 1993–2025, University of Washington, Seattle. GeneReviews is a registered trademark of the University of Washington, Seattle. All rights reserved.; 1993.

48. A 12-year-old boy with Neurofibromatosis Type 1 presents to neurology clinic for follow-up. Which of the following should be included in his health maintenance exams?
   A. Annual pulmonary function testing
   B. School assessments
   C. Routine EEG
   D. Echocardiogram
   Correct answer: B

Explanation

Close monitoring of development and school progress is important to identify any developmental challenges, as approximately 50% of people with NF1 will experience learning difficulties and up to 75–80% are diagnosed with attention-deficit/hyperactivity disorder. Other routine testing should include blood pressure monitoring, scoliosis evaluation, skin examinations, and ophthalmology follow up. Echocardiograms and EEG are not indicated in routine care of children with NF1.

References

Baudou E, Chaix Y. The value of screening tests in children with neurofibromatosis type 1 (NF1). Childs Nerv Syst. 2020;36(10):2311–9. https://doi.org/10.1007/s00381-020-04711-6.

Copyright © 1993–2025, University of Washington, Seattle. GeneReviews is a registered trademark of the University of Washington, Seattle. All rights reserved.; 1993.

Friedman JM. Neurofibromatosis 1. In: Adam MP, Feldman J, Mirzaa GM, Pagon RA, Wallace SE, Amemiya A, editors. GeneReviews(®). Seattle (WA): University of Washington, Seattle

49. A 2-year-old patient with Alexander Disease dies, and an autopsy is performed. The histological findings seen on her brain autopsy are shown below. Which of the following describes the histologic findings?

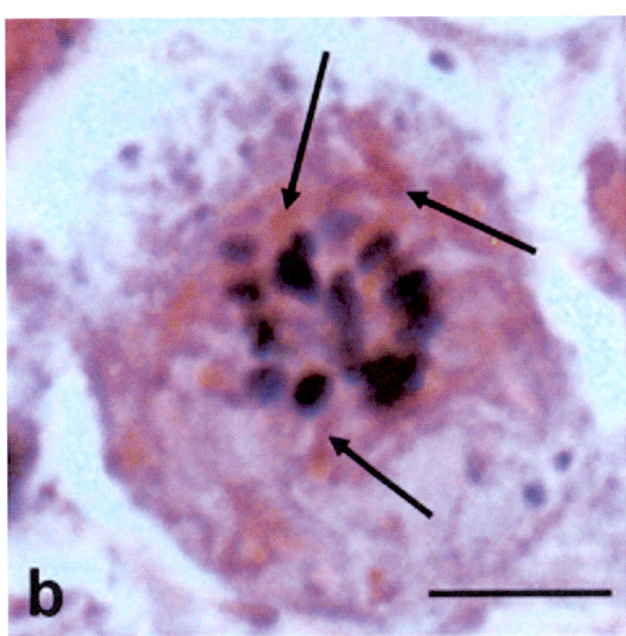

Microscopy with hematoxylin and eosin staining. (Source: Sosunov, A., McKhann, G M., Goldman, J. E. CC-BY 4.0 (https://creativecommons.org/licenses/by/4.0/), via *Acta Neuropathologica Communications*. Image has been cropped from source. Please see full attribution with citation below in references section for this question.)

   A. Rosenthal fibers
   B. Cells with round nuclei and clear cytoplasm
   C. Non-caseating granulomas
   D. Perivascular pseudorosettes
   Correct answer: A

Explanation

Alexander disease is an autosomal-dominant leukodystrophy that causes progressive destruction to the white matter in the brain. It is caused by mutations in the glial fibrillary acidic protein (GFAP). The destruction of the white matter is accompanied by fibrous eosinophilic bundles called Rosenthal fibers, which are shown by the arrows in the image. These fibers are also seen in patients with pilocytic astrocytomas,

Parkinson disease, and ALS. Answer choice B describes the classic "fried egg" appearance seen in oligodendrogliomas. Non-caseating granulomas are seen in conditions including sarcoidosis and tuberculosis. Answer choice D describes a common histologic feature seen in ependymomas.

References

Copyright © 1993–2025, University of Washington, Seattle. GeneReviews is a registered trademark of the University of Washington, Seattle. All rights reserved.; 1993.

Reichard EA, Ball WS, Jr., Bove KE. Alexander disease: a case report and review of the literature. Pediatr Pathol Lab Med. 1996;16(2):327–43.

Sosunov AA, McKhann GM, 2nd, Goldman JE. The origin of Rosenthal fibers and their contributions to astrocyte pathology in Alexander disease. Acta Neuropathol Commun. 2017;5(1):27. https://doi.org/10.1186/s40478-017-0425-9.

Srivastava S, Waldman A, Naidu S. Alexander Disease. In: Adam MP, Feldman J, Mirzaa GM, Pagon RA, Wallace SE, Amemiya A, editors. GeneReviews(®). Seattle (WA): University of Washington, Seattle

Wippold FJ, 2nd, Perry A, Lennerz J. Neuropathology for the neuroradiologist: Rosenthal fibers. AJNR Am J Neuroradiol. 2006;27(5):958–61.

50. Which of the statements regarding Chiari malformations is false?
    A. Sudden cardiorespiratory failure can be the cause of the death in patients with Chiari II malformation
    B. Hyperreflexia and spasticity in the legs can be notable findings on exam in Chiari I malformation
    C. Myelomeningocele and hydrocephalus are associated findings seen in Chiari II malformation
    D. Chiari I malformations are usually an incidental finding on MRI and are often the cause of pediatric headaches

Correct answer: D

Explanation

Most type I malformations are incidentally found on MRI. Although headache is the most common symptom of Chiari malformations (when symptoms occur), patients are usually asymptomatic, and these are found incidentally. A malformation should be considered in patients with an occipital headache that worsens with valsalva maneuvers (coughing, sneezing). A type II malformation should be suspected in children with myelomeningocele. Respiratory distress including episodes of apnea or Cheyne-Stokes respirations can be evidence of brainstem compression due to cerebellar herniation.

Reference

Swaiman, K. F., Ashwal, S., Ferriero, D. M., Schor, N. F., Finkel, R. S., Gropman, A. L., & Pearl, P. L. (2017). *Swaiman's pediatric neurology e-book: Principles and practice*. Elsevier Health Science

51. A child presents to the clinic for his 2-year-old well-child visit. His mother reports concern regarding his behaviors, as he will often go up to strangers with no sense of danger. Labs are significant for hypercalcemia. On exam he has a wide mouth, large ears, aortic murmur, and an unsteady gait. What condition does this child most likely have?
    A. Prader-Willi Syndrome
    B. Fragile X Syndrome
    C. Williams Syndrome
    D. Noonan Syndrome

Correct answer: C

Explanation

This patient's presentation is most consistent with Williams Syndrome. This syndrome is caused by a deletion in chromosome 7. Notable features include developmental delay, difficulty with identifying strangers, and excessive empathy. Common facial features may include large ears, prominent cheeks and lips, small jaw, and short stature. Hypercalcemia is a common endocrine abnormality, but the exact pathophysiology is unknown.

References

Morris, C. A., & Mervis, C. B. (2021). Williams syndrome. Cassidy and Allanson's Management of Genetic Syndromes, 1021–1038.

Morris CA, Demsey SA, Leonard CO, Dilts C, Blackburn BL. Natural history of Williams syndrome: physical characteristics. J Pediatr. 1988;113(2):318–26. https://doi.org/10.1016/s0022-3476(88)80272-5.

52. Which of the following statements regarding Prader-Willi Syndrome and Angelman Syndrome is correct?
    A. Both conditions are caused by microdeletions on chromosome 17
    B. Prader-Willi Syndrome is associated with hypotonia while Angelman Syndrome is associated with seizures and ataxic gait
    C. Developmental delay is more severe in Prader-Willi Syndrome
    D. Prader-Willi Syndrome is associated with a deletion on the maternal gene while Angelman Syndrome is caused by a deletion on the paternal gene

Correct answer: B

Explanation

Prader-Willi Syndrome is caused by a deletion in paternal chromosome 15 while Angelman Syndrome is caused by a deletion in the maternal chromosome 15. Developmental delay is more severe in Angelman Syndrome. Other characteristic findings include hyperphagia and endocrine abnormalities in Prader-Willi Syndrome and paroxysms of laughter in Angelman Syndrome

References

Buiting K. Prader-Willi syndrome and Angelman syndrome. Am J Med Genet C Semin Med Genet. 2010;154c(3):365–76. https://doi.org/10.1002/ajmg.c.30273.

Swaiman, K. F., Ashwal, S., Ferriero, D. M., Schor, N. F., Finkel, R. S., Gropman, A. L., & Pearl, P. L. (2017). Swaiman's pediatric neurology e-book: Principles and practice. Elsevier Health Sciences.

53. A 4-year-old boy presents to developmental pediatrics clinic for expressive speech delay and behavioral difficulties. Family history is significant for a maternal uncle with developmental delay and similar facial features to this child. The patient also has an older brother with similar features who has a diagnosis of autism spectrum disorder. Which of the following is correct regarding this patient's likely condition?
    A. The condition is autosomal recessive
    B. Notable associated facial features include almond shaped eyes, upward slanted eyes, and small ears
    C. The mutation involves an expansion of the DNA sequence CGG
    D. The condition has a decreased lifespan
    Correct answer: C

Explanation

The patient's family history of developmental delay suggests a genetic neurodevelopmental disorder. Given the male predominance in this family, an X-linked disorder should be suspected. The language delays, facial features, and the autism spectrum disorder diagnosis in his brother are most consistent with Fragile X Syndrome. This is caused by an expansion of CGG repeats in the fragile X messenger ribonucleoprotein 1 (FMR1) gene and is the most common known genetic cause of autism. Classic physical features of Fragile X syndrome include long face, prominent jaw and ears, hypertelorism, and a prominent forehead. The features described in B are consistent with Down Syndrome.

References

Bagni C, Tassone F, Neri G, Hagerman R. Fragile X syndrome: causes, diagnosis, mechanisms, and therapeutics. J Clin Invest. 2012;122(12):4314–22. https://doi.org/10.1172/jci63141.

Kidd SA, Lachiewicz A, Barbouth D, Blitz RK, Delahunty C, McBrien D, et al. Fragile X syndrome: a review of associated medical problems. Pediatrics. 2014;134(5):995–1005. https://doi.org/10.1542/peds.2013-4301.

54. Which of the following statements is correct regarding the condition depicted on MRI?
    A. Respiratory distress can be a severe clinical presentation
    B. It occurs as an isolated findings usually with no other associated anomalies
    C. The condition can be diagnosed postnatally
    D. Hydrocephalus is usually present on birth
    Correct answer: A

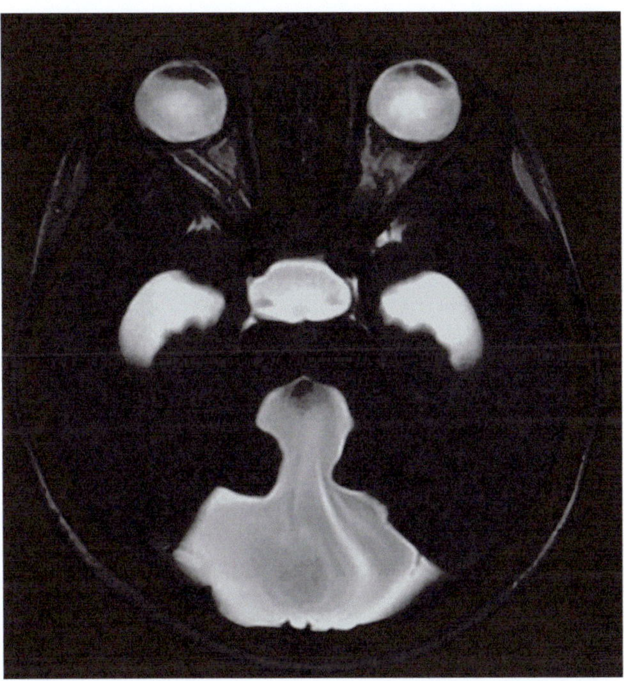

T2-weighted axial MRI brain. (Source: Jadhav, S. S., Dhok, A., Mitra, K., Khan, S., Khandaitkar, S. CC-BY 4.0 (https://creativecommons.org/licenses/by/4.0/) via *Cureus*. Image has not been modified. Please see full attribution with citation below in references section for this question.)

Explanation

The MRI depicted shows hypoplasia of the cerebellar vermis with dilation of the fourth ventricle and posterior fossa, which is consistent with Dandy-Walker malformation (DWM). Dandy-Walker variant also involves hypoplasia of the cerebellar vermis; however, it lacks the posterior fossa enlargement. DWM is usually diagnosed within the first year of life due to signs of hydrocephalus, but hydrocephalus is not usually present at birth. Prenatal ultrasound can also reveal this diagnosis as early as 14 weeks of gestation. It is associated with congenital heart defects, encephalocele, agenesis of the corpus callosum, and ocular abnormalities. Severe forms may include macrocephaly secondary to hydrocephalus, feeding, and respiratory dysfunction.

References

Jadhav SS, Dhok A, Mitra K, Khan S, Khandaitkar S. Dandy-Walker Malformation With Hydrocephalus: Diagnosis and Its Treatment. Cureus. 2022;14(5):e25287. https://doi.org/10.7759/cureus.25287.

Stambolliu E, Ioakeim-Ioannidou M, Kontokostas K, Dakoutrou M, Kousoulis AA. The Most Common Comorbidities in Dandy-Walker Syndrome Patients: A Systematic Review of Case Reports. J Child Neurol. 2017;32(10):886–902. https://doi.org/10.1177/0883073817712589.

55. A 12-year-old boy presents to neurology clinic for headache follow-up. He has a history of pressure-like headaches for many years with associated vision changes. His MRI shows a hyperintense T1 lesion in the midline parasellar region. What condition does this child likely have?
    A. Pituitary adenoma
    B. Dermoid cyst
    C. Colloid cyst
    D. Schwannoma
    Correct answer: B

Explanation

Dermoid cysts are most often found in the posterior fossa. On MRI, dermoid cysts resemble lipomas as they demonstrate T1 hyperintensity and variable T2 signal. If patients are symptomatic, surgical resection can be considered. Dermoid cysts are often incidental findings but can present with headaches, seizures, or vision changes due to compression of the optic chiasm.

References

Badri M, Gader G, Bahri K, Zammel I. Atypical imaging features of posterior fossa's dermoid cyst: Case report and review of literature. Surg Neurol Int. 2018;9:97. https://doi.org/10.4103/sni.sni_411_17.

Swaiman, K. F., Ashwal, S., Ferriero, D. M., Schor, N. F., Finkel, R. S., Gropman, A. L., & Pearl, P. L. (2017). Swaiman's pediatric neurology e-book: Principles and practice. Elsevier Health Science

56. Which of the following is not a risk factor for the development of craniosynostosis?
    A. Gestational diabetes
    B. Maternal hypothyroidism
    C. Maternal use of levetiracetam
    D. Maternal smoking
    Correct answer: C

Explanation

Craniosynostosis describes the process of premature sutural fusion. The most common cause is constraint of the fetal head in utero. This may result from macrosomia and maternal uterine malformations. Thyroid hormones play an important role in fetal bone development. Many antiepileptic medications can cause congenital malformations. However, there is no established relationship between the development of craniosynostosis and levetiracetam use. Valproate monotherapy, however, significantly increases the risk for congenital malformations including craniosynostosis.

References

Carmichael SL, Ma C, Rasmussen SA, Cunningham ML, Browne ML, Dosiou C, et al. Craniosynostosis and risk factors related to thyroid dysfunction. Am J Med Genet A. 2015;167a(4):701–7. https://doi.org/10.1002/ajmg.a.36953.

Swaiman, K. F., Ashwal, S., Ferriero, D. M., Schor, N. F., Finkel, R. S., Gropman, A. L., & Pearl, P. L. (2017). Swaiman's pediatric neurology e-book: Principles and practice. Elsevier Health Science

57. Which of the following characteristics would not support a diagnosis of Septic-optic dysplasia?
    A. Optic tract hypoplasia
    B. Absence of the septum pellucidum
    C. Hypothalamic-dysfunction
    D. Hydrocephalus
    Correct answer: D

Explanation

Septic-optic dysplasia, also known as de Morsier syndrome, is a disorder characterized by the midline brain defects, underdevelopment of the optic nerves, and pituitary gland abnormalities. 50% of children also have an association with schizencephaly, which is sometimes referred to as septic-optic dysplasia plus.

Reference

Sataite I, Cudlip S, Jayamohan J, Ganau M. Septo-optic dysplasia. Handb Clin Neurol. 2021;181:51–64. https://doi.org/10.1016/b978-0-12-820683-6.00005-1.

Linked questions: 58–59

58. A 6-year-old girl presents to neurology clinic for evaluation of gait instability. Her parents report sudden attacks of generalized loss of balance that are associated with muscle stiffening, vomiting, and slurred speech. These episodes often are exacerbated during the heat. What condition does this child likely have?

A. Seizures
B. Episodic ataxia
C. Hartnup disease
D. Maple syrup urine disease

Correct answer: B

Explanation

Episodic ataxia describes a group of inherited conditions associated with impaired coordination and balance. These attacks may be triggered by stress, fever, hot temperatures, or sudden movements. The episodes last from a few minutes up to a few days depending on the subtype of episodic ataxia. Episodes are characterized by sudden attacks of generalized ataxia, dysarthria, muscle stiffening, and dizziness.

Reference

Singhvi JP, Prabhakar S, Singh P. Episodic ataxia: a case report and review of literature. Neurol India. 2000;48(1):78–80.

Linked question

59. Which of the following medications may be recommended for the condition described in question 58?
A. Acetazolamide
B. Levetiracetam
C. Gabapentin
D. Steroids

Correct answer: A

Explanation

Acetazolamide works as a carbonic anhydrase inhibitor, which results in decreased levels of lactate and pyruvate. High levels of these substrates in the cerebrospinal fluid are hypothesized to contribute to the acute attacks of ataxia. Additional medications that may be used include phenytoin and carbamazepine.

Reference

Zasorin NL, Baloh RW, Myers LB. Acetazolamide-responsive episodic ataxia syndrome. Neurology. 1983;33(9):1212–4. https://doi.org/10.1212/wnl.33.9.1212.

Vascular Neurology

Sean Kelly, Levi Dygert, Amanda Bilski, Cen Zhang,
and Alexandra Kvernland

1. A 70-year-old man with a history of hypertension presents with sudden-onset left-sided weakness and facial droop that began 45 min ago. On exam, he is alert but has a dense left hemiparesis. Blood pressure is 145/90 mm Hg. Non-contrast head CT shows no hemorrhage or early infarct signs. He takes no medications and has no known medical allergies. Before proceeding with IV thrombolysis, which of the following is the most critical laboratory test to obtain?
   A. Platelet count
   B. Coagulation panel (PT/INR, aPTT)
   C. Serum creatinine
   D. Serum glucose
   E. Troponin
   Correct answer: D

Explanation

Hypoglycemia can mimic acute ischemic stroke, and it must be excluded prior to administration of IV thrombolytics. A blood glucose level is fast, essential, and always required before thrombolysis. Although coagulation labs are also typically checked, they are not required to delay tissue plasminogen activator (tPA) in most patients not on anti-coagulation. Creatinine is not urgently needed unless contrast imaging is planned. Troponin and platelet count are not required prior to alteplase administration. According to the American Heart Association guidelines IV, thrombolytics are recommended in otherwise eligible patients with initial glucose levels >50 mg/dL.

2. A 56-year-old woman with type 2 diabetes presents to the hospital after having an episode of right arm and leg weakness with slurred speech that resolved after 20 min. Her blood pressure on arrival is 155/100. MRI brain reveals no acute infarct or hemorrhage, while MR angiogram reveals mild narrowing of the right middle cerebral and posterior cerebral arteries. She has no history of atrial fibrillation, and echocardiogram is unremarkable.
   What is the patient's ABCD2 score?
   A. 2
   B. 3
   C. 4
   D. 5
   E. 6
   Correct answer: D

Explanation

The ABCD2 score is a clinically validated tool used to help triage acute TIA for short-term risk of stroke based on various risk factors.

Component	Value	Points
Age ≥60 years	Yes/No	+1
BP ≥140/90 mmHg	Yes/No	+1
Clinical features of the TIA	Unilateral Weakness	+2
	Speech disturbance without weakness	+1
	Other symptoms	0
Duration of symptoms	<10 min	0
	10–59 min	+1
	≥60 min	+2
History of diabetes	Yes/No	+1

S. Kelly (✉) · A. Bilski
Department of Neurology, New York University School
of Medicine, New York, NY, USA
e-mail: sean.kelly2@nyulangone.org;
amanda.bilski@nyulangone.org

L. Dygert · C. Zhang
Department of Neurology, New York University Grossman School
of Medicine, New York, NY, USA
e-mail: levi.dygert@nyulangone.org; cen.zhang@nyulangone.org

A. Kvernland
Department of Neurology, NYU Langone Medical Center,
New York, NY, USA
e-mail: alexandra.kvernland@nyulangone.org

© The Author(s), under exclusive license to Springer Nature Switzerland AG 2026
T. E. Smith, V. Arena (eds.), *Essential Neurology Board Review Q & A*, https://doi.org/10.1007/978-3-032-17213-6_3

The patient in the question vignette scores for initial blood pressure >140/90 (1), unilateral weakness (2), Duration 10–59 min (1), and history of diabetes (1).

Reference

Johnston, S. C., Rothwell, P. M., Nguyen-Huynh, M. N., Giles, M. F., Elkins, J. S., Bernstein, A. L., & Sidney, S. (2007). Validation and refinement of scores to predict very early stroke risk after transient ischaemic attack. The Lancet, 369(9558), 283–292

3. Which approach to medical management is best supported by literature to reduce the prior patient's risk of recurrent stroke in the short term?
   A. Initiation of a high intensity statin
   B. Blood pressure lowering to a strict goal of <140/90
   C. Initiation of aspirin and plavix for a period of 21–30 days
   D. Initiation of aspirin and plavix for a period of 90 days
   E. Initiation of aspirin monotherapy
   Correct answer: C

Explanation

he patient presents with a high-risk TIA (ABCD2 score >4). In such patients, the risk of recurrent stroke or TIA is significantly elevated in the short term. Two prospective randomized controlled trials (POINT and CHANCE) demonstrated a significant reduction in recurrent stroke for patients who were treated with aspirin and plavix for a period of 21 or 30 days following such an event compared to aspirin monotherapy. While initiation of a high intensity statin is appropriate, the specific impact on short-term stroke risk is unknown, and rapid or strict reduction of blood pressure in the immediate period following stroke has not been shown to be a safe intervention for all patients. Though the patient does have some intracranial artery narrowing, it is reported as mild and in vessels not directly relevant to the patient's TIA, thus would not recommend a more prolonged course of dual antiplatelet treatment.

References

Johnston SC, Easton JD, Farrant M, et al. Clopidogrel and Aspirin in Acute Ischemic Stroke and High-Risk TIA. N Engl J Med. 2018;379(3):215–225. https://doi.org/10.1056/NEJMoa1800410c

Wang Y, Wang Y, Zhao X, et al. Clopidogrel with aspirin in acute minor stroke or transient ischemic attack. N Engl J Med. 2013;369(1):11–19. https://doi.org/10.1056/NEJMoa1215340

4. A 68-year-old woman with heart failure with reduced ejection fraction, hypertension, and chronic kidney disease presents to the emergency room at 8:30 AM with new aphasia and right- sided weakness on waking at 8 AM. Her last known well was 11 PM. The results from which of the following trials support the safe use of thrombolysis in this patient?
   A. DAWN
   B. EXTEND-IA
   C. WAKE-UP
   D. DEFUSE 3
   E. SAMMPRISTERY
   Correct answer: C

Explanation

The WAKE-UP trial studied patients with acute ischemic stroke who had an unknown time of onset (such as wake-up strokes) and were therefore outside the standard 4.5-h thrombolysis window based on clock time. Patients were selected using MRI with diffusion-weighted imaging (DWI)–fluid-attenuated inversion recovery (FLAIR) mismatch, which suggests the stroke is likely within 4.5 h of onset. The trial found that intravenous alteplase given to these imaging-selected patients improved functional outcomes without a significantly increased risk of symptomatic intracerebral hemorrhage compared to placebo.

Other trials:

- DAWN and DEFUSE 3: Extended mechanical thrombectomy window using perfusion imaging for large-vessel occlusion.
- EXTEND-IA: Thrombectomy trial for large-vessel occlusion within 6 h.
- SAMMPRIS: Compared aggressive medical therapy vs stenting for symptomatic intracranial atherosclerosis

Reference

Thomalla G, Simonsen CZ, Boutitie F, et al. MRI-Guided Thrombolysis for Stroke with Unknown Time of Onset. N Engl J Med. 2018;379(7):611-622. https://doi.org/10.1056/NEJMoa1804355

5. A 68-year-old man with a history of hypertension, type 2 diabetes, and smoking presents with sudden onset of right arm weakness and expressive aphasia. CT angiography reveals a chronic appearing high-grade stenosis of the left internal carotid artery at its origin. B1000 diffusion sequence on MRI brain is shown below. He is not in atrial fibrillation and echocardiogram is normal.

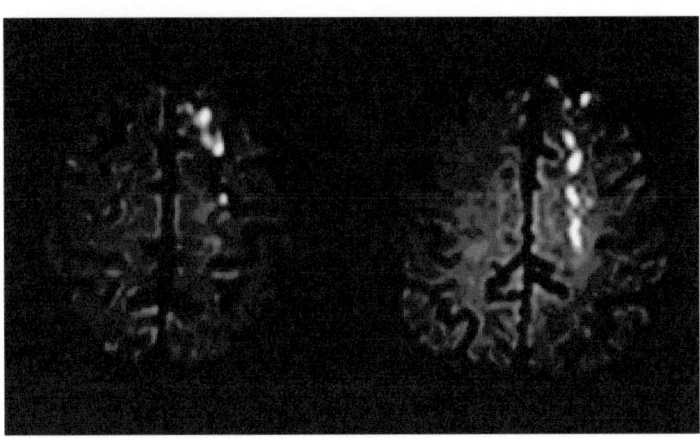

Axial MRI DWI sequences. (Source: Cuadrado-Godia E, Ois A, Roquer J via Current cardiology reviews (2010). CC-BY 2.5 (https://creativecommons.org/licenses/by/2.5/). Image has not been modified. Please see full attribution with citation below in references section for this question.)

Which of the following is the most likely mechanism of his stroke?

A. Cardioembolism
B. Artery-to-artery embolism from atherosclerotic plaque
C. Lipohyalinosis of perforating arteries
D. Left hemisphere hypoperfusion
E. Symptomatic intracranial atherosclerosis

Correct answer: D

Explanation

The representative MRI image shown depicts multiple areas of acute infarction confined to the border zones, or watershed areas, between multiple vascular territories, including the ACA/MCA and PCA/MCA cortical border zones, as well as the internal border zones. This radiographic pattern is consistent with failure of blood flow originating from the internal carotid artery, which is also known to be significantly narrowed in this patient. Cardioembolism would likely send multiple clots to different cortical territories more stochastically and not confined to the border zones. Lipohyalinosis typically leads to isolated lacunar infarcts in subcortical locations. Intracranial atherosclerosis would lead to acute infarcts within specific single vessel territories, not along watershed territories.

Reference

Cuadrado-Godia E, Ois A, Roquer J. Heart failure in acute ischemic stroke. Curr Cardiol Rev. 2010;6(3):202–213. https://doi.org/10.2174/157340310791658776

6. A 33-year-old woman with a history of asthma and nosebleeds is 8 weeks postpartum after an uncomplicated delivery. She develops a large acute right parietal stroke with an NIHSS of 8 and is admitted for further evaluation. Her workup shows normal cerebral vasculature, negative hypercoagulable serologies, and no DVTs in her lower extremities. Her echocardiogram with bubble shows a large intrapulmonary shunt. Which of the following is the next course of treatment?

A. Refer to cardiology for PFO closure
B. Start heparin infusion
C. Obtain CTA chest
D. Obtain cardiac MRI
E. Load with aspirin and plavix

Correct answer: C

Explanation

This patient's presentation is most consistent with a paradoxical embolic stroke due to an intrapulmonary right-to-left shunt, likely from pulmonary arteriovenous malformations (PAVMs) in the setting of hereditary hemorrhagic telangiectasia (HHT). The clinical clues include her young age, history of asthma (which may represent misdiagnosed dyspnea from shunting), recurrent nosebleeds (epistaxis is the most common symptom of HHT), and a postpartum state, which increases thromboembolic risk. The echocardiogram with bubble confirming a large intrapulmonary shunt makes a cardiac source such as a PFO less likely, so PFO closure is not indicated. The appropriate next step is to obtain a CTA of the chest to identify and localize the PAVMs. This is important because PAVMs can be treated with transcatheter embolization, which reduces the risk of recurrent paradoxical emboli and brain abscess.

Reference

Topiwala KK, Patel SD, Saver JL, Streib CD, Shovlin CL. Ischemic Stroke and Pulmonary Arteriovenous Malformations: A Review. Neurology. 2022;98(5):188–198. https://doi.org/10.1212/WNL.0000000000013169

7. A 68-year-old man undergoing aortic aneurysm repair is noted after post-operative recovery to have new flaccid paralysis of both lower extremities. Sensation to pain and temperature is absent below the umbilicus, but proprioception is intact. His patellar and achilles reflexes are absent.

What vascular territory is most likely affected?

A. Posterior spinal artery
B. Artery of Adamkiewicz
C. Anterior spinal artery
D. Posterior inferior cerebellar artery
E. Anterior spinal vein

Correct answer: C

Explanation

The patient has presented with a sudden onset myelopathy after aortic surgery, most consistent with acute infarction of the thoracic spinal cord. Based on the described exam, the affected tracts of the spinal cord include motor pathways as well as the spinothalamic tract, carrying pain and temperature sensation signals to the brain. These structures are located in the ventral spinal cord, supplied by the anterior spinal artery. Other structures, such as the proprioceptive sensory tracts known to be in the dorsal spinal cord, are spared.

References

Kumral E, Polat F, Güllüoglu H, Uzunköprü C, Tuncel R, Alpaydın S. Spinal ischaemic stroke: clinical and radiological findings and short-term outcome. Eur J Neurol. 2011;18(2):232-239. https://doi.org/10.1111/j.1468-1331.2010.02994.

Sandoval JI, De Jesus O. Anterior Spinal Artery Syndrome. [Updated 2024 Jun 7]. In: StatPearls [Internet]. Treasure Island (FL): StatPearls Publishing; 2025 Jan-. Available from: https://www.ncbi.nlm.nih.gov/books/NBK560731/

Zalewski, N. L., Rabinstein, A. A., Krecke, K. N., Brown, R. D. Jr., Wijdicks, E. F. M., Weinshenker, B. G., & Flanagan, E. P. (2019). Characteristics of spontaneous spinal cord infarction and proposed diagnostic criteria. JAMA Neurology, 76(1), 56–63. https://doi.org/10.1001/jamaneurol.2018.2734

8. A 38-year-old man was walking around at home when he felt a strange painful constrictive sensation around the center of his abdomen. Over the next hour, he noticed that both of his legs became progressively numb and weak to the point that he could no longer walk, leading him to activate EMS to take him to the emergency department. In the ED, he is noted to have almost complete flaccid paralysis of the legs, reduced pinprick sensation below the waist, and absent reflexes in the bilateral patellas and achilles. Straight catheterization was required after bladder scan identified 780 cc of urine. He is admitted to the hospital with further testing completed over 2 days. CSF: protein 38, glucose 60, with no nucleated cells and 4 RBCs noted, no detected infectious organisms on meningitis-encephalitis panel. Erythrocyte sedimentation rate (ESR) is not elevated.

MRI spine 36 hours later shows the following:

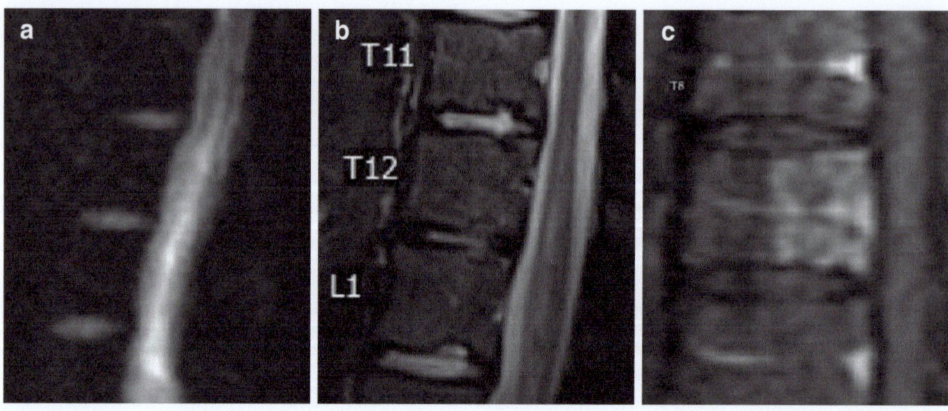

From Left to right: (**a**) Sagittal b1000 diffusion of spinal cord, (**b**) Sagittal T2/STIR of spinal cord, (**c**) Sagittal T1 post contrast of vertebral bodies and spinal cord. (Source: Chornay et al. via Stroke (2025).

Which of the following is the most likely cause of the patient's clinical presentation?

A. Acute immune-mediated demyelinating polyneuropathy (AIDP)
B. Transverse myelitis
C. Anterior spinal artery occlusion
D. Spinal dural arteriovenous fistula
E. Spinal canal hemorrhage
F. Cauda equina syndrome

Correct answer: C

Explanation

The patient's constellation of symptoms includes a bandlike pain sensation with worsening weakness, numbness, reflex changes, and urinary retention that suggest a syndrome localizing to the spinal cord. The sudden onset over less than a few hours with associated discomfort in addition to the neurologic exam findings are most suggestive of an acute spinal cord infarction rather than a transverse myelitis or demyelinating polyneuropathy. AIDP also would likely not include a sensory level or urinary retention. The MR imaging presented shows diffusion restriction and abnormal T2 signal involving the central portion of the spinal cord itself, with no evidence of extra-axial hemorrhage or abnormal vasculature, while the third panel shows evidence of a vertebral body infarction on post-contrast imaging. These findings are all supportive of the diagnosis of acute infarction of the spinal cord, which can result from anterior spinal artery occlusion.

References

Chornay, C., Ahmed, H., Kvernland, A., Nossek, E., & Kelly, S. M. (2025). Spontaneous spinal cord infarction in a young patient: An overview of clinical features and management. Stroke, 56(2), e58–e61. https://doi.org/10.1161/STROKEAHA.124.049502

Faig J, Busse O, Salbeck R. Vertebral body infarction as a confirmatory sign of spinal cord ischemic stroke: report of three cases and review of the literature. Stroke. 1998;29:239–243. https://doi.org/10.1161/01.str.29.1.239

Kumral E, Polat F, Güllüoglu H, Uzunköprü C, Tuncel R, Alpaydın S. Spinal ischaemic stroke: clinical and radiological findings and short-term outcome. Eur J Neurol. 2011;18(2):232–239. https://doi.org/10.1111/j.1468-1331.2010.02994.x

Zalewski, N. L., Rabinstein, A. A., Krecke, K. N., Brown, R. D. Jr., Wijdicks, E. F. M., Weinshenker, B. G., & Flanagan, E. P. (2019). Characteristics of spontaneous spinal cord infarction and proposed diagnostic criteria. JAMA Neurology, 76(1), 56–63. https://doi.org/10.1001/jamaneurol.2018.2734

9. A 32-year-old woman with no significant past medical history presents to the emergency department with transient numbness and weakness of her right hand and arm. Lipid panel and hemoglobin A1C are within normal limits, and echocardiogram is normal. Her cerebral angiogram is shown below.

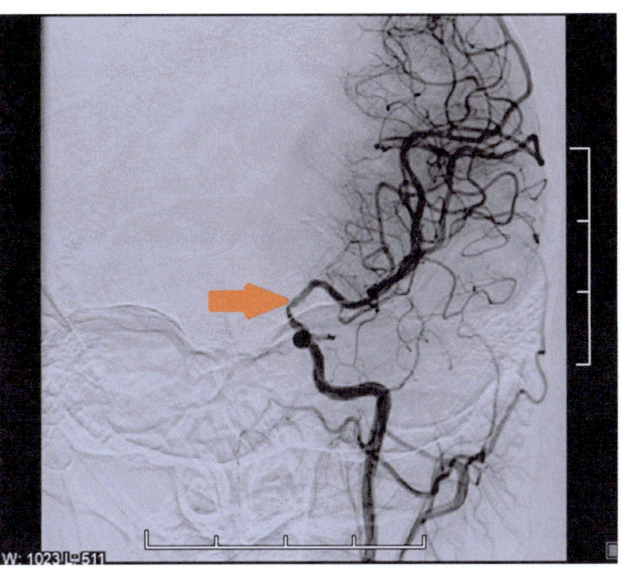

Digital Subtraction Angiogram. (Source: McDonald, A. Via Cureus (2020). CC-BY 4.0 (https://creativecommons.org/licenses/by/4.0/). Image has not been modified. Please see full attribution with citation in the references section below)

What is the cause of the condition that most likely led to the patient's presentation?

A. Abberant electrical activity in the atrium of the heart overtaking the sinus node
B. Intra-arterial wall deposition of lipids with subsequent plaque rupture
C. Abnormal fibroblast proliferation in segments of the arterial tunica media
D. Lipohyalinosis of intracranial small penetrating arterioles

Correct answer: C

Explanation

The patient has presented with symptoms suggestive of right hemispheric TIA centered around the hand knob of the right precentral gyrus. The patient's diagnostic angiogram shows multifocal irregularities of the proximal segments of both internal carotid arteries. In such a young patient with no known history of hyperlipidemia or heart disease, atrial fibrillation (A) and cervical atherosclerotic plaque rupture (B) are significantly less likely to be the cause of the patient's TIA. Lipohyalinosis can result from chronic hypertension, which the patient is not known to have. Therefore, the most likely underlying cause is Fibromuscular dysplasia. The underlying pathology includes abnormal fibroblast proliferation in segments of the arterial tunica media.

Reference

McDonald A. A Case of Isolated Intracranial Fibromuscular Dysplasia. Cureus. 2020;12(6):e8755. https://doi.org/10.7759/cureus.8755.

10. A 45-year-old woman with migraines undergoes magnetic resonance angiography of the head and neck. Her MRA neck shows alternating narrowing and dilatation in the extracranial vasculature. Which of the following vessels is most commonly affected by this condition?
    A. Vertebral artery
    B. Internal carotid artery
    C. Subclavian artery
    D. External carotid artery
    E. Basilar artery
    Correct answer: B

Explanation

This patient's imaging description of alternating narrowing and dilatation in the extracranial vasculature is classic for fibromuscular dysplasia. The internal carotid artery, particularly in its mid to distal cervical segment, is the most frequently involved vessel in cerebrovascular FMD, followed by the vertebral arteries. Involvement can also occur in renal arteries, where it may cause renovascular hypertension.

References

Cardounell SZ, Gonzalez L. Carotid Artery Fibromuscular Dysplasia. [Updated 2023 Aug 8]. In: StatPearls [Internet]. Treasure Island (FL): StatPearls Publishing; 2025 Jan-. Available from: https://www.ncbi.nlm.nih.gov/books/NBK538199/

Kesav P, Manesh Raj D, John S. Cerebrovascular Fibromuscular Dysplasia - A Practical Review. Vasc Health Risk Manag. 2023;19:543-556. Published 2023 Aug 28. https://doi.org/10.2147/VHRM.S388257

11. A 38-year-old man with no significant past medical history presents with sudden onset of left-sided neck pain and Horner's syndrome. Within hours, he develops right-sided hemiparesis. MRI brain reveals an infarct in the left lateral medulla and cerebellum. MRA of the neck shows tapering stenosis of the left vertebral artery.
    What is the most likely cause of his stroke?
    A. Atherosclerosis of the vertebral artery
    B. Intracranial arterial aneurysm rupture
    C. Arterial dissection of the vertebral artery
    D. Small vessel lacunar infarct
    E. Arterial dissection of the carotid artery
    Correct answer: C

Explanation

In a younger patient who experiences stroke symptoms associated with neck pain, cervical artery dissection is the most likely cause of stroke. Both carotid artery dissection and vertebral artery dissection can lead to Horner's syndrome, however, the findings and location of the described infarct would only be consistent with a vertebral artery dissection. Below is the patient's T2 weighted MRI showing bright signal in the right vertebral indicating an intramural hematoma (clot within the vessel wall) and complete blockage of the artery. There is no intraluminal hematoma.

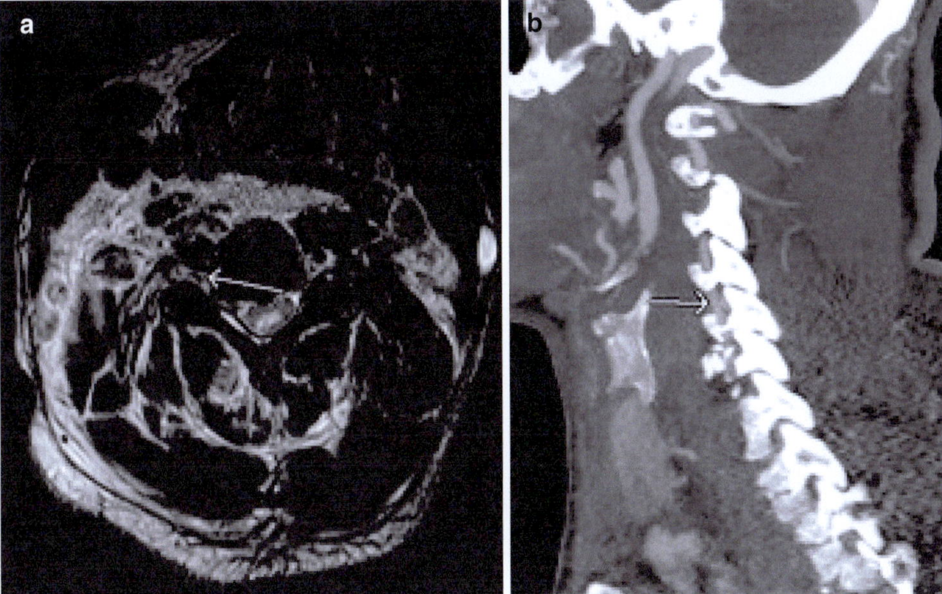

(**a**) Axial T2 weighted image. (**b**) Subsequent CT angiogram of the neck. (Source: Kumar Y and Hayashi D via BMC musculoskeletal disorders (2016). CC-BY 4.0 (https://creativecommons.org/licenses/by/4.0/). Image has been cropped to show only panels A and B. Kumar Y, Hayashi D. Role of magnetic resonance imaging in acute spinal trauma: a pictorial review. BMC Musculoskelet Disord. 2016;17:310. Published 2016 Jul 22. https://doi.org/10.1186/s12891-016-1169-6)

Reference

Kumar Y, Hayashi D. Role of magnetic resonance imaging in acute spinal trauma: a pictorial review. BMC Musculoskelet Disord. 2016;17:310. Published 2016 Jul 22. https://doi.org/10.1186/s12891-016-1169-6

12. A 75-year-old man with hypertension and coronary artery disease presents to the hospital with an acute left posterior circulation stroke. His cerebral vasculature is patent. He undergoes echocardiogram the following day. Which of the following, if present, represents a high-risk source of ischemic stroke?
    A. Papillary fibroelastoma
    B. Left ventricular hypertrophy
    C. Mitral annular calcification
    D. Patent foramen ovale
    E. Wall motion abnormality
    Correct answer: A

Explanation

A papillary fibroelastoma is a benign cardiac tumor, most often found on heart valves, and is a recognized high-risk source of cardioembolic stroke. Even though it is histologically benign, it can cause embolism via tumor fragments or thrombus formation on its surface. Because of this high embolic potential, surgical removal is often recommended in appropriate candidates, especially if the lesion is mobile or symptomatic.

Reference

Kernan WN, Ovbiagele B, Black HR, et al. "Guidelines for the prevention of stroke in patients with stroke and transient ischemic attack." Stroke. 2014;45(7):2160–2236. See Table 4 ("High-risk" vs "Potential" cardioembolic sources).

13. A 67-year-old woman presents to the ophthalmology clinic with sudden, painless vision loss in her right eye that began 2 h ago. She describes it as a "curtain coming down" over her vision. Past medical history includes hypertension and hyperlipidemia. Fundoscopic exam shows a pale retina with a cherry-red spot at the fovea.

    Which of the following questions is most important to ask at this time?
    A. "Have you had any recent head trauma?"
    B. "Do you have any pain when chewing or tenderness of the scalp?"
    C. "Does anyone in your family have glaucoma?"
    D. "Have you noticed any light sensitivity or eye discharge?"
    E. "Do you wear contact lenses?"
    Correct answer: B

Explanation

This presentation is consistent with central retinal artery occlusion (CRAO), a form of acute monocular vision loss.

CRAO is most commonly due to embolism into the central retinal artery (non-arteritic variety) or, less commonly, to vasculitis involving the central retinal artery (arteritic variety), most commonly Giant Cell Arteritis (GCA). In patients over 50, it's essential to evaluate for giant cell arteritis (GCA) as a potential cause. GCA can present with symptoms such as jaw claudication, scalp tenderness, new headaches, and constitutional symptoms. Prompt diagnosis is critical, as untreated GCA can lead to irreversible bilateral blindness. Asking about these symptoms during history-taking helps identify the need for immediate corticosteroid therapy and temporal artery biopsy. Other answer choices are less immediately relevant.

Reference

Tripathy K, Shah SS, Waymack JR. Central Retinal Artery Occlusion. [Updated 2024 May 2]. In: StatPearls [Internet]. Treasure Island (FL): StatPearls Publishing; 2025 Jan-. Available from: https://www.ncbi.nlm.nih.gov/books/NBK470354/

14. A 77-year-old man presents with a 15-min episode of painless vision loss in his left eye, which he describes as "a curtain descending over the eye." His medical history includes hypertension, type 2 diabetes mellitus, and hyperlipidemia, all managed with medication. On arrival, his vital signs are: BP 170/100 mm Hg and HR 70/min, regular. Laboratory studies reveal a blood glucose level of 160 mg/dL and an LDL cholesterol of 140 mg/dL. Neurologic examination and noncontrast head CT are normal.

 Which of the following diagnostic tests is most likely to identify the cause of this event?
 A. Dilated ophthalmologic examination
 B. Erythrocyte sedimentation rate
 C. CT angiography of the neck
 D. Outpatient cardiac monitoring
 E. Transthoracic echocardiography
 Correct answer: C

Explanation

This patient's transient monocular vision loss—described as a "curtain falling" —is characteristic of amaurosis fugax, often due to retinal ischemia. In older adults with vascular risk factors, the most common etiology is embolism from carotid artery atherosclerosis. Therefore, vascular imaging (such as CT angiography or carotid duplex ultrasound) is the most appropriate next step to evaluate for carotid stenosis, a known source of emboli to the ophthalmic artery.

 Although cardiac sources of embolism (e.g., atrial fibrillation or valvular disease) are possible, carotid disease is more likely in this scenario, making echocardiography or prolonged rhythm monitoring less immediately useful. An ophthalmologic exam may reveal retinal emboli but cannot determine the ischemia source. ESR would be appropriate if giant cell arteritis were suspected (e.g., progressive visual loss, headache, jaw claudication), but this patient lacks those features.

Reference

Tripathy K, Shah SS, Waymack JR. Central Retinal Artery Occlusion. [Updated 2024 May 2]. In: StatPearls [Internet]. Treasure Island (FL): StatPearls Publishing; 2025 Jan-. Available from: https://www.ncbi.nlm.nih.gov/books/NBK470354/

15. Which of the following statements is true regarding the blood supply to the retina and the pathophysiology of the cherry-red spot seen in central retinal artery occlusion (CRAO)?
 A. The retina is exclusively supplied by the central retinal artery, which explains the uniform pallor seen in CRAO
 B. The fovea appears as a cherry-red spot in CRAO because it receives collateral blood flow from the choroidal circulation.
 C. The fovea appears red in CRAO because it is thinner and overlying the pigmented retinal epithelium
 D. The ciliary arteries primarily supply the inner retina and are responsible for vision
 E. CRAO affects only the outer retina, which is why central vision is often preserved
 Correct answer: B

Explanation

The retina has a dual blood supply: the central retinal artery supplies the inner retina, while the choroidal circulation, derived from the posterior ciliary arteries, supplies the outer retina, including the fovea. In CRAO, ischemia of the inner retina causes retinal whitening, but the fovea, which is thinner and avascular (receiving nutrients from the intact choroidal supply), remains red against the pale surrounding retina—producing the classic cherry-red spot. C is partially true anatomically (the fovea is thinner and sits over pigmented epithelium), but the key reason for the cherry-red spot is preserved choroidal flow.

Reference

Tripathy K, Shah SS, Waymack JR. Central Retinal Artery Occlusion. [Updated 2024 May 2]. In: StatPearls [Internet]. Treasure Island (FL): StatPearls Publishing; 2025 Jan-. Available from: https://www.ncbi.nlm.nih.gov/books/NBK470354/

16. A 65-year-old man develops left-sided weakness and is found to have scattered right hemispheric strokes in a watershed distribution with 90% stenosis of the right internal carotid artery. He is started on aspirin and atorvastatin. Three days later, he undergoes revascularization with carotid endarterectomy. The procedure is uncomplicated, and his neurologic exam is unchanged. Overnight, he develops severe headaches and becomes more somnolent. A stat CT head does not show new infarct or hemorrhage, and his CTA shows patent right internal carotid artery. His vitals are: blood pressure 180/90 mm Hg, heart rate 80. His fingerstick is 92. Which of the following most likely explains his symptoms?

    A. Hypoglycemia
    B. Hemorrhagic transformation of ischemic strokes
    C. Watershed strokes
    D. Reperfusion syndrome
    E. Subclinical seizures

    Correct answer: D

Explanation

Cerebral hyperperfusion (reperfusion) syndrome occurs after sudden restoration of blood flow to chronically hypoperfused brain tissue, usually within days of carotid endarterectomy or stenting. Chronic hypoperfusion leads to impaired autoregulatory vasoconstriction; when flow is restored, the ipsilateral hemisphere is exposed to high perfusion pressures, resulting in increased capillary permeability, cerebral edema, and symptoms such as headache, confusion, seizures, or focal deficits.

Reference

Lin YH, Liu HM. Update on cerebral hyperperfusion syndrome. J Neurointerv Surg. 2020;12(8):788-793. https://doi.org/10.1136/neurintsurg-2019-015621

17. A 59-year-old man presents to the clinic reporting a series of episodes over the past week during which he experiences vertigo, gait instability, difficulty controlling his left arm, slurred speech, blurred or double vision, and a tingling sensation in his right arm and left side of the face. These episodes last 10–30 min and resolve completely. He has no history of seizures or migraines. Neurological exam between episodes is unremarkable. He has a 40-pack-year smoking history.

    Which artery is most likely involved?

    A. Left anterior cerebral artery
    B. Right middle cerebral artery
    C. Posterior communicating artery
    D. Left vertebral artery
    E. Left anterior choroidal artery
    F. Right vertebral artery

    Correct answer: D

Explanation

Based on the description, the patient is experiencing episodes of dizziness, dysarthria, double vision, and dysmetria that are most consistent with a posterior circulation vascular syndrome. More specifically, the crossed body sensory loss with cerebellar signs and eye movement control that could very likely reflect a lateral medullary syndrome (Wallenberg syndrome). This syndrome is most often precipitated by disease of the vertebral artery (or less commonly occlusion of PICA). An infarction of the lateral medulla and cerebellum from a vertebral artery occlusion will cause IPSILATERAL cerebellar signs and facial numbness, and CONTRALATERAL sensory loss of the body, in this case localizing the event to the LEFT vertebral artery, which may be stenotic in the setting of atherosclerosis rather than fully occluded based on the fluctuating symptoms.

18. A 72-year-old right-handed woman with a history of poorly controlled hypertension and atrial fibrillation presents with sudden onset of right-sided hemiplegia, right-sided hemisensory loss, and aphasia. MRI reveals a hyperintense signal on DWI in the left MCA territory, including the basal ganglia, frontal, and parietal lobes. Which of the following additional findings is most likely present?

    A. Apraxia of the left hand
    B. Conduction aphasia
    C. Alexia without agraphia
    D. Gerstmann syndrome

    Correct answer: A

Explanation

A left MCA territory infarct involves the dominant hemisphere, affecting the supplementary motor area (SMA) and parietal cortex, key regions for motor planning. Damage here disrupts connections between the parietal and motor cortices, leading to ideomotor apraxia, particularly in the contralateral (right) hand but potentially affecting the left hand due to interhemispheric connections. A conduction aphasia typically results from damage to the arcuate fasciculus, a white matter tract linking Broca's and Wernicke's areas. This infarct involves broader frontal and parietal regions, producing more global language deficits rather than isolated conduction aphasia. Alexia without agraphia occurs with PCA infarcts involving the splenium of the corpus callosum and occipital lobe, not the MCA territory. Gerstmann Syndrome involves the angular gyrus and presents with agraphia, acalculia, finger agnosia, and left-right disorientation. This patient's deficits are more extensive, indicating a larger MCA territory infarct rather than a focal parietal lesion.

19. A 68-year-old right-handed woman with a history of diabetes and hypertension presents with difficulty writing and calculating and inability to distinguish her left from her right. She is otherwise alert and oriented. MRI reveals an infarct involving the left angular gyrus and supramarginal gyrus. Which of the following findings may also be present?
    A. Dyslexia
    B. Finger agnosia
    C. Visual field impairment
    D. Right arm and leg numbness
    E. Ideomotor apraxia
    Correct answer: B

Explanation

Gerstmann syndrome involves a lesion in the dominant parietal lobe, particularly the angular gyrus, leading to a tetrad of agraphia, acalculia, finger agnosia, and left-right disorientation. The patient already exhibits agraphia, acalculia, and left-right disorientation; finger agnosia, the inability to identify or distinguish individual fingers, would complete the syndrome. Dyslexia is typically associated with lesions in the temporo-parietal region rather than the angular gyrus. Right arm and leg numbness would be more indicative of sensory cortex involvement rather than the angular gyrus.

Reference

Altabakhi IW, Liang JW. Gerstmann Syndrome. [Updated 2023 Aug 28]. In: StatPearls [Internet]. Treasure Island (FL): StatPearls Publishing; 2025 Jan-. Available from: https://www.ncbi.nlm.nih.gov/books/NBK519528/

20. A 62-year-old man with poorly controlled hypertension presents with sudden-onset right-sided hemiplegia, right-sided hemisensory loss, and homonymous hemianopia. Head CT reveals a small infarct in the posterior limb of the internal capsule. Which of the following arterial territories is most likely involved?
    A. Lenticulostriate arteries
    B. Anterior choroidal artery
    C. Posterior cerebral artery
    D. Middle cerebral artery
    E. Anterior cerebral artery
    Correct answer: B

Explanation

The anterior choroidal artery, a branch of the internal carotid artery, supplies key structures including the posterior limb of the internal capsule, globus pallidus, optic tract, lateral geniculate body, and parts of the thalamus and hippocampus. Infarcts in this territory often present with the classic triad of contralateral hemiplegia, hemisensory loss, and homonymous hemianopia.

21. A 76-year-old woman with a history of hypertension and prior occipital stroke presents to the emergency department with confusion. She can accurately describe the shape, color, and texture of a key but cannot name it until she holds it and feels its distinct features. This deficit is most likely due to a disconnection between which of the following?
    A. Temporal lobe from the angular gyrus
    B. Parietal lobe from the frontal lobe
    C. Occipital lobe from the parietal lobe
    D. Occipital lobe from the temporal lobe
    E. Temporal lobe from the Broca area
    Correct answer: D

Explanation

The patient exhibits visual object agnosia, characterized by the inability to recognize objects by sight while other sensory modalities (e.g., touch) remain intact. This occurs due to a disconnection between the occipital lobe (visual processing) and the temporal lobe (object identification and semantic processing). The occipitotemporal pathway (ventral stream), often referred to as the "what" pathway, is crucial for object recognition. In cases where visual information cannot effectively reach the temporal lobe, the patient can still identify objects by tactile input, which accesses the temporal lobe through alternative sensory pathways.

22. An 85-year-old right-handed man develops a stroke affecting the left occipital lobe and splenium of the corpus callous. On exam, he is able to speak in full sentences, follow commands, repeat phrases, and write a sentence about the weather. However, he cannot read the sentence he wrote or other words on the NIHSS stroke card. Which of the following conditions does this patient most likely have?
    A. Conduction aphasia
    B. Pure word deafness
    C. Transcortical motor aphasia
    D. Alexia without agraphia
    E. Aphemia
    Correct answer: D

Explanation

This patient's stroke involves the left occipital lobe and the splenium of the corpus callosum, a classic lesion location for alexia without agraphia. In this condition, the left primary visual cortex is damaged, resulting in right homonymous hemianopia, and the splenial involvement interrupts visual information transfer from the right occipital cortex to the left angular gyrus, which is critical for reading. Because the angular gyrus in the dominant hemisphere cannot access visual input, the patient is unable to read words, even those he has just written. However, his language production, comprehension, naming, repetition, and writing remain intact, explaining why he can speak fluently, follow commands, and write sentences normally. This syndrome is sometimes referred to as pure alexia and is most often caused by a left posterior cerebral artery (PCA) stroke that also involves the splenium.

Other answer choices are incorrect because conduction aphasia presents with impaired repetition, pure word deafness results from bilateral temporal lesions affecting speech perception, transcortical motor aphasia features nonfluent speech with preserved repetition, and aphemia is a disorder of speech articulation with preserved writing and reading comprehension.

Reference

Carranza-Rentería O, Swerdloff MA. Clinicoradiological Features of Alexia Without Agraphia. Cureus. 2024;16(4):e58309. Published 2024 Apr 15. https://doi.org/10.7759/cureus.58309

23. A 55-year-old man sees you in clinic after he sustained a stroke 3 weeks ago. His MRI brain shows scattered strokes in the right frontal lobe and the right occipital lobe, all of the same age. On exam he has mild left sided weakness and a left homonymous visual field cut. He explains that all of his symptoms came on at the same time. You decide to order an MRA of the head and neck. Which of the following anatomical variant is most likely to be seen on his MRA?
    A. Azygous anterior cerebral artery
    B. Fetal right posterior cerebral artery
    C. Hypoplastic right vertebral artery
    D. Persistent trigeminal artery
    E. Fenestrated basilar artery
    Correct answer: B

Explanation

This patient has acute infarcts in both the right anterior circulation (frontal lobe) and right posterior circulation (occipital lobe) that occurred at the same time, suggesting a single vascular event affecting both territories simultaneously. The most likely mechanism is an embolus lodging in a vessel that supplies both regions, which can occur if there is a fetal origin of the right posterior cerebral artery (PCA). In this common anatomical variant, the PCA originates from the internal carotid artery via a large posterior communicating artery, rather than from the basilar artery. This means that the right ICA supplies both the right MCA/ACA territory and the right PCA territory. An embolus in the right ICA can therefore cause simultaneous anterior and posterior circulation infarcts on the same side.

24. A 28-year-old man is involved in a car accident in which he is the driver. Three days later, he notes vertigo. On exam, he is noted to have left ptosis, absent sensation to pinprick on his left cheek. Which additional findings are NOT expected on the remainder of his exam.
    A. Hoarse voice
    B. Hiccups
    C. Left sided ataxia
    D. Right arm weakness
    E. Nystagmus
    Correct answer: D

Explanation

The findings localize to a left lateral medullary infarct, classically a PICA territory or vertebral artery lesion. Ipsilateral facial pain and temperature loss arises from involvement of the spinal trigeminal nucleus and tract, and ipsilateral ptosis reflects Horner syndrome from disruption of descending sympathetic fibers. Vertigo and nystagmus are due to vestibular nuclei involvement, and hiccups and a hoarse voice result from nucleus ambiguus dysfunction. Ipsilateral limb ataxia comes from injury to the inferior cerebellar peduncle. The corticospinal tract lies more anterior and is typically spared in lateral medullary syndrome, so contralateral limb weakness would not be expected. Therefore, right arm weakness is the least likely additional finding.

25. A 68-year-old man develops a headache while sitting at home. Minutes later, he notices he has slurred speech and rapidly worsening weakness of the right arm and leg. His family calls EMS and he is taken to the ED. On arrival, he is increasingly lethargic and having difficulty speaking full sentences. His blood pressure is 194/115, initial CT scan is shown below. He is admitted to the ICU for close monitoring and further care.

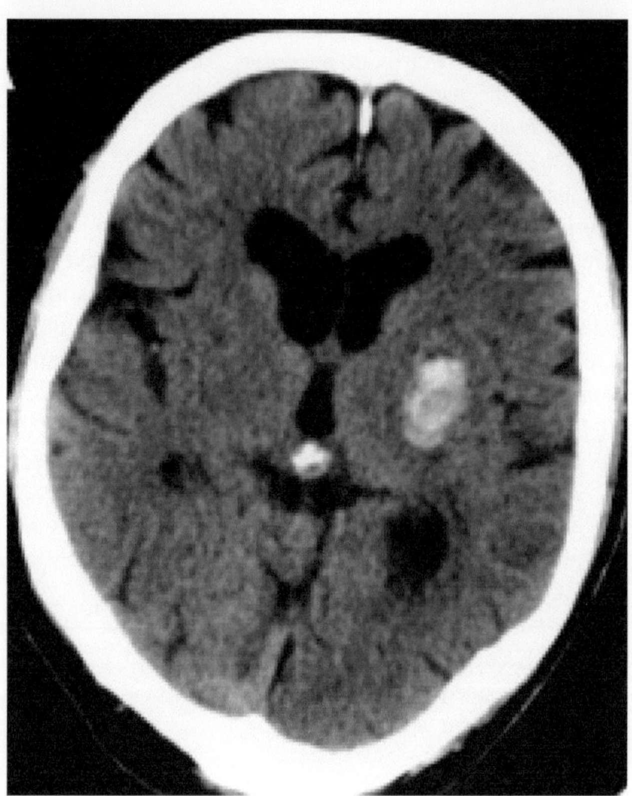

Axial CT scan of the brain. (Source: Ovesen C, Havsteen I, Rosenbaum S, Christensen H via Frontiers in Neurology (2014). CC-BY 4.0 (https://creativecommons.org/licenses/by/4.0/). Image has been cropped to include only panel A of the original. Please see full attribution with citation below in references section for this question.)

What is the most likely underlying risk factor that precipitated the patient's stroke?

   A. AV malformation
   B. Amyloid angiopathy
   C. Hypertension
   D. Ischemic stroke
   E. Tumor

Correct answer: C

Explanation

The patient has presented with acute onset neurologic symptoms localizing to the left MCA territory. His head CT reveals and acute hyperdensity of the left putamen consistent with an acute intracranial hemorrhage (ICH). The putamen is the most common location for a hypertensive ICH to occur, and the head CT shows a well circumscribed hyperdensity without significant surrounding hypodensity or irregularity, more consistent with hypertension than underlying tumor or stroke. AV malformation is a significantly less common cause of ICH than hypertensive vasculopathy. Other com-mon locations for hypertensive hemorrhage include other basal ganglia nuclei, the thalamus, pons, or cerebellum.

References

Biller, J., & Sacco, R. L. (2023). Cerebrovascular diseases. In A. H. Ropper, M. A. Samuels, J. P. Klein, & S. Prasad (Eds.), Adams and Victor's principles of neurology (12th ed., pp. 660–770). McGraw Hill.

Ovesen C, Havsteen I, Rosenbaum S, Christensen H. Prediction and observation of post-admission hematoma expansion in patients with intracerebral hemorrhage. Front Neurol. 2014;5:186. Published 2014 Sep 29. https://doi.org/10.3389/fneur.2014.00186

26. An 82-year-old man arrives in the ED by ambulance after being found at home to be lethargic and weak on the left side. On arrival, his blood pressure is 183/110. On exam, he opens eyes to voice, but cannot follow commands and only speaks with inappropriate words and does not maintain alertness. He localizes to touch or painful stimuli when needed. His CT scan is shown below. Radiology reviews it and reports the hemorrhagic findings shown, measuring a total volume of 7 cc.

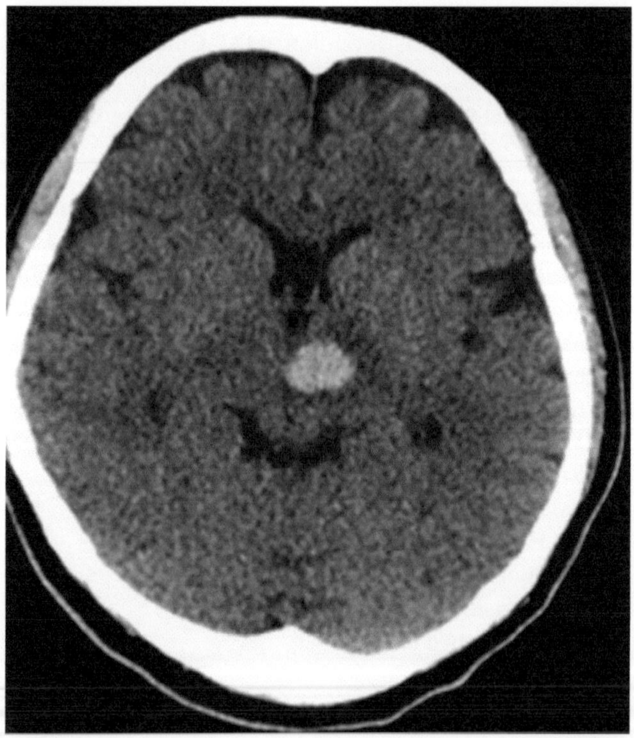

Axial CT scan of the brain. (Source: de Oliveira Manoel AL, Goffi A, Zampieri FG, et al. via Crit Care (2016). CC-BY 4.0 (https://creativecommons.org/licenses/by/4.0/). Image has been cropped to include only select image. Please see full attribution with citation below in references section for this question.)

What is the patient's ICH score?

A. 2
B. 3
C. 4
D. 5
E. 6

Correct answer: A

Explanation

The ICH score is a clinical grading scale for intracerebral hemorrhage that has been validated in multiple studies as a means to estimate ICH severity and 30-day mortality. The components include the following: Glasgow coma scale (GCS) 3–4 (2 points), 5–12 (1 point), 13–15 (0 points); Age >80 (1 point); ICH volume >30 cc (1 point); Intraventricular hemorrhage (1 point); Infratentorial origin of hemorrhage (1 point). The patient scores 2 points for GCS ~10 and age 82.

References

de Oliveira Manoel AL, Goffi A, Zampieri FG, et al. The critical care management of spontaneous intracranial hemorrhage: a contemporary review. Crit Care. 2016;20:272. Published 2016 Sep 18. https://doi.org/10.1186/s13054-016-1432-0

Hemphill JC 3rd, Bonovich DC, Besmertis L, Manley GT, Johnston SC. The ICH score: a simple, reliable grading scale for intracerebral hemorrhage. Stroke. 2001;32(4):891-897. https://doi.org/10.1161/01.str.32.4.891

27. An 85-year-old woman exhibits forgetfulness and mood changes over 3 years. She develops sudden blurry vision and presents to the ER where her CT head shows an acute left occipital lobar hemorrhage. CTA does not show underlying vascular malformation. Her MRI brain additionally shows numerous peripheral and subcortical microhemorrhages, extensive subcortical white matter disease, and three areas of cortical superficial siderosis. Which of the following carries the highest risk of recurrent intracerebral hemorrhage in this patient?

A. Lobar hemorrhage
B. Peripheral micro hemorrhages
C. White matter disease
D. Cortical superficial siderosis
E. Subcortical microhemorrhages

Correct answer: D

Explanation

This patient has probable cerebral amyloid angiopathy (CAA) per Boston Criteria 2.0: age >55, lobar hemorrhage, and supportive MRI findings (peripheral microhemorrhages, cSS, white matter disease). Multiple studies show that corti-

cal superficial siderosis (especially disseminated or bilateral) is the strongest MRI predictor of future hemorrhage in CAA. It reflects prior bleeding into the subarachnoid space from fragile amyloid-laden cortical vessels, indicating advanced vascular pathology and instability.

Reference

Biller, J., & Sacco, R. L. (2023). Cerebrovascular diseases. In A. H. Ropper, M. A. Samuels, J. P. Klein, & S. Prasad (Eds.), Adams and Victor's principles of neurology (12th ed., pp. 660–770). McGraw Hill.

28. A 72-year-old woman presents after falling in the bathroom and hitting her head. There is no loss of consciousness. Her CT head scan is unremarkable. She complains of headache and double vision. An MRI brain with contrast is obtained with the T1 post-contrast sequence hown below. What is the structure pointed out by the white arrow?

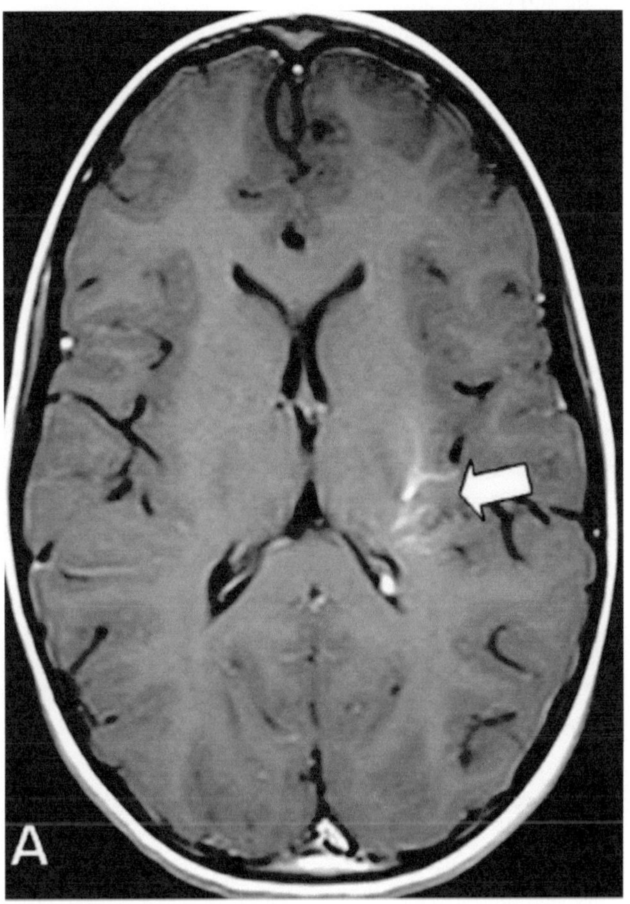

Axial T1 contrast enhanced MRI. (Source: Abdelgawd, MS and Aly, RA via Egypt J Radiol Nucl (2020). CC-BY 4.0 (https://creativecommons.org/licenses/by/4.0/deed.en). Image has been cropped to show only panel A. Please see full attribution in references section below)

A. Cerebral contusion
B. Arteriovenous malformation
C. Cerebral cavernoma
D. Developmental venous anomaly
E. Berry aneurysm
Correct answer: D

Explanation

A developmental venous anomaly is a benign, congenital vascular variant caused by anomalous medullary veins that converge into a central draining vein. On MRI with susceptibility-weighted imaging (SWI) or post-contrast T1, DVAs appear as a "caput medusae" (head of Medusa) pattern—multiple small medullary veins radiating to a larger collector vein, which then drains into a dural sinus or deep vein.

References

Abdelgawad, M.S., Aly, R.A. Value of susceptibility-weighted MR imaging (SWI) in the detection of developmental venous anomaly. Egypt J Radiol Nucl Med 51, 90 (2020). https://doi.org/10.1186/s43055-020-00216-z

Lee C, Pennington MA, Kenney CM. MR evaluation of developmental venous anomalies: medullary venous anatomy of venous angiomas. AJNR Am J Neuroradiol. 1996;17(1): 61–70.

29. A 25-year-old right-handed male presents with his third seizure and is found to have a 2 cm cavernous malformation in the right temporal lobe. EEG shows his seizures emanate from this lesion. He is on three anti-seizure medications, is adherent to all medications, and his levels are therapeutic. His MRI brain shows acute hemorrhage within the right temporal lobe. A CT scan from 3 years ago when he was hospitalized for another seizure shows acute hemorrhage in the right temporal lobe. Which of the following would be the strongest indication for surgical resection of this cavernous malformation?
A. The size of the cavernous malformation
B. Location in non-eloquent hemisphere
C. Patient's age
D. Family history of cavernous
E. Medically refractory seizures
Correct answer: E

Explanation

This patient has drug-resistant focal epilepsy with clear lesion–symptom concordance: seizures arise from a right temporal cavernous malformation, he is on three appropriately dosed antiseizure medications without control, and he has had recurrent hemorrhage from the same region. For cavernous malformations, the strongest indication for surgery is medically refractory seizures when the epileptogenic focus localizes to the lesion, because lesionectomy with removal of the hemosiderin rim and involved cortex offers the highest chance of seizure freedom and prevents further hemorrhage from the offending lesion. Size alone does not mandate resection, location in a non-eloquent hemisphere simply makes surgery safer rather than necessary, patient age does not by itself determine the need for surgery, and a family history may suggest multiplicity but is not an indication to operate on an otherwise stable lesion. Here, persistent seizures despite optimal medical therapy is the decisive reason to proceed with surgical resection.

Reference

Akers, A., Al-Shahi Salman, R., A Awad, I., Dahlem, K., Flemming, K., Hart, B., Kim, D. S., Kondziolka, D., Lee, C., Morrison, L., Ogilvy, C., Pojoga, L., Porter, P. J., Whitehead, K. J., Zabramski, J. M., & CCM Care Guidelines Consortium. (2017). Synopsis of guidelines for the clinical management of cerebral cavernous malformations: Consensus recommendations based on systematic literature review by the Angioma Alliance Scientific Advisory Board Clinical Experts Panel. Neurosurgery, 80(5), 665–680.

30. A 73-year-old woman presents with severe headache and is found to have subarachnoid hemorrhage due to a ruptured 9 mm anterior communicating aneurysm. Her medical history includes hypertension, diabetes, COPD, and heart failure with reduced ejection fraction. Which of the following characteristics favors aneurysm coiling over clipping in this patient?
A. Aneurysm has a wide neck
B. Lower rate of recurrent aneurysm growth
C. Longer recovery time
D. Avoids need for antithrombotics
E. Avoids need for craniotomy
Correct answer: E

Explanation

In this patient with significant medical comorbidities, minimizing surgical stress and recovery time is important. Endovascular coiling treats the aneurysm from within the vessel and does not require a craniotomy, which reduces perioperative morbidity, shortens hospitalization, and is generally better tolerated in older or medically fragile patients. While coiling has certain limitations, such as higher recurrence rates compared to clipping and potential difficulty with wide-neck aneurysms, it offers a less invasive approach that is advantageous here.

Reference

Ferreira, M. Y., et al. (2024). Comparing surgical clipping with endovascular treatment for unruptured middle cerebral artery aneurysms: A systematic review and updated meta-analysis. Journal of Neurosurgery, 142(1), 116–126

31. Which of the following risk factors is responsible for the largest number of stroke deaths?
    A. Diabetes
    B. Smoking cigarettes
    C. Hypertension
    D. Hyperlipidemia
    E. Coronary artery disease
    Correct answer: C

Explanation

Hypertension is the single most important modifiable risk factor for both ischemic and hemorrhagic stroke worldwide, and it accounts for the largest number of stroke-related deaths. Chronically elevated blood pressure accelerates atherosclerosis, promotes small vessel lipohyalinosis, and increases the risk of intracerebral hemorrhage by weakening vessel walls. Multiple large epidemiologic studies, including the INTERSTROKE study, have shown that hypertension has the highest population-attributable risk for stroke, meaning that controlling blood pressure would prevent more strokes and stroke deaths than targeting any other individual risk factor.

Reference

O'Donnell MJ, Chin SL, Rangarajan S, et al. Global and regional effects of potentially modifiable risk factors associated with acute stroke in 32 countries (INTERSTROKE): a case-control study. Lancet. 2016;388(10046):761-775. https://doi.org/10.1016/S0140-6736(16)30506-2

32. A 65-year-old man presents to the clinic with mild memory loss over the past 3 years. Which of the following risk factors have been linked with cognitive decline?
    A. Consumption of polyunsaturated fatty acids
    B. Atrial fibrillation
    C. College-level education
    D. Low homocysteine level
    E. Elevated high-density lipoprotein (HDL) levels
    Correct answer: B

Explanation

Atrial fibrillation (AF) is strongly associated with an increased risk of both overt stroke and subclinical cerebral infarcts, which in turn contribute to cognitive decline and dementia. AF can lead to chronic cerebral hypoperfusion, microembolization, and inflammation, all of which can impair cognitive function even in the absence of clinically apparent strokes. Several longitudinal cohort studies have confirmed that patients with AF have a higher incidence of cognitive decline compared to age-matched controls, and anticoagulation in AF reduces but does not eliminate this risk. The other options are not linked to increased cognitive decline.

The other options are not associated with increased cognitive decline. Consumption of polyunsaturated fatty acids is generally considered beneficial for cardiovascular and brain health. College-level education is protective due to the concept of cognitive reserve, which allows individuals to better tolerate age-related brain changes or pathology before manifesting clinical symptoms. Low homocysteine levels are not harmful; in fact, it is elevated homocysteine that has been linked to vascular cognitive impairment. Similarly, elevated high-density lipoprotein levels are typically protective for cardiovascular health and may confer some protection against cognitive decline.

Reference

Alonso A, Arenas de Larriva AP. Atrial Fibrillation, Cognitive Decline And Dementia. Eur Cardiol. 2016;11(1):49-53. https://doi.org/10.15420/ecr.2016:13:2

33. Which of the following is not a known risk factor for cerebral venous sinus thrombosis?
    A. Oral contraceptive use
    B. Inflammatory bowel disease
    C. Polycythemia vera
    D. Carotid artery dissection
    E. Pregnancy
    Correct answer: D

Explanation

Carotid artery dissection is a well-established cause of arterial ischemic stroke, especially in younger adults, but it is not a risk factor for cerebral venous sinus thrombosis (CVST). CVST involves thrombus formation in the dural venous sinuses, which is pathophysiologically distinct from arterial dissection. In contrast, oral contraceptive use, pregnancy, inflammatory bowel disease, and polycythemia vera all contribute to hypercoagulable states that directly increase the risk of venous thrombosis, including in the cerebral venous system.

References

Ferro, J. M., & Bousser, M.-G. (2017). Cerebral venous thrombosis. Nature Reviews Neurology, 13(9), 555–565

Yaghi, S., Engelter, S., Del Brutto, V. J., Field, T. S., Jadhav, A. P., Kicielinski, K., Madsen, T. E., … on behalf of the American Heart Association Stroke Council; Council on Cardiovascular and Stroke Nursing; Council on Clinical Cardiology; and Council on Peripheral Vascular Disease. (2024). Treatment and outcomes of cervical artery dissection in adults: A scientific statement from the American Heart Association. Stroke, 55(3), e91–e106.

34. A 35-year-old woman with a history of Crohn's disease and oral contraceptive use presents to the emergency department after a generalized tonic-clonic seizure. She has no prior history of epilepsy. Head CT reveals an intraparenchymal hemorrhage in the right temporal lobe. MRI and contrast-enhanced MRV show absence of contrast filling in the left transverse sinus.

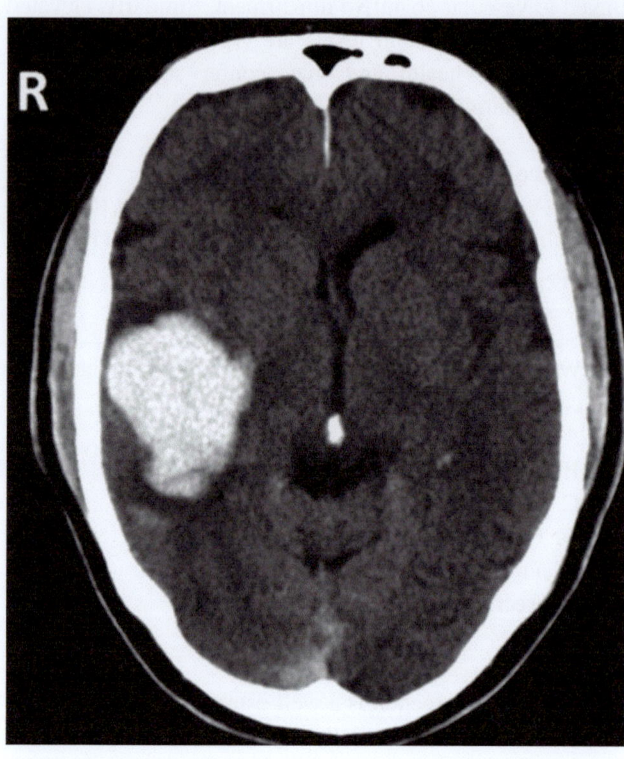

Axial CT scan of the brain. (Source: Cope TE, Baguley DM, and Griffiths TD via Practical neurology. (2015). CC-BY 4.0 (https://creativecommons.org/licenses/by/4.0/). Image has not been modified. Cope TE, Baguley DM, Griffiths TD. The functional anatomy of central auditory processing. Pract Neurol. 2015;15(4):302–308. https://doi.org/10.1136/practneurol-2014-001073)

What is the next best step in management?
A. Decompressive craniectomy
B. Heparin infusion
C. Platelet transfusion
D. Oral warfarin immediately
E. Observation
Correct answer: B

Explanation

This patient has multiple risk factors for Cerebral Venous Sinus Thrombosis (CVST), including inflammatory bowel disease (Crohn's) and oral contraceptive use, both of which contribute to a hypercoagulable state. The absence of contrast opacification in the left transverse sinus on MRV confirms the diagnosis. Despite the presence of intraparenchymal hemorrhage, anticoagulation with heparin (typically intravenous unfractionated heparin or low molecular weight heparin) remains the mainstay of treatment for CVST. The underlying problem is ongoing venous outflow obstruction, which, if left untreated, can worsen edema, venous infarction, and lead to further hemorrhagic transformation. Several studies and clinical guidelines (e.g., AHA/ASA and ESO) support anticoagulation even in the setting of hemorrhagic lesions unless there is a separate contraindication. Delaying treatment out of concern for bleeding risks may result in a worse outcome due to propagation of the thrombus.

References

Cope TE, Baguley DM, Griffiths TD. The functional anatomy of central auditory processing. Pract Neurol. 2015;15(4):302–308. https://doi.org/10.1136/practneurol-2014-001073

Ferro, J. M., & Bousser, M.-G. (2017). Cerebral venous thrombosis. Nature Reviews Neurology, 13(9), 555–565

Ropper AH, Klein JP. Cerebral Venous Thrombosis. N Engl J Med. 2021;385(1):59–64. https://doi.org/10.1056/NEJMra2106545

35. Which of the following is most strongly associated with a poor prognosis in CVST?
A. Isolated headache without focal deficits
B. Deep venous system thrombosis
C. Female sex
D. Oral contraceptive use
E. Dural arteriovenous fistula
Correct answer: B

Explanation

Thrombosis involving the deep cerebral venous system (such as the internal cerebral veins, vein of Galen, or straight sinus) is strongly associated with poor prognosis due to its anatomic involvement of critical deep brain structures like the thalami and basal ganglia. These areas are less tolerant of ischemia and edema, and their involvement often leads to altered consciousness, seizures, and high ICP, which are poor prognostic signs. In contrast, other factors like female sex, oral contraceptive use, or even isolated headache are more common presentations but typically correlate with a better clinical outcome. Dural arteriovenous fistulas may be a sequela of chronic CVST but are not themselves a primary prognostic indicator.

Reference

Lin L, Liu S, Wang W, He XK, Romli MH, Rajen Durai R. Key prognostic risk factors linked to poor functional outcomes in cerebral venous sinus thrombosis: a systematic review and meta-analysis. BMC Neurol. 2025;25(1):52. Published 2025 Feb 6. https://doi.org/10.1186/s12883-025-04059-x

36. A 12-year-old female suddenly develops transient episode of right face and hand weakness after a prolonged crying episode. Her MRI brain shows diffusion restriction in the left frontal lobe. Her MRA shows severe narrowing of the terminal left internal carotid artery. Which of the following conditions has been shown to be associated with this finding?
    A. African heritage
    B. Tuberous sclerosis
    C. Cranial irradiation
    D. Prader-Willi syndrome
    E. Parahyperthyroidism
    Correct answer: C

Explanation

This patient's presentation is most consistent with moyamoya syndrome, characterized by progressive stenosis of the terminal internal carotid arteries and their proximal branches, often with prominent basal collateral vessels. Moyamoya can be idiopathic or secondary to other conditions. Secondary causes include prior cranial irradiation, sickle cell disease, Down syndrome, neurofibromatosis type 1, and certain vasculitides. Cranial irradiation is a well-recognized risk factor because it causes progressive radiation-induced vasculopathy, which can manifest years after treatment for brain tumors, leukemia, or other malignancies.

References

Gonzalez, N. R., Derdeyn, C. P., McDougall, C. G., Smith, E. E., Sciacca, R. R., Albuquerque, F. C., … & American Heart Association/American Stroke Association Stroke Council; Council on Cardiovascular and Stroke Nursing; Council on Clinical Cardiology. (2023). Adult moyamoya disease and syndrome: Current perspectives and future directions: A scientific statement from the American Heart Association/American Stroke Association. Stroke, 54(e1–e14).

Smith J.L., Scott R.M. & Wakefield D. (2009). Understanding and treating moyamoya disease in children. J Neurosurg: Pediatrics, 4(6), 481–91.

37. A 10-year-old girl presents with recurrent episodes of right arm weakness and speech arrest lasting several minutes, consistent with transient ischemic attacks. MRI shows multiple small acute cortical infarcts in the left MCA distribution and some separate chronic appearing ischemic lesions. CTA reveals bilateral stenosis of the terminal internal carotid arteries and M1 MCA segments, with extensive basal collateral vessels. Direct surface angiography shows delayed filling of distal branches of the left MCA.

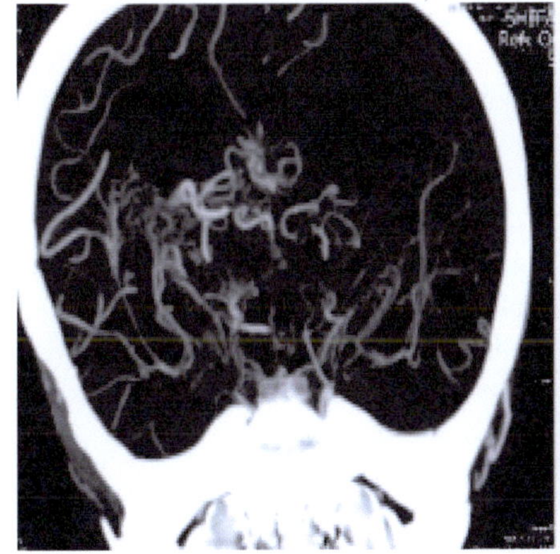
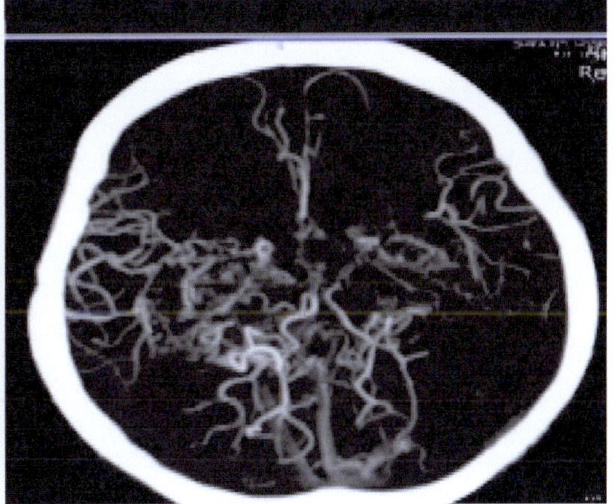

CT angiography of the head. (Source: Magsi, S et al. via Case Reports in Neurological Medicine. CC-BY 4.0 (https://creativecommons.org/licenses/by/4.0/). Image has not been modified. Please see full attribution with citation below in references section for this question.)

What is the most appropriate next step in management?

A. Begin dual antiplatelet therapy and monitor for recurrence

B. Initiate high-dose statin therapy and monitor perfusion

C. Recommend direct surgical revascularization (e.g., STA-MCA bypass)

D. Recommend indirect surgical bypass (Encephaloduroarteriosynangiosis or "EDAS")

E. Treat with therapeutic anticoagulation

Correct answer: D

Explanation

Given the multiple symptomatic episodes consistent with TIA, evidence of established infarcts on imaging and apparently advanced stenocclusive disease with poor left hemisphere perfusion, it is reasonable to plan for surgical treatment of the patient's Moya Moya disease. In pediatric patients, with symptomatic ischemia, evidence of infarcts, and hemodynamic compromise, indirect revascularization (like EDAS) is the treatment of choice. Children typically respond better to indirect methods due to having a robust angiogenic response.

References

Griessenauer C.J., et al. (2023). Surgical revascularizations for pediatric moyamoya: a systematic review and meta-analysis. Child's Nervous System, (2023) 39:353–364.

Magsi S, Khoja A, Rameez MA, Khan A, Ishaque N. Bilateral Moyamoya Disease in a 2-Year-Old Pakistani Male Treated with Bilateral Encephaloduroarteriosynangiosis: A Positive Outcome. Case Rep Neurol Med. 2016;2016:1467582. https://doi.org/10.1155/2016/1467582

Smith J.L., Scott R.M. & Wakefield D. (2009). Understanding and treating moyamoya disease in children. J Neurosurg: Pediatrics, 4(6), 481–91.

38. A 26-year-old male with a history of sickle cell anemia (confirmed homozygous mutations, hemoglobin typically 8–9 g/dL) presents to the hospital with moderate weakness of the left face arm and leg that began 1 day prior. Hemoglobin is 7 g/dL on admission lab testing. The patient is given intravenous fluids and blood transfusion for hemoglobin stabilization and exchange. Which of the following would be the most appropriate therapy to initiate for secondary stroke prevention moving forward.

A. Aspirin monotherapy

B. Colchicine

C. Aspirin and plavix

D. Hydroxyurea

E. Plasmapharesis

F. IVIG infusions

Correct answer: D

Explanation

In patients with SCD and prior ischemic stroke or TIA, hydroxyurea is a reasonable approach for reduction of hemoglobin S by increasing the production of fetal hemoglobin. This is in turn thought to lower the probability of forming intravascular clots or occlusions leading to stroke.

Reference

Yawn, B. P., Buchanan, G. R., Afenyi-Annan, A. N., Ballas, S. K., Hassell, K. L., James, A. H., … & American Society of Hematology (2019). 2019 American Society of Hematology (ASH) guideline for sickle cell disease: Vaso-occlusive pain and other complications. Blood Advances, 3(23), 3867–3897.

39. Which of the following has NOT been shown to reduce risk of ischemic stroke in patients with sickle cell disease?

A. Long-term anticoagulation

B. Routine transcranial doppler ultrasound screening

C. Red blood cell transfusion

D. Hydroxyurea

E. Hematopoietic stem-cell transplantation

Correct answer: A

Explanation

In patients with sickle cell disease, the primary mechanisms of ischemic stroke are related to chronic vasculopathy of large intracranial vessels and recurrent sickling-induced vascular injury, not cardioembolism or atrial fibrillation, so long-term anticoagulation has no established role in primary stroke prevention for this population.

Evidence-based strategies that do reduce stroke risk in sickle cell disease include:

- Routine transcranial Doppler (TCD) screening in children to identify elevated flow velocities indicating high stroke risk, allowing for early intervention.

- Chronic red blood cell transfusion therapy to maintain HbS levels below 30 percent, which reduces sickling and vascular injury.

- Hydroxyurea to increase fetal hemoglobin and reduce vaso-occlusive episodes; while less potent than transfusion for primary prevention in children, it does lower stroke risk.

- Hematopoietic stem-cell transplantation as a curative option in selected patients, which can eliminate sickling entirely and prevent future strokes.

Reference

Light J, Boucher M, Baskin-Miller J, Winstead M. Managing the Cerebrovascular Complications of Sickle Cell Disease: Current Perspectives. J Blood Med. 2023;14:279–293. Published 2023 Apr 14. https://doi.org/10.2147/JBM.S383472

40. A 42-year-old woman with a remote history of DVT who previously completed a course of anticoagulation and switched to aspirin monotherapy is admitted to the hospital with an acute cortical stroke in right MCA territory causing left arm weakness and slurred speech, with partial left-sided hemineglect. MRI brain shows an isolated acute infarct in the right hemisphere. Her CT angiogram demonstrates no evidence of atherosclerotic changes and no significant intracranial stenoses or occlusions. Her carotid arteries are widely patent without plaque. EKG and telemetry show normal sinus rhythm, and a transthoracic echocardiogram shows no significant cardiac abnormalities. Her INR is 1.0 and aPTT is 48. Screening tests for thrombophilia are sent, with Activated protein C and Factor V Leiden tests found to be normal. Anticardiolipin IgM is positive and DRVVT is elevated to 1.5.

As the patient prepares for discharge from the hospital, which of the following is the most correct interpretation of her test results and approach for management?

A. The patient's stroke mechanism is unclear, and she should be continued on aspirin monotherapy
B. Cardioembolism is possible, and outpatient cardiac monitoring for atrial fibrillation should be completed while the patient continues to take aspirin monotherapy
C. The patient's results confirm a diagnosis of antiphospholipid syndrome (APLS), and she should be continued on therapeutic anticoagulation lifelong with lovenox (low molecular weight heparin injections)
D. The patient's serology is suggestive of probable APLS, and she should be initiated on warfarin and planned for repeat serologic testing in 3 months.
E. The patient's serology is suggestive of probable APLS, and she should continue taking aspirin until repeat serologic testing is completed at 3 months.

Correct answer: D

Explanation

The patient's history of both venous AND arterial thrombosis events as well as a two positive serologies on initial screen raises significant concern that she has underlying antiphospholipid syndrome (APLS). Her elevated aPTT is also consistent with this. Technically, serologic criteria for diagnosis of APLS requires two positive serologic tests at least 12 weeks apart, which she does not formally meet at this time. However, given her apparent high risk, it would be prudent to treat her empirically for the most likely stroke mechanism, and warfarin has been shown to be the most effective treatment for APLS.

References

Adelhelm, J. B., Heim, A., Schmidt, H., & Lehman, L. (2023). A systematic review and meta-analysis of randomized trials: direct oral anticoagulants versus vitamin K antagonists in antiphospholipid syndrome. Lupus, 10(2), e001018.

Pengo V, Denas G, Zoppellaro G, et al. Rivaroxaban vs warfarin in high-risk patients with antiphospholipid syndrome. Blood. 2018;132(13):1365–1371. https://doi.org/10.1182/blood-2018-04-848333.

41. A 23-year-old woman with a history of sensorineural hearing loss and a history of frequent headaches presents to the emergency department 1 day after developing acute-onset confusion, right arm weakness, and expressive aphasia. MRI brain shows areas of cortical hyperintensity on diffusion-weighted imaging that do not conform to a vascular territory. Labs reveal elevated lactate levels. Her mother and maternal aunt have a history of similar episodes in early adulthood.

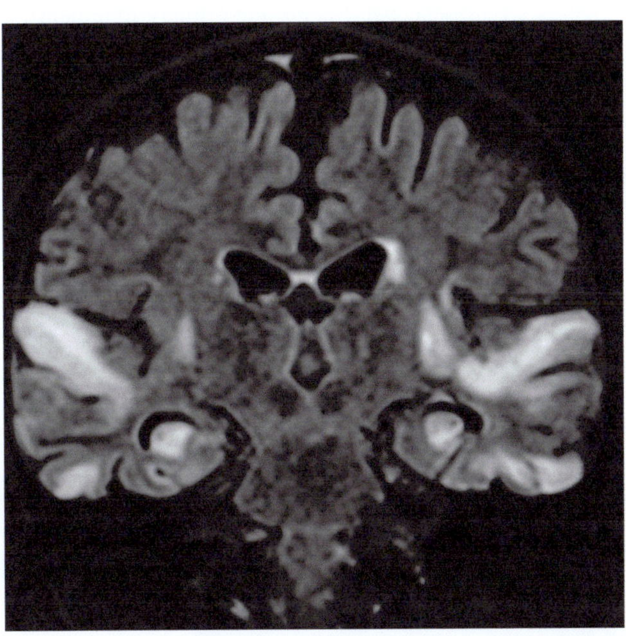

MRI brain, Coronal FLAIR. (Source: Pittet MP, Idan RB, Kern I, Guinand N, Van HC, Toso S, Fluss J via Journal of inherited metabolic disease (2016). CC-BY 4.0 (https://creativecommons.org/licenses/by/4.0/). Image has been cropped. See full reference in references section below)

Which of the following is the most appropriate acute treatment to consider in this patient?

A. High-dose intravenous corticosteroids
B. Thrombolytic therapy with intravenous alteplase
C. Intravenous L-arginine
D. Intravenous mannitol
E. Antiepileptic therapy with levetiracetam

Correct answer: C

Explanation

This patient presents with several of the classic features of mitochondrial encephalomyopathy with lactic acidosis and stroke-like episodes (MELAS) syndrome, a mitochondrial disorder often caused by a point mutation in the mitochondrial DNA (e.g., m.3243A>G mutation in the MT-TL1 gene). Clinical features include stroke-like episodes (typically not confined to vascular territories), lactic acidosis, hearing loss, and migraine-like headaches.

During acute stroke-like episodes, IV L-arginine is used as treatment because it is thought to improve cerebral perfusion through its role as a nitric oxide precursor, potentially mitigating the stroke-like process. Some protocols recommend a loading dose followed by maintenance infusion. A. Corticosteroids are not effective for mitochondrial stroke-like episodes and are not part of MELAS treatment. B. Thrombolysis is not appropriate here because the imaging findings do not follow a vascular distribution, and this is a metabolic stroke, not an ischemic infarct. D. Mannitol is used for elevated intracranial pressure but is not standard for MELAS attacks. E. Antiepileptic therapy may be needed if seizures are present, but it is not the primary treatment for stroke-like episodes in MELAS.

References

Pittet MP, Idan RB, Kern I, et al. Acute cortical deafness in a child with MELAS syndrome. J Inherit Metab Dis. 2016;39(3):465–466. https://doi.org/10.1007/s10545-016-9929-x

Zhao Y, Xu Z, Yan C, Ji K. Unraveling the Diagnostic Puzzle: Minor Stroke-like Lesions and Normal Muscle Histopathology in MELAS Syndrome. Stroke. 2024;55(4):e127–e130. https://doi.org/10.1161/STROKEAHA.123.045984

42. A 38-year-old man with history of migraines becomes gradually withdrawn and inattentive. His neurologic exam is notable for MOCA of 15. His lumbar puncture is unremarkable. His TSH, B12, RPR are within normal limits. Over the next 2 years, he becomes forgetful and is unable to work and care for his family. There is no family history of neurodegenerative disease, stroke, or autoimmune disease. An MRI brain is show below. Which of the following is NOT associated with this condition?

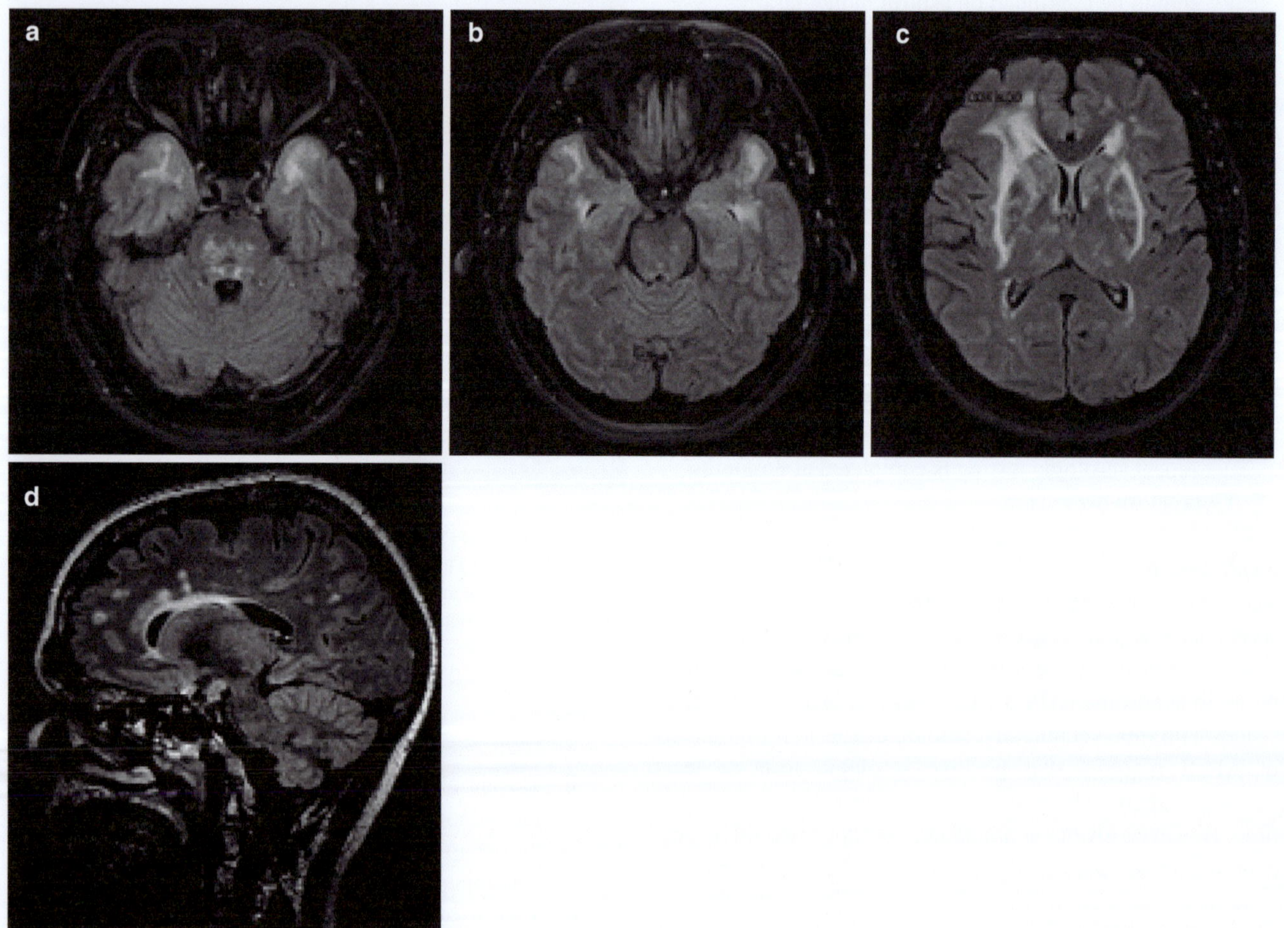

(**a–c**) Axial FLAIR MRI brain; (**d**) Sagittal FLAIR MRI brain. (Source: Di Donato et al. via BMC Med (2017). CC BY 4.0. (https://creativecommons.org/licenses/by/4.0/). Image has not been modified. Please see full attribution in references section below)

A. Alopecia
B. Dementia
C. Cervical stenosis
D. Peripheral neuropathy
E. Mood disor.ders
Correct answer: D

Explanation

This patient's presentation is most consistent with CADASIL, or Cerebral Autosomal-Dominant Arteriopathy with Subcortical Infarcts and Leukoencephalopathy, a hereditary small vessel disease caused by pathogenic variants in the NOTCH3 gene. The key clinical clues include onset in the late 30 s, a history of migraines with aura often being the earliest manifestation, progressive cognitive decline over a few years, and mood or behavioral changes. The workup is unrevealing for metabolic, infectious, or inflammatory causes, and MRI in CADASIL typically shows confluent T2 or FLAIR hyperintensities involving the anterior temporal lobes and external capsules, which is highly characteristic. The question asks for the feature not associated with this condition, and peripheral neuropathy is the correct choice because CADASIL pathology is confined to the cerebral small vessels and does not involve the peripheral nervous system. In contrast, dementia, mood disorders, and even premature alopecia have been reported as part of the disease spectrum, and areas of spinal stenosis have also been reported in CADASIL patients. The absence of peripheral nervous system involvement helps distinguish CADASIL from other hereditary vasculopathies or leukodystrophies that can present with both central and peripheral features.

References

Chabriat H, Joutel A, Dichgans M, Tournier-Lasserve E, Bousser MG. Cadasil. Lancet Neurol. 2009;8(7):643–653. https://doi.org/10.1016/S1474-4422(09)70127-9

Cramer J, Lui F, White ML. Cerebral Autosomal Dominant Arteriopathy. [Updated 2024 Mar 21]. In: StatPearls [Internet]. Treasure Island (FL): StatPearls Publishing; 2025 Jan-. Available from: https://www.ncbi.nlm.nih.gov/books/NBK470293/

Di Donato, I., Bianchi, S., De Stefano, N. et al. Cerebral Autosomal Dominant Arteriopathy with Subcortical Infarcts and Leukoencephalopathy (CADASIL) as a model of small vessel disease: update on clinical, diagnostic, and management aspects. BMC Med 15, 41 (2017). https://doi.org/10.1186/s12916-017-0778-8

Hack RJ, Rutten J, Lesnik Oberstein SAJ. CADASIL. 2000 Mar 15 [Updated 2019 Mar 14]. In: Adam MP, Feldman J, Mirzaa GM, et al., editors. GeneReviews® [Internet]. Seattle (WA): University of Washington, Seattle; 1993–2025. Available from: https://www.ncbi.nlm.nih.gov/books/NBK1500/

43. Which of the following medications is used for secondary stroke prevention in patients with atrial fibrillation and directly inhibits factor Xa?
    A. Apixaban
    B. Dabigatran
    C. Clopidogrel
    D. Warfarin
    E. Acetylsalicylic acid (aspirin)
    Correct answer: A

Explanation

Several anticoagulant medications are approved for secondary stroke prevention in patients with nonvalvular atrial fibrillation, each with distinct mechanisms of action. Apixaban and rivaroxaban are direct factor Xa inhibitors. Warfarin works by inhibiting the synthesis of vitamin K–dependent clotting factors II, VII, IX, and X, as well as the anticoagulant proteins C and S. Dabigatran is a direct thrombin (factor IIa) inhibitor. Clopidogrel and aspirin (acetylsalicylic acid) are antiplatelet agents, not anticoagulants, and are generally not recommended alone for stroke prevention in atrial fibrillation.

44. A 68-year-old right-handed man presents with sudden onset of global aphasia and dense right hemiplegia. He has a history of nonvalvular atrial fibrillation treated with dabigatran. His daughter, who witnessed symptom onset 15 min prior to arrival, is unsure whether he took his morning dose or the prior evening dose. Which of the following laboratory studies best evaluates the anticoagulant activity of dabigatran in this scenario?
    A. Anti-Xa activity
    B. aPTT
    C. Dilute Russell viper venom time (dRVVT)
    D. PT
    E. Thrombin time
    Correct answer: E

Explanation

Dabigatran is a direct thrombin (factor IIa) inhibitor used to reduce the risk of thromboembolic events in patients with atrial fibrillation. Both aPPT (activated partial thromboplastin time) and PT (prothrombin time) can be affected by dabigatran, but these changes are variable and not reliably correlated with plasma concentrations, especially outside peak levels. Thrombin time (TT) is the most sensitive readily available test to assess dabigatran activity. A normal TT suggests little to no anticoagulant effect. According to the American Heart Association, thrombolytics may be administered in patients on dabigatran if the last dose was taken more than 48 h prior or, if the timing is unknown, a normal thrombin time can be used to guide treatment decisions. Anti-Xa activity is used to monitor factor Xa inhibitors (e.g., apixaban, rivaroxaban), not dabigatran. dRVVT is primarily used for diagnosing lupus anticoagulant.

Reference

Powers WJ, et al. 2023 AHA/ASA Guideline for the Early Management of Patients With Acute Ischemic Stroke: A Guideline From the American Heart Association/American Stroke Association. Stroke. 2023;54:e199–e300. https://doi.org/10.1161/STR.0000000000000434

45. A 79-year-old man with atrial fibrillation, a mechanical aortic valve, and a prior embolic stroke is on warfarin. His INR is 2.6, and he is scheduled to undergo a tooth extraction next week. What is the most appropriate recommendation for peri-procedural anticoagulation management?
    A. Substitute warfarin with low-molecular-weight heparin and stop 12 h prior
    B. Reduce warfarin dose by half until after the procedure
    C. Hold warfarin now and restart after extraction
    D. Continue warfarin at the current dose
    E. Temporarily switch to aspirin and resume warfarin post-procedure
    Correct answer: D

Explanation

Minor dental procedures such as single-tooth extraction have a low bleeding risk. If the INR is within therapeutic range, anticoagulation is not typically interrupted, especially given the high thromboembolic risk. Local hemostatic techniques (e.g., gauze pressure, topical agents) are preferred to changing systemic anticoagulation.

46. Which of the following agents specifically reverses the anticoagulant effects of dabigatran?
    A. Idarucizumab
    B. Protamine sulfate
    C. Recombinant factor VIIa
    D. Vitamin K
    E. Tranexamic acid
    Correct answer: A

Explanation

Idarucizumab is a monoclonal antibody fragment that binds dabigatran with high affinity and rapidly neutralizes its anticoagulant effect. It is the reversal agent of choice for dabigatran in cases of bleeding or emergency surgery. Andexanet reverses factor Xa inhibitors, while protamine sulfate reverses heparin. Tranexamic acid is an antifibrinolytic but not a specific antidote.

47. A 65-year-old woman with hypertension and type 2 diabetes mellitus presents 1 h after acute onset of left hemiplegia and visuospatial neglect. CT shows a hyperdense right MCA sign but is otherwise unremarkable. She receives IV Tenecteplase (TNK) in the emergency department. When is it safe to initiate subcutaneous DVT prophylaxis?
    A. Immediately
    B. 24 h post-TNK
    C. 48 h post-TNK
    D. 72 h post-TNK
    E. 1 week post-TNK
    Correct answer: B

Explanation

Patients with acute ischemic stroke who receive IV TNK should not receive anticoagulants (even for DVT prophylaxis) within the first 24 h due to bleeding risk. After 24 h, if follow-up neuroimaging shows no hemorrhage, subcutaneous heparin or enoxaparin should be started for DVT prophylaxis.

48. A 75-year-old man with a history of atrial fibrillation and chronic kidney disease (eGFR 25 mL/min/1.73 m^2) presents with an acute ischemic stroke. He is not currently on anticoagulation. Which of the following is the most appropriate oral anticoagulant for secondary stroke prevention in this patient?
    A. Dabigatran
    B. Rivaroxaban
    C. Apixaban
    D. Edoxaban
    E. Warfarin
    Correct answer: C

Explanation

In patients with nonvalvular atrial fibrillation and moderate to severe chronic kidney disease (CKD), anticoagulant selection requires careful consideration of both efficacy and bleeding risk. Apixaban is the direct oral anticoagulant (DOAC) with the most favorable safety and efficacy profile in CKD and is approved for use down to an eGFR of 15 mL/min. In contrast, dabigatran, which is primarily renally excreted, is not recommended in patients with advanced renal dysfunction due to accumulation and increased bleeding risk. Rivaroxaban and edoxaban are also renally cleared and should be used cautiously or avoided depending on the degree of renal impairment. Although warfarin remains an option across all stages of renal function and is often used in end-stage kidney disease, it requires regular INR monitoring and carries a higher risk of vascular calcification and hemorrhage in advanced CKD.

A 2019 meta-analysis of 45 trials demonstrated that, in patients with mild to moderate CKD, DOACs were associated with a lower risk of stroke compared to warfarin (RR 0.79; 95% CI 0.66–0.93) without a significant increase in major bleeding (RR 0.80; 95% CI 0.61–1.04). Notably, patients with end-stage kidney disease (eGFR <15 mL/min) were largely excluded from these trials, so data in that population remain limited.

Reference

Ha JT, Neuen BL, Cheng LP, et al. Benefits and harms of oral anticoagulant therapy in chronic kidney disease: a systematic review and meta-analysis. Ann Intern Med. 2019;171(3):181–189. https://doi.org/10.7326/M19-0832

49. A 75-year-man presents with aphasia and is found to have a left frontal stroke. Workup reveals 80% stenosis of the left internal carotid artery with ulcerated plaque. His echocardiogram is normal. He undergoes revascularization with a carotid stent. He is started on aspirin, ticagrelor, rosuvastatin, and amlodipine. He returns to the office a week later complaining of shortness of breath. Which of the following is the most likely reason for his symptoms?

A. Aspirin
B. Ticagrelor
C. Rosuvastatin
D. Amlodipine
E. Carotid stent

Correct answer: B

Explanation

Ticagrelor, a reversible P2Y12 receptor antagonist, is well known to cause dyspnea in up to 20 percent of patients. The mechanism is not due to bronchospasm but is believed to involve increased extracellular adenosine levels (by inhibition of adenosine uptake via equilibrative nucleoside transporter 1), stimulating vagal C-fibers in the lungs. This symptom typically occurs within the first week of therapy and is unrelated to cardiac or pulmonary disease. Aspirin does not cause isolated dyspnea in otherwise stable patients without allergic reaction or bronchospasm.

Linked questions: 50–51

50. A 54-year-old man with history of hypertension and active tobacco use presented with severe onset headache, double vision, and lethargy. Head CT obtained with the below findings.

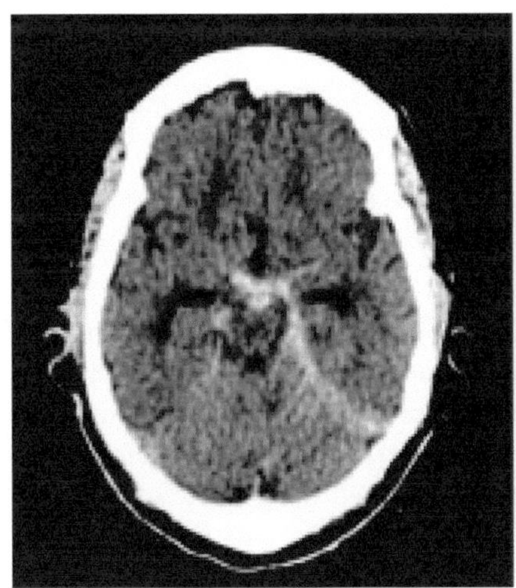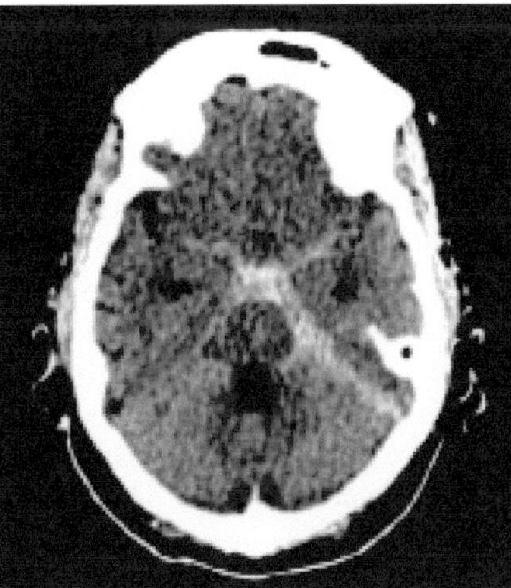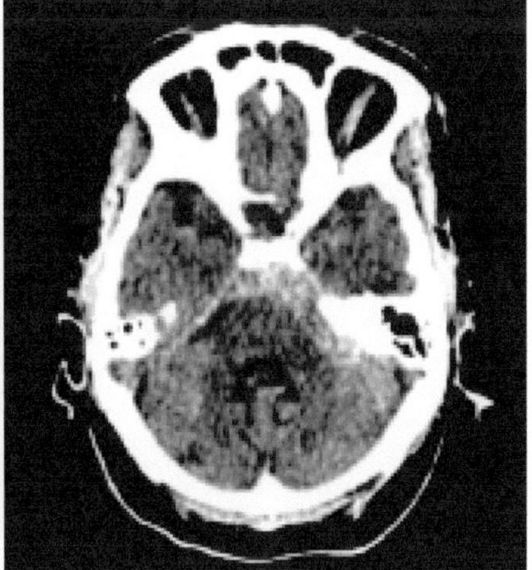

Axial CT scans of brain. (Source. Marupudi NI, Mittal S via Journal of clinical medicine. (2015). CC-BY 4.0 (https://creativecommons.org/licenses/by/4.0/). Image has not been modified. Please see full attribution in the references section below)

Which of the following is an incorrect statement?

A. Vasospasm will most likely occur starting 2 weeks after the bleed
B. The most likely etiology is a ruptured aneurysm
C. Hydrocephalus is a possible complication
D. Oral nimodipine use is associated with improved functional outcome
E. Induced hypertension is sometimes used as a management option later on in the clinical course

Correct answer: A

Explanation

Vasospasm after aneurysmal subarachnoid hemorrhage typically occurs between 4 and 14 days post-hemorrhage and peaks between days 5 and 7 post-hemorrhage. It involves narrowing of cerebral blood vessels and can caused delayed cerebral ischemia (DCI) and ischemic stroke if not reversed. Treatment involves oral nimodipine (a calcium channel blocker), maintaining euvolemia, induced hypertension, and at times endovascular therapy (balloon angioplasty and intra-arterial vasodilators).

References

Hoh BL, Ko NU, Amin-Hanjani S, et al. 2023 Guideline for the Management of Patients With Aneurysmal Subarachnoid Hemorrhage: A Guideline From the American Heart Association/American Stroke Association. Stroke. 2023;54(7):e314-e370. https://doi.org/10.1161/STR.0000000000000436

Marupudi NI, Mittal S. Diagnosis and Management of Hyponatremia in Patients with Aneurysmal Subarachnoid Hemorrhage. J Clin Med. 2015;4(4):756–767. https://doi.org/10.3390/jcm4040756

Linked question

51. He is admitted to the neurologic intensive care unit for further management. He was found to have a ruptured aneurysm of the right middle cerebral artery, and it was embolized. On day 5 of hospitalization, his nurse noticed that he has new onset left-sided weakness. Which of the following is the most appropriate next step in management?

A. Obtain an electroencephalogram
B. Obtain a CT angiogram and perfusion study
C. Give lorazepam for presumed seizure
D. Decrease his blood pressure with antihypertensives due to concern for re-rupture of the aneurysm

Correct answer: B

Explanation

Acute onset focal neurologic deficit in the days following subarachnoid hemorrhage secondary to a ruptured aneurysm should raise suspicion for cerebral vasospasm and prompt an emergent CT angiogram (CTA) and CT perfusion (CTP). CTA has high sensitivity (91%) for detecting vasospasm when symptoms develop, and CTP allows early prediction of perfusion abnormalities. Early detection and intervention are essential for optimal patient outcomes as vasospasm is a major cause of morbidity and mortality after aneurysmal SAH.

Reference

Hoh BL, Ko NU, Amin-Hanjani S, et al. 2023 Guideline for the Management of Patients With Aneurysmal Subarachnoid Hemorrhage: A Guideline From the American Heart Association/American Stroke Association. Stroke. 2023;54(7):e314–e370. https://doi.org/10.1161/STR.0000000000000436

52. A 65-year-old female is admitted to the neuro-ICU after coil embolization of a ruptured anterior communicating artery aneurysm. Her exam is stable. According to current guidelines, which of the following is correct regarding the use of nimodipine?

A. It is only indicated in patients with known symptomatic cerebral vasospasm
B. It can be routinely substituted for other calcium channel blockers (nicardipine, verapamil)
C. It should be combined with hypervolemia and hemodilution (triple H therapy)
D. It reduces the incidence of delayed cerebral ischemia and improves neurologic outcomes

Correct answer: D

Explanation

Nimodipine is a dihydropyridine calcium channel blocker and recommended for all patients with aneurysmal subarachnoid hemorrhage unless contraindicated, not just those with symptomatic cerebral vasospasm. It is administered orally for 21 days (IV use is not recommended due to hypotension and lack of benefit) and is the only calcium channel blocker with proven benefit in patients with aneurysmal SAH. It does not reliably prevent angiographic vasospasm, but is associated with reduced incidence of delayed cerebral ischemia (DCI) and improves long-term neurologic functional outcomes. Triple H therapy is no longer recommended, rather treatment focuses on maintaining euvolemia.

References

Hoh BL, Ko NU, Amin-Hanjani S, et al. 2023 Guideline for the Management of Patients With Aneurysmal Subarachnoid Hemorrhage: A Guideline From the American Heart Association/American Stroke Association. Stroke. 2023;54(7):e314-e370. https://doi.org/10.1161/STR.0000000000000436

Pickard JD, Murray GD, Illingworth R, et al. Effect of oral nimodipine on cerebral infarction and outcome after subarachnoid haemorrhage: British Aneurysm Nimodipine Trial. BMJ. 1989;298(6674):636–642. https://doi.org/10.1136/bmj.298.6674.636

53. A 54-year-old man is admitted to the neuro-ICU after aneurysmal SAH s/p coil embolization. On day 6, he develops lethargy and hypotension. Labs are notable for serum sodium 123, urine sodium >60 mEq/L (normal <20 mEq/L), and urine osmolality 340 mOsm/kg. (normal 50–1200 mOsm/kg) Which of the following is the most likely etiology?
    A. Central diabetes insipidus (DI)
    B. Syndrome of inappropriate antidiuretic hormone secretion (SIADH)
    C. Cerebral salt wasting (CSW)
    D. Osmotic diuresis
    Correct answer: C

Explanation

Cerebral salt wasting is a relatively common complication after aneurysmal SAH and is characterized by hyponatremia with high urine sodium/osmolality and hypovolemia. Treatment is with sodium and volume replacement, and delays in diagnosis and treatment can increase the risk of delayed cerebral ischemia. SIADH has similar lab findings but is characterized by euvolemia or hypervolemia and is treated with fluid restriction. Central DI is characterized by hypernatremia and polyuria with dilute urine and osmotic diuresis and is associated with high urine output in the setting of mannitol use or hyperglycemia.

Reference

Sherlock M, O'Sullivan E, Agha A, et al. The incidence and pathophysiology of hyponatremia after subarachnoid hemorrhage. Clin Endocrinol (Oxf). 2006;64(3):250–254. https://doi.org/10.1111/j.1365-2265.2006.02432.x

54. A 37-year-old woman with no significant past medical history presents with acute onset thunderclap headache. Noncontrast head CT is unremarkable. CTA of the head and neck is shown below. What is the most likely diagnosis?

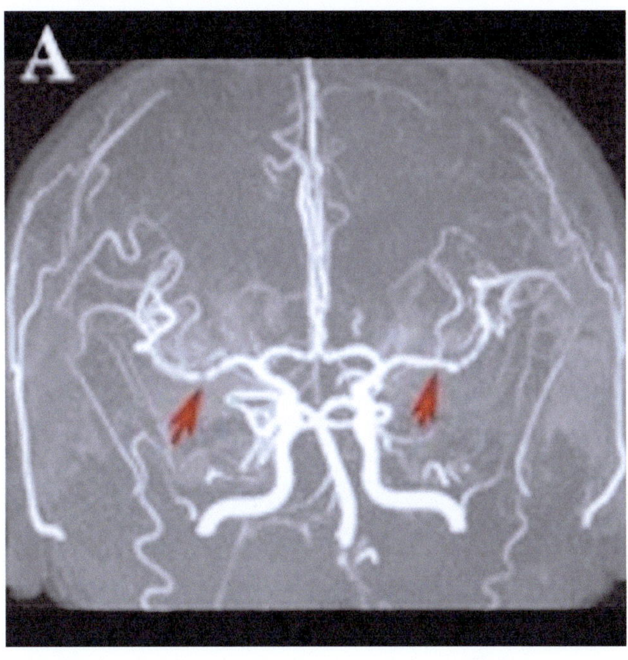

MR angiogram of cerebral vasculature. (Source: Liang H, Xu Z, Zheng Z, Lou H, Yue W via Orphanet Journal of Rare Diseases (2015). CC-BY 4.0 (https://creativecommons.org/licenses/by/4.0/). Image has been cropped to include only panel A. Please see full citation in references section below)

    A. Intracranial atherosclerotic disease
    B. Moyamoya disease
    C. Reversible cerebral vasoconstriction syndrome (RCVS)
    D. Migraine with aura
    E. Primary CNS vasculitis
    Correct answer: C

Explanation

Reversible cerebral vasoconstriction syndrome is characterized clinically by acute onset recurrent thunderclap headache and can cause ischemic stroke or intracranial hemorrhage (cortical SAH, ICH). Radiographically it is characterized by segmental vasoconstriction of cerebral arteries. It is monophasic and typically resolves within 12 weeks. Common triggers include SSRIs, cannabis, sympathomimetics, postpartum statin, exertion/sexual activity. The other listed conditions are not characterized by acute onset thunderclap headache.

References

Liang H, Xu Z, Zheng Z, Lou H, Yue W. Reversible cerebral vasoconstriction syndrome following red blood cells transfusion: a case series of 7 patients. Orphanet J Rare Dis. 2015;10:47. Published 2015 Apr 22. https://doi.org/10.1186/s13023-015-0268-z

Miller TR, Shivashankar R, Mossa-Basha M, Gandhi D. Reversible Cerebral Vasoconstriction Syndrome, Part 1. AJNR Am J Neuroradiol. 2015;36(8):1392–1399. https://doi.org/10.3174/ajnr.A4214

55. A 23-year-old female presents with acute onset thunderclap headache and is found to have convexity subarachnoid hemorrhage on CT head. CTA head shows multifocal narrowing of distal middle cerebral and anterior cerebral arteries. Which of the following is most appropriate management?
    A. Aspirin
    B. Calcium channel blockers (nimodipine, verapamil) and supportive care
    C. Endovascular angioplasty and stenting of the affected vessels
    D. High-dose glucocorticoids
    E. Anticoagulation
    Correct answer: B

Explanation

The clinical presentation and imaging are classic for reversible cerebral vasoconstriction syndrome (RCVS). Calcium channel blockers such as nimodipine and verapamil are first-line empiric therapy in RCVS in addition to supportive care and avoidance of triggers. Steroids can worsen clinical outcomes in RCVS and should be avoided.

Reference

Natbony, L. R., & Ray, C. N. (2024). Headache Horizons: Reversible cerebral vasoconstriction syndrome: Presentation, diagnosis, and treatment of a complex neurovascular disorder. Practical Neurology.

56. A 43-year-old man presents with sudden onset thunderclap headache after exercising. CT head is obtained and normal. CTA shows multifocal narrowing of medium and distal intracranial arteries in both the anterior and posterior circulation. LP is also obtained and shows normal cell counts and protein. He is admitted and upon reassessment exam is notable for left hemiparesis. MRI is obtained and shows multifocal acute cortical infarcts. Which statement is most accurate?
    A. The patient should be started on anticoagulation for secondary stroke prevention
    B. The headache is most likely migrainous and a triptan should be initiated
    C. The patient most likely has primary CNS vasculitis and steroids should be initiated

D. The patient most likely has RCVS and should be started on a calcium channel blocker
E. The patient should be started on dual antiplatelet therapy for secondary stroke prevention
Correct answer: D

Explanation

Reversible cerebral vasoconstriction syndrome (RCVS) is characterized by recurrent thunderclap headache and multifocal, reversible arterial narrowing on CTA or DSA. Whereas CSF in primary CNS vasculitis is abnormal (elevated protein, pleocytosis), CSF in RCVS is normal. Accurate diagnosis is key as steroids, and triptans can both worsen RCVS and are contraindicated.

References

Burton, T. M., & Bushnell, C. D. (2019). Reversible cerebral vasoconstriction syndrome. Stroke, 50(8), 2253–2258.

Kraayvanger, L., Sluzewski, M., & Holl, J. (2018). Cerebrospinal fluid findings in reversible cerebral vasoconstriction syndrome. Journal of the Neurological Sciences, 387, 59–62.

57. A 38-year-old female presents with sudden onset severe thunderclap headache. She is 2 weeks postpartum with no headache history. CT head is normal. CTA head shows multifocal narrowing of the distal cerebral arteries. Which of the following is NOT a known trigger for her condition?
    A. Triptans
    B. Postpartum state
    C. Chronic NSAID use
    D. Cannabis
    E. Selective serotonin reuptake inhibitors (SSRIs)
    Correct answer: C

Explanation

Common RCVS triggers include postpartum state, vasoactive drugs (including triptans, SSRIs/SNRIs, nasal decongestants, cocaine, amphetamines, ergot derivatives), physical exertion, sexual activity, and catecholamine-secreting tumors.

Reference

Ducros A. Reversible cerebral vasoconstriction syndrome. Lancet Neurol. 2012;11(10):906–917. https://doi.org/10.1016/S1474-4422(12)70135-7

58. A 35-year-old male with recent kidney transplant on tacrolimus presents with confusion after a generalized tonic-clonic seizure. His blood pressure is 220/110. MRI is obtained with the below findings. Which of the following is the most likely diagnosis?

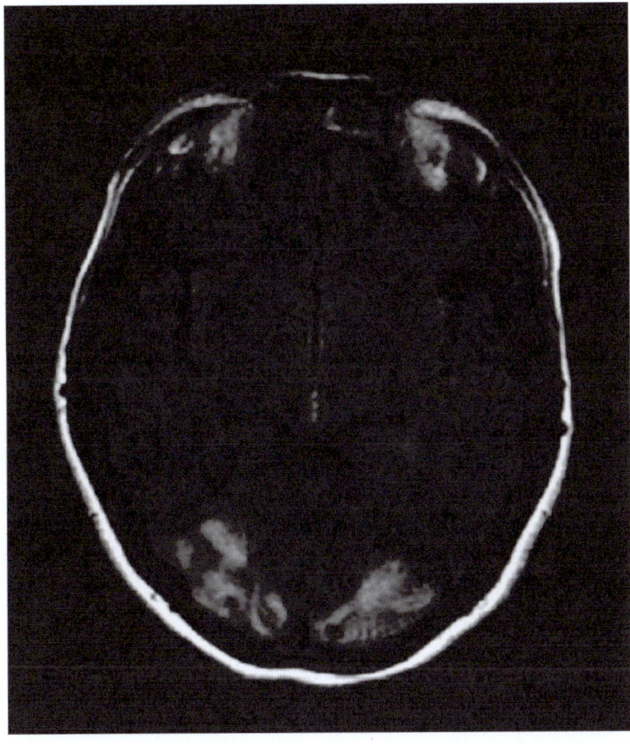

Axial FLAIR MRI Brain. (Source: Ural UM, Balik G, Sentürk S, Ustüner I, Cobanoğlu U, Sahin FK via Case Reports in Obstetrics and Gynecology (2014). CC-BY 3.0 (https://creativecommons.org/licenses/by/3.0/). Image has not been modified. Please see full citation in references section below)

A. Meningoencephalitis
B. Acute ischemic stroke
C. Posterior reversible encephalopathy syndrome (PRES)
D. Primary CNS vasculitis
E. MRI changes secondary to seizure

Correct answer: C

Explanation

Posterior reversible encephalopathy syndrome often presents with a clinical triad of encephalopathy, seizures, and visual disturbances and is characterized by vasogenic edema (T2/FLAIR hyperintensity without diffusion restriction) in the parieto-occipital regions. Common triggers including hypertensive crisis, eclampsia/pre-eclampsia, cytotoxic drugs (tacrolimus, cyclosporine, chemotherapeutic agents), renal failure, and autoimmune disease.

References

Ural UM, Balik G, Sentürk S, Ustüner I, Cobanoğlu U, Sahin FK. Posterior Reversible Encephalopathy Syndrome in a Postpartum Preeclamptic Woman without Seizure. Case Rep Obstet Gynecol. 2014;2014:657903. https://doi.org/10.1155/2014/657903

Zelaya JE, Al-Khoury L. Posterior Reversible Encephalopathy Syndrome. [Updated 2024 Oct 11]. In: StatPearls [Internet]. Treasure Island (FL): StatPearls Publishing; 2025 Jan-. Available from: https://www.ncbi.nlm.nih.gov/books/NBK554492/

59. A 46-year-old female with history of lupus nephritis on cyclophosphamide presents with headache and blurry vision. Blood pressure is 180/110. MRI brain shows bilateral parieto-occipital FLAIR hyperintensities as well as areas of frontal and basal ganglia FLAIR hyperintensity. LP is obtained and shows mild protein elevation with normal cell count. Which of the following is the most likely diagnosis?
A. Primary CNS vasculitis
B. HSV encephalitis
C. Lupus cerebritis
D. Acute disseminated encephalomyelitis (ADEM)
E. PRES associated with lupus and immunosuppression

Correct answer: E

Explanation

The clinical history, imaging findings, and CSF analysis are most suggestive of PRES related to lupus and cyclophosphamide use which are both known risk factors. While PRES classically involves the parieto-occipital lobes, it can extend to the frontal lobes, basal ganglia, and cerebellum (atypical PRES). CNS vasculitis is associated with abnormal CSF (pleocytosis, elevated protein) and ischemic infarcts. HSV encephalitis and lupus cerebritis are both associated with abnormal CSF findings. ADEM is classically characterized by asymmetric multifocal white matter lesions and is associated with mild lymphocytic pleocytosis and mildly elevated CSF protein.

References

Fischer M, Schmutzhard E. Posterior reversible encephalopathy syndrome. J Neurol. 2017;264(8):1608-1616. https://doi.org/10.1007/s00415-016-8377-8

Zelaya JE, Al-Khoury L. Posterior Reversible Encephalopathy Syndrome. [Updated 2024 Oct 11]. In: StatPearls [Internet]. Treasure Island (FL): StatPearls Publishing; 2025 Jan-. Available from: https://www.ncbi.nlm.nih.gov/books/NBK554492/

60. A 36-year-old woman with systemic lupus erythematosus presents with acute onset confusion, headache, and generalized seizure. Blood pressure is 200/120 mmHg. A rapid MRI is obtained which shows FLAIR hyperintensities in the parieto-occipital regions. Which of the following is the best next management step?
    A. Start oral nimodipine
    B. Administer IV TNK
    C. Start high dose glucocorticoids
    D. Administer IV labetalol to lower blood pressure
    E. Start empiric broad spectrum antibiotics
    Correct answer: D

Explanation

Acute management of PRES involves timely blood pressure control, withdrawal of the offending agent (ex tacrolimus, cyclosporine, chemotherapy, etc.) and seizure control. IV antihypertensives (labetalol, nicardipine) are preferred with the goal of reducing mean arterial blood pressure by approximately 25% in the first few hours in patients with hypertensive emergency.

Reference

Fischer M, Schmutzhard E. Posterior reversible encephalopathy syndrome. J Neurol. 2017;264(8):1608–1616. https://doi.org/10.1007/s00415-016-8377-8

61. A 62-year-old man with no significant past medical history presents with headache and acute onset confusion. CT head shows a right frontal intraparenchymal hemorrhage. Subsequent MRI shows a hemorrhagic right frontal ring-enhancing lesion. Which of the following primary brain tumors is most likely?
    A. Atypical meningioma
    B. Oligodendroglioma
    C. Glioblastoma multiforme
    D. Pilocytic astrocytoma
    Correct answer: C

Explanation

Glioblastoma multiforme are the most common primary hemorrhagic brain tumors. Meningiomas are extra-axial tumors that rarely bleed. Oligodendrogliomas can be calcified but are rarely associated with hemorrhage. Pilocytic astrocytomas are cystic but rarely hemorrhagic.

Reference

Ostrowski RP, He Z, Pucko EB, Matyja E. Hemorrhage in brain tumor – an unresolved issue. Brain Hemorrhages. 2022;3(2):98–102. https://doi.org/10.1016/j.hest.2022.01.005

62. A 45-year-old female with metastatic melanoma presents with acute onset headache and focal seizure. CT head shows a left frontal intraparenchymal hemorrhage. Which of the following is the most likely underlying mechanism of her intratumoral hemorrhage?
    A. Coagulopathy
    B. Lipohyalinosis of small surrounding cerebral blood vessels
    C. Invasion of dural venous sinuses
    D. Neovascularization with abnormal thin-walled vessels
    E. Increased intracranial pressure
    Correct answer: D

Explanation

Metastatic hemorrhagic brain tumors promote abnormal angiogenesis leading to formation of new, thin-walled vessels that lack adequate blood–brain barrier due to poor pericyte support and are prone to rupture and hemorrhage. Cancers that are associated with hemorrhagic metastases include melanoma, renal cell carcinoma (RCC), choriocarcinoma, thyroid carcinoma, and lung adenocarcinoma.

References

Kondziolka D, Bernstein M, Resch L, et al. Significance of hemorrhage into brain tumors: clinicopathological study. J Neurosurg. 1987;67(6):852–857. https://doi.org/10.3171/jns.1987.67.6.0852

Louis DN, Perry A, Wesseling P, et al. The 2021 WHO Classification of Tumors of the Central Nervous System: a summary. Neuro Oncol. 2021;23(8):1231–1251. https://doi.org/10.1093/neuonc/noab106

63. A 60-year-old male with atrial fibrillation on apixaban presents with acute onset aphasia and right hemiparesis. CT scan shows a left MCA hemorrhage with surrounding edema. MRI brain shows restricted diffusion in the left MCA territory extending beyond the area of hemorrhage. Which of the following is the most likely diagnosis?
    A. Brain tumor
    B. Hypertensive hemorrhage
    C. Cerebral amyloid angiopathy
    D. Hemorrhagic transformation of an ischemic infarct
    E. Arteriovenous malformation
    Correct answer: D

Explanation

Hemorrhage location and MRI features are helpful in distinguishing underlying etiology. Hemorrhages that are confined to an arterial vascular territory with restricted diffusion that often extends beyond the area of GRE/SWI should raise suspicion for hemorrhagic transformation of an ischemic infarct. Primary ICH (hypertensive, CAA) often have small areas of adjacent ischemia, however, there is no restricted diffusion within the hematoma itself.

Reference

Siddiqui FM, Bekker SV, Qureshi AI. Neuroimaging of hemorrhage and vascular defects. Neurotherapeutics. 2011;8(1):28–38. https://doi.org/10.1007/s13311-010-0009-x

64. A 54-year-old male with no significant past medical history presents with acute onset dizziness and mild gait instability. CT head shows a small left cerebellar hemorrhage. Subsequent MRI shows a rounded, well circumscribed lesion on GRE with a T2 hypointense rim. Which of the following is the most likely diagnosis?
    A. Hypertensive hemorrhage
    B. Cerebral amyloid angiopathy
    C. Cavernous malformation
    D. Arteriovenous malformation
    E. Hemorrhagic transformation of an ischemic infarct
    Correct answer: C

Explanation

Cerebral cavernous malformations (cavernomas) are vascular malformations made up of clusters of thin-walled capillaries without intervening brain parenchyma. They classically appear as "popcorn" lesions on MRI (due to mixed T1/2 signal of different ages of blood) with a hemosiderin rim.

65. A 66-year-old woman is admitted to the neuro-ICU after coil embolization of a ruptured anterior choroidal artery aneurysm. On hospital day 7, she develops acute onset right arm weakness and expressive aphasia. CT head is unchanged from prior. CTA shows diffuse narrowing of the left MCA concerning for vasospasm. Which is the most appropriate initial management step?
    A. Start high dose glucocorticoid
    B. Induce hypertension with intravenous vasopressors
    C. Endovascular angioplasty of the left MCA
    D. Triple H therapy (hypervolemia, hypertension, hemodilution)
    E. Intra-arterial injection of calcium channel blocker
    Correct answer: B

Explanation

First-line treatment for symptomatic vasospasm after aneurysmal subarachnoid hemorrhage is induced hypertension with vasopressors to help augment cerebral perfusion to ischemic territory. If symptoms persist despite induced hypertension, rescue therapy includes endovascular treatment with angioplasty and intra-arterial injection of calcium channel blockers. Triple H therapy is no longer recommended.

Reference

Hoh BL, Ko NU, Amin-Hanjani S, et al. 2023 Guideline for the Management of Patients With Aneurysmal Subarachnoid Hemorrhage: A Guideline From the American Heart Association/American Stroke Association. Stroke. 2023;54(7):e314–e370. https://doi.org/10.1161/STR.0000000000000436

66. A 34-year-old man with a history of intravenous heroin use presents with 2 days of fever, headache, and new left-sided weakness. Examination reveals temperature 39.2 °C, disorientation to time and place, a grade 3/6 holosystolic murmur at the apex, and mild photophobia. Neurologic exam shows left hemiparesis, left visual field cut, and left facial weakness. Fundoscopy reveals multiple retinal hemorrhages with pale centers. Brain MRI shows multiple small, restricted diffusion lesions in the right frontal, parietal, and occipital lobes, as well as punctate hemorrhages in the cerebellum and bilateral cortical sulci on GRE sequences. Blood cultures are pending. Which of the following findings would most strongly support the diagnosis of septic emboli due to infective endocarditis?
    A. Transesophageal echocardiogram revealing mitral valve vegetation
    B. Positive anti-neutrophil cytoplasmic antibody (ANCA) serologies
    C. Lumbar puncture showing neutrophilic pleocytosis and low glucose
    D. Vessel wall enhancement on brain MRA suggestive of vasculitis
    E. MRI showing confluent white matter hyperintensities in the periventricular and temporal lobes
    Correct answer: A

Explanation

This patient's fever, neurologic deficits, new murmur, IV drug use, and multiple infarcts in different vascular territories with associated hemorrhagic lesions strongly suggest septic embolic strokes from infective endocarditis (IE). Retinal hemorrhages with pale centers (Roth spots) further support a systemic embolic process. Among the diagnostic tests listed, transesophageal echocardiogram (TEE) is the most definitive for confirming IE, especially in patients with suspected left-sided involvement (e.g., mitral valve). TEE is more sensitive than transthoracic echo, particularly in detecting small vegetations or abscesses.

67. A 66-year-old man presents to the emergency department 6 h after the onset of mild right facial droop and clumsiness of his right hand. His symptoms have improved but are still present. Neurologic examination shows subtle right pronator drift and mild dysarthria. NIH Stroke Scale score is 2. CT head is unremarkable, and CT angiography reveals no large vessel occlusion. MRI confirms a small acute infarct in the left frontal lobe. He has no history of atrial fibrillation and is not on any antithrombotic therapy. Which of the following is the most appropriate next step in management to reduce early risk of stroke recurrence?
    A. Initiate aspirin monotherapy
    B. Initiate apixaban
    C. Initiate high-dose statin and defer antiplatelets until cardiac workup is completed
    D. Initiate dual antiplatelet therapy with aspirin and clopidogrel
    E. Initiate intravenous thrombolysis
    Correct answer: D

Explanation

In patients with minor non-cardioembolic ischemic stroke (NIHSS ≤3) or high-risk transient ischemic attack, early initiation of dual antiplatelet therapy (DAPT) with aspirin and clopidogrel has been shown to reduce the risk of early recurrent stroke. Trials such as CHANCE and POINT demonstrated that starting DAPT within 24 h of symptom onset and continuing for 21 days significantly reduces stroke recurrence without a major increase in bleeding risk.

References

Johnston SC, Easton JD, Farrant M, et al. Clopidogrel and Aspirin in Acute Ischemic Stroke and High-Risk TIA. N Engl J Med. 2018;379(3):215–225. https://doi.org/10.1056/NEJMoa1800410

Wang Y, Wang Y, Zhao X, et al. Clopidogrel with aspirin in acute minor stroke or transient ischemic attack. N Engl J Med. 2013;369(1):11–19. https://doi.org/10.1056/NEJMoa1215340

68. A 62-year-old man with a history of hypertension presents with sudden-onset vertigo, nausea, left-sided facial weakness, and unsteadiness. He also reports decreased hearing in his left ear and tinnitus that began at the same time as his other symptoms. On examination, he has left horizontal nystagmus, left peripheral facial palsy, dysmetria of the left arm, and a wide-based gait. Audiometry confirms sensorineural hearing loss on the left. Brain MRI shows an infarct in the lateral pons and cerebellar peduncle. Which of the following arteries is most likely involved?

    A. Posterior inferior cerebellar artery (PICA)
    B. Anterior inferior cerebellar artery (AICA)
    C. Superior cerebellar artery (SCA)
    D. Basilar artery
    E. Vertebral artery
    Correct answer: B

Explanation

The patient's symptoms are classic for an AICA territory infarct, which affects the lateral caudal pons, inferior cerebellar peduncle, and may involve the internal auditory artery, a branch of AICA that supplies the cochlea and vestibular apparatus. Key features of AICA stroke include ipsilateral hearing loss (sensorineural); vertigo, nausea; peripheral facial palsy; gait ataxia; and ipsilateral limb dysmetria. This is distinct from PICA stroke, which does not cause hearing loss, and from basilar or vertebral artery infarcts, which may have more diffuse or bilateral findings.

Reference

Lee H, Kim JS, Chung EJ, et al. Infarction in the territory of anterior inferior cerebellar artery: spectrum of audiovestibular loss. Stroke. 2009;40(12):3745–3751. https://doi.org/10.1161/STROKEAHA.109.564682

69. A 41-year-old woman presents with recurrent episodes of left-sided weakness and expressive aphasia lasting 10–15 min. MRI reveals multiple chronic watershed infarcts in the right hemisphere. MR angiography shows bilateral stenosis of the distal internal carotid arteries and a network of basal collateral vessels. Conventional angiography confirms the diagnosis of Moyamoya disease. Which of the following is the most appropriate next step in management to reduce the risk of future ischemic events?
    A. High-dose corticosteroids
    B. Dual antiplatelet therapy with aspirin and clopidogrel
    C. Direct or indirect revascularization surgery
    D. Endovascular stenting of the internal carotid arteries
    E. Long-term anticoagulation with warfarin
    Correct answer: C

Explanation

Moyamoya disease is a progressive, non-atherosclerotic arteriopathy characterized by stenosis or occlusion of the distal internal carotid arteries and proximal circle of Willis, with subsequent formation of abnormal basal collateral vessels that appear as a "puff of smoke" on angiography (hence the name moyamoya in Japanese). Patients typically present with TIAs, ischemic strokes, or intracerebral hemorrhages, depending on the pattern of disease progression and the extent of collateral circulation. In this patient, recurrent ischemic symptoms and chronic watershed infarcts reflect hypoperfusion, not embolism. The most effective treatment to reduce future ischemic events in symptomatic Moyamoya disease is surgical revascularization, either direct (e.g., superficial temporal artery to middle cerebral artery [STA-MCA] bypass) or indirect (e.g., encephaloduroarteriosynangiosis [EDAS]). These procedures improve cerebral perfusion and have been shown to reduce the risk of recurrent strokes and TIAs.

References

Berry JA, Cortez V, Toor H, Saini H, Siddiqi J. Moyamoya: An Update and Review. Cureus. 2020;12(10):e10994. Published 2020 Oct 16. https://doi.org/10.7759/cureus.10994

Ihara M, Yamamoto Y, Hattori Y, et al. Moyamoya disease: diagnosis and interventions. Lancet Neurol. 2022;21(8):747–758. https://doi.org/10.1016/S1474-4422(22)00165-X

Kappel AD, Feroze AH, Torio E, Sukumaran M, Du R. Management of moyamoya disease: a review of current and future therapeutic strategies. J Neurosurg. 2024;141(4):975–982. Published 2024 Apr 19. https://doi.org/10.3171/2024.1.JNS221977

70. A 27-year-old woman presents with acute-onset right-sided weakness and expressive aphasia. She reports no history of trauma but mentions that she had a sudden sharp neck pain while turning her head in bed that morning. MRI shows acute infarcts in the left frontal and parietal lobes. CTA reveals a tapered stenosis of the left internal carotid artery just distal to the bifurcation with a surrounding crescentic hyperdensity. Notably, she has a history of spontaneous pneumothorax and reports that her mother died suddenly at age 38 of a "ruptured artery." Which of the following is the most likely underlying etiology of this patient's stroke?
    A. Fabry disease
    B. Antiphospholipid antibody syndrome
    C. Mitochondrial encephalopathy with lactic acidosis and stroke-like episodes (MELAS)
    D. Ehlers-Danlos syndrome, vascular type (type IV)
    E. Cerebral autosomal dominant arteriopathy with subcortical infarcts and leukoencephalopathy
    Correct answer: D

Explanation

This is a classic presentation of arterial dissection in a young patient, most likely due to an underlying connective tissue disorder, specifically vascular Ehlers-Danlos syndrome (vEDS). Key clues include: internal carotid artery dissection causing stroke at a young age; sudden neck pain, often preceding neurologic symptoms in dissection; history of spontaneous pneumothorax (suggesting fragile connective tissue); and family history of arterial rupture in a first-degree relative at a young age. vEDS (type IV Ehlers-Danlos) is caused by mutations in the COL3A1 gene (type III collagen), leading to arterial, intestinal, and uterine fragility. Patients may have vascular dissections, spontaneous organ rupture, and family history of sudden death.

Reference

Byers PH. Vascular Ehlers-Danlos Syndrome. 1999 Sep 2 [Updated 2025 Apr 10]. In: Adam MP, Feldman J, Mirzaa GM, et al., editors. GeneReviews® [Internet]. Seattle (WA): University of Washington, Seattle; 1993–2025. Available from: https://www.ncbi.nlm.nih.gov/books/NBK1494/

71. A 45-year-old man presents with a history of recurrent migraines with aura since his 30 s, and more recently, progressive cognitive decline and gait instability. His father had early-onset dementia and died at age 55. Neurologic exam reveals mild dysarthria and executive dysfunction. MRI of the brain shows confluent T2 hyperintensities in the periventricular white matter, external capsules, and anterior temporal lobes, with multiple lacunar infarcts in the basal ganglia. Which of the following diagnostic tests is most likely to confirm the suspected diagnosis?
    A. CSF analysis showing elevated neurofilament light chain
    B. Brain biopsy with Congo red staining
    C. APOE genotyping
    D. Anti-aquaporin-4 antibody testing
    E. Skin biopsy with electron microscopy for granular osmiophilic material
    Correct answer: E

Explanation

This patient presents with a classic clinical and radiographic picture of CADASIL (Cerebral Autosomal-Dominant Arteriopathy with Subcortical Infarcts and Leukoencephalopathy): autosomal dominant inheritance, migraine with aura often precedes other symptoms, patients experience subcortical ischemic events, dementia, gait impairment, and mood disturbances. MRI features include white matter T2 hyperintensities in the periventricular region, anterior temporal lobes, and external capsules, as well as lacunar infarcts in deep gray structures. CADASIL is caused by NOTCH3 mutations leading to deposition of granular osmiophilic material (GOM) in the walls of small arteries, which can be detected by electron microscopy of a skin biopsy, a less invasive alternative to brain biopsy.

References

Chabriat H, Joutel A, Dichgans M, Tournier-Lasserve E, Bousser MG. Cadasil. Lancet Neurol. 2009;8(7):643–653. https://doi.org/10.1016/S1474-4422(09)70127-9

Cramer J, Lui F, White ML. Cerebral Autosomal Dominant Arteriopathy. [Updated 2024 Mar 21]. In: StatPearls [Internet]. Treasure Island (FL): StatPearls Publishing; 2025 Jan-. Available from: https://www.ncbi.nlm.nih.gov/books/NBK470293/

Hack RJ, Rutten J, Lesnik Oberstein SAJ. CADASIL. 2000 Mar 15 [Updated 2019 Mar 14]. In: Adam MP, Feldman J, Mirzaa GM, et al., editors. GeneReviews® [Internet]. Seattle (WA): University of Washington, Seattle; 1993–2025. Available from: https://www.ncbi.nlm.nih.gov/books/NBK1500/

72. A 68-year-old man presents with acute-onset left-sided weakness and visual neglect. His symptoms began abruptly this morning. Two months ago, he developed a vesicular rash over his right forehead and scalp that resolved with oral acyclovir. MRI of the brain shows multiple small cortical and subcortical infarcts in the right parietal and occipital lobes. MRA of the head and neck shows no significant stenosis or large-vessel occlusion. CSF analysis reveals 52 WBC/μL (lymphocytic), protein 78 mg/dL, and normal glucose.

    Which of the following is the most appropriate next diagnostic step?
    A. Lumbar puncture for CSF bacterial and fungal cultures
    B. Serum rapid plasma reagin (RPR)
    C. Lumbar puncture for CSF varicella-zoster virus PCR and IgG
    D. Serum HIV and hepatitis panel
    E. Temporal artery biopsy

Correct answer: C

Explanation

This patient likely has varicella-zoster virus (VZV) vasculopathy, a form of infectious central nervous system vasculitis that can occur weeks to months after herpes zoster, especially involving the ophthalmic (V1) branch of the trigeminal nerve. Key features include history of shingles in the V1 distribution, delayed neurologic symptoms (stroke, encephalopathy, focal deficits), lymphocytic pleocytosis and elevated protein in CSF, and multiple infarcts in various vascular territories (suggesting small- and medium-vessel involvement). The best diagnostic test is CSF VZV PCR and CSF VZV IgG antibody testing which has higher sensitivity than the PCR.

Reference

Gilden D, Cohrs RJ, Mahalingam R, Nagel MA. Varicella zoster virus vasculopathies: diverse clinical manifestations, laboratory features, pathogenesis, and treatment. Lancet Neurol. 2009;8(8):731–740. https://doi.org/10.1016/S1474-4422(09)70134-6

73. A 72-year-old woman is hospitalized following a left middle cerebral artery infarct. On exam, she has dense right hemiparesis, nonfluent aphasia, and right visual field deficit. She is medically stable on hospital day 6 and has begun early mobilization. She requires moderate assistance for transfers and maximal assistance for dressing and toileting. Cognitive testing shows intact comprehension but significant expressive language deficits. She is motivated to participate in therapy. She lives alone in a single-level home with a few front steps and has no local family support. She was fully independent prior to her stroke. Which of the following is the most appropriate discharge plan?
    A. Discharge home with home health services and outpatient therapy
    B. Admit to an inpatient rehabilitation facility with speech, PT, and OT
    C. Transfer to skilled nursing facility with low-intensity rehabilitation
    D. Refer to long-term acute care hospital for prolonged medical management
    E. Discharge home with full-time private caregiver and outpatient speech therapy only

Correct answer: B

Explanation

This patient has significant functional impairments after a left MCA stroke, including right hemiparesis, expressive aphasia, and visual field cut. Despite these impairments, she is medically stable, cognitively intact aside from expressive language, and motivated to participate in therapy. She meets criteria for inpatient rehabilitation, which includes medical stability, capacity to participate in ≥3 h of therapy per day, need for multidisciplinary rehab (PT, OT, and SLP), and potential for functional improvement.

74. A 59-year-old man is admitted for rehabilitation after a left middle cerebral artery infarct. He has right hemiparesis, expressive aphasia, and mild right visual field deficit. He is able to sit unsupported and stand with minimal assistance. Comprehension is intact, and he participates actively in therapy. He was independent in all activities of daily living prior to the stroke. Brain MRI shows a large cortical and subcortical infarct without hemorrhagic transformation. Which of the following factors is most predictive of favorable functional recovery at 6 months?
    A. Location of the infarct in the dominant hemisphere
    B. Initial presence of expressive aphasia
    C. Ability to sit unsupported in the first week after stroke
    D. Extent of MRI lesion on diffusion-weighted imaging
    E. Involvement of the internal capsule
    Correct answer: C

Explanation

In stroke rehabilitation, early functional status such as the ability to sit unsupported, stand, or participate in therapy within the first days to week after stroke is one of the strongest predictors of long-term functional outcome. This patient's ability to sit unsupported suggests intact postural control and early motor recovery, both of which are highly correlated with better ADL independence at 3–6 months.

Reference

Vargas P, Maldonado-Diaz M, Gutiérrez-Panchana T. Early prediction of functional mobility severity after stroke: two key milestones. J Neurol Sci. 2024;466:123278. https://doi.org/10.1016/j.jns.2024.123278

75. A 54-year-old man with a history of hypertension presents to the emergency department with sudden-onset severe headache, nausea, and visual disturbances. On examination, he is found to have bitemporal hemianopsia and right-sided ptosis with ophthalmoplegia. Laboratory studies reveal hyponatremia and low morning cortisol. NCHCT shows the following:

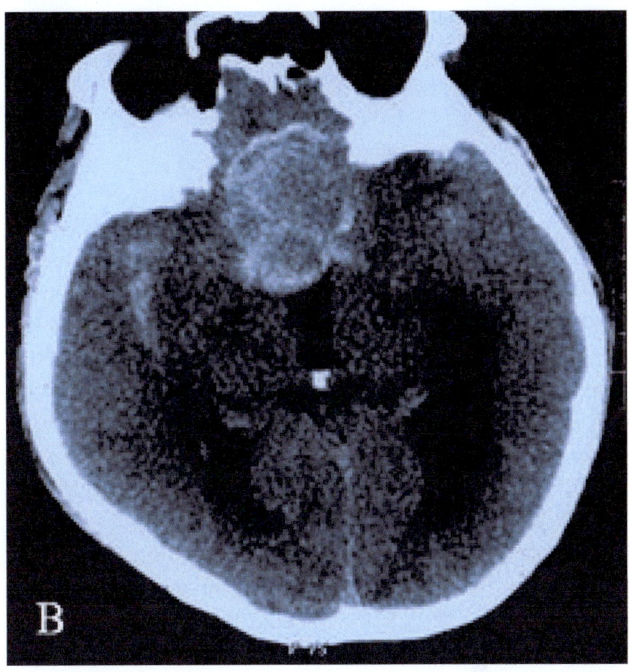

Axial CT brain. (Source: Xu et al. via World Journal of Surgical Oncology (2015). CC-BY 4.0 (https://creativecommons.org/licenses/by/4.0/). Image has been cropped to show only panel B. Please see full attribution in references section below)

Which of the following is the most appropriate next step in management?
    A. Start high-dose corticosteroids and urgent neurosurgical consultation
    B. Begin dopamine agonist therapy
    C. Schedule transsphenoidal resection in 4–6 weeks
    D. Initiate intravenous antibiotics and obtain blood cultures
    E. Refer for radiation therapy
    Correct answer: A

Explanation

This patient presents with classic features of pituitary apoplexy, including sudden headache, visual field deficits (bitemporal hemianopsia), cranial nerve palsies, and signs of adrenal insufficiency (e.g., low cortisol, hyponatremia). Immediate management includes stress-dose corticosteroids to address potential adrenal crisis and reduce inflammation/edema, and urgent neurosurgical evaluation for possible decompression, especially in the presence of visual or neurologic deficits.

References

Baldeweg SE, Vanderpump M, Drake W, et al. SOCIETY FOR ENDOCRINOLOGY ENDOCRINE EMERGENCY GUIDANCE: Emergency management of pituitary apoplexy in adult patients. Endocr Connect. 2016;5(5):G12-G15. https://doi.org/10.1530/EC-16-0057

Mayol Del Valle M, De Jesus O. Pituitary Apoplexy. [Updated 2023 Aug 23]. In: StatPearls [Internet]. Treasure Island (FL): StatPearls Publishing; 2025 Jan-. Available from: https://www.ncbi.nlm.nih.gov/books/NBK559222/

Xu K, Yuan Y, Zhou J, Yu J. Pituitary adenoma apoplexy caused by rupture of an anterior communicating artery aneurysm: case report and literature review. World J Surg Oncol. 2015;13:228. Published 2015 Jul 30. https://doi.org/10.1186/s12957-015-0653-z

76. A 74-year-old woman is brought to the emergency department with acute onset of word-finding difficulty and confusion. She has no history of hypertension, trauma, or anticoagulant use. Neurologic exam reveals fluent aphasia and right upper visual field deficit. Non-contrast CT of the head reveals a left temporoparietal lobar hemorrhage without intraventricular extension. MRI with susceptibility-weighted imaging (SWI) shows multiple small hypointense foci in the cortex of the occipital and parietal lobes bilaterally. Which of the following is the most likely underlying pathophysiology of this patient's hemorrhage?
    A. Hyaline arteriolosclerosis affecting penetrating arteries
    B. Beta-amyloid deposition in leptomeningeal and cortical vessels
    C. High-flow arteriovenous shunting through fragile venous channels
    D. Reperfusion injury due to thrombolysis of a cortical infarct
    E. Capillary telangiectasia with hemosiderin-laden macrophages

Correct answer: B

Explanation

This is a classic presentation of cerebral amyloid angiopathy (CAA), a leading cause of non-traumatic lobar hemorrhage in elderly, normotensive patients. Key features in this vignette include age, cortical/lobar location of hemorrhage, no hypertension or coagulopathy, MRI showing cortical microhemorrhages, and clinical signs pointing to cortical involvement. CAA involves beta-amyloid deposition in the walls of small-to-medium-sized leptomeningeal and cortical vessels, leading to vessel fragility and a high risk of hemorrhage.

Reference

Malhotra K, Theodorou A, Katsanos AH, et al. Prevalence of Clinical and Neuroimaging Markers in Cerebral Amyloid Angiopathy: A Systematic Review and Meta-Analysis. Stroke. 2022;53(6):1944–1953. https://doi.org/10.1161/STROKEAHA.121.035836

77. A 62-year-old man with poorly controlled hypertension presents with sudden-onset right hemiplegia and gaze deviation to the left. CT of the head shows an acute hemorrhage centered in the left internal capsule extending into the adjacent basal ganglia and deep white matter. MRI susceptibility-weighted imaging reveals multiple small hypointense foci in the basal ganglia and thalamus bilaterally. Which of the following is the most likely underlying cause of this patient's hemorrhage?
    A. Cerebral amyloid angiopathy
    B. Hypertensive lipohyalinosis of deep perforating arteries
    C. Embolic infarction with hemorrhagic transformation
    D. Cavernous malformation of the basal ganglia
    E. Arteriovenous malformation involving the lenticulostriate vessels

Correct answer: B

Explanation

This patient presents with a deep (subcortical) hemorrhage, specifically affecting the internal capsule and basal ganglia, which are classic locations for hypertensive intracerebral hemorrhage (ICH). The underlying pathology is lipohyalinosis and fibrinoid necrosis of the small penetrating arteries (e.g., lenticulostriate arteries), which become prone to rupture due to chronic hypertension. The presence of microbleeds on MRI in deep structures (basal ganglia, thalamus) supports a hypertensive vasculopathy, distinguishing it from amyloid-related bleeding, which typically shows lobar microbleeds.

Reference

Biller, J., & Sacco, R. L. (2023). Cerebrovascular diseases. In A. H. Ropper, M. A. Samuels, J. P. Klein, & S. Prasad (Eds.), Adams and Victor's principles of neurology (12th ed., pp. 660–770). McGraw Hill.

78. A 65-year-old man presents with new-onset headache, nausea, and right-sided weakness. CT of the head shows a left parietal intracerebral hemorrhage with surrounding vasogenic edema. MRI of the brain with contrast demonstrates a heterogeneously enhancing cortical lesion with central hemorrhage and adjacent edema. Gradient-echo sequences reveal multiple hypointense foci suggestive of hemorrhage. Which of the following is the most likely primary cancer responsible for this patient's brain lesion?
    A. Hepatocellular carcinoma
    B. Non-small cell lung carcinoma
    C. Renal cell carcinoma
    D. Prostate adenocarcinoma
    E. Pancreatic adenocarcinoma
    Correct answer: C

Explanation

Renal cell carcinoma (RCC) is one of the classic malignancies known to cause hemorrhagic brain metastases, along with melanoma, lung cancer, choriocarcinoma, and thyroid carcinoma. RCC is highly vascular and prone to bleeding, both at the primary site and in metastases. The imaging features of a hemorrhagic brain lesion (edema, ring enhancement, GRE blooming) in conjunction with a hypervascular renal mass strongly point to RCC as the source.

Reference

Ostrowski RP, He Z, Pucko EB, Matyja E. Hemorrhage in brain tumor – an unresolved issue. Brain Hemorrhages. 2022;3(2):98–102. https://doi.org/10.1016/j. hest.2022.01.005

79. A 42-year-old woman presents with a 5-day history of worsening headache, fever, and right-sided periorbital swelling. She reports double vision and pain with eye movements. On exam, her temperature is 38.5 °C. Right eye shows proptosis, chemosis, and ophthalmoplegia with impaired abduction and ptosis. Pupils are equal and reactive. Sensation is decreased over the right forehead and cheek. Fundoscopic exam reveals no papilledema. MRI brain and orbits with and without contrast below:

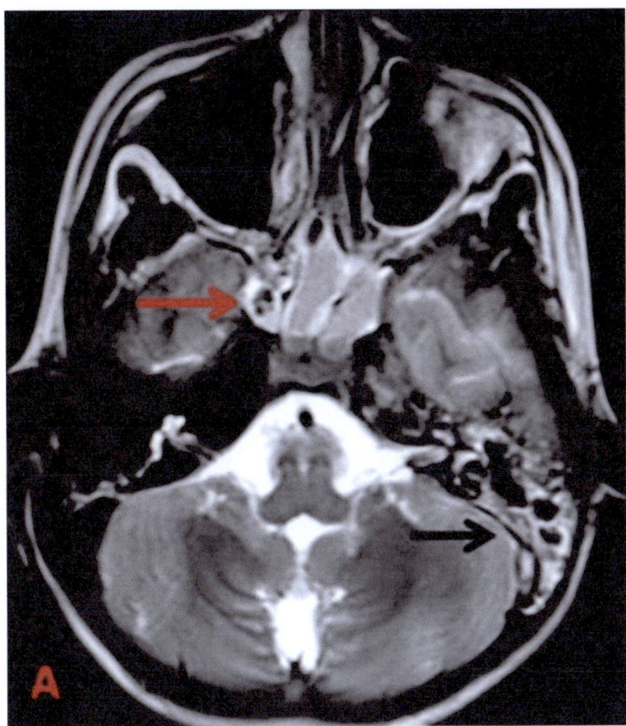

Axial T2 MRI. (Source: Khaladkar et al. via Cureus (2024). CC-BY 4.0. (https://creativecommons.org/licenses/by/4.0/deed.en). Image has been cropped to show only panel A. Please see full attribution with citation below in references section for this question.)

Which of the following cranial nerves is most likely affected first in this patient's condition?
    A. Cranial nerve III
    B. Cranial nerve IV
    C. Cranial nerve V1
    D. Cranial nerve VI
    E. Cranial nerve VII
    Correct answer: D

Explanation

This patient has cavernous sinus thrombosis (CST), suggested by fever, periorbital edema, proptosis, ophthalmoplegia, and trigeminal sensory loss. The abducens nerve (CN VI) lies centrally within the cavernous sinus and is therefore the first cranial nerve to be affected by thrombosis or inflammation, causing impaired lateral gaze (difficulty abducting the eye). Other cranial nerves in the lateral wall (III, IV, V1, V2) are affected later. Facial nerve (CN VII) is not involved as it is anatomically distant.

Reference

Khaladkar S M, Julakanti S, Pandey A, et al. (August 05, 2024) Vascular and Neurological Complications in Sphenoid Sinusitis. Cureus 16(8): e66181. https://doi.org/10.7759/cureus.66181

80. A 29-year-old woman, gravida 2 para 1, presents to the emergency department with a 4-day history of progressive headache, nausea, and blurry vision. She is currently 3 weeks postpartum. On examination, she is alert but has bilateral papilledema and mild right-sided weakness. MRI of the brain with MR venography reveals thrombosis of the superior sagittal sinus and right transverse sinus. Which of the following best explains this patient's increased risk for cerebral venous sinus thrombosis?
    A. Increased platelet destruction and thrombocytopenia during pregnancy
    B. Dehydration due to postpartum diuresis
    C. Reduced venous tone in cerebral vessels due to progesterone
    D. Hypercoagulable state induced by pregnancy and the postpartum period
    E. Cerebral autoregulation failure due to peripartum blood pressure changes

Correct answer: D

Explanation

This patient's clinical presentation and imaging are classic for cerebral venous sinus thrombosis (CVST), a form of stroke more common in young women, especially during pregnancy and the postpartum period. Pregnancy is a well-established hypercoagulable state, which persists for up to 6 weeks postpartum. Physiologic changes include increased levels of procoagulant factors (e.g., fibrinogen, factor VII, VIII, X), reduced fibrinolytic activity, and decreased levels of anticoagulant proteins (e.g., protein S). These changes are adaptive for reducing hemorrhage during delivery, but they also significantly increase the risk of venous thromboembolism, including CVST.

Reference

Algahtani H, Bazaid A, Shirah B, Bouges RN. Cerebral venous sinus thrombosis in pregnancy and puerperium: A comprehensive review. Brain Circ. 2022;8(4):180–187. Published 2022 Dec 6. https://doi.org/10.4103/bc.bc_50_22

81. A 48-year-old man is brought to the emergency department after a motor vehicle accident. He was restrained but struck his head against the window. On arrival, his Glasgow Coma Scale (GCS) score is 14. He is alert but reports a severe headache. CT of the head reveals thin linear hyperdensities in the left Sylvian and interhemispheric fissures without mass effect, midline shift, or intraparenchymal hemorrhage. No skull fracture is identified. Which of the following is the most appropriate next step in management?
    A. Observation with neurologic checks and repeat head CT in 6 h
    B. Emergent neurosurgical evacuation of the hemorrhage
    C. Lumbar puncture to assess for aneurysmal rupture
    D. CT angiography of the head to evaluate for cerebral vasospasm
    E. Initiation of nimodipine to reduce delayed ischemic deficits

Correct answer: A

Explanation

This patient has a traumatic subarachnoid hemorrhage (tSAH), as evidenced by the linear subarachnoid hyperdensities after head trauma. tSAH is common after blunt head trauma and often occurs in sulci over the convexities, unlike aneurysmal SAH, which typically involves the basal cisterns or Sylvian fissures bilaterally. In a patient who is neurologically stable with no signs of increased intracranial pressure or mass effect, the standard management is observation, frequent neurologic checks, and repeat head CT in 6 h to monitor for progression. Routine angiographic workup for aneurysm or vasospasm is not indicated unless there's a high suspicion of aneurysmal SAH (e.g., basal cistern hemorrhage, no trauma, or severe presentation).

References

Cooper SW, Bethea KB, Skrobut TJ, Gerardo R, Herzing K, Torres-Reveron J, Ekeh AP. Management of traumatic subarachnoid hemorrhage by the trauma service: is repeat CT scanning and routine neurosurgical consultation necessary? Trauma Surg Acute Care Open. 2019 Nov 17;4(1):e000313. https://doi.org/10.1136/tsaco-2019-000313. PMID: 31799413; PMCID: PMC6861109.

Hoh BL, Ko NU, Amin-Hanjani S, et al. 2023 Guideline for the Management of Patients With Aneurysmal Subarachnoid Hemorrhage: A Guideline From the

American Heart Association/American Stroke Association. Stroke. 2023;54(7):e314–e370. https://doi.org/10.1161/STR.0000000000000436

Wu Z, Li S, Lei J et-al. Evaluation of traumatic subarachnoid hemorrhage using susceptibility-weighted imaging. AJNR Am J Neuroradiol. 2010;31 (7): 1302–10.

Goursaud S, Martinez de Lizarrondo S, Grolleau F, et al. Delayed Cerebral Ischemia After Subarachnoid Hemorrhage: Is There a Relevant Experimental Model? A Systematic Review of Preclinical Literature. Front Cardiovasc Med. 2021;8:752769. Published 2021 Nov 15. https://doi.org/10.3389/fcvm.2021.752769

82. A 58-year-old woman is admitted to the neurocritical care unit with a diagnosis of aneurysmal subarachnoid hemorrhage (aSAH) following rupture of a left anterior communicating artery aneurysm. She underwent successful endovascular coiling on hospital day 1. On day 7 of hospitalization, she develops new-onset right-sided weakness and expressive aphasia. Her temperature is 37.2 °C, blood pressure is 155/90 mmHg, and her white blood cell count is normal. CT head shows no new hemorrhage or hydrocephalus. CT angiography reveals narrowing of the left middle cerebral artery branches. Which of the following is the most likely cause of her new neurologic deficits?

   A. Acute rebleeding of the aneurysm
   B. Cerebral vasospasm with delayed cerebral ischemia
   C. Hydrocephalus due to impaired CSF absorption
   D. Seizure with postictal Todd's paresis
   E. Hyponatremia from syndrome of inappropriate antidiuretic hormone (SIADH)

   Correct answer: B

Explanation

The patient presents on day 7 after aneurysmal SAH (aSAH) with focal neurologic deficits and CT angiography showing arterial narrowing, strongly suggestive of cerebral vasospasm leading to delayed cerebral ischemia, a common and serious complication of aSAH, typically occurring between days 3 and 14, peaking around days 5–10. Vasospasm causes arterial narrowing, reducing cerebral perfusion and resulting in ischemia if untreated. This is a leading cause of morbidity and mortality after the initial hemorrhage in aSAH patients.

References

Dodd WS, Laurent D, Dumont AS, et al. Pathophysiology of Delayed Cerebral Ischemia After Subarachnoid Hemorrhage: A Review. J Am Heart Assoc. 2021;10(15):e021845. https://doi.org/10.1161/JAHA.121.021845

83. A 56-year-old previously healthy man presents with sudden-onset severe headache that began while walking. He did not lose consciousness and has no history of trauma. He is alert and oriented, with a normal neurologic exam. A non-contrast head CT performed within 6 h of symptom onset reveals blood localized to the interpeduncular cistern and ambient cisterns, without extension into the Sylvian fissures, interhemispheric fissure, ventricles, or cortical sulci. CT angiography shows no vascular abnormalities. MRI brain and MR venography are unremarkable. Which of the following is the most appropriate next step in management?

   A. Schedule digital subtraction angiography to evaluate for a small, ruptured aneurysm
   B. Discharge home with headache precautions and outpatient follow-up
   C. Initiate nimodipine and ICU-level monitoring for vasospasm risk
   D. Begin empiric anticoagulation for possible cerebral venous sinus thrombosis
   E. Repeat MRI brain with susceptibility-weighted imaging to evaluate for cavernous malformation

   Correct answer: A

Explanation

This patient's CT pattern suggests non-aneurysmal perimesencephalic subarachnoid hemorrhage with blood centered in interpeduncular and ambient cisterns and no extension into classic aneurysmal regions (Sylvian fissures, interhemispheric fissure, ventricles). Although CT angiography (CTA) is often sufficient, digital subtraction angiography (DSA) remains the gold standard when initial imaging is suggestive of SAH but no aneurysm is found, especially in younger or atypical cases. Even in perimesencephalic SAH, first-time bleeds should receive one formal DSA to rule out a small, thrombosed, or posterior circulation aneurysm.

Neuromuscular Disorders

Sakinah Sabadia, Vanessa Dwairi, Marissa Ilardi, and Arielle Matalon

4

1. A 36-year-old woman is admitted to the Labor and Delivery service. One day prior, she had a normal spontaneous vaginal delivery of an 8.5-pound infant boy. She had an epidural catheter placed for anesthesia approximately 6 h prior to delivery, and it was removed shortly after. She developed numbness and weakness in her left leg 2 h after placement of the epidural, which persisted until the following day. The Neurology service is called for a consultation for persistent symptoms.

   On examination, she has a flaccid foot drop. She has full strength in the left iliopsoas and quadriceps. The left hamstring is 4+/5. The left tibialis anterior, peroneus longus, tibialis posterior, gastrocnemius, and extensor hallucis longus (EHL) are 0/5. Strength is 5/5 throughout the right lower extremity. The left ankle jerk is absent, reflexes are otherwise 2+ in both legs with absent Babinski sign. Sensation is reduced to light touch and pinprick throughout the left foot and in the lateral left calf.

   What is the most likely localization of these deficits?
   A. L5 nerve root
   B. Common peroneal nerve
   C. Neuromuscular junction
   D. Sciatic nerve
   E. Femoral nerve
   Correct answer: D

Explanation

The L5 nerve root contributes to ankle dorsiflexion, eversion, inversion, and toe extension. Ankle plantarflexion which is predominantly powered by the gastrocnemius is primarily S1. Thus, gastrocnemius weakness would not be expected in L5 radiculopathy. Additionally, severe weakness to this degree would not be expected in an isolated single radiculopathy as all of the muscles involved have at least dual root-innervation. The common peroneal nerve divides into the superficial and deep peroneal nerves. The superficial peroneal nerve innervates the peroneus longus and brevis and supplies sensation to the lateral calf, dorsum of the foot sparing the first dorsal web space. The deep peroneal nerve innervates the tibialis anterior and extensor hallucis longus and provides sensation to the first dorsal web space. The common peroneal nerve does not innervate the gastrocnemius. Neuromuscular junction disorders can cause fluctuating weakness but would not cause numbness. The femoral nerve innervates hip flexors and quadriceps muscles and would not be expected to cause this particular set of deficits.

References

Preston DC, Shapiro BE. Sciatic Neuropathy. In: *Electromyography and Neuromuscular Disorders: Clinical-Electrophysiologic-Ultrasound Correlations.* 3rd ed. Elsevier; 2013:518.

Preston DC, Shapiro BE. Radiculopathy. In: *Electromyography and Neuromuscular Disorders: Clinical-Electrophysiologic-Ultrasound Correlations.* 3rd ed. Elsevier; 2013:448, 451.

Preston DC, Shapiro BE. Femoral neuropathy. In: *Electromyography and Neuromuscular Disorders: Clinical-Electrophysiologic-Ultrasound Correlations.* 3rd ed. Elsevier; 2013:357.

2. What are the two major branches of the sciatic nerve?
   A. Femoral and obturator
   B. Common peroneal and tibial
   C. Common peroneal and femoral
   D. Sural and tibial
   E. Femoral and saphenous
   Correct answer: B

S. Sabadia (✉) · V. Dwairi · M. Ilardi · A. Matalon
Department of Neurology, New York University Langone Health, New York City, NY, USA
e-mail: sakinah.sabadia@nyulangone.org; vanessa.dwairi@nyulangone.org; marissa.ilardi@nyulangone.org; arielle.matalon@nyulangone.org

Explanation

The sciatic nerve divides into the common peroneal nerve and tibial nerve above the level of the popliteal fossa.

Reference

Preston DC, Shapiro BE. Peroneal Neuropathy. In: *Electromyography and Neuromuscular Disorders: Clinical-Electrophysiologic-Ultrasound Correlations.* 3rd ed. Elsevier; 2013:346.

3. Which nerve provides cutaneous innervation to the dorsal aspect of the foot *sparing* the first dorsal web space?

A. Sural
B. Saphenous
C. Femoral
D. Superficial peroneal
E. Deep peroneal

Correct answer: D

Explanation

The superficial peroneal nerve supplies sensation to the lateral calf and dorsum of the foot sparing the first dorsal web space. The deep peroneal nerve supplies sensation to the first dorsal web space.

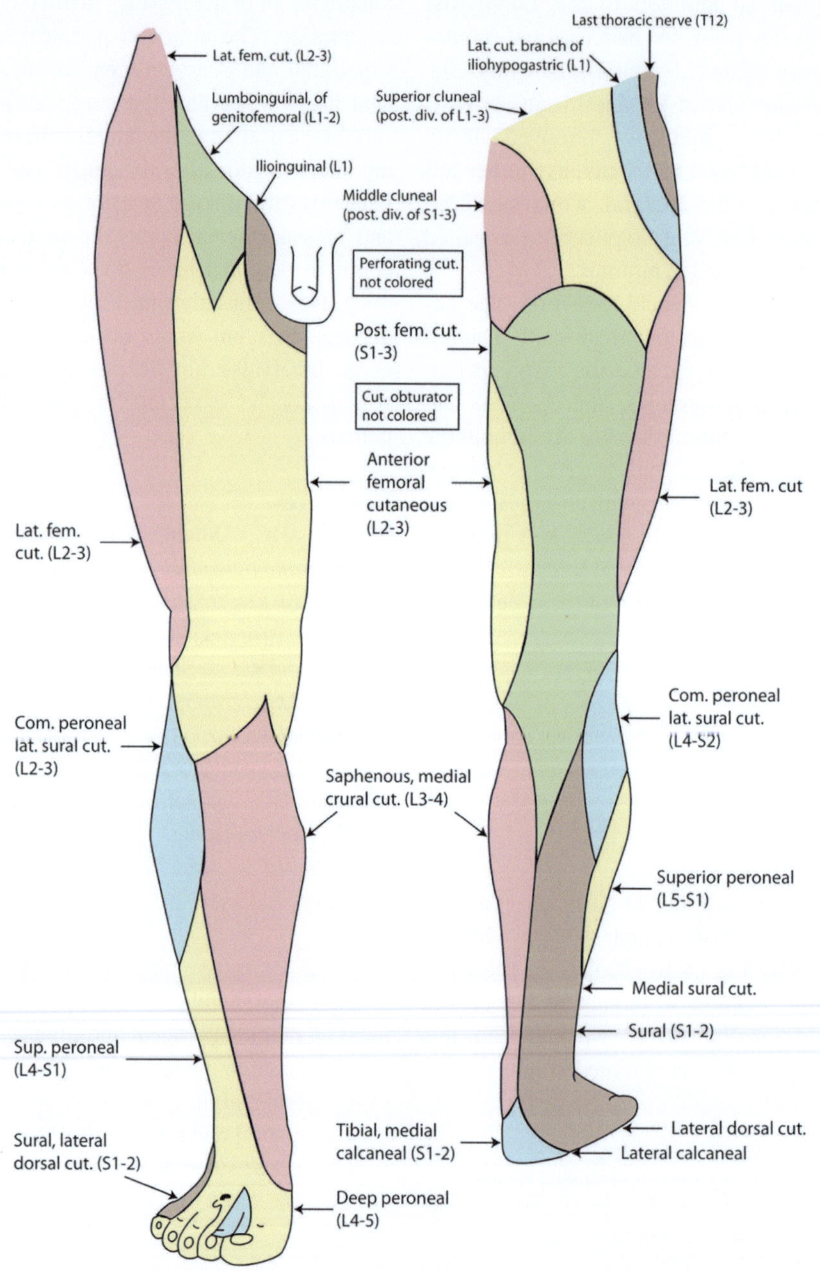

Cutaneous innervation of the lower limb, anterior and posterior view. (Source: Wikimedia Commons. *Modified from Gray H. Anatomy of the Human Body. 20th ed. Philadelphia, PA: Lea & Febiger; 1918*: Plate 826 and 831. Public Domain (https://creativecommons.org/public-domain/zero/1.0/). Image has not been further modified. https://commons.wikimedia.org/wiki/File:Gray826and831.svg)

Reference

Preston DC, Shapiro BE. Peroneal Neuropathy. In: *Electromyography and Neuromuscular Disorders: Clinical-Electrophysiologic-Ultrasound Correlations.* 3rd ed. Elsevier; 2013:347.

4. You are on the inpatient Neurology consult service. You receive a consult to see a 65-year-old man who is post-op day 3 from an elective right total hip arthroplasty with persistent right leg weakness and numbness since the surgery. A femoral neuropathy is expected. Which of the following examination findings would *not* be seen in an isolated femoral neuropathy?
   A. Absent patellar reflex
   B. Numbness in the medial calf
   C. Weakness in ankle dorsiflexion
   D. Preserved hip abduction strength
   E. Weakness in knee extension

Correct answer: C

Explanation

The femoral nerve supplies the iliopsoas which flexes the hip. It also innervates all of the quadriceps muscles which primarily function to extend the knee. With quadriceps weakness in femoral neuropathy, the patellar reflex is affected. The cutaneous distribution is as indicated in the image below (anterior femoral cutaneous nerve, saphenous nerve). Ankle dorsiflexion is not a function of the femoral nerve.

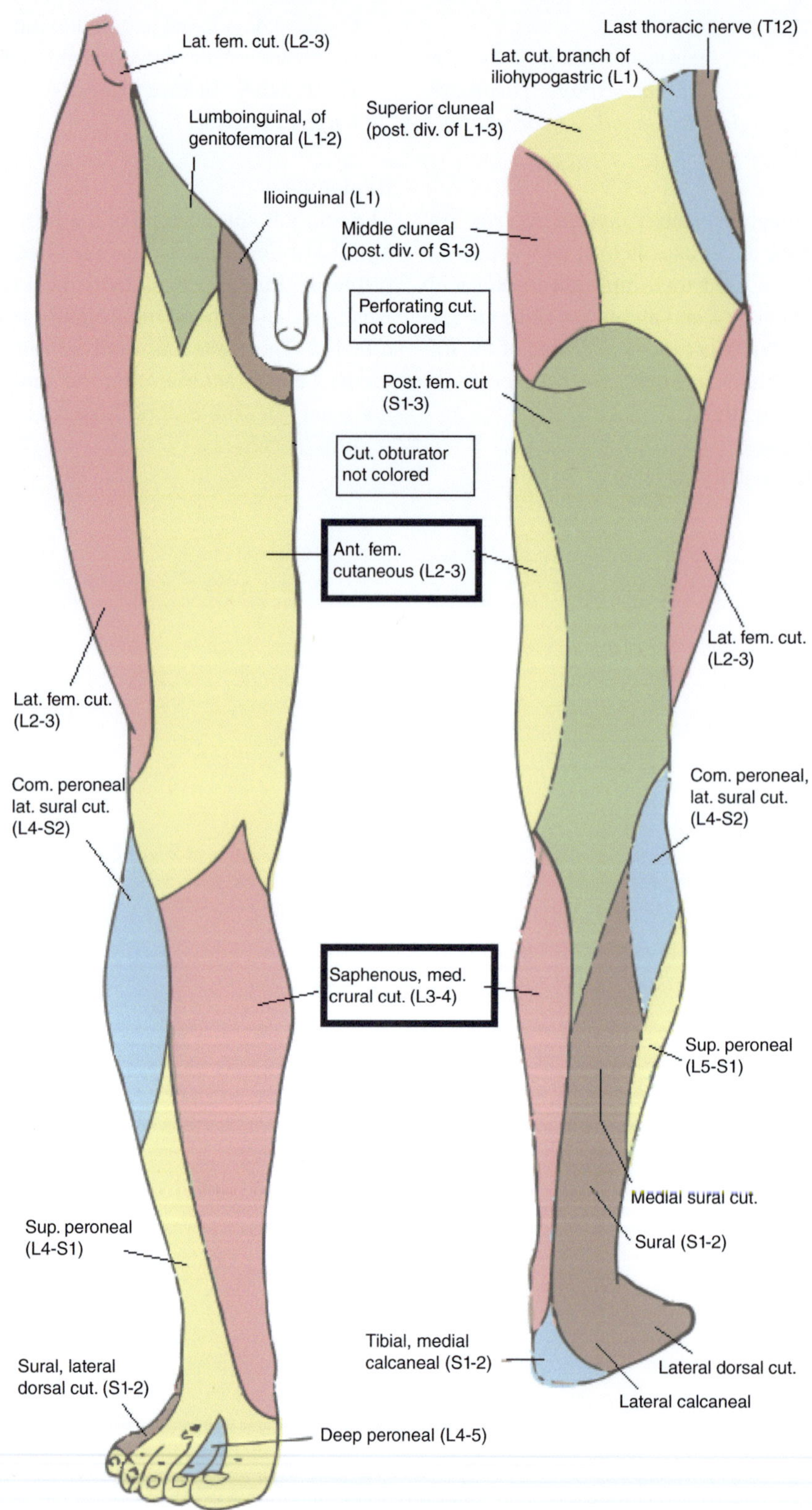

Cutaneous innervation of the lower limb, anterior and posterior view. (Source: Wikimedia Commons. *Modified from Gray H. Anatomy of the Human Body. 20th ed. Philadelphia, PA: Lea & Febiger; 1918*: Plate 826 and 831. Public Domain (https://creativecommons.org/public-domain/zero/1.0/). Modified with boxes to highlight Ant. Femoral cutaneous nerve and saphenous nerve. https://en.wikipedia.org/wiki/Cutaneous_innervation_of_the_lower_limbs#/media/File:Gray826and831.svg)

Reference

Preston DC, Shapiro BE. Femoral Neuropathy. In: *Electromyography and Neuromuscular Disorders: Clinical-Electrophysiologic-Ultrasound Correlations.* 3rd ed. Elsevier; 2013:357–358.

5. A 52-year-old woman develops left shoulder weakness immediately following left-sided mastectomy and radical neck dissection for breast cancer. On examination, she is unable to shrug her left shoulder and has weakness with head turn to the right. What is the most likely explanation?
   A. Parsonage-Turner syndrome (neuralgic amyotrophy)
   B. Cervical radiculopathy
   C. Right MCA territory stroke
   D. Spinal accessory neuropathy
   E. Axillary neuropathy
   Correct answer: D

Explanation

The pattern of weakness describes fits with the spinal accessory nerve or cranial nerve XI. This is a pure motor nerve that innervates the trapezius and sternocleidomastoid. The trapezius functions to shrug the ipsilateral shoulder and the sternocleidomastoid contributes to neck flexion and turns the head to the contralateral side.

Reference

Preston DC, Shapiro BE. Proximal Neuropathies of the Shoulder and Arm. In: *Electromyography and Neuromuscular Disorders: Clinical-Electrophysiologic-Ultrasound Correlations.* 3rd ed. Elsevier; 2013:494–495.

6. What is the origin of the suprascapular nerve from the brachial plexus?
   A. Lower (inferior) trunk
   B. Posterior cord
   C. Lateral cord
   D. Upper (superior) trunk
   Correct answer: D

Explanation

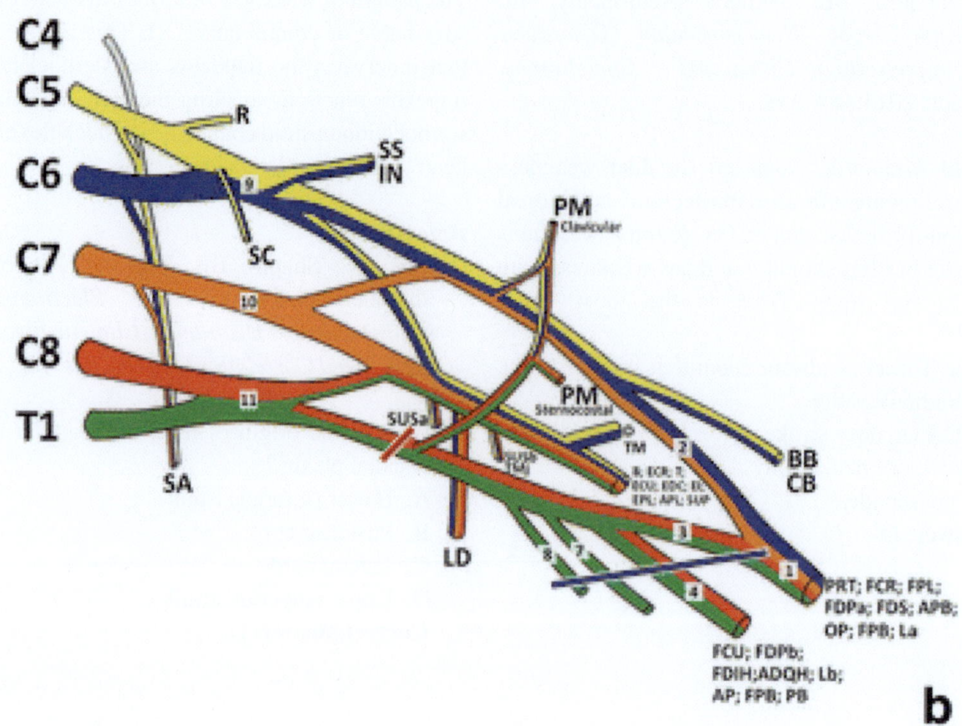

Graphic illustration of the brachial plexus, roots, trunks, divisions, cords, terminal branches, and the muscles (m.) they innervate. 1, median nerve; 2, median nerve root side; 3, medial root of the median nerve; 4, ulnar nerve; 5, axillary artery; 6, axillary vein; 7, medial cutaneous nerve of the arm; 8, medial cutaneous nerve of the forearm; 9, upper trunk of the brachial plexus; 10, middle trunk of the brachial plexus; 11, lower trunk of the brachial plexus. SA serratus anterior m., SC subclavius m., R rhomboids m., SS supraspinatus m., IN infraspinatus m., PM pectoralis major m., SUSa subscapularis m. (upper half), LD latissimus dorsi m., SUSb subscapularis m. (lower half), TMj teres major m., D deltoid m., TM teres minor m., B brachioradialis m., ECR extensor carpi radialis m., T triceps m., ECU extensor carpi ulnaris m., EDC extensor digitorum communis m., EI extensor indicis proprius m., EPL extensor policis longus m., APL abductor pollicis longus m., SUP supinator m., BB biceps brachii m., CB coracobrachialis m., PRT pronator teres m., FCR flexor carpi radialis m., FPL flexor pollicis longus m., FDPa flexor digitorum profundus m. [bellies for the index and middle finger], FDS flexor digitorum superficialis m., APB abductor pollicis brevis m., OP opponens pollicis m., FPB flexor pollicis brevis m., La first and second lumbricals m., FCU flexor carpi ulnaris m., FDPb Flexor digitorum profundus m. [bellies for the ring and small fingers], FDIH first dorsal interosseous m., ADQH abductor digiti quinti m., Lb third and fourth lumbricals m., AP adductor pollicis m., FPB flexor pollicis brevis m. (deep head), PB palmaris brevis m. . (Source: Casal et al via Journal of Medical Case Reports. 2017. CC-BY 4.0 (https://creativecommons.org/licenses/by/4.0/). Image has been cropped to show only panel B. Please see full attribution with citation below in references section for this question)

References

Casal et al via Journal of Medical Case Reports. 2017. CC-BY 4.0 (https://creativecommons.org/licenses/by/4.0/). Image has been cropped to show only panel B.

Casal D, Cunha T, Pais D, et al. A stab wound to the axilla illustrating the importance of brachial plexus anatomy in an emergency context: a case report. *J Med Case Rep.* 2017;11(1):6. Published 2017 Jan 4. https://doi.org/10.1186/s13256-016-1162-6

Linked questions: 7–9

7. A 55-year-old man with a history of hypertension, hyperlipidemia, and diabetes was started on a lipid lowering agent by his primary care doctor. He developed diffuse myalgias within 2 weeks of starting this medication. Upon discussion with his primary care doctor, his dose was lowered by half. However, he continued to experience myalgias, thus he stopped it altogether. He returned to the clinic 3 months later with a moderate degree of weakness in all extremities, proximal more than distal. He has no rash or constitutional symptoms. He had started using a walker a few weeks prior after sustaining multiple falls. What serum test would be the most appropriate to be sent as a screen for the suspected condition?
   A. Creatinine kinase
   B. Hemoglobin A1c
   C. Erythrocyte sedimentation rate
   D. Triglycerides
   Correct answer: A

Explanation

This history is highly concerning for an inflammatory myopathic process, specifically related to statin use. Of the labs listed, creatine kinase is the most high-yield, as a marked elevation of CK is supportive of myositis.

Reference

Doughty CT, Amato AA. Toxic myopathies. *Continuum (Minneap Minn).* 2019;25(6):1712–1731. https://doi.org/10.1212/CON.0000000000000806

Linked question

8. His primary care doctor sent a creatinine kinase level which results at 4000 IU/L (normal: 22–198). He is sent into the emergency department for expedited Neurology evaluation. He is admitted to the Neurology service and further workup including EMG/NCS is conducted. Which

of the following findings would be unexpected in this suspected condition?
   A. Preserved sensory nerve action potentials
   B. High amplitude motor unit action potentials
   C. Fibrillations and positive sharp waves
   D. Early and full recruitment of motor unit action potentials
   E. Short duration motor unit action potentials
   Correct answer: B

Explanation

This history is most suspicious for an inflammatory myopathy. In myopathies, nerve conductions would be expected to show normal to low amplitude compound muscle action potentials (CMAPs) and intact sensory nerve action potentials (SNAPs)—unless there is a separate process affecting SNAPs such as diabetes mellitus. Needle electromyography classically demonstrates fibrillations and positive sharp waves, and early and full recruitment of polyphasic, low amplitude, and short duration motor unit action potentials (MUAPs). High amplitude MUAPs are usually seen in chronic neurogenic processes.

Reference

Doughty CT, Amato AA. Toxic myopathies. *Continuum (Minneap Minn).* 2019;25(6):1712–1731. https://doi.org/10.1212/CON.0000000000000806

Linked question

9. EMG/NCS demonstrates low amplitude motor unit action potentials, preserved sensory nerve action potentials, and diffuse fibrillations and positive sharp waves with early recruitment of polyphasic, short duration, and low amplitude motor unit action potentials, consistent with an irritable myopathic process. Which study is most likely to yield the suspected diagnosis?
   A. Anti-nuclear antibody
   B. Anti-Jo-1 antibody
   C. HMG CoA reductase antibody
   D. Anti-MDA-5 antibody
   E. Anti-dsDNA antibody
   Correct answer: C

Explanation

Given the history of an inflammatory myositis starting weeks after beginning a lipid lowering agent, the most likely diagnosis is immune mediated necrotizing myopathy related to statin use. HMG CoA reductase antibody is highly specific and sensitive for immune-mediated necrotizing myopathy.

References

Doughty CT, Amato AA. Toxic myopathies. *Continuum (Minneap Minn).* 2019;25(6):1712–1731. https://doi.org/10.1212/CON.0000000000000806

Mammen AL, Pak K, Williams EK, et al. Rarity of anti–3-hydroxy–3-methylglutaryl–coenzyme A reductase antibodies in statin users, including those with self-limited musculoskeletal side effects. *Arthritis Care Res (Hoboken).* 2012;64(2):269–272. https://doi.org/10.1002/acr.20662

10. A 40-year-old man with acetylcholine receptor positive generalized myasthenia gravis establishes care in Neurology clinic 10 years after diagnosis. He was initially diagnosed by a primary care doctor out of state who prescribed him escalating doses of prednisone and pyridostigmine. He has since moved around and seen different providers who processed his refills, but he has not had any consistent follow up. He has been taking 35 mg of prednisone daily for the last 6 months which is the highest dose he has been prescribed. He also takes pyridostigmine 60 mg three times a day. He does not have any other medical conditions and takes no other medications or supplements. He initially felt nearly asymptomatic on this regimen, but for the last 3 months, he has had difficulty washing his hair, reaching for objects on high shelves, and climbing stairs. He does not have any ptosis, diplopia, dyspnea, or bulbar symptoms. On examination, he has 4/5 strength in proximal muscles in all extremities without any fatigability. Reflexes are reduced throughout, and sensation is intact. What is likely to be found on workup for the suspected diagnosis?
    A. Markedly elevated creatine kinase level
    B. Increase in compound motor action potential amplitude after 10 s of maximal exercise
    C. Electromyography with fibrillations and positive sharp waves in the affected muscles
    D. Nerve conduction study with low amplitude compound motor action potentials
    E. Muscle biopsy with preferential atrophy of type 2 fibers

    Correct answer: E

Explanation

This patient has developed subacute proximal weakness on prednisone. In a myasthenia gravis exacerbation, fatigable weakness would be expected on exam. This is most consistent with a steroid induced myopathy. This process preferentially affects type 2 fibers which is demonstrated on muscle biopsy. Nerve conductions, needle electromyography, and CK level are normal in these cases.

Reference

Doughty CT, Amato AA. Toxic myopathies. *Continuum (Minneap Minn).* 2019;25(6):1712–1731. https://doi.org/10.1212/CON.0000000000000806.

11. Which of the following drugs are not known to cause toxic myopathy?
    A. Hydroxychloroquine
    B. Amiodarone
    C. PCSK9 inhibitors
    D. Colchicine
    E. Zidovudine

    Correct answer: C

Explanation

All the other listed drugs are known to cause toxic myopathy. PCSK9 inhibitors have not been linked to myopathy and can be used as an alternative lipid lowering agent in patients with statin-induced myopathies.

Reference

Doughty CT, Amato AA. Toxic myopathies. *Continuum (Minneap Minn).* 2019;25(6):1712–1731. https://doi.org/10.1212/CON.0000000000000806.

12. A 55-year-old woman underwent gastric bypass surgery 2 years ago for morbid obesity. She lost 150 pounds and has been maintaining a vegan diet. She stopped taking her prescribed supplements 6 months ago. In the last 3 months, she has developed paresthesias in her hands and feet and progressive gait instability. Her examination is notable for reduced vibration in the hands and feet, impaired proprioception, diffuse hyperreflexia with positive Babinski sign bilaterally, and inability to tandem. Deficiency in which vitamin is most likely responsible for her symptoms?
    A. Vitamin D
    B. Vitamin E
    C. Vitamin B6
    D. Vitamin B12
    E. Vitamin B1

    Correct answer: D

Explanation

Deficiency in vitamin B12 can cause subacute combined degeneration (demyelination of the dorsal columns and corticospinal tracts), peripheral neuropathy, and cognitive impairment. The combination of subacute combined degeneration and peripheral neuropathy produces examination findings consistent with myeloneuropathy.

References

Holroyd KB, Berkowitz AL. Metabolic and toxic myelopathies. *Continuum (Minneap Minn)*. 2024;30(1):199–223. https://doi.org/10.1212/CON.0000000000001376.

Saji AM, Lui F, De Jesus O. Spinal cord subacute combined degeneration. In: *StatPearls* [Internet]. Treasure Island (FL): StatPearls Publishing; 2025 Jan.

13. A previously healthy 60-year-old man has a prolonged ICU admission for pneumonia and sepsis with respiratory failure requiring IV antibiotics and invasive mechanical ventilation for 10 days. After successful extubation, he noted decreased grip strength when trying to hold a cup of water and numbness in his hands and feet. Examination is notable for 4/5 strength in all extremities distally, diffuse hyporeflexia, and decreased sensation to vibration in the feet. What is the most likely explanation for these symptoms?
    A. New onset diabetes with peripheral neuropathy
    B. Critical illness polyneuropathy
    C. Critical illness myopathy
    D. Mononeuropathy multiplex
    E. B12 deficiency
    Correct answer: B

Explanation

Critically ill patients are at risk of developing weakness due to critical illness polyneuropathy (CIP) and myopathy (CIM). The examination is more consistent with CIP given the decreased sensation to vibration, which would not be affected in CIM. CIP is a distal, axonal sensorimotor peripheral neuropathy. It can present as an inability to wean from the ventilator.

Reference

Kress JP, Hall JB. ICU-acquired weakness and recovery from critical illness. *N Engl J Med.* 2014;370(17):1626–1635. https://doi.org/10.1056/NEJMra1209390.

Linked questions: 14–15

14. A 52-year-old female with type 2 diabetes diagnosed 15 years ago presents to Neurology clinic with progressive painful paresthesias in her lower extremities for 5 years. She has not been taking any prescription medications to manage her diabetes, and instead has been seeing a naturopath for herbal supplements to reduce her blood sugar. Her A1c is 13.2. She is ordered for an NCS/EMG of the lower extremities. What findings can be expected to be seen on this study? *(select all that apply)*
    A. Reduced amplitude or absent sensory nerve action potential (SNAP) amplitudes
    B. Severely slowed motor conduction velocities
    C. Motor conduction block
    D. Fibrillations and positive sharp waves in distal muscles
    E. Reduced recruitment of high amplitude and long duration motor unit action potentials
    Correct answer: A, D, and E

Explanation

This patient has a length dependent polyneuropathy due to diabetes. Diabetic neuropathy is axonal, thus demyelinating features such as severely slowed conduction velocities and conduction block are not expected to be seen on electrodiagnostic studies. Reduced SNAP amplitudes reflect axon loss of large sensory fibers. D and E are findings expected with motor axon loss.

Reference

Elafros MA, Callaghan BC. Diabetic Neuropathies. *Continuum (Minneap Minn)*. 2023;29(5):1401–1417. https://doi.org/10.1212/CON.0000000000001291

Linked question

15. Her NCS/EMG demonstrates a severe, symmetric, length-dependent sensorimotor axonal polyneuropathy with fibrillations and positive sharp waves and reduced recruitment of high amplitude and long duration motor unit action potentials in the tibialis anterior and gastrocnemius. In patients with severe peripheral neuropathy secondary to diabetes, what is another possible complication?
    A. Bradycardia
    B. Orthostatic hypotension
    C. Increased appetite
    D. Hypertension
    E. Increased libido
    Correct answer: B

Explanation

Autonomic neuropathy, including cardiovascular autonomic neuropathy can occur in diabetes. Orthostatic hypotension is a symptom of autonomic neuropathy in patients with long-standing diabetes due to vasomotor dysfunction affecting peripheral vasoconstriction.

Reference

Elafros MA, Callaghan BC. Diabetic Neuropathies. *Continuum (Minneap Minn)*. 2023;29(5):1401–1417. https://doi.org/10.1212/CON.0000000000001291

Linked questions: 16–17

16. A 42-year-old man presents to a Neurology clinic with progressive, bilateral hand numbness, and weakness for 1 year. A focused examination is notable for thenar eminence atrophy, weakness in the abductor pollicis brevis bilaterally, and reduced sensation in the thumb, index and middle fingers. What findings would *not* be expected to be seen in the suspected diagnosis?
    A. Weakness of flexor digitorum superficialis (FDS)
    B. Tinel's sign over the wrists
    C. Preserved sensation over the fifth digit and medial half of the fourth digit
    D. Prolonged distal motor latency of the median nerve compound muscle action potential (CMAP) on motor nerve conductions
    E. Preserved upper extremity deep tendon reflexes

Correct answer: A

Explanation

The suspected diagnosis is median neuropathy at the wrist or carpal tunnel syndrome. B-E can all be seen in carpal tunnel syndrome. A is incorrect, as the FDS is innervated by the median nerve proximal to the wrist, and thus is spared in carpal tunnel syndrome.

References

Preston DC, Shapiro BE. Median Neuropathy at the Wrist. In: *Electromyography and Neuromuscular Disorders: Clinical-Electrophysiologic-Ultrasound Correlations.* 3rd ed. Elsevier; 2013:269.

Preston DC, Shapiro BE. Proximal Median Neuropathy. In: *Electromyography and Neuromuscular Disorders: Clinical-Electrophysiologic-Ultrasound Correlations.* 3rd ed. Elsevier; 2013:290.

Linked question

17. On general examination, you notice peripheral leg edema, which started over one year ago. He has also had dyspnea and orthopnea. He recalls his father passed away in his 50s from heart failure. On further examination of his legs, he has severely reduced vibration in the toes and absent ankle jerks. Laboratory testing including complete blood count, basic metabolic panel, hepatic panel, vitamin B12 level, hemoglobin A1c, thyroid function tests, heavy metal screen, serum and urine protein electrophoresis, serum and urine immunofixation, and serum-free light chains are all within normal limits. What is the most likely diagnosis?
    A. Diabetic polyneuropathy
    B. Hirayama disease

    C. AL amyloidosis
    D. Neuropathic hereditary transthyretin amyloidosis
    E. Chronic inflammatory demyelinating polyradiculoneuropathy

Correct answer: D

Explanation

This constellation of findings of severe bilateral carpal tunnel syndrome, peripheral neuropathy, and signs of heart failure should raise concern for amyloidosis. AL amyloidosis is the most common cause of systemic amyloidosis, and it is an acquired form of amyloidosis. Workup for this would demonstrate a monoclonal gammopathy. Transthyretin amyloidosis is the most common form of hereditary amyloidosis. The lack of monoclonal gammopathy and family history favors answer D over AL amyloidosis.

Reference

Kaku M, Berk JL. Neuropathy associated with systemic amyloidosis. *Semin Neurol.* 2019;39(5):578–588. https://doi.org/10.1055/s-0039-1688994.

18. Which of the following statements regarding chronic inflammatory demyelinating polyradiculoneuropathy (CIDP) and Guillain-Barré syndrome (GBS) is false?
    A. Progressive sensorimotor deficits over 8 weeks is supportive of CIDP over GBS
    B. Steroids are beneficial in both CIDP and GBS
    C. Both syndromes exhibit albuminocytological dissociation in the cerebrospinal fluid
    D. Both CIDP and GBS can be treated with intravenous immunoglobulins (IVIg)
    E. Both CIDP and GBS can be treated with plasmapharesis

Correct answer: B

Explanation

Steroids can be used as maintenance treatment for CIDP, however, there is no data to support any benefit of steroids in GBS.

References

Hughes RAC, Brassington R, Gunn AA, van Doorn PA. Corticosteroids for Guillain-Barré syndrome. *Cochrane Database Syst Rev.* 2016 Jan 18;2016(1):CD001446. https://doi.org/10.1002/14651858.CD001446.pub6.

Lin J, Gao Q, Xiao K, Tian D, Hu W, Han Z. Efficacy of therapies in the treatment of Guillain-Barré syndrome: A network meta-analysis. *Medicine* (Baltimore). 2021;100(41):e27351. https://doi.org/10.1097/MD.0000000000027351.

19. Which antibody is associated with Miller-Fisher syndrome?
    A. GM1
    B. GD1a
    C. GM2
    D. GQ1b
    Correct answer: D

Explanation

Miller–Fisher syndrome is a variant of Guillain-Barré syndrome characterized by ophthalmoplegia, sensory ataxia, and areflexia. The GQ1b antibody is present in 83% of cases of Miller–Fisher syndrome.

Reference

Zhu W, Li K, Cui T, Yan Y. Detection of anti-ganglioside antibodies in Guillain-Barré syndrome. *Ann Transl Med.* 2023;11(7):289. https://doi.org/10.21037/atm-20-2285.

20. A 65-year-old man presents with 3 months of progressive right-sided wrist drop, followed by left-sided wrist drop. He then started to trip over his left foot and has since been using a cane. There is no associated numbness or pain. Examination is notable for asymmetric muscle atrophy predominantly in the distal upper extremities, weakness in bilateral wrist extension and finger extension, and mild weakness of left ankle dorsiflexion. Reflexes are normal to reduced throughout. Babinski sign is absent. Sensation to all modalities is intact. Of the following, what is the most likely diagnosis?
    A. Chronic inflammatory demyelinating polyradiculoneuropathy
    B. Polyradiculitis
    C. Multifocal motor neuropathy
    D. Motor neuron disease
    E. Hereditary neuropathy with liability to pressure palsies
    Correct answer: C

Explanation

Multifocal motor neuropathy (MMN) is an immune-mediated motor neuropathy characterized by progressive asymmetric weakness and atrophy without sensory changes. It can be differentiated from chronic inflammatory demyelinating polyradiculoneuropathy (CIDP) which additionally causes sensory deficits. MMN can be confused with motor neuron disease given the progressive weakness and atrophy, however, MMN would not be expected to have upper motor neuron signs as seen in motor neuron disease. Hereditary

neuropathy with liability to pressure palsies (HNPP) similarly presents with peripheral nerve palsies, however, the sensory axons are additionally involved in HNPP.

Reference

Garg N, Park SB, Vucic S, Yiannikas C, Spies J, Howells J, Huynh W, Matamala JM, Krishnan AV, Pollard JD, Cornblath DR, Reilly MM, Kiernan MC. Differentiating lower motor neuron syndromes. *J Neurol Neurosurg Psychiatry.* 2017 Jun;88(6):474–483. https://doi.org/10.1136/jnnp-2016-313526. Epub 2016 Dec 21.

21. A 55-year-old man presents to the emergency department with 3 weeks of dizziness. He first started to experience lightheadedness with standing. This has progressively worsened and in the last weeks, he has had multiple syncopal episodes. On review of systems, he also has early satiety and alternating diarrhea and constipation. On examination, supine blood pressure is 130/75. Upon standing after 1 min, his blood pressure drops to 70/40, and he experiences lightheadedness. His pupils are 6 mm and unreactive to light. The remainder of his neurological exam is unremarkable. He was diagnosed and treated with high-dose intravenous methylprednisolone followed by oral prednisone with significant improvement in his symptoms. Which test was most likely to be abnormal in his case?
    A. Ganglionic acetylcholine receptor antibody
    B. Acetylcholine receptor binding antibody
    C. Creatinine kinase
    D. CSF protein
    E. Serum protein electrophoresis
    Correct answer: A

Explanation

This is a case of autoimmune autonomic ganglionopathy (AAG). Manifestations of AAG include orthostatic hypotension, pupillary response abnormalities, gastrointestinal motility dysfunction, and hypohydrosis. The ganglionic acetylcholine receptor antibody is elevated in approximately half of patients with AAG. These patients typically respond well to immunotherapy.

References

Lu Z, Cao X, Wang M, Peng F, Chen L, Yin Z, Zheng B, Fan J, Zhang M. A case of relapsed gAChR-positive autoimmune autonomic ganglionopathy treated by plasma exchange and mycophenolate mofetil. *Front Neurol.* 2025 Jan 10;15:1533840. https://doi.org/10.3389/

fneur.2024.1533840. PMID: 39866515; PMCID: PMC11757093.

Nakane S, Mukaino A, Higuchi O, Watari M, Maeda Y, Yamakawa M, Nakahara K, Takamatsu K, Matsuo H, Ando Y. Autoimmune autonomic ganglionopathy: an update on diagnosis and treatment. Expert Rev Neurother. 2018 Dec;18(12):953–965. https://doi.org/10.1080/1473 7175.2018.1540304. Epub 2018 Nov 1. PMID: 30352532.

22. A 42-year-old woman presents to Neurology clinic with 6 months of progressive numbness. She first noted numbness around her lips and patchily in her face. This then progressed to involve her left arm, then right arm, then both lower extremities. She has had difficulty grasping objects, and her balance has become progressively impaired. She has also experienced lightheadedness with standing, and on multiple occasions has nearly lost consciousness. She also has early satiety, and alternating diarrhea and constipation. Her examination is notable for patchily decreased sensation to all modalities diffusely in her face, trunk, and extremities, with severe reduction in vibration in the hands and feet. Strength was preserved. There are writhing movements in her fingers with her arms outstretched, which worsens with eyes closed. On review of systems, she has had several months of dry eyes and dry mouth. What is the likely cause of the symptoms and underlying diagnosis?
    A. Mononeuritis multiplex in systemic lupus erythematosus
    B. Sensory and autonomic ganglionopathy in Sjogren syndrome
    C. Dysautonomia in chronic inflammatory polyradiculoneuropathy
    D. Peripheral neuropathy due to vitamin B12 deficiency
    E. Peripheral neuropathy due to diabetes mellitus type 2

Correct answer: B

Explanation

This patient is experiencing a constellation of symptoms that fit with a ganglionopathy due to Sjogren syndrome. The effect of the sensory ganglia, which contain the cell bodies of sensory neurons, causes a non-length dependent pattern of sensory dysfunction (typically involving both large and small fiber modalities) with preservation of strength. Facial numbness in particular is due to involvement of the trigeminal ganglia. The autonomic ganglia can also be affected and cause symptoms such as orthostatic hypotension and gastrointestinal dysmotility described in this case.

Reference

Amato AA, Ropper AH. Sensory ganglionopathy. *N Engl J Med*. 2020;383(17):1657–1662. https://doi.org/10.1056/NEJMra2023935.

23. What is the finding expected in postural orthostatic tachycardia syndrome (POTS)?
    A. Drop in systolic blood pressure of >20 mmHg within 3 min of standing
    B. Drop in heart rate with head-up tilt on tilt table testing
    C. Increase in heart rate by 30 beats per minute within 10 min of standing
    D. Generalized spike-and-wave discharges on routine EEG
    E. Long pauses on Holter monitoring

Correct answer: C

Explanation

In unaffected individuals, standing produces 5–10 mmHg drop in systolic blood pressure, 5–10 mmHg rise in diastolic blood pressure, and 10–20 bpm rise in heart rate. In POTS, blood pressure does not change with standing, but heart rate rises by 30 or more bpm within 10 min.

Reference

Cutsforth-Gregory JK. Postural Tachycardia Syndrome and Neurally Mediated Syncope. *CONTINUUM: Lifelong Learning in Neurology*. 2020;26(1):93–115. https://doi.org/10.1212/CON.0000000000000818.

Linked questions: 24–25

24. A 32-year-old woman presents to the emergency department with 1 week of progressive weakness and paresthesias in all extremities, with 2 days of dysphagia and diplopia. Two weeks prior to onset of symptoms, she had a flu-like illness with diarrhea. On examination, she is using accessory muscles to breathe. She has dysarthric speech, a left abducens palsy, diffuse weakness, distal predominant sensory loss, and hyporeflexia. She is intubated and admitted to the Neurocritical care unit. Which test would be most useful at this time?
    A. Lumbar puncture
    B. Serum creatine kinase level
    C. Acetylcholine receptor binding, blocking and modulating antibodies
    D. Hemoglobin A1c

Correct answer: A

Explanation

This presentation is most consistent with Guillain-Barré syndrome (GBS). A lumbar puncture may demonstrate albuminocytological dissociation (elevated protein with normal WBC) and can also help to rule out other potential etiologies. CK level is not typically affected in GBS, but can be elevated in myositis. Sensory loss and cranial neuropathy in this case are not consistent with myositis. Acetylcholine receptor antibodies are used to diagnose myasthenia gravis. Nearly all the noted symptoms can be seen in myasthenia gravis except sensory loss. Hemoglobin A1c is not helpful, as diabetic neuropathy is not this fulminant.

Reference

Bellanti R, Rinaldi S. Guillain-Barré syndrome: a comprehensive review. Eur J Neurol. 2024 Aug;31(8):e16365. https://doi.org/10.1111/ene.16365. Epub 2024 May 30. PMID: 38813755; PMCID: PMC11235944.

Linked question

25. A lumbar puncture is performed and demonstrates 0 WBC, 2 RBC, and 140 protein. She was started on intravenous immunoglobulin (IVIg) for treatment of Guillain-Barré syndrome. Within 48 h of admission, she developed periods of hypotension down to 80s/40s, and variable heart rate from 40 to 140 bpm. Which of the following is the most likely cause of these vital sign changes?
    A. Allergic reaction to IVIg
    B. Intracranial hypertension
    C. Pulmonary embolus
    D. Dysautonomia
    Correct answer: D

Explanation

Patients with severe GBS who require mechanical ventilation are more likely to have autonomic dysfunction with labile blood pressures and arrhythmias. They can also experience vasomotor and gastrointestinal motility dysfunction.

Reference

Zaeem Z, Siddiqi ZA, Zochodne DW. Autonomic involvement in Guillain–Barré syndrome: an update. *Clin Auton Res.* 2019;29(3):289–299. https://doi.org/10.1007/s10286-018-0542-y

26. A 24-year-old woman presents to the Emergency Department for a dilated pupil. She woke up in the morning and noted photophobia and blurred vision in her right eye. When she looked in the mirror, she noticed her right pupil was substantially larger than her left. There was no associated ocular pain, redness, tearing, or headache. There was no preceding trauma to her eye. On examination in ambient light, her left pupil is 3 mm and right pupil is 7 mm. With light directly shone into either eye, only the left pupil constricts, and the right pupil remains fixed at 7 mm. With accommodation, both pupils constrict to 2 mm. What diagnostic test would help you confirm the suspected condition?
    A. MRI of the brain and orbits
    B. Chest CT
    C. MRA neck
    D. Lumbar puncture
    E. Instill pilocarpine diluted to 0.125% into the right eye
    Correct answer: E

Explanation

This is a case of Adie's pupil. It is usually unilateral, in which case the affected pupil is substantially dilated compared to the unaffected pupil. The affected pupil has weak or absent direct and consensual response to light and preserved constriction to accommodation. It typically occurs in women between the ages of 20 and 40. The underlying pathophysiology is parasympathetic denervation from the ciliary ganglion. The affected eye is sensitive to dilute pilocarpine which causes rapid pupillary constriction.

References

Kanzaria HK, Farzan N, Coralic Z. Adie's tonic pupil. *West J Emerg Med.* 2012;13(6):543. https://doi.org/10.5811/westjem.2012.7.12923

Xu SY, Song MM, Li L, Li CX. Adie's pupil: a diagnostic challenge for the physician. *Med Sci Monit.* 2022;28:e934657. https://doi.org/10.12659/MSM.934657.

Linked questions: 27–28

27. A 37-year-old woman with systemic lupus erythematosus is referred from her rheumatologist to Neurology clinic for 3 months of leg pain and paresthesias. The symptoms initially started in her left leg distal to the knee, then a few days later involved her right leg in the same distribution with associated burning pain. A few weeks later, she developed a wrist drop on the right. On examination, right wrist and finger extension is 0/5 with reduced sensation to light touch and pinprick over the dorsal aspect of the hand. There is mild weakness in bilateral toe extension, ankle dorsiflexion, and eversion, with reduced sensation to light touch and pinprick over the lateral calves and dorsal aspects of the feet. Gait is steppage.

    With this condition, what would you expect to see on histopathology?

A. Apple-green birefringence on Congo red staining on skin biopsy
B. Vasculitis involving the endoneurial blood vessels (vasa nervorum) with axonal degeneration
C. Perifascicular muscle fiber atrophy and endomysial fibrosis
D. Endomysial inflammation with rimmed vacuoles in muscle fibers

Correct answer: B

Explanation

This is a case of vasculitic mononeuritis multiplex due to lupus. In mononeuritis multiplex, individual nerves are affected in a multifocal rather than a diffuse or length-dependent nature. Typically, there is associated pain. Nerve biopsies show axonal degeneration and vasculitis of the vasa nervorum.

Reference

Leone P, Prete M, Malerba E, Bray A, Susca N, Ingravallo G, Racanelli V. Lupus vasculitis: an overview. Biomedicines. 2021;9(11):1626. https://doi.org/10.3390/biomedicines9111626.

Linked question

28. Which peripheral nerves are clinically affected in this case? (select all that apply)
    A. Median nerve
    B. Radial nerve
    C. Common peroneal nerve
    D. Sciatic nerve
    E. Tibial nerve

Correct answer: B, C

Explanation

Weakness of wrist and finger extension can be attributed to the radial nerve at the spiral groove. The common peroneal nerve splits into the deep and superficial peroneal nerves. It dorsiflexes and everts the ankle and extends the toes. The figure below shows the cutaneous distribution of these nerves.

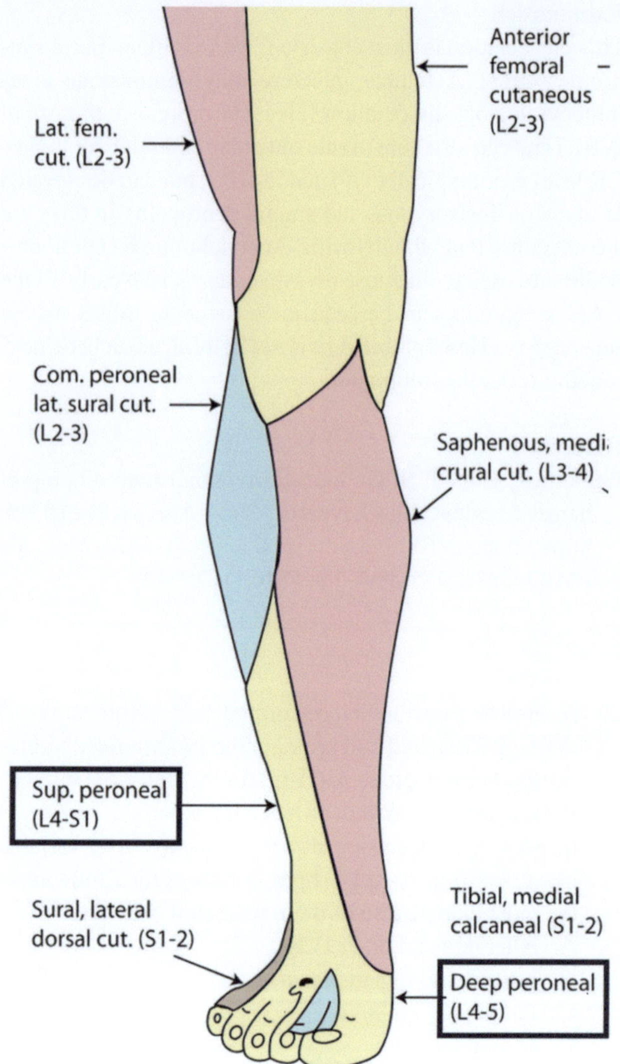

Cutaneous innervation of the lower limb, anterior view. (Source: Wikimedia Commons. *Modified from Gray H. Anatomy of the Human Body. 20th ed. Philadelphia, PA: Lea & Febiger; 1918*: Plate 826. Public Domain (https://creativecommons.org/publicdomain/zero/1.0/). Modified to highlight Superficial Peroneal nerve and deep peroneal nerve. https://commons.wikimedia.org/wiki/File:Gray826and831.svg)

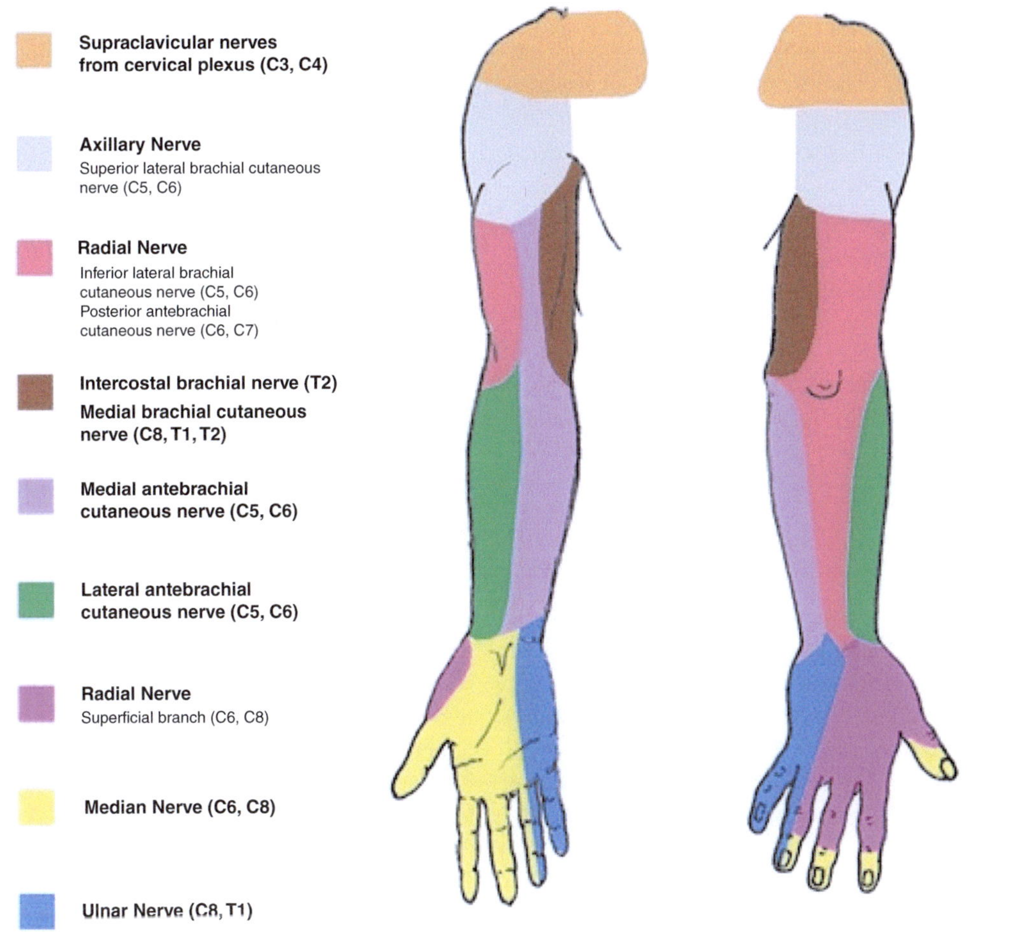

Cutaneous innervation of upper limb. (Source: Casal et al via Journal of Medical Case Reports. 2017. CC-BY 4.0. (https://creativecommons.org/licenses/by/4.0/). Image has not been modified.)

References

Casal D, Cunha T, Pais D, et al. A stab wound to the axilla illustrating the importance of brachial plexus anatomy in an emergency context: a case report. *J Med Case Rep.* 2017;11(1):6. Published 2017 Jan 4. https://doi.org/10.1186/s13256-016-1162-6

Preston DC, Shapiro BE. Radial Neuropathy. In: *Electromyography and Neuromuscular Disorders: Clinical-Electrophysiologic-Ultrasound Correlations.* 3rd ed. Elsevier; 2013:335.

Preston DC, Shapiro BE. Peroneal Neuropathy. In: *Electromyography and Neuromuscular Disorders: Clinical-Electrophysiologic-Ultrasound Correlations.* 3rd ed. Elsevier; 2013:348.

Linked questions: 29–30

29. A 30-year-old woman presents to Neurology clinic with a foot drop. She has a tendency to cross her legs, and 3 days prior, after sitting for 2 hours at work with her right leg crossed over her left, she stood up and noted right foot weakness and numbness which has persisted. On examination, strength is 0/5 in the right ankle dorsiflexion and eversion. Sensation is reduced in the right dorsal foot and lateral calf. Reflexes are 1+ throughout. She is prescribed physical therapy and an ankle foot orthosis, and she has complete recovery in her strength after 1 month. Over the subsequent years, she is diagnosed with bilateral carpal tunnel syndrome, cubital tunnel syndrome, with recurrence of the right foot drop with incomplete recovery. What is the likely diagnosis?

A. Charcot Maric Tooth Type 1A
B. Multifocal motor neuropathy
C. Hereditary neuropathy with liability to pressure palsies (HNPP)
D. Chronic inflammatory demyelinating polyradiculoneuropathy (CIDP)
E. Myotonic dystrophy type 1

Correct answer: C

Explanation

This patient has had multiple and recurrent episodes of compressive neuropathies concerning for HNPP. Answer A would present as progressive distal weakness, atrophy, and numbness. With answer B, there is progressive asymmetric weakness without numbness. With answer D, there is progressive, numbness and weakness, both proximally and distally, generally with disability if left untreated. With answer E, there is progressive weakness without numbness.

Reference

Attarian S, Fatehi F, Rajabally YA, Pareyson D. Hereditary neuropathy with liability to pressure palsies. *J Neurol.* 2020;267(8):2198–2206. https://doi.org/10.1007/s00415-019-09319-8

Linked question

30. She later recalls that her mother had also been diagnosed with carpal tunnel syndrome and has had recurrent wrist and foot drops which she was never worked up for. Her younger sister who recently turned 20 years old had a wrist drop which spontaneously recovered after 1 week. What would be expected to be found on genetic testing for all of the affected individuals?
    A. PMP22 deletion
    B. PMP22 duplication
    C. SOD1 mutation
    D. GJB1 mutation
    E. C9orf72 mutation
    Correct answer: A

Explanation

PMP22 deletion is seen in genetic testing for HNPP. PMP22 duplication seen in Charcot-Marie-Tooth type 1A, the most common CMT subtype. Answers C and D are mutations found in familial forms of amyotrophic lateral sclerosis. Answer D is seen in CMT1X.

Reference

Amato AA, Russell JA. Testing in Neuromuscular Disease. In: *Neuromuscular Disorders*. 2nd ed. New York, NY: McGraw-Hill Education; 2015:65–67.

31. A 44-year-old man with longstanding untreated HIV infection presents with progressive weakness and numbness in his right foot and left hand over the past 2 weeks. He describes sharp, burning pain in the affected areas. On examination, there is decreased pinprick sensation in the distribution of the right peroneal and left ulnar nerves, with associated distal motor weakness. His labs are notable for CD4 count of 160 cells/mm^3 and elevated HIV viral load. What do you expect to see on nerve conductions of the upper extremities?
    A. Slowed sensory and motor nerve conduction velocities with multifocal conduction block.
    B. Absent sensory responses with normal motor responses
    C. Absent motor responses with normal sensory responses
    D. Diffusely low amplitude motor and sensory responses with normal velocities.
    E. Axon loss affecting multiple peripheral nerves in a non-length-dependent pattern.
    Correct answer: E

Explanation

Mononeuropathy multiplex is often due to immune-mediated vasculitis affecting the vasa nervorum of peripheral nerves. In this case, it is attributed to severe immunosuppression from AIDS. The presentation is classically asymmetric, painful, and multifocal, consistent with axonal damage seen on nerve conduction studies. CMV infection is also commonly seen in these cases and should be tested for. Treatment should include highly active anti-retroviral therapy and antiviral therapy for CMV if active infection is detected.

Reference

Robinson-Papp J, Simpson DM, Stucky S. Neuromuscular diseases associated with HIV-1 infection. Muscle Nerve. 2009;40(6):1043–1053. https://doi.org/10.1002/mus.21465.

32. A 55-year-old woman presents to your clinic with complaints of weakness in her right leg. She reports difficulty crossing her legs and notices that she cannot bring her right thigh in toward her midline as easily as she used to. She denies any pain but mentions some occasional numbness in the inner aspect of her thigh. On examination, you observe that she has weakness in hip adduction on the right side, while her other lower limb functions, including knee extension and foot movement, remain intact. Which of the following is the most likely diagnosis?
    A. Femoral nerve mononeuropathy
    B. Sciatic nerve mononeuropathy
    C. Obturator nerve mononeuropathy
    D. Common peroneal nerve mononeuropathy
    Correct answer C

Explanation

The patient's difficulty with adducting her right thigh and associated sensory changes in the medial thigh suggest obturator nerve mononeuropathy. The obturator nerve innervates the adductor muscles of the thigh, and damage to this nerve leads to weakness or inability to perform hip adduction. The other options describe conditions involving different nerves that do not produce the same symptoms of hip adduction weakness and medial thigh sensory loss.

References

Kuhn, J. R. (2021). Neuropathy and mononeuropathies: Clinical presentation and diagnosis. *Manual of Neurologic Therapeutics* (9th ed.), 507–520.

Nag, M., & Anwar, M. (2019). Obturator nerve mononeuropathy: A case report. *Journal of Clinical Neuromuscular Disease*, 21(4), 293–295.

33. A 42-year-old man presents with sudden-onset weakness of the right side of his face. He reports that he went to sleep in his usual state of health and noticed his right eye feeling dry and his mouth drooping when he smiled this morning. On examination, there is complete paralysis of the right side of his face, including the forehead, lower eyelid, and mouth. He is unable to close his right eye tightly, and there is no wrinkle on the right side of his forehead. The remainder of the neurological examination is normal. Which of the following is the most appropriate initial treatment for this patient?
    A. Intravenous tenecteplase
    B. Intravenous immunoglobulin (IVIg)
    C. Oral corticosteroids and antiviral medications
    D. Surgical decompression of the facial nerve
    Correct answer: C

Explanation

The most appropriate initial treatment for Bell's palsy is the administration of oral corticosteroids (i.e., prednisone). Corticosteroids help reduce inflammation and improve the chances of recovery, particularly if started within 72 h of symptom onset. Antiviral medications like valacyclovir are used as adjunctive therapy for patients with severe facial palsy at presentation. Intravenous tenecteplase would not be used as this is not a stroke given that the pattern of facial weakness is of a lower motor neuron pattern, where the entire hemi-face is weak, unlike in the case of an upper motor neuron pattern where the forehead musculature is spared and only the lower face is weak. In addition, the patient would be out of the window for that IV tenecteplase treatment. IVIg would also not be indicated in this case as this is unlikely a presentation of AIDP. Surgical decompression is not a first-line treatment and is usually reserved for specific or severe cases of Bell's palsy that have not improved with time.

References

Baugh, R. F., et al. (2013). Clinical practice guideline: Bell's palsy. *Otolaryngology–Head and Neck Surgery*, 149(3_suppl), S1-S27.

Gilden, D. H. (2004). Bell's palsy. *New England Journal of Medicine*, 351(11), 1131–1133.

Maggioni, F., et al. (2019). Corticosteroid therapy in Bell's palsy: A systematic review and meta-analysis. *JAMA Otolaryngology–Head & Neck Surgery*, 145(3), 259–265.

UpToDate. Bell's palsy: Treatment and prognosis in adults. Available at: https://www.uptodate.com/contents/bells-palsy-treatment-and-prognosis-in-adults

34. A 62-year-old woman presents with a 3-week history of severe, paroxysmal, unilateral facial pain localized to the right cheek, along the V2 (maxillary) distribution of the trigeminal nerve. The pain is described as stabbing and electric shock-like, triggered by light touch such as brushing her teeth. MRI of the brain reveals a vascular loop near the right trigeminal nerve root, consistent with trigeminal neuralgia (TN). After confirming the diagnosis, you initiate first-line treatment. Which of the following side effects should you closely monitor for while she is on that therapy?
    A. Hypertension and weight gain
    B. Skin rash and blood dyscrasias
    C. Hepatotoxicity and electrolyte imbalances
    D. Cognitive impairment and ataxia
    Correct answer: B

Explanation

Carbamazepine is the first-line treatment for trigeminal neuralgia. While generally effective, it can be associated with significant side effects, including skin rash (i.e., Stevens-Johnson syndrome) and blood dyscrasias (i.e., leukopenia, thrombocytopenia, aplastic anemia). This requires monitoring for any dermatologic reactions and monitoring of complete blood counts while on the medication. The other correct answer choices are not common side effects of carbamazepine.

References

Marangell, L. B., & Renshaw, P. F. (2001). Carbamazepine in the treatment of trigeminal neuralgia: A review of the pharmacology and adverse effects. *Journal of Clinical Psychiatry*, 62(6), 449–454.

UpToDate. Trigeminal neuralgia: Treatment and prognosis. Available at: https://www.uptodate.com/contents/trigeminal-neuralgia-treatment-and-prognosis

35. A 31-year-old woman who is 36 weeks pregnant presents with numbness and tingling in her left upper outer thigh. She endorses intermittent pain in that region, but denies weakness in her lower extremities. She admits to habitual leg crossing as well as recent weight gain of 55 pounds related to her pregnancy. She has continued practicing yoga during her pregnancy, which includes frequent squatting. She also spends time working in the garden when she is able to. Which of the following habits puts her at risk of developing these neurological symptoms?

   A. Leg crossing
   B. Weight gain
   C. Yoga
   D. Gardening

Correct answer: B

Explanation

This question describes lateral femoral cutaneous neuropathy, also known as meralgia paresthetica. The lateral femoral cutaneous nerve branches off the lumbar plexus and is composed of fibers from L2 and L3 nerve roots. It courses through the pelvis and enters the leg through the inguinal ligament, which is a common site of compression. The nerve is purely sensory, responsible for sensation to the anterolateral and lateral thigh. Lateral femoral cutaneous neuropathy alone should not cause weakness. Risk factors include obesity, pregnancy, tight belts or waistbands, groin trauma. The other habits listed in the question would put the patient at risk of developing peroneal neuropathy at the fibular head.

References

David, W. S. (2021). Meralgia paresthetica (lateral femoral cutaneous nerve entrapment). *UpToDate*. Retrieved December 17, 2021, from https://www.uptodate.com/contents/meralgia-paresthetica-lateral-femoral-cutaneous nerve-entrapment:contentReference[oaicite:5]{index=5}

Mayo Clinic. (2023). *Meralgia paresthetica*. Retrieved from https://www.mayoclinic.org/diseases-conditions/meralgia-paresthetica/symptoms-causes/syc-20355635

36. A 35-year-old agricultural worker presents to the clinic with progressive weakness in his lower limbs and difficulty walking, two weeks after being hospitalized for acute organophosphate poisoning. Neurological examination reveals distal muscle weakness and decreased deep tendon reflexes. Which of the following best describes the underlying pathophysiology of his condition?

   A. Demyelination of peripheral nerves due to immune-mediated attack

   B. Delayed axonal degeneration of long peripheral nerves
   C. Acute cholinergic excess at neuromuscular junctions
   D. Mitochondrial dysfunction in motor neurons
   E. Inhibition of voltage-gated sodium channels

Correct answer: B

Explanation

Organophosphate-induced delayed polyneuropathy is a well-documented complication that typically develops 1–3 weeks after acute organophosphate exposure. It is caused by axonal degeneration, particularly in long motor nerves, and is associated with inhibition of neuropathy target esterase (NTE) rather than acetylcholinesterase. This is distinct from the acute cholinergic crisis seen immediately after exposure.

References

Roberts DM, Karunarathna A, et al. (2007). *"Investigations into the mechanism of organophosphate-induced delayed polyneuropathy."* Clinical Toxicology, 45(4), 367–370. [https://doi.org/10.1080/15563650701357799]

Vale JA. (2005). *"Toxicokinetics and toxicodynamics of organophosphates."* In: Handbook of Pesticide Toxicology. 2nd ed.

World Health Organization (WHO). *"Health implications of organophosphorus pesticides."* WHO Environmental Health Criteria 63. https://www.who.int/publications/i/item/9241542630

37. A 67-year-old man with a past medical history of HIV infection presents with burning pain in his feet as well as progressive numbness and tingling over the past 6 months. He is currently on antiretroviral therapy including stavudine, laminvudine, and efavirenz. On neurological examination, there is decreased pinprick and vibration sensation in a stocking distribution up to the bilateral ankles with hyporeflexia in the bilateral ankles and knees. Which of the following is the most likely cause of his symptoms?

   A. Cytomegalovirus infection of the dorsal root ganglia
   B. Direct neurotoxicity from antiretroviral therapy
   C. Autoimmune demyelination of peripheral nerves
   D. Vascular ischemia due to HIV-associated vasculitis
   E. Vitamin B12 deficiency secondary to malabsorption

Correct answer: B

Explanation

HIV-associated distal symmetric polyneuropathy is one of the most common neurological complications in patients with HIV. It can result from both HIV itself and neurotoxic effects of certain antiretroviral drugs. Symptoms typically include distal sensory loss, paresthesia, and burning pain, predominantly in the feet. This condition is characterized histologically by axonal degeneration of sensory fibers. While HIV can cause vasculitis leading to mononeuritis multiplex or central nervous system infarcts, this usually presents as asymmetric, patchy neuropathy, or strokes instead of a symmetric distal sensory polyneuropathy.

References

Centers for Disease Control and Prevention (CDC) – *HIV Neurological Complications Overview.* https://www.cdc.gov/hiv/clinicians/treatment/complications.html

Ellis RJ, Rosario D, Clifford DB, et al. (2010). *"Continued high prevalence and adverse clinical impact of human immunodeficiency virus–associated sensory neuropathy in the era of combination antiretroviral therapy."* Arch Neurol. 67(5):552–558. https://doi.org/10.1001/archneurol.2010.76

Schifitto G, McDermott MP, et al. (2002). *"Incidence of and risk factors for HIV-associated distal sensory polyneuropathy."* Neurology. 58(12):1764–1768.

38. A 13-year-old boy presents with progressive gait ataxia, loss of proprioception, and absent deep tendon reflexes in the lower limbs. He also shows signs of hypertrophic cardiomyopathy and scoliosis. Genetic testing reveals GAA trinucleotide repeat expansion in the FXN gene. Which of the following best explains the underlying pathological mechanism responsible for his sensory deficits?
    A. Demyelination of peripheral nerves due to autoimmune inflammation
    B. Neuronal loss in dorsal root ganglia causing degeneration of peripheral sensory neurons
    C. Motor neuron degeneration in the anterior horn of the spinal cord
    D. Demyelination of the corticospinal tracts in the spinal cord
    E. Autoimmune destruction of muscle fibers causing sensory loss

    Correct answer: B

Explanation

Friedreich ataxia is a hereditary ataxia caused by GAA repeat expansions in the FXN gene leading to deficiency of frataxin, a mitochondrial protein. The disease primarily affects dorsal root ganglia neurons, resulting in sensory neuronopathy (ganglionopathy). This leads to degeneration of large sensory neurons that are responsible for mediating propriocep-

tion and vibratory sensation. This leads to an ataxic gait and loss of reflexes. Other systemic findings include cardiomyopathy, which is a major cause of morbidity and mortality, as well as scoliosis and diabetes mellitus due to pancreatic involvement.

References

Delatycki MB, Corben LA. (2012). *"Friedreich ataxia: clinical features, pathogenesis and management."* Neurogenetics. 13(3):217–26. [https://doi.org/10.1007/s10048-012-0313-9]

Koeppen AH. (2011). *"The pathogenesis of Friedreich ataxia."* J Neuropathol Exp Neurol. 70(5): 353–361. [https://doi.org/10.1097/NEN.0b013e31821a6187]

National Institute of Neurological Disorders and Stroke (NINDS): Friedreich Ataxia Information Page. https://www.ninds.nih.gov/health-information/disorders/friedreich-ataxia

39. A 32-year-old woman with a past medical history of Sjogren's Syndrome presents with painful numbness and tingling involving her feet. On neurological exam, there is decreasing pinprick and temperature sensation distally in the lower extremities, vibration, and proprioception are intact, strength is 5/5 throughout, and reflexes are 2+ and symmetric throughout. Nerve conduction study and electromyography is obtained and demonstrates no evidence of mononeuropathy, large fiber polyneuropathy, or radiculopathy. What is the next best step in determining the etiology of this patient's symptoms?
    A. Lumbar puncture
    B. MRI of the brain
    C. Skin biopsy
    D. EEG

    Correct answer: C

Explanation

Sjogren's syndrome is one of the most common rheumatologic causes of small fiber neuropathy. In the case of small fiber neuropathy, patients usually present with sensory symptoms, including painful distal paresthesias, allodynia, and hyperesthesia. Strength and deep tendon reflexes are preserved as the large nerve fibers are spared. Patients may also exhibit autonomic symptoms, such as dry eyes or mouth, orthostatic hypotension, urinary symptoms, and sexual dysfunction. Nerve conduction study and electromyography does not demonstrate evidence of large fiber neuropathy in these cases. To assess the small nerve fibers, a skin biopsy should be pursued where the epidermal nerve fiber density can be evaluated.

References

Dollfus C, et al. "Small fiber neuropathy in Sjögren syndrome." *Medicine (Baltimore)*. 1999;78(5):278–287.

Figueroa JJ, et al. "Small Fiber Neuropathy: Clinical Features, Diagnosis, and Management." *Curr Neurol Neurosci Rep.* 2021;21(10):49.

40. A 63-year-old woman presents with complaints of muscle weakness, cramps, and stiffness. She also endorses hair loss and weight gain over the last 5 months. On exam she is noted to have proximal muscle weakness and delayed relaxation of deep tendon reflexes. Work-up demonstrates elevated thyroid stimulating hormone (TSH) and low T4 hormone. She is started on levothyroxine therapy. Which of the following outcomes is most likely regarding her muscle symptoms?

    A. Muscle weakness will worsen initially due to thyroid hormone side effects

    B. Immunosuppressive therapy is required to reverse muscle weakness

    C. Muscle symptoms are permanent and will not respond to therapy

    D. Muscle symptoms will gradually improve as metabolic function normalizes

    E. Physical therapy alone is sufficient without hormonal treatment

    Correct answer: D

Explanation

This is an example of hypothyroidism leading to an acquired metabolic muscle disorder. Deficiency of thyroid hormone leads to decreased mitochondrial oxidative metabolism and glycosaminoglycan accumulation. Treatment is with thyroid hormone replacement, levothyroxine, which corrects the underlying metabolic disturbance. Symptoms including muscle weakness, cramps, and stiffness usually gradually improve over weeks to months with appropriate therapy.

Reference

Duyff RF, et al. (2000). "Neuromuscular findings in thyroid dysfunction: a prospective clinical and electrodiagnostic study." *Journal of Neurology, Neurosurgery & Psychiatry, 68(6), 750–755.*

41. A 72-year-old man with a history of well-controlled hypertension and hyperlipidemia presents with a 2-week history of muscle pain and weakness in his legs. He states that he recently initiated rigorous spinning classes after several months of inactivity during the winter. He denies recent travel or medication changes. On exam there is 4/5 strength in bilateral hip flexors, with normal sensation and 2+ deep tendon reflexes. There is tenderness upon palpation of the thigh muscles. Laboratory studies reveal:

    - Creatine kinase (CK): 2500 U/L (normal <200)
    - Serum thyroid stimulating hormone (TSH): 1.6 mIU/L (normal)
    - Erythrocyte sedimentation rate (ESR): 13 mm/h (normal)
    - Serum electrolytes and renal function: within normal limits
    - Urinalysis: negative for myoglobin

    Which of the following is the most likely diagnosis?

    A. Statin-associated necrotizing autoimmune myopathy

    B. Hypothyroid myopathy

    C. Inclusion body myositis

    D. Polymyalgia rheumatica

    E. Exercise-induced rhabdomyolysis

    Correct answer: E

Explanation

This is an example of exercise-induced rhabdomyolysis. This patient presents with subacute proximal lower extremity weakness after vigorous exercise following multiple months of being sedentary. In the case of rhabdomyolysis patients may present with the triad of myalgia, muscle weakness, and dark-colored urine, however, few patients have all three classic symptoms. The lack of medication changes, normal TSH, lack distal upper extremity weakness, and normal inflammatory markers make the other answer choices less likely to be correct.

References

Huerta-Alardín AL, Varon J, Marik PE. (2005). *"Bench-to-bedside review: Rhabdomyolysis — an overview for clinicians."* Crit Care, 9(2);158–69.

Miller, R. (2025). *Rhabdomyolysis: Clinical manifestations and diagnosis*. UpToDate. Retrieved June 2, 2025, from https://www.uptodate.com/contents/rhabdomyolysis-clinical-manifestations-and-diagnosis

42. In the case of paraneoplastic autonomic neuropathy associated with small cell lung cancer, what is the mechanism of action by which neuronal damage occurs?

    A. Malignant cells directly invading neurons

    B. Deposition of immune complexes in autonomic ganglia

    C. Antibody mediated disruption of voltage-gated calcium channels at the neuromuscular junction

D. Autoimmune attack on neuronal antigens shared between tumor and autonomic neurons

E. Ischemic injury due to paraneoplastic vasculitis

Correct answer: D

Explanation

In paraneoplastic autonomic neuropathy, the immune system produces antibodies (i.e., anti-Hu in the case of small cell lung cancer) that target antigens shared between tumor cells and neurons. As a result, there is immune-mediated neuronal injury, rather than direct tumor invasion or vascular pathology. The neurons that are targeted are often involved in the autonomic nervous system, leading to symptoms such as orthostatic hypotension, gastrointestinal dysmotility, and sexual dysfunction.

References

Graus F, Dalmau J. Paraneoplastic neurological syndromes: diagnosis and treatment. *Curr Opin Neurol.* 2012;25(6):795–801.

Pittock SJ, Lucchinetti CF, Parisi JE, et al. Paraneoplastic autonomic neuropathy and small cell lung carcinoma: clinical and immunologic features. *Neurology.* 2001;56(12):1741–7.

43. A 15-year-old boy presents with constant discomfort of his hands and feet, described as burning pain involving his palms and soles. He also endorses poor exercise tolerance and decreased sweating when attempting to exercise. On physical examination he is noted to have small, raised, dark red papules clustered throughout his torso. What is the pathophysiologic mechanism of action of the disease he most likely has?

    A. Mutation in voltage-gated sodium channels causing abnormal nerve excitability

    B. Autoimmune destruction of acetylcholine receptors at the neuromuscular junction

    C. Deficiency of alpha-galactosidase A resulting in accumulation of glycosphingolipids

    D. Mutation in keratin genes leading to abnormal skin keratinization

    E. Impaired glucose-6-phosphate dehydrogenase activity causing red blood cell hemolysis

    Correct answer: C

Explanation

This patient's symptoms of burning pain in the hands and feet (acroparesthesias), poor exercise tolerance, decreased sweating (hypohidrosis), with the presence of dark red papules (angiokeratomas), is characteristic of Fabry disease. Fabry disease is an X-linked glycolipid storage disease caused by deficient activity of the lysosomal enzyme alpha-galactosidase A. This causes accumulation of glycosphingolipids in lysosomes of various cell types, including endothelial cells and neurons. Neurologic manifestations include small-fiber peripheral neuropathy. The painful paresthesias are sometimes misdiagnosed as "growth pain." As patients age the pain tends to decrease secondary to progressive nerve fiber loss.

References

Cruse R, Schiffmann R. Fabry disease: Neurologic manifestations. In: Kopp J, ed. *UpToDate.* Waltham, MA: UpToDate; 2025. Available at: https://www.uptodate.com/contents/fabry-disease-neurologic-manifestations?search=Fabry%20disease&topicRef=7195&source=see_link. Accessed June 3, 2025.

Michaud M, Mauhin W, Belmatoug N, Bedreddine N, Garnotel R, Catros F, Lidove O, Gaches F. Maladie de Fabry : quand y penser ? [Fabry disease: A review]. Rev Med Interne. 2021 Feb;42(2):110–119. French. https://doi.org/10.1016/j.revmed.2020.08.019. Epub 2020 Nov 7. PMID: 33172708.

44. A 26-year-old male who recently immigrated from Mexico presents with progressive weakness and numbness in his hands and feet. On examination he has thickened peripheral nerves and muscle wasting in the affected limbs. His dermatologic examination reveals hypopigmented, anesthetic patches with well-defined borders. What would you expect to be demonstrated on nerve biopsy?

    A. Demyelination and axonal loss with lymphocytic infiltration and *Mycobacterium leprae* bacilli within Schwann cells

    B. Segmental demyelination and onion bulb formation without infectious organisms

    C. Necrotizing vasculitis with immune complex deposition

    D. Axonal degeneration with intracellular viral inclusions

    E. Granulomatous inflammation with caseous necrosis

    Correct answer: A

Explanation

This patient's presentation is consistent with leprosy, also known as Hansen's disease. Leprosy is a chronic disease caused by *Mycobacterium leprae* that involves the skin, mucosa of the upper respiratory tract, and peripheral nerves. Within the United States, most cases of leprosy affect immigrants from endemic areas such as Mexico and Southeast Asia. Neurologic manifestation occurs due to bacterial invasion of the Schwann cells in the peripheral nerves.

Consequently, there is both segmental demyelination and axonal degeneration. Sensory and potentially motor loss tends to occur in the distribution of the nerves that are in close vicinity to the tuberculoid lesion.

References

Cruse R. Overview of acquired peripheral neuropathies in children. In: Kopp J, ed. *UpToDate*. Waltham, MA: UpToDate; 2025. Available at: https://www.upto-date.com/contents/overview-of-acquired-peripheral-neuropathies-in-children?search=diphtheria%20 neurology&source=search_result&selectedTitle=4~150 &usage_type=default&display_rank=4#H8. Accessed June 3, 2025.

Gilmore A, Roller J, Dyer JA. Leprosy (Hansen's disease): An Update and Review. Mo Med. 2023 Jan-Feb;120(1):39–44. PMID: 36860602; PMCID: PMC9970335.

45. A 68-year-old man presents with a 6-month history of progressive burning pain and numbness in his feet, along with episodes of dizziness upon standing, early satiety, and urinary difficulties. On physical examination, he has orthostatic hypotension and decreased pinprick and temperature sensation in a stocking distribution over his lower extremities, but proprioception and vibration sense are preserved. Reflexes are normal. Nerve conduction studies and electromyography reveal no abnormalities in large myelinated fibers. A skin punch biopsy is performed to evaluate small fiber neuropathy. What histopathologic finding do you expect to observe on the skin biopsy?
    A. Markedly decreased epidermal nerve fiber density with Congo red-positive amyloid deposits surrounding small nerve fibers
    B. Demyelination with onion bulb formation around large nerve fibers
    C. Perivascular lymphocytic infiltration with deposition of immune complexes in vessel walls
    D. Presence of viral cytopathic changes within Schwann cells
    E. Fibrinoid necrosis and inflammation of vasa nervorum causing ischemic nerve injury

Correct answer: A

Explanation

This is an example of small fiber neuropathy caused by amyloidosis. In the case of amyloidosis, amyloid fibrils deposit in peripheral nerves, especially small unmyelinated fibers responsible for pain and autonomic function. Early on the large fiber nerves may not be affected, hence the normal

nerve conduction study and electromyography. Skin biopsy demonstrates decreased epidermal nerve fiber density and Congo red staining may reveal amyloid deposits.

References

Gertz MA. Immunoglobulin light chain amyloidosis: 2018 update on diagnosis, prognosis, and treatment. *Am J Hematol*. 2018;93(9):1169–1180. https://doi.org/10.1002/ ajh.25111

Gibbons CH, Freeman R. Diagnosis of small fiber neuropathy: a comparative study of methodologies. *Neurology*. 2010;75(11):998–1004. https://doi.org/10.1212/ WNL.0b013e3181f13d80

46. A 47-year-old woman presents with an 8-month history of progressive burning pain and tingling in her feet. She reports episodic lightheadedness when going from sitting to standing as well as decreased sweating. On examination there is loss of pinprick sensation in a stocking distribution in the lower extremities, with normal vibration and proprioception. Motor strength is 5/5 throughout and reflexes are 2+. Nerve conduction studies are normal. Which of the following is the most appropriate diagnostic test to confirm the suspected diagnosis?
    A. Nerve conduction study and electromyography
    B. Skin punch biopsy to measure intraepidermal nerve fiber density
    C. Serum vitamin B12 and methylmalonic acid levels
    D. MRI of the total spine
    E. Lumbar puncture with cerebrospinal fluid analysis

Correct answer: B

Explanation

The patient's presentation of distal pinprick sensation loss, orthostatic hypotension, and hypohidrosis are concerning for small fiber neuropathy. The lack of involvement of vibration and proprioception, normal strength, normal reflexes, in conjunction with the normal nerve conduction studies makes large fiber neuropathy less likely. The diagnostic test for small fiber neuropathy is a skin punch biopsy. This test enables the quantification of intraepidermal nerve fiber density. Reduced density ultimately confirms the diagnosis.

References

Devigili G, Tugnoli V, Penza P, et al. The diagnostic criteria for small fibre neuropathy: from symptoms to neuropathology. *Brain*. 2008;131(7):1912–1925. https://doi. org/10.1093/brain/awn093

Lauria G, Hsieh ST, Johansson O, et al. European Federation of Neurological Societies/Peripheral Nerve Society guideline on the use of skin biopsy in the diagnosis of small fiber neuropathy. *Eur J Neurol*. 2010;17(7):903–912. https://doi.org/10.1111/j.1468-1331.2010.02999.x

47. A 50-year-old woman with breast cancer is receiving chemotherapy. After multiple rounds of chemotherapy treatments, she develops painful numbness and tingling in her hands and feet. Her oncologist is reviewing her treatment regimen to identify the likely cause of her symptoms. Which of the following chemotherapy agents is *least likely* to cause peripheral neuropathy as a side effect?
    A. Paclitaxel
    B. Vincristine
    C. Cisplatin
    D. Doxorubicin
    E. Bortezomib
    Correct answer: D

Explanation

Doxorubicin is most commonly associated with cardio-toxicity, myelosuppression, and mucositis. It is not commonly linked to peripheral neuropathy. The other answer choices are commonly associated with chemotherapy-induced peripheral neuropathy (CIPN). Sensory, motor, and autonomic nerves can be affected. While there is no cure for CIPN, various neuropathic pain medications are used to help manage symptoms. There are no proven methods to prevent CIPN, but dose adjustment may help to minimize risk.

References

Park SB, Goldstein D, Krishnan AV, et al. Chemotherapy-induced peripheral neurotoxicity: a critical analysis. *CA Cancer J Clin*. 2013;63(6):419–437. https://doi.org/10.3322/caac.21146

Thompson AM. Overview of side effects of chemotherapy for early-stage breast cancer. In: UpToDate, Post TW (Ed), UpToDate, Waltham, MA. Updated May 9, 2024. Available from: https://www.uptodate.com/contents/overview-of-side-effects-of-chemotherapy-for-early-stage-breast-cancer. Accessed June 3, 2025.

48. A 58-year-old man develops progressive difficulty in climbing stairs and intermittent choking on liquids. Examination shows tongue fasciculations, hyperreflexia, and EMG with widespread fibrillations and fascicula-tions. He is diagnosed with ALS and you plan on initiating Riluzole. Which of the following is the mechanism of action of that medication?
    A. Inhibition of presynaptic glutamate release
    B. Scavenging of free radicals and reduction of oxidative stress

C. Stabilization of mitochondrial and endoplasmic reticulum function
    D. Inhibition of acetylcholinesterase activity
    E. Enhancement of GABA-A receptor transmission
    Correct answer: A

Explanation

Riluzole is an FDA-approved medication for ALS that modestly extends survival by approximately 2–3 months. Its primary mechanism is *inhibition of presynaptic glutamate release*, thus reducing glutamate-mediated excitotoxicity in both upper and lower motor neurons. While riluzole also has some sodium channel blocking properties, its main clinical benefit stems from decreasing excessive glutamatergic neurotransmission, a key driver of neuronal injury in ALS.

Option B describes edaravone, which acts as a free radical scavenger and combats oxidative stress to preserve motor neurons. Option C refers to sodium phenylbutyrate and taurursodiol, believed to stabilize mitochondrial and endoplasmic reticulum function to delay neuronal death.

Option D, inhibition of acetylcholinesterase, is the mechanism of drugs used in Alzheimer's disease (e.g., donepezil), not ALS. Option E, enhancement of GABA-A receptor transmission, describes the action of benzodiazepines and is unrelated to ALS disease-modifying therapies.

References

Bensimon G, Lacomblez L, Meininger V, et al; ALS/Riluzole Study Group. A controlled trial of riluzole in amyotrophic lateral sclerosis. *N Engl J Med*. 1994;330(9):585–591. https://doi.org/10.1056/NEJM199403033300901.

Paganoni S, Macklin EA, Hendrix S, et al. Trial of Sodium Phenylbutyrate-Taurursodiol for Amyotrophic Lateral Sclerosis. *N Engl J Med*. 2020;383(10):919–930. https://doi.org/10.1056/NEJMoa1916945

49. A 45-year-old woman with a family history of ALS in her father presents with progressive limb weakness, muscle atrophy, and brisk reflexes. Genetic testing reveals a pathogenic variant in SOD1. What is the inheritance pattern of SOD1-related ALS?
    A. Autosomal recessive
    B. X-linked recessive
    C. Autosomal dominant
    D. Mitochondrial
    E. Digenic
    Correct answer: C

Explanation

About 20% of familial ALS cases are due to autosomal-dominant mutations in the SOD1 gene, which encodes superoxide dismutase 1. Penetrance is high but age-related, and the clinical course resembles sporadic ALS.

Reference

Renton AE, Chio A, Traynor BJ. State of play in amyotrophic lateral sclerosis genetics. *Nat Neurosci.* 2014;17(1):17–23. https://doi.org/10.1038/nn.3584.

50. A 6-month-old girl with hypotonia and poor head control is diagnosed with SMA type 1. Parents ask about the mechanism of the first-line therapy. Which describes how nusinersen works?
    A. Gene replacement via AAV9 vector
    B. Antisense oligonucleotide enhancing SMN2 exon 7 inclusion
    C. Small-molecule SMN2 splicing modulator
    D. CRISPR-Cas9 correction of SMN1
    E. Stabilization of SMN protein
    Correct answer: B

Explanation

Nusinersen is an intrathecal 2′-O-methoxyethyl antisense oligonucleotide that binds SMN2 pre-mRNA, promoting exon 7 inclusion and increasing full-length SMN protein. In the ENDEAR trial, nusinersen led to significant improvements in motor milestones and event-free survival in infants with SMA type 1 ($p < 0.001$).

Reference

Finkel RS, Mercuri E, Darras BT, et al. Nusinersen versus sham control in infantile-onset spinal muscular atrophy. *N Engl J Med.* 2017;377(18):1723–1732. https://doi.org/10.1056/NEJMoa1702752.

51. A 50-year-old man presents with slowly progressive limb and bulbar weakness, gynecomastia, and a fine tremor. Neurologic examination reveals mild facial weakness and diffuse muscle fasciculations; EMG demonstrates chronic denervation in multiple myotomes. Which type of genetic mutation underlies his condition?
    A. Missense point mutation
    B. CAG trinucleotide repeat expansion
    C. Large gene deletion
    D. Exonic duplication
    E. Promoter hypermethylation
    Correct answer: B

Explanation

The combination of adult-onset bulbar and limb weakness with endocrine manifestations (gynecomastia) is characteristic of spinal and bulbar muscular atrophy (Kennedy disease). SBMA is an X-linked recessive motor neuron disease caused by a CAG trinucleotide repeat expansion >35 in exon 1 of the androgen receptor gene. Longer repeats correlate inversely with age at onset but not rate of progression.

Reference

La Spada AR, Wilson EM, Lubahn DB, Harding AE, Fischbeck KH. Androgen receptor gene mutations in X-linked spinal and bulbar muscular atrophy. *Nature.* 1991;352(6330):77–79. https://doi.org/10.1038/352077a0.

52. A 6-month-old Ashkenazi Jewish infant presents with developmental regression, exaggerated startle, and a cherry-red macula. Which enzyme deficiency causes this disease?
    A. Beta-glucocerebrosidase
    B. Alpha-L-iduronidase
    C. Beta-hexosaminidase A
    D. Arylsulfatase A
    E. Glucosylceramide synthase
    Correct answer: C

Explanation

Tay-Sachs disease is an autosomal recessive lysosomal storage disorder caused by deficiency of *beta-hexosaminidase A*, leading to accumulation of GM2 ganglioside in neurons. It typically presents between 3 and 6 months of age with *developmental regression, exaggerated startle, hypotonia*, and the classic *cherry-red spot* on the macula. It is more common in Ashkenazi Jewish populations and does *not involve hepatosplenomegaly*, which helps differentiate it from other storage disorders like Gaucher disease.

Reference

Myerowitz R. Tay-Sachs disease-causing mutations and neutral polymorphisms in the Hex A gene. Hum Mutat. 1997;9(3):195–208. https://doi.org/10.1002/(SICI)1098-1004(1997)9:3<195::AID-HUMU1>3.0.CO;2-7. PMID: 9090523.

Linked questions: 52–53

52. A 19-year-old male presents with progressive weakness and atrophy of his right hand and wrist over the past two years. The symptoms have now stabilized. There is no sensory loss or upper motor neuron signs. Cervical spine MRI in the neutral position is unremarkable. What is the most likely diagnosis?
    A. Cervical spondylotic myelopathy
    B. Multifocal motor neuropathy
    C. Hirayama disease
    D. Spinal muscular atrophy
    E. Charcot-Marie-Tooth disease
    Correct answer: C

Explanation

This presentation is classic for *Hirayama disease (monomelic amyotrophy)*, a rare cervical myelopathy affecting young males. It typically presents with *unilateral distal upper limb weakness and wasting*, most often in the *C7–T1 myotomes*, which stabilizes after a few years. The absence of sensory findings and upper motor neuron signs, along with normal neutral MRI, are distinguishing features.

Reference

Hirayama K. [Juvenile muscular atrophy of unilateral upper extremity (Hirayama disease)--half-century progress and establishment since its discovery]. Brain Nerve. 2008 Jan;60(1):17–29. Japanese. PMID: 18232329.

Linked question

53. Which of the following findings on flexion cervical MRI would confirm the diagnosis?

    A. Anterior cord compression by osteophytes
    B. Forward displacement of posterior dural sac
    C. Intramedullary T2 hyperintensity at C4
    D. Laminar hypertrophy of facet joints
    E. Syrinx formation
    Correct answer: B

Explanation

Flexion MRI in Hirayama disease demonstrates *anterior displacement of the posterior dura*, leading to a crescent-shaped enlarged *posterior epidural space*, often with prominent *engorged epidural veins*. This dynamic compression transiently reduces blood flow and causes chronic ischemia of the anterior horn cells in the lower cervical spinal cord. The key radiologic sign is *an increased laminodural space*, typically more than 6 mm during flexion.

Reference

Hirayama K. [Juvenile muscular atrophy of unilateral upper extremity (Hirayama disease)--half-century progress and establishment since its discovery]. Brain Nerve. 2008 Jan;60(1):17–29. Japanese. PMID: 18232329.

54. A 21-year-old man presents with progressive weakness and atrophy of his right hand and forearm over the past two years. He denies sensory symptoms or bowel/bladder dysfunction. Neurological exam reveals decreased grip strength and visible muscle wasting of the intrinsic hand muscles on the right, without fasciculations or spasticity. Cervical spine MRI in neutral position is normal. A *flexion MRI* is obtained and shown below:

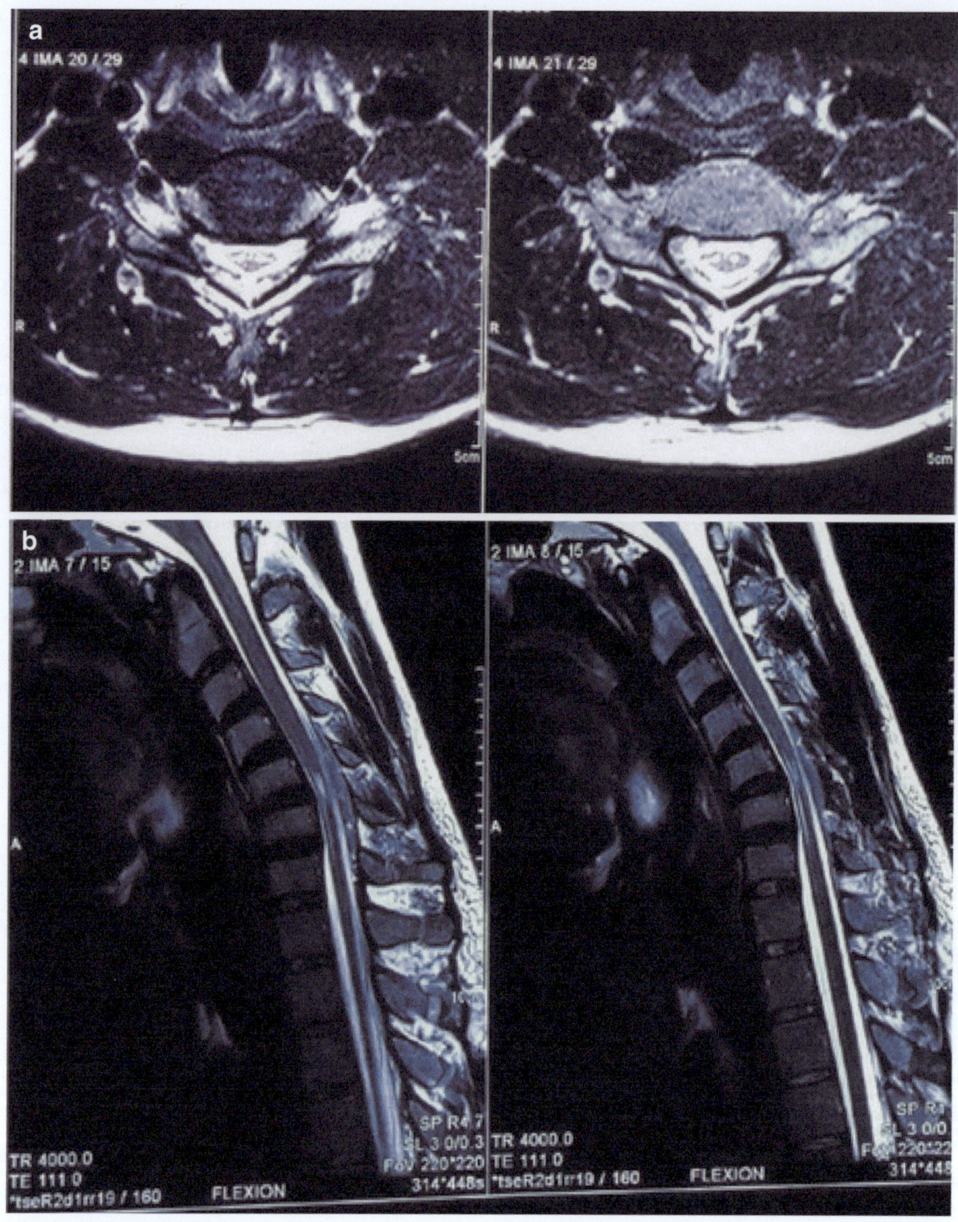

(**a**) Axial and (**b**) sagittal MRI of the cervical spine. (Source: Anuradha S, Fanai via Case Reports in Neurological Medicine (2016). CC-BY 4.0. (https://creativecommons.org/licenses/by/4.0/). Images have not been modified. Please see full attribution with citation below in references section for this question)

What is the most likely diagnosis?
    A. Cervical spondylotic myelopathy
    B. Hirayama disease
    C. Spinal muscular atrophy
    D. Multifocal motor neuropathy
    E. Multiple sclerosis
    Correct answer: B

Explanation

The image shows *anterior displacement of the posterior dura* during neck flexion with a crescent-shaped *posterior epidural space*, characteristic of *Hirayama disease*. This dynamic myelopathy predominantly affects young males and causes slowly progressive, unilateral distal upper limb weakness, and wasting (monomelic amyotrophy). Flexion MRI is essential for diagnosis, as neutral imaging may appear normal.

References

Anuradha S, Fanai via Case Reports in Neurological Medicine (2016). CC-BY 4.0 (https://creativecommons.org/licenses/by/4.0/). Images have not been modified.

Anuradha S, Fanai V. Hirayama Disease: A Rare Disease with Unusual Features. *Case Rep Neurol Med.* 2016;2016:5839761. https://doi.org/10.1155/2016/5839761

Boruah DK, Prakash A, Gogoi BB, Yadav RR, Dhingani DD, Sarma B. The Importance of Flexion MRI in Hirayama Disease with Special Reference to Laminodural Space Measurements. *AJNR Am J Neuroradiol.* 2018;39(5):974–980. https://doi.org/10.3174/ajnr.A5577

55. A 67-year-old smoker develops subacute progressive limb weakness with EMG evidence of denervation. Anti-Hu antibodies are positive; a lung mass is found. What is the most likely underlying tumor?
    A. Squamous cell carcinoma of lung
    B. Small-cell lung cancer
    C. Adenocarcinoma of colon
    D. Breast carcinoma
    E. Ovarian teratoma
    Correct answer: B

Explanation

Anti-Hu (ANNA-1) paraneoplastic syndrome is most often associated with limited-stage small-cell lung cancer and may present as sensory neuropathy, encephalomyelitis, or lower motor neuron syndrome.

Reference

Graus F, Dalmau J. Paraneoplastic neurological syndromes: diagnosis and treatment. Curr Opin Neurol. 2007 Dec;20(6):732–7. https://doi.org/10.1097/WCO.0b013e3282f189dc. PMID: 17992098.

Linked questions: 56–57

56. A 64-year-old man presents with rapidly progressive weakness and muscle atrophy in the right hand and forearm, followed by slurred speech and difficulty swallowing over 6 weeks. Neurologic exam reveals asymmetric distal wasting of the upper limbs, tongue fasciculations, and hyperreflexia. He has no sensory deficits. EMG shows diffuse fibrillation potentials and fasciculations in bulbar and cervical segments without sensory involvement. Brain and cervical spine MRI are unremarkable. A chest CT reveals a right perihilar mass with mediastinal adenopathy.

    What is the most likely diagnosis?
    A. Sporadic ALS
    B. West Nile virus–associated poliomyelitis

C. Paraneoplastic lower motor neuronopathy
    D. Adult-onset SMA type IV
    E. Multifocal motor neuropathy
    Correct answer: C

Explanation

This presentation is most consistent with a paraneoplastic motor neuron syndrome. The red flags here are the acute-to-subacute onset, the presence of bulbar symptoms, the rapid progression, and most importantly, the discovery of a lung mass—suggestive of small cell lung carcinoma. These syndromes mimic ALS but progress more rapidly and may improve with treatment of the underlying malignancy or immunotherapy.

Sporadic ALS is typically more insidious in onset and not usually associated with malignancy. West Nile virus poliomyelitis can cause acute flaccid paralysis but is often associated with fever, meningitis, or encephalitis, and wouldn't present with isolated bulbar symptoms in this age group. Adult-onset SMA is a slowly progressive pure lower motor neuron syndrome with no known association with cancer. Multifocal motor neuropathy does not fit the full clinical picture here.

Linked question

57. Which of the following antibodies is most classically associated with this paraneoplastic motor neuron presentation?
    A. Anti-GAD65
    B. Anti-SOX1
    C. Anti-Hu (ANNA-1)
    D. Anti-GM2
    E. Anti-Zic4
    Correct answer: C

Explanation

Anti-Hu (ANNA-1) antibodies are strongly associated with paraneoplastic motor neuron syndromes, especially in patients with small cell lung cancer. These antibodies target neuronal nuclear antigens and are markers of a cytotoxic T-cell–mediated autoimmune process affecting anterior horn cells and other parts of the nervous system. Clinical presentations may mimic ALS, particularly in the presence of bulbar symptoms, and antibody testing can guide diagnosis and prompt cancer screening.

Anti-GAD65 antibodies are typically linked to stiff-person syndrome and some cerebellar syndromes. Anti-SOX1 is associated with Lambert-Eaton myasthenic syndrome and sometimes paraneoplastic cerebellar degeneration, but not with motor neuronopathies. Anti-GM2 is not a clinically relevant paraneoplastic antibody; ganglioside antibodies (like anti-GM1 or GD1a) are more relevant in neuropathies, not motor neuron disease. Anti-Zic4 is primarily associated with paraneoplastic cerebellar degeneration, particularly in association with small cell lung cancer, but not with motor neuronopathy.

Reference

Lancaster E. Paraneoplastic Disorders. Continuum (Minneap Minn). 2017 Dec;23(6, Neuro-oncology):1653–1679. https://doi.org/10.1212/CON.0000000000000542. PMID: 29200116.

58. A 34-year-old man from South Asia presents with gradually progressive leg stiffness and difficulty walking over several months. He reports consuming large quantities of grass pea as a dietary staple during the past year due to limited food availability. On examination, he has bilateral lower extremity spasticity, brisk reflexes, and extensor plantar responses. There is no sensory involvement or sphincter dysfunction. His upper limbs and cranial nerves are unaffected.

    Which neurotoxin is the most likely cause of his condition?
    A. β-methylamino-L-alanine (BMAA)
    B. β-N-oxalylamino-L-alanine (β-ODAP)
    C. Aflatoxin B1
    D. Cyanide
    E. Ochratoxin A
    Correct answer: B

Explanation

This clinical presentation is consistent with *neurolathyrism*, a neurodegenerative disease seen in populations relying heavily on *Lathyrus sativus* (grass pea) during food shortages. The responsible neurotoxin is *β-ODAP*, a glutamate analog that induces excitotoxicity by activating AMPA/kainate receptors. This leads to selective *upper motor neuron damage*, presenting with isolated spastic paraparesis, preserved sensory function, and no bladder involvement.

Other options:

- *BMAA* is linked to ALS-parkinsonism-dementia in Guam but not to lathyrism.
- *Aflatoxin B1* causes hepatotoxicity and is a known carcinogen.
- *Cyanide* causes acute mitochondrial toxicity and encephalopathy.
- *Ochratoxin A* is nephrotoxic and carcinogenic, not linked to motor neuron syndrome

Reference

Spencer PS, Roy DN, Ludolph A, Hugon J, Dwivedi MP, Schaumburg HH. Lathyrism: evidence for role of the neuroexcitatory aminoacid BOAA. Lancet. 1986 Nov 8;2(8515):1066–7. https://doi.org/10.1016/s0140-6736(86)90468-x. PMID: 2877226.

59. A 29-year-old unvaccinated man presents with progressive trismus, opisthotonus, and painful generalized muscle spasms after stepping on a rusty nail. Which of the following best explains the pathogenic mechanism of the responsible neurotoxin?
    A. Cleavage of SNARE proteins at the neuromuscular junction, blocking acetylcholine release
    B. Cleavage of synaptobrevin in inhibitory interneurons, blocking GABA, and glycine release
    C. Direct destruction of anterior horn cells leading to flaccid paralysis
    D. Immune-mediated demyelination of motor fibers
    E. Excessive presynaptic glutamate release causing excitotoxicity
    Correct answer: B

Explanation

Tetanospasmin, produced by *Clostridium tetani*, is internalized at the wound site and transported retrogradely into the CNS. There, it specifically targets inhibitory interneurons in the spinal cord and brainstem. It cleaves synaptobrevin (a SNARE complex protein essential for vesicular neurotransmitter release), inhibiting the release of the inhibitory neurotransmitters GABA and glycine. The loss of inhibition leads to continuous motor neuron activation, manifesting clinically as muscle rigidity, trismus, and spasms.

- *Option A* describes *botulinum toxin* action, which blocks acetylcholine release at the neuromuscular junction, leading to *flaccid paralysis*, not the spasticity seen in tetanus.
- *Option C* refers to the mechanism of poliomyelitis, which selectively destroys anterior horn cells, again causing *flaccid paralysis*.
- *Option D* describes autoimmune processes such as Guillain-Barré syndrome, characterized by peripheral demyelination and weakness, not toxin-mediated spasticity.
- *Option E* (glutamate excitotoxicity) is relevant to some neurodegenerative diseases but not to the pathophysiology of tetanus.

Reference

Pellizzari R, Rossetto O, Schiavo G, Montecucco C. Tetanus and botulinum neurotoxins: mechanism of action and therapeutic uses. Philos Trans R Soc Lond B Biol Sci. 1999 Feb 28;354(1381):259–68. https://doi.org/10.1098/rstb.1999.0377. PMID: 10212474; PMCID: PMC1692495.

60. A previously healthy 8-year-old develops sudden arm weakness and MRI shows spinal gray matter lesions. EV-D68 is detected in respiratory swab. Which best describes the pathogenesis?
    A. Molecular mimicry causing autoimmune axonal damage
    B. Direct infection and injury of anterior horn cells
    C. Demyelination of peripheral nerves
    D. Blockade of acetylcholine receptors
    E. Cerebral vasculitis
    Correct answer: B.

Explanation

EV-D68 can cause acute flaccid myelitis by direct invasion and replication in anterior horn motor neurons, producing poliomyelitis-like paralysis. Option A (molecular mimicry) is more typical of post-infectious syndromes like Guillain-Barré syndrome. Option C (peripheral nerve demyelination) describes acute inflammatory demyelinating polyneuropathy (AIDP). Option D (acetylcholine receptor blockade) refers to the pathogenesis of myasthenia gravis.

Option E (cerebral vasculitis) is not a feature of EV-D68-related acute flaccid myelitis.

Reference

Messacar K, Asturias EJ, Hixon AM, Van Leer-Buter C, Niesters HGM, Tyler KL, Abzug MJ, Dominguez SR. Enterovirus D68 and acute flaccid myelitis-evaluating the evidence for causality. Lancet Infect Dis. 2018 Aug;18(8):e239-e247. https://doi.org/10.1016/S1473-3099(18)30094-X. Epub 2018 Feb 23. PMID: 29482893; PMCID: PMC6778404.

Linked questions: 61–62

61. A 23-year-old woman presents with slowly progressive foot drop and intrinsic hand weakness without sensory symptoms. Nerve conduction studies reveal reduced compound muscle action potentials (CMAPs) with normal sensory nerve action potentials (SNAPs).
    Which diagnosis is most likely?
    A. Charcot-Marie-Tooth disease type 1 (CMT1)
    B. Chronic inflammatory demyelinating polyneuropathy (CIDP)
    C. Distal hereditary motor neuropathy (dHMN)
    D. Multifocal motor neuropathy (MMN)
    E. Amyotrophic lateral sclerosis (ALS)
    Correct answer: C

Explanation

Distal hereditary motor neuropathies (dHMNs) are *pure motor* inherited neuropathies that cause progressive weakness, particularly in the distal limbs, while *sparing sensory fibers*—hence normal sensory nerve action potentials. CMT1 would typically show both motor and sensory involvement with demyelination. CIDP presents with sensory symptoms and demyelination. MMN also causes pure motor deficits but usually shows conduction block rather than simple axonal loss. ALS involves both upper and lower motor neurons and often shows EMG evidence of widespread denervation and reinnervation rather than isolated peripheral nerve findings.

Linked question

62. Based on the diagnosis, which nerve conduction study feature is most characteristic of distal hereditary motor neuropathy?
    A. Demyelinating pattern
    B. Pure motor axonal loss
    C. Uniform slowing of conduction
    D. Conduction block
    E. Abnormal F waves
    Correct answer: B

Explanation

Distal hereditary motor neuropathies (dHMNs) are a heterogeneous group of inherited neuropathies characterized by slowly progressive, length-dependent pure motor axonal degeneration with normal sensory conduction studies. Clinically, they resemble axonal Charcot-Marie-Tooth type 2 (CMT2) but crucially lack sensory involvement.

- Option A (demyelinating pattern) would suggest CMT1 or CIDP.
- Option C (uniform slowing) is typical for demyelinating diseases like CMT1.
- Option D (conduction block) is associated with MMN.
- Option E (abnormal F-waves) may be seen in various motor neuron disorders but is nonspecific and not the hallmark finding for dHMN.

Reference

Tazir M, Nouioua S. Distal hereditary motor neuropathies. Rev Neurol (Paris). 2024 Dec;180(10):1031–1036. https://doi.org/10.1016/j.neurol.2023.09.005. Epub 2024 May 3. PMID: 38702287.

Linked questions: 63–64

63. A 64-year-old man with type 2 diabetes presents with 3 weeks of progressive left thigh pain followed by weakness. He now requires a cane to walk due to knee buckling. On exam, he has atrophy and weakness of the left quadriceps and an absent left patellar reflex. Sensation is intact. EMG/NCS shows active denervation in the left iliopsoas and quadriceps muscles, with normal sural sensory responses.

    What is the most likely diagnosis?
    A. Femoral neuropathy
    B. L2–L4 lumbar plexopathy
    C. Lumbosacral radiculoplexus neuropathy
    D. Anterior horn cell disease
    E. Neuromuscular junction disorder
    Correct answer: C

Explanation

This patient presents with diabetic lumbosacral radiculoplexus neuropathy (DLRPN), also known as diabetic amyotrophy. It begins with severe proximal leg pain followed by weakness and atrophy, often asymmetrical. EMG findings of denervation in proximal muscles with preserved sural sensory responses suggest a *radiculopathy* rather than peripheral nerve involvement. In DLRPN, ischemic injury affects multiple roots (most often L2–L4), resulting in a polyradiculopathy pattern. Other conditions, such as *femoral neuropathy*, typically affect only one nerve and would not explain the diffuse muscle involvement. *Lumbar plexopathy* could involve multiple muscles, but it would present with a more *diffuse weakness* and would not spare sensation in this way. *Anterior horn cell diseases*, like ALS, would cause *widespread* weakness and *upper motor neuron signs*, which are absent here. Finally, *neuromuscular junction disorders* such as myasthenia gravis would not cause the *persistent muscle atrophy* or specific EMG findings seen in DLRPN.

Linked question

64. What is the most appropriate first-line management?
    A. High-dose corticosteroids
    B. IV immunoglobulin
    C. Conservative supportive care
    D. Plasma exchange
    E. Surgical decompression
    Correct answer: C

Explanation

The primary management for diabetic lumbosacral radiculoplexus neuropathy (DLRPN) is supportive care, including optimal glycemic control, pain management (typically with neuropathic agents like gabapentin or duloxetine), and physical and occupational therapy to maintain strength and mobility. Although small studies and case series have suggested that corticosteroids or immunotherapy (like IVIG) might accelerate early symptom improvement by reducing presumed inflammation, high-quality randomized controlled trials have not proven a consistent benefit. Therefore, routine use of steroids or immunomodulatory therapy is not universally recommended. Most patients gradually recover strength and function over 6–18 months with conservative therapy alone.

Reference

Dyck PJ, Windebank AJ. Diabetic and nondiabetic lumbosacral radiculoplexus neuropathies: new insights into pathophysiology and treatment. Muscle Nerve. 2002 Apr;25(4):477–91. https://doi.org/10.1002/mus.10080. PMID: 11932965.

65. A 47-year-old man presents with a 3-week history of right foot drop. On examination, you find weakness in dorsiflexion and inversion of the foot. The ankle jerk reflex is normal, and there is no weakness in hip flexion or knee extension. Sensory examination reveals hypoesthesia over the dorsum of the foot and lateral aspect of the lower leg.

    What is the most likely localization of the lesion?
    A. Peroneal neuropathy at the fibular head
    B. L5 radiculopathy
    C. Sciatic neuropathy
    D. Lumbosacral plexopathy
    Correct answer: B.

Explanation

The patient's symptoms of foot drop, weakness in dorsiflexion, and inversion, along with sensory changes in the *L5 dermatome* (dorsum of the foot and lateral lower leg), point to *L5 radiculopathy* as the most likely diagnosis. The *normal ankle reflex* and absence of other significant weaknesses (such as in hip flexion or knee extension) further support this, indicating a *nerve root* issue at the *L5 level*. *Peroneal neuropathy* typically affects *foot dorsiflexion and eversion*, but does not cause significant weakness in inversion, which is more indicative of *L5 involvement*. *Sciatic neuropathy* would affect *hip extension and knee flexion*, but not selective weakness in dorsiflexion or inversion. *Lumbosacral plexopathy* could present with more generalized weakness, but this case is more confined to the L5 root.

Reference

Preston, D. C., & Shapiro, B. E. (2013). **Electromyography and Neuromuscular Disorders: Clinical-Electrophysiologic Correlations** (3rd ed.). Elsevier

66. A 52-year-old man presents with a 3-week history of right foot drop and numbness over the dorsum of the foot. On examination, you observe weakness in dorsiflexion and difficulty lifting the toes during gait. The ankle reflexes are normal, and there is no weakness in hip flexion or knee extension. Sensory examination reveals hypoesthesia over the L5 dermatome. Given the clinical presentation, you suspect L5 radiculopathy.

    Which group of muscles is most likely to show abnormalities on EMG?
    A. Extensor hallucis longus, tibialis anterior, and gluteus maximus
    B. Extensor hallucis longus, tibialis anterior, and hamstrings
    C. Extensor hallucis longus, tibialis posterior, and gastrocnemius
    D. Extensor hallucis longus, flexor hallucis longus, and tibialis posterior
    E. Gluteus medius, vastus lateralis, and hamstrings
    Correct answer: B

Explanation

In L5 radiculopathy, the L5 nerve root is involved, which supplies motor function to muscles including the extensor hallucis longus (responsible for great toe dorsiflexion), tibialis anterior (which controls foot dorsiflexion), and the hamstrings (specifically the biceps femoris). These muscles are expected to show abnormalities on EMG, including denervation or reduced motor action potentials. The gluteus maximus and gastrocnemius (involved in hip and plantarflexion, respectively) are more associated with other nerve roots like L4 and S1, not L5. The flexor hallucis longus are innervated by the tibial nerve with S1 and S2 contribution, not directly by the L5 root.

Reference

Preston DC, Shapiro BE. *Electromyography and Neuromuscular Disorders: Clinical-Electrophysiologic Correlations*. 3rd ed. Elsevier Saunders; 2013.

67. A 58-year-old woman with a history of diabetes mellitus, hypertension and chronic alcoholism presents with a 6-month history of progressive numbness and weakness in her lower extremities, particularly difficulty walking and frequent falls. On examination, she has bilateral lower extremity weakness, mainly in ankle dorsiflexion and hip flexion, with hyperreflexia and positive Babinski signs. Sensory examination reveals loss of vibration and proprioception in the lower limbs, while pain and temperature sensation are preserved. An MRI of the spine shows T2 hyperintensities in the posterior columns of the thoracic and cervical spinal cord.

    Which of the following deficiencies is most likely responsible for the patient's findings?
    A. Vitamin B12 deficiency
    B. Vitamin E deficiency
    C. Folate deficiency
    D. Copper deficiency
    E. Vitamin D deficiency
    Correct answer: A

Explanation

This patient's clinical presentation and MRI findings of T2 hyperintensities in the posterior columns of the thoracic and cervical spinal cord, along with bilateral lower extremity weakness and sensory changes (loss of vibration and proprioception), are consistent with B12 deficiency myeloneuropathy and subacute combined degeneration (SCD) of the spinal cord. Vitamin B12 deficiency leads to demyelination of the dorsal columns and corticospinal tracts, resulting in sensory ataxia, hyperreflexia, and lower extremity weakness. This condition is most often seen in patients with chronic alcoholism, pernicious anemia, or malnutrition, as in this case.

Vitamin E deficiency (B) can cause sensory and motor deficits due to spinocerebellar ataxia, but it typically involves progressive ataxia, dysarthria, and vision problems, with no characteristic dorsal column involvement seen on MRI. Vitamin E deficiency is also rarely associated with posterior column demyelination like in B12 deficiency.

Folate deficiency (C) can lead to peripheral neuropathy and myelopathy, but it typically causes megaloblastic anemia and peripheral neuropathy rather than subacute combined degeneration of the spinal cord. Folate deficiency does not generally cause the posterior column changes or hyperreflexia seen in B12 deficiency.

Copper deficiency (D) can cause a myeloneuropathy similar to B12 deficiency, resulting in subacute combined degeneration. However, copper deficiency is typically associated with hypopigmentation (i.e., Menke's disease in children or idiopathic copper deficiency in adults) and would present with additional signs like anemia and neutropenia. MRI findings in copper deficiency may also not have the classic posterior column pattern seen in B12 deficiency.

Vitamin D deficiency (E) can lead to muscle weakness and bone pain, particularly in the context of osteomalacia, but it does not typically cause myeloneuropathy or posterior column demyelination. The neurological manifestations of vitamin D deficiency are usually limited to proximal muscle weakness rather than sensory and motor deficits with spinal cord involvement.

Reference

Saji AM, Lui F, De Jesus O. Spinal Cord Subacute Combined Degeneration. [Updated 2024 Apr 21]. In: StatPearls [Internet]. Treasure Island (FL): StatPearls Publishing; 2025 Jan-. Available from: https://www.ncbi.nlm.nih.gov/books/NBK560728/

68. A 58-year-old man presents with neck pain radiating into his right arm for the past 3 weeks. He reports tingling in the right thumb and mild weakness when lifting objects. On examination, he has weakness in elbow flexion and decreased sensation in the lateral forearm and thumb. What is the most likely affected nerve root?
    A. C5
    B. C6
    C. C7
    D. C8
    E. T1
    Correct answer: B

Explanation

This patient presents with symptoms localizing to the *C6* nerve root, which commonly affects the biceps reflex, elbow flexion, wrist extension, and sensation over the lateral forearm and thumb. C5 radiculopathy would typically involve deltoid weakness and lateral upper arm sensory loss. C7 affects triceps, wrist flexion, and the middle finger. C8 and T1 more commonly involve hand muscles and medial forearm/hand sensory deficits.

Reference

Preston DC, Shapiro BE. *Electromyography and Neuromuscular Disorders: Clinical-Electrophysiologic-Ultrasound Correlations*. 4th ed. Elsevier; 2020. Chapter 32.

69. A 47-year-old man presents with right-sided neck and shoulder pain following a recent lifting injury. He reports difficulty lifting his arm and performing overhead activities. Cervical MRI reveals a right C4–C5 disc herniation compressing the exiting nerve root. Electromyography

is ordered to support the diagnosis. Which of the following muscle groups would most likely show active denervation?
    A. First dorsal interosseous, flexor carpi ulnaris, abductor digiti minimi
    B. Triceps brachii, pronator teres, extensor carpi radialis
    C. Deltoid, biceps brachii, infraspinatus
    D. Abductor pollicis brevis, opponens pollicis, flexor pollicis longus
    E. Brachioradialis, extensor digitorum, supinator
    Correct answer: C

Explanation

This patient presents with classic signs of a *C5 radiculopathy*, including weakness in shoulder abduction and elbow flexion, diminished biceps reflex, and sensory loss over the lateral upper arm. The C5 nerve root provides motor input to several muscles, most notably the *deltoid* (via the axillary nerve), *biceps brachii* (via the musculocutaneous nerve), and *infraspinatus* (via the suprascapular nerve). These muscles are typically sampled during EMG when evaluating suspected C5 radiculopathy. Denervation in these muscles would support involvement of the C5 root. The other options contain muscles innervated by different roots or nerves: choice A includes ulnar-innervated muscles (C8–T1), choice B involves C6–C7 muscles, choice D includes median-innervated hand muscles (C8–T1), and choice E involves radial-innervated forearm muscles (C6–C7). Therefore, only the group in option C is correctly localized to the C5 myotome.

Reference

Preston DC, Shapiro BE. *Electromyography and Neuromuscular Disorders: Clinical-Electrophysiologic-Ultrasound Correlations*. 4th ed. Elsevier; 2020. Chapter 32.

Linked questions: 70–71

70. *Part 1*: A 28-year-old woman presents with new onset fluctuating diplopia and ptosis, more pronounced at the end of the day. Neurologic examination reveals fatigable weakness of the extraocular muscles. To confirm the diagnosis, several diagnostic tests are considered. Which of the following is the most sensitive diagnostic test for generalized myasthenia gravis?
    A. Repetitive nerve stimulation
    B. Single-fiber electromyography (SFEMG)
    C. Chest CT for thymoma
    D. Serum anti-AChR antibody testing
    E. Ice pack test
    Correct answer: B

Linked question

71. She undergoes a single fiber electromyography testing. What finding would most likely be observed in the affected muscle?
    A. Decreased recruitment of motor units
    B. High-frequency repetitive discharges
    C. Increased jitter and blocking
    D. Long-duration motor unit potentials
    E. Increased spontaneous fibrillations and positive sharp waves

    Correct answer: C

Explanation

Single-fiber electromyography (SFEMG) is the most *sensitive* test for detecting defects in neuromuscular transmission and can identify subclinical involvement. In generalized MG, SFEMG has a sensitivity of *up to 99%*, although its specificity is lower since it can be abnormal in other neuromuscular junction disorders. *Anti-AChR antibody testing* (choice D) is highly *specific* (close to 100%), but less *sensitive* (positive in about 80–85% of generalized MG cases and only ~50% in ocular MG). Therefore, *SFEMG* is the most *sensitive and specific combined* neurophysiologic test for MG. Repetitive nerve stimulation (choice A) has lower sensitivity, particularly in ocular MG. The ice pack test (choice E) is a helpful bedside tool but lacks the diagnostic rigor of SFEMG. Chest CT (choice C) is essential for thymoma evaluation but not diagnostic for MG itself. The most characteristic finding on SFEMG is *increased jitter*, which refers to *variation in the time between muscle action potentials*. This is due to the impairment of neuromuscular transmission caused by the *autoantibodies* targeting acetylcholine receptors at the postsynaptic membrane. *Blocking* occurs when an action potential fails to transmit across the neuromuscular junction. These findings are highly suggestive of MG and are often seen even in the absence of clinical weakness.

Reference

Preston DC, Shapiro BE. *Electromyography and Neuromuscular Disorders: Clinical-Electrophysiologic-Ultrasound Correlations*. 4th ed. Elsevier; 2020. Chapter 37.

72. A 50-year-old woman with a known history of generalized myasthenia gravis presents to the emergency department with worsening shortness of breath, inability to speak in full sentences, and difficulty swallowing. She has been feeling progressively more fatigued over the past 48 hours and reports increased weakness in the extremities. On examination, she is unable to lift her head from the pillow, and her respiratory rate is elevated to 28 breaths per minute. Her *vital capacity* is 0.9 L, and *forced vital capacity (FVC)* is 0.8 L. What is the next best step in management?
    A. Start IV immunoglobulin (IVIG) and monitor closely
    B. Start non-invasive positive pressure ventilation (NIPPV) and assess response
    C. Intubate and initiate mechanical ventilation
    D. Initiate plasmapheresis immediately
    E. Increase acetylcholinesterase inhibitors and monitor closely

    Correct answer: C

Explanation

This patient is experiencing *myasthenic crisis*, a potentially life-threatening condition characterized by respiratory failure and severe weakness of the respiratory muscles. The patient has signs of severe respiratory distress, including inability to speak in full sentences, elevated respiratory rate, and severe weakness. Her vital capacity (0.9 L) and FVC (0.8 L) are significantly reduced, indicating respiratory muscle weakness. In this scenario, intubation and mechanical ventilation (choice C) are required to secure the airway and manage respiratory failure. Non-invasive positive pressure ventilation (NIPPV) (choice B) may be used initially in patients with mild to moderate respiratory distress, but this patient is exhibiting severe respiratory failure that is unlikely to improve with NIPPV alone. IVIG (choice A) and plasmapheresis (choice D) are important treatments for myasthenic crisis, but these interventions should be performed after securing the airway and ensuring adequate ventilation. Increasing acetylcholinesterase inhibitors (choice E) would not be beneficial in this situation and may exacerbate respiratory failure.

Reference

Preston DC, Shapiro BE. *Electromyography and Neuromuscular Disorders: Clinical-Electrophysiologic-Ultrasound Correlations*. 4th ed. Elsevier; 2020. Chapter 37.

Linked questions: 73–74

73. A 62-year-old man with a past medical history of hypertension, hyperlipidemia, coronary artery disease, and tobacco use presents with progressive proximal muscle weakness, particularly in the legs, that worsens throughout the day. On further questions, he also reports new onset constipation and erectile dysfunction. On examination, deep tendon reflexes are markedly reduced, but there is improvement in strength after brief exercise. Which of the following antibody tests is most likely to confirm the diagnosis of his condition?
    A. Anti-acetylcholine receptor antibody

B. Anti-voltage-gated calcium channel antibody
C. Anti-titin antibody
D. Anti-striated muscle antibody
E. Anti-dipeptidyl peptidase 4 (DPP-4) antibody
Correct answer: B

Linked question

74. His anti-voltage-gated calcium channel antibody came back positive, what is the next required diagnostic step?
    A. Proceed with a single fiber EMG test
    B. Obtain an MRI of his lumbosacral plexus
    C. CT scan of the chest to evaluate for an underlying malignancy
    D. Nerve conduction studies to assess neuromuscular transmission
    E. Lumbar puncture to analyze cerebrospinal fluid (CSF)
    Correct answer: C

Explanation

This patient's presentation, with progressive proximal muscle weakness, autonomic symptoms (such as dry mouth and constipation), and reduced deep tendon reflexes, strongly suggests Lambert-Eaton Myasthenic Syndrome (LEMS), particularly in the context of small cell lung cancer (SCLC), a common cause of paraneoplastic LEMS. The first step in confirming the diagnosis is to perform anti-voltage-gated calcium channel antibody testing (choice B), as these antibodies are present in LEMS and target the presynaptic calcium channels at the neuromuscular junction. The presence of these antibodies disrupts the release of acetylcholine, which leads to the characteristic symptoms of LEMS. Although single fiber EMG testing (choice A) is also useful for diagnosing LEMS, the antibody test is more specific and should be done first to confirm the diagnosis.

Given the high likelihood of paraneoplastic syndrome in this patient with a history of SCLC, the next best step is to obtain a CT scan of the chest (choice C) to evaluate for an underlying malignancy. LEMS is often associated with SCLC, and addressing the underlying cancer can lead to significant improvement in the patient's neuromuscular symptoms. MRI of the lumbosacral plexus (choice B) is more appropriate for evaluating plexopathies, which is not consistent with this case. Nerve conduction studies (choice D) can help assess neuromuscular transmission but are not diagnostic for LEMS, especially in the absence of cancer screening. Finally, a lumbar puncture (CSF analysis) (choice E) is unnecessary, as LEMS is a peripheral neuro-muscular disorder and not a central nervous system problem.

Reference

Preston DC, Shapiro BE. *Electromyography and Neuromuscular Disorders: Clinical-Electrophysiologic-Ultrasound Correlations*. 4th ed. Elsevier; 2020. Chapter 37.

75. A 3-month-old infant presents with hypotonia, poor feeding, and ptosis since birth. The mother has no history of autoimmune disease. Physical examination reveals fatigable weakness, particularly in the facial and bulbar muscles. Electromyography (EMG) shows a significant decremental response on low-frequency repetitive nerve stimulation. Genetic testing identifies a mutation in the *CHRNE* gene. Which of the following is the most appropriate next step in management?
    A. Initiate corticosteroid therapy
    B. Begin treatment with pyridostigmine
    C. Administer intravenous immunoglobulin (IVIG)
    D. Start plasmapheresis
    E. Recommend thymectomy
    Correct answer: B

Explanation

This infant's presentation is characteristic of a *congenital myasthenic syndrome (CMS)*, particularly one associated with a mutation in the *CHRNE* gene, which encodes the epsilon subunit of the acetylcholine receptor. CMS are inherited disorders of the neuromuscular junction that typically present in infancy or early childhood with symptoms like hypotonia, ptosis, and feeding difficulties. Unlike autoimmune myasthenia gravis, CMS is not caused by antibodies and therefore does not respond to immunosuppressive therapies such as corticosteroids, IVIG, or plasmapheresis. *Pyridostigmine*, an acetylcholinesterase inhibitor, is often the first line treatment for many types of CMS, especially those involving postsynaptic defects like CHRNE mutations. It works by increasing the concentration of acetylcholine at the neuromuscular junction, thereby improving neuromuscular transmission. *Thymectomy* is not indicated in CMS, as the thymus is not involved in the pathogenesis of this genetic disorder.

Reference

Preston DC, Shapiro BE. *Electromyography and Neuromuscular Disorders: Clinical-Electrophysiologic-Ultrasound Correlations*. 4th ed. Elsevier; 2020. Chapter 37.

76. A 6-month-old boy presents with ptosis, feeding difficulty, and respiratory distress since birth. Examination reveals nasal speech and fatigable weakness. EMG shows a >10% decrement in the compound muscle action potential (CMAP) on low-frequency repetitive nerve stimulation. Acetylcholine receptor (AChR) and MuSK antibody tests are negative. His mother has no autoimmune history, and there is no thymic enlargement on imaging. What is the most likely diagnosis?
    A. Seronegative autoimmune myasthenia gravis
    B. Congenital myasthenic syndrome
    C. Neonatal transient myasthenia
    D. Myotonic dystrophy
    E. Spinal muscular atrophy type 1
    Correct answer: B

Explanation

This infant's presentation—ptosis, bulbar symptoms (feeding difficulty, nasal speech), and fatigable weakness beginning in early infancy—combined with negative acetylcholine receptor (AChR) and MuSK antibodies and a decremental response on low-frequency repetitive nerve stimulation is most consistent with *congenital myasthenic syndrome (CMS)*. Unlike autoimmune myasthenia gravis, CMS is caused by inherited defects in neuromuscular transmission and does not involve autoantibodies. Therefore, antibody tests are typically negative and immunotherapies such as steroids or IVIG are ineffective. Diagnosis is confirmed through genetic testing, often identifying mutations in genes such as *CHRNE, RAPSN,* or *DOK7*. CMS must be distinguished from neonatal myasthenia (which is transient and occurs in infants of mothers with MG), autoimmune seronegative MG (which typically presents later), and other neuromuscular disorders, such as spinal muscular atrophy or myotonic dystrophy, which have distinct clinical and electrophysiologic features.

Reference

Engel AG, Shen XM, Selcen D, Sine SM. Congenital myasthenic syndromes: pathogenesis, diagnosis, and treatment. Lancet Neurol. 2015 Apr;14(4):420–34. https://doi. org/10.1016/S1474-4422(14)70201-7. Erratum in: Lancet Neurol. 2015 May;14(5):461. https://doi.org/10.1016/ S1474-4422(15)00010-1. PMID: 25792100; PMCID: PMC4520251.

Linked questions: 77–78

77. A 3-month-old infant with no prior medical history is brought to the emergency department for poor feeding, weak cry, and constipation for 3 days. On examination, she has hypotonia, bilateral ptosis, sluggish pupillary reflexes, and diminished deep tendon reflexes. Her parents report no history of recent illness or fever, and they have continued attempting to feed her small amount of infant formula and homemade pureed fruits sweetened with honey.
    Which of the following is the most likely diagnosis?
    A. Spinal muscular atrophy type 1
    B. Infant botulism
    C. Congenital myasthenic syndrome
    D. Guillain-Barré syndrome
    E. Myasthenia gravis
    Correct answer: B

Linked question

78. Which of the following best describes the pathophysiology of this condition?
    A. Autoantibodies targeting presynaptic voltage-gated calcium channels
    B. Complement-mediated postsynaptic acetylcholine receptor destruction
    C. Toxin-mediated blockade of acetylcholine release via SNARE protein cleavage
    D. Genetic mutation in choline acetyltransferase
    E. Antibodies to muscle-specific kinase (MuSK)
    Correct answer: C

Explanation

This infant presents with hallmark signs of infant botulism: hypotonia, ptosis, poor cry, constipation, and diminished reflexes in the absence of fever or infection. Though several foods are mentioned, honey-sweetened puree stands out as a risk factor due to its potential contamination with *Clostridium botulinum* spores. In infants, these spores colonize the gut, producing botulinum toxin, which cleaves SNARE proteins and prevents presynaptic acetylcholine release, leading to descending flaccid paralysis.

Alternative diagnoses are less likely:

- SMA type 1 causes hypotonia but not constipation or cranial nerve findings like ptosis.
- Congenital myasthenic syndrome is genetic and does not typically present acutely.
- Guillain-Barré syndrome is rare in infants and often follows infection.
- Neonatal myasthenia gravis occurs soon after birth in infants of myasthenic mothers and resolves spontaneously.

Reference

Engel AG, Shen XM, Selcen D, Sine SM. Congenital myasthenic syndromes: pathogenesis, diagnosis, and treatment. Lancet Neurol. 2015 Apr;14(4):420–34. https://doi. org/10.1016/S1474-4422(14)70201-7. Erratum in: Lancet

Neurol. 2015 May;14(5):461. https://doi.org/10.1016/S1474-4422(15)00010-1. PMID: 25792100; PMCID: PMC4520251.

79. A 58-year-old woman with non-small cell lung cancer (NSCLC) is undergoing treatment with the immune checkpoint inhibitor nivolumab. She has a history of rheumatoid arthritis, for which she has been on methotrexate and hyperlipidemia for which she has been on atorvastatin for years. The patient presents to the clinic with progressive weakness over the past two weeks. She describes increasing fatigue and difficulty climbing stairs and lifting objects. Additionally, she reports ptosis, which worsens later in the day. On examination, she has bilateral ptosis, proximal muscle weakness, and normal deep tendon reflexes. There is no family history of neuromuscular disorders. Her acetylcholine receptor antibody test is negative. Which of the following is the most likely cause of her symptoms?
    A. Immune checkpoint inhibitor-induced myasthenia gravis
    B. Methotrexate-induced myasthenia gravis
    C. Botulism induced by clostridium toxin
    D. Medically induced Lambert-Eaton Myasthenic Syndrome (LEMS)
    E. Statin-induced myopathy
    Correct answer: A

Explanation

This patient's symptoms of progressive muscle weakness, ptosis, and proximal muscle weakness that is fatigable, are highly suggestive of myasthenia gravis. Given her recent treatment with nivolumab, an immune checkpoint inhibitor (ICI), the most likely cause of her symptoms is immune checkpoint inhibitor-induced myasthenia gravis (Choice A). ICIs, such as nivolumab, can trigger autoimmune responses, including the development of myasthenia gravis, by promoting T-cell activation that attacks the neuromuscular junction. Myasthenia gravis caused by ICIs is often seronegative, meaning that tests for acetylcholine receptor (AChR) antibodies may be negative, which is consistent with this patient's presentation.

- Methotrexate-induced myasthenia gravis (Choice B) is less likely because methotrexate is not commonly associated with myasthenia gravis, and its toxicity usually manifests as hematologic or hepatic dysfunction rather than neuromuscular symptoms.
- Botulism (Choice C), caused by Clostridium botulinum toxin, usually presents with acute flaccid paralysis and is associated with gastrointestinal symptoms such as nausea, vomiting, and diarrhea, which are not present in this case.

- Medically-induced Lambert-Eaton Myasthenic Syndrome (LEMS) (Choice D) is unlikely since LEMS is more commonly associated with small cell lung cancer, not non-small cell lung cancer, and typically presents with autonomic symptoms (e.g., dry mouth, constipation) along with proximal weakness.
- Statin-induced myopathy (Choice E) generally causes generalized muscle pain, elevated creatine kinase levels, and weakness, but it does not typically cause the specific pattern of ptosis and fluctuating weakness observed in this patient.

Reference

Marco C, Simó M, Alemany M, Casasnovas C, Domínguez R, Vilariño N, Calvo M, Martín-Liberal J, Brenes J, Sabater-Riera J, Bruna J, Velasco R. Myasthenia Gravis Induced by Immune Checkpoint Inhibitors: An Emerging Neurotoxicity in Neuro-Oncology Practice: Case Series. J Clin Med. 2022 Dec 24;12(1):130. https://doi.org/10.3390/jcm12010130. PMID: 36614930; PMCID: PMC9821391.

Linked questions: 80–82

80. A 45-year-old woman presents with a 6-month history of progressive muscle stiffness and pain. She describes the stiffness as worsening primarily in her lower back and legs, making it difficult to walk. She reports episodes of spasms, especially during emotional stress, which are accompanied by severe pain and difficulty moving. On examination, there is marked stiffness of the trunk and proximal limbs, with increased tone and hyperreflexia. The rest of her neurological examination is otherwise normal. Laboratory tests reveal no signs of inflammation or infection. Based on her clinical presentation, which of the following is the most likely diagnosis?
    A. Stiff Person Syndrome (SPS)
    B. Multiple sclerosis
    C. Neuroleptic malignant syndrome
    D. Paroxysmal dyskinesia
    E. Hereditary spastic paraplegia
    Correct answer: A

Linked question

81. Given the strong clinical suspicion for Stiff Person Syndrome (SPS), which antibody would most likely be found in this patient?
    A. Anti-acetylcholine receptor antibody
    B. Anti-glutamic acid decarboxylase (GAD) antibody
    C. Anti-demyelinating antibody
    D. Anti-voltage-gated potassium channel antibody
    E. Anti-ribonucleoprotein antibody
    Correct answer: B

Linked question

82. What is the first-line treatment for *Stiff Person Syndrome (SPS)*?
    A. Beta-blockers
    B. Immunosuppressive therapy (e.g., corticosteroids)
    C. Plasmapheresis
    D. Benzodiazepines (e.g., diazepam)
    E. Acetylcholinesterase inhibitors
    Correct answer: D

Explanation

80: The patient's *progressive muscle stiffness*, *pain*, and *episodic spasms* in the context of *hypertonia* and *hyperreflexia* are highly suggestive of *Stiff Person Syndrome (SPS)*. SPS is a *rare, autoimmune, neurological disorder* characterized by *muscle stiffness*, *spasms*, and *impaired mobility*, often worsened by emotional stress. The key feature of SPS is *extrapyramidal rigidity*, particularly affecting the *trunk and proximal limbs*. The other options are less likely based on her clinical presentation. Multiple sclerosis (MS) typically presents with relapsing-remitting neurological deficits, such as optic neuritis, and sensory deficits—which are absent here. Neuroleptic malignant syndrome usually presents with fever, autonomic instability, and altered mental status, which are not described here. Paroxysmal dyskinesia usually involves sudden, brief movements, and not continuous stiffness. Hereditary spastic paraplegia primarily presents with progressive leg spasticity but lacks the painful spasms seen in SPS.

81: Anti-glutamic acid decarboxylase (GAD) antibodies are the most commonly found in patients with Stiff Person Syndrome (SPS), especially in classic SPS and SPS associated with diabetes mellitus. GAD is an enzyme involved in the synthesis of gamma-aminobutyric acid (GABA), a key inhibitory neurotransmitter in the brain. Anti-GAD antibodies disrupt GABAergic function, leading to the muscle stiffness and spasms characteristic of SPS. The other antibodies listed are not typically associated with SPS. Anti-acetylcholine receptor antibodies are seen in myasthenia gravis. Anti-demyelinating antibodies are more commonly seen in multiple sclerosis. Anti-voltage-gated potassium channel antibodies are seen in Lambert-Eaton myasthenic syndrome (LEMS). Anti-ribonucleoprotein antibodies are associated with mixed connective tissue diseases and Sjögren's syndrome.

82: The first-line treatment for Stiff Person Syndrome (SPS) is typically aimed at muscle relaxation and spasm control. Benzodiazepines, such as diazepam, are commonly used due to their muscle relaxant properties and their ability to reduce spasms and anxiety, which often exacerbate symptoms. Immunosuppressive therapy (e.g., corticosteroids) may be used in patients with autoimmune-related SPS but is generally not the first-line treatment. Plasmapheresis may be considered in severe, refractory cases, especially in patients with high anti-GAD antibody titers. Beta-blockers and acetylcholinesterase inhibitors are not effective in managing SPS symptoms.

Reference

Bose S, Jacob S. Stiff-person syndrome. Pract Neurol. 2025 Jan 16;25(1):6–17. https://doi.org/10.1136/pn-2023-003974. PMID: 39222980.

83. A 45-year-old man presents with a 6-month history of progressive muscle stiffness, cramping, and myokymia, especially in the calves and thighs. He notes that symptoms persist during sleep and are worsened by activity. Neurologic exam reveals delayed muscle relaxation after contraction and visible rippling muscle movements at rest. Reflexes are brisk but symmetric. There is no sensory loss or upper motor neuron involvement.

    EMG reveals spontaneous, high-frequency discharges of single motor unit potentials in a semirhythmic, continuous pattern even at rest. Which of the following best explains this patient's condition?
    A. Loss of acetylcholine receptor function at the neuromuscular junction
    B. Autoantibodies targeting voltage-gated potassium channels (VGKCs)
    C. Mutation in the DMPK gene causing RNA toxicity
    D. Abnormal expansion of polyglutamine repeats in motor neurons
    E. Autoimmune demyelination of peripheral motor axons
    Correct answer: B

Explanation

This patient's symptoms and EMG findings are characteristic of Isaac syndrome (acquired neuromyotonia), a rare peripheral nerve hyperexcitability disorder. It is most often associated with autoantibodies against VGKCs, particularly Caspr2 or LGI1, leading to sustained depolarization and spontaneous discharges of motor nerves. Option A describes myasthenia gravis, which causes fatigable weakness rather than stiffness or myokymia. Option C refers to myotonic dystrophy type 1, which includes systemic features and delayed relaxation but not continuous myokymia. Option D refers to spinal and bulbar muscular atrophy (Kennedy disease), which presents differently and does not involve peripheral nerve hyperexcitability. Option E could describe conditions like Guillain-Barré, but those typically involve areflexia, sensory changes, and acute progression—not persistent myokymia.

Reference

Ahmed, A. and Simmons, Z. (2015), Isaacs syndrome: A review. Muscle Nerve, 52: 5–12. https://doi.org/10.1002/mus.24632

Linked questions: 84–85

84. A 62-year-old man presents with several months of progressive muscle twitching, cramping, and stiffness. He notes frequent involuntary jerks in his limbs that persist during sleep, along with new-onset confusion and short-term memory impairment. On exam, he has visible myokymia in the calves and perioral region, but no weakness or sensory loss. Brain MRI shows increased signal in the mesial temporal lobes, and EMG demonstrates spontaneous discharges including multiplets and fasciculations. Which autoantibody is most likely responsible for this patient's condition?
    A. Acetylcholine receptor antibody
    B. GAD65 antibody
    C. LGI1 antibody
    D. CASPR2 antibody
    E. Anti-Hu antibody
    Correct answer: C

Linked question

85. What is the most appropriate initial treatment for this patient's condition?
    A. Pyridostigmine
    B. IVIG or corticosteroids
    C. Riluzole
    D. Acetazolamide
    E. Carbamazepine monotherapy
    Correct answer: B

Explanation

This patient has *autoimmune encephalitis with peripheral nerve hyperexcitability*, most consistent with *LGI1 antibody–associated Isaac syndrome*. LGI1 is part of the voltage-gated potassium channel (VGKC) complex and is linked to both neuromyotonia and limbic encephalitis. *CASPR2* is also part of the VGKC complex and can cause neuromyotonia, but is more commonly associated with Morvan syndrome and thymomas, and less so with encephalopathy. *GAD65* is seen in stiff-person syndrome. *Anti-Hu* suggests paraneoplastic neuropathy. *Acetylcholine receptor antibodies* are specific to myasthenia gravis.

Treatment typically begins with *immunotherapy* (steroids, IVIG, or plasmapheresis), which addresses the autoimmune mechanism. Symptomatic therapies like carbamazepine may help with twitching, but they do not modify the underlying immune process and are not first-line.

Reference

Ahmed, A. and Simmons, Z. (2015), Isaacs syndrome: A review. Muscle Nerve, 52: 5–12. https://doi.org/10.1002/mus.24632

Linked questions: 86–90

86. You are seeing a 52-year-old right-handed male in the clinic for right-sided shoulder pain and weakness. Two weeks ago, he developed severe right-sided shoulder and scapular pain without preceding injury, described as constant, sharp, and stabbing. He was seen in the emergency department where they performed right shoulder x rays which were unremarkable. Subsequently, he was sent home with ibuprofen and referral to neurology. In your office, he reports continued pain that has not responded to ibuprofen or tylenol as well as the development of weakness in lifting his right arm. His exam is notable for weakness in right shoulder abduction, external rotation and elbow flexion, atrophy of the right deltoid, supraspinatus and infraspinatus, and decreased sensation to light touch in a patch over her right deltoid. He has no significant past medical history. His only medication is as needed ibuprofen. What is your suspected diagnosis?
    A. Parsonage-Turner syndrome
    B. Neurogenic thoracic outlet syndrome (TOS)
    C. Hirayama disease
    D. Chronic inflammatory demyelinating polyradiculoneuropathy (CIDP)
    E. Erb's Palsy
    Correct answer: A

Explanation

Parsonage-Turner syndrome (PTS), also known as neuralgic amyotrophy, idiopathic brachial plexus neuropathy, or brachial plexus neuritis is a multifocal, inflammatory peripheral nervous system disorder that involves the brachial plexus and individual nerves of the upper limbs and shoulders. Typically, there is acute-onset of shoulder and arm pain as well as arm weakness. The pain usually resolves within a few weeks, although sometimes milder pain, like a dull aching, can persist for longer. Numbness can be seen but is less common. There is typically early onset (within the first few weeks) of muscle atrophy. The pattern of weakness and atrophy varies based on which part of the brachial plexus or peripheral nerves are involved. Frequently nerves composed solely or predominantly of motor axons are involved. Proximal involvement typically includes the long thoracic, suprascapular, axillary, and musculocutaneous nerves. Distally the anterior and posterior interosseous nerves or the motor branches to individual muscles are most commonly involved. The upper trunk of the brachial plexus is also frequently involved. Any age or gender can be affected but parsonage turner syndrome is most frequently seen in middle-aged men.

Neurogenic thoracic outlet syndrome is a rare disorder caused by compression of the lower brachial plexus by congenital abnormalities such as cervical ribs or fibrous bands originating from a cervical rib, and more rarely scalene hypertrophy. Typically, patients will report chronic sensory disturbance like aching and paresthesia along the medial aspect of the arm and forearm and will present with progressive forearm and hand weakness. T1 axons are typically affected more than C8 axons. Thenar muscles, which are heavily T1-innervated, will be the most affected.

Hirayama disease (HD) also known as juvenile muscular atrophy of the distal upper extremity or monomelic amyotrophy is characterized by asymmetric weakness and atrophy of the hand and forearm muscles. It typically affects young males, particularly Asian populations. In affected individuals, movement of the dural sac in the cervical region during neck flexion and extension has been observed, and it is hypothesized that with these movements the anterior horn cells of the lower cervical spine become injured leading to the clinical presentation. Typically, there is initial progression of symptoms with periods of stability. If patients have progressive disability, cervical decompression, and fusion can be considered.

CIDP is a chronic autoimmune neuropathy. Patients present with numbness, weakness, and sensory changes. Typical CIDP manifests as symmetric distal and proximal weakness, length dependent sensory loss, and areflexia. While there are variants that can present more acutely and asymmetrically, this presentation of acute pain, weakness, and muscle atrophy is more consistent with Parsonage-Turner.

Erb's palsy, a form of perinatal brachial plexus palsy, is an upper plexus palsy affecting the C5, C6, and or C7 nerve roots. This condition is typically due to traumatic injury of the brachial plexus during delivery due to excessive traction applied to the infant's neck. The most commonly affected muscles include the external rotators and abductors of the shoulders, flexors of the elbows, and supinators of the forearm. The wrist extensors can also be affected. This pattern of weakness leads to the classic "waiter's tip" posture: internal rotation and adduction of the shoulder, extension of the elbow, pronation of the forearm, and flexion at the wrist.

References

Bhattacharyya S. Spondylotic and Other Structural Myelopathies. Continuum (Minneap Minn). 2021 Feb 1;27(1):163–184. https://doi.org/10.1212/CON.0000000000000975. PMID: 33522741.

Dodds SD, Wolfe SW. Perinatal brachial plexus palsy. Curr Opin Pediatr. 2000 Feb;12(1):40–7. https://doi.org/10.1097/00008480-200002000-00009. PMID: 10676773.

Ferrante MA. Brachial plexopathies. Continuum (Minneap Minn). 2014 Oct;20(5 Peripheral Nervous System Disorders):1323–42. https://doi.org/10.1212/01.CON.0000455878.60932.37. PMID: 25299285.

Gwathmey K. Chronic Inflammatory Demyelinating Polyradiculoneuropathy and Its Variants. Continuum (Minneap Minn). 2020 Oct;26(5):1205–1223. https://doi.org/10.1212/CON.0000000000000907. Erratum in: Continuum (Minneap Minn). 2021 Apr 1;27(2):553. https://doi.org/10.1212/CON.0000000000001030. [dosage error in article text]. PMID: 33002999.

Meiling JB, Boon AJ, Niu Z, Howe BM, Hoskote SS, Spinner RJ, Klein CJ. Parsonage-Turner Syndrome and Hereditary Brachial Plexus Neuropathy. Mayo Clin Proc. 2024 Jan;99(1):124–140. https://doi.org/10.1016/j.mayocp.2023.06.011. PMID: 38176820.

Panther EJ, Reintgen CD, Cueto RJ, Hao KA, Chim H, King JJ. Thoracic outlet syndrome: a review. J Shoulder Elbow Surg. 2022 Nov;31(11):e545-e561. https://doi.org/10.1016/j.jse.2022.06.026. Epub 2022 Aug 10. PMID: 35963513.

van Alfen N. Clinical and pathophysiological concepts of neuralgic amyotrophy. Nat Rev Neurol. 2011 May 10;7(6):315–22. https://doi.org/10.1038/nrneurol.2011.62. PMID: 21556032.

Wang H, Tian Y, Wu J, Luo S, Zheng C, Sun C, Nie C, Xia X, Ma X, Lyu F, Jiang J, Wang H. Update on the Pathogenesis, Clinical Diagnosis, and Treatment of Hirayama Disease. Front Neurol. 2022 Feb 1;12:811943. https://doi.org/10.3389/fneur.2021.811943. PMID: 35178023; PMCID: PMC8844368.

Linked question

87. You suspect Parsonage-Turner syndrome and send the patient for further workup with imaging of the cervical spine and brachial plexus, ultrasound of the brachial plexus, and electromyography, and nerve conduction study. All of the following are expected findings, *except*?

    A. Normal nerve conduction studies of routine nerves (median motor and sensory, radial sensory, ulnar motor, and sensory)
    B. Hyperintensity of individual nerves of the brachial plexus and hourglass constrictions on contrast enhanced study of the brachial plexus
    C. Normal non-contrast study of the brachial plexus
    D. Focal nerve enlargements on ultrasound
    E. Homogenous and diffuse sensory and motor nerve conduction slowing on nerve conduction studies

    Correct answer: E

Explanation

In Parsonage-Turner syndrome (PTS) electrodiagnostic testing can reveal broader abnormalities than indicated by the clinical exam which can help support a multifocal process. Often the nerves surveyed on routine nerve conduction studies including the median, ulnar, and radial nerve are unaffected, and these will be normal. Axon loss may more commonly be seen in suprascapular motor, axillary motor, and lateral antebrachial cutaneous sensory studies. Needle electromyography (EMG) is often a more helpful tool for surveying proximal musculature and can show patchy findings. Depending on the time after injury, you may see reduced recruitment of motor unit action potentials (acutely, 1–2 weeks), membrane instability with fibrillation potentials and positive sharp waves as well as polyphasic, long duration, and tall amplitude motor unit action potentials (subacute to chronic). These studies can be helpful to distinguish Parsonage-Turner syndrome from cervical radiculopathy when you would expect changes in a root distribution, rather than patchy nerve distribution.

Contrast enhanced MRI imaging of the brachial plexus will often reveal affected nerves with a hyperintense signal indicating inflammation or "hourglass constrictions." Ultrasound can reveal focal or diffuse nerve enlargement, constriction of nerves, and torsion of nerve fascicles. Homogenous and diffuse sensory and motor nerve conduction slowing is more consistent with an inherited demyelinating neuropathy such as Charcot-Marie-Tooth disease type 1A.

References

Al Khalili Y, Jain S, Lam JC, DeCastro A. Brachial Neuritis. 2024 Feb 2. In: StatPearls [Internet]. Treasure Island (FL): StatPearls Publishing; 2025 Jan–. PMID: 29763017.

Meiling JB, Boon AJ, Niu Z, Howe BM, Hoskote SS, Spinner RJ, Klein CJ. Parsonage-Turner Syndrome and Hereditary Brachial Plexus Neuropathy. Mayo Clin Proc. 2024 Jan;99(1):124–140. https://doi.org/10.1016/j.mayocp.2023.06.011. PMID: 38176820.

van Paassen BW, van der Kooi AJ, van Spaendonck-Zwarts KY, Verhamme C, Baas F, de Visser M. PMP22 related neuropathies: Charcot-Marie-Tooth disease type 1A and Hereditary Neuropathy with liability to Pressure Palsies. Orphanet J Rare Dis. 2014 Mar 19;9:38. https://doi.org/10.1186/1750-1172-9-38. PMID: 24646194; PMCID: PMC3994927.

Linked question

88. Further workup with imaging of the brachial plexus and nerve conduction studies is consistent with Parsonage-Turner syndrome. What would be the next most appropriate step in treating the patient?
    A. Referral for surgical evaluation
    B. Corticosteroids
    C. Plasma exchange
    D. Rituximab
    Correct answer: B

Explanation

Typically, conservative therapy should be tried initially as symptoms can spontaneously resolve. Initial management focuses on treating pain which is typically more responsive to steroids than non-steroidal anti-inflammatory drugs (NSAIDs). Neuropathic pain medications and narcotic pain medications can also be considered. Once pain is controlled physical or occupational therapy can be recommended for strengthening and stretching exercises. IVIG has been tried in the treatment of Parsonage-Turner syndrome, but the effectiveness of this and other immunomodulatory therapy has not been established. If symptoms do not improve after several months, surgical referral for neurolysis or nerve transfer can be considered.

References

Al Khalili Y, Jain S, Lam JC, DeCastro A. Brachial Neuritis. 2024 Feb 2. In: StatPearls [Internet]. Treasure Island (FL): StatPearls Publishing; 2025 Jan–. PMID: 29763017.

Ferrante MA. Brachial plexopathies. Continuum (Minneap Minn). 2014 Oct;20(5 Peripheral Nervous System Disorders):1323–42. https://doi.org/10.1212/01.CON.0000455878.60932.37. PMID: 25299285.

Meiling JB, Boon AJ, Niu Z, Howe BM, Hoskote SS, Spinner RJ, Klein CJ. Parsonage-Turner Syndrome and Hereditary Brachial Plexus Neuropathy. Mayo Clin Proc. 2024 Jan;99(1):124–140. https://doi.org/10.1016/j.mayocp.2023.06.011. PMID: 38176820.

Linked question

89. If the patient had presented findings in the ulnar nerve distribution, which of the following findings on electromyography and nerve conduction study would be supportive of involvement of the medial cord of the brachial plexus, rather than the ulnar nerve itself?
    A. Decreased or absent lateral antebrachial cutaneous nerve sensory nerve action potential (SNAP)
    B. Membrane instability (fibrillations and positive sharp waves) in the supraspinatus
    C. Decreased or absent medial antebrachial cutaneous nerve SNAP
    D. Decreased or absent radial nerve compound muscle action potential (CMAP) as recorded over the extensor indicis proprius
    E. Membrane instability (fibrillations and positive sharp waves) noted in the brachioradialis
    Correct answer: C

Linked question

90. All of the following nerves arise from the posterior cord
    of the brachial plexus except?
    A. Axillary nerve
    B. Radial nerve
    C. Subscapular nerve
    D. Thoracodorsal nerve
    E. Dorsal scapular nerve
    Correct answer: E

Explanation

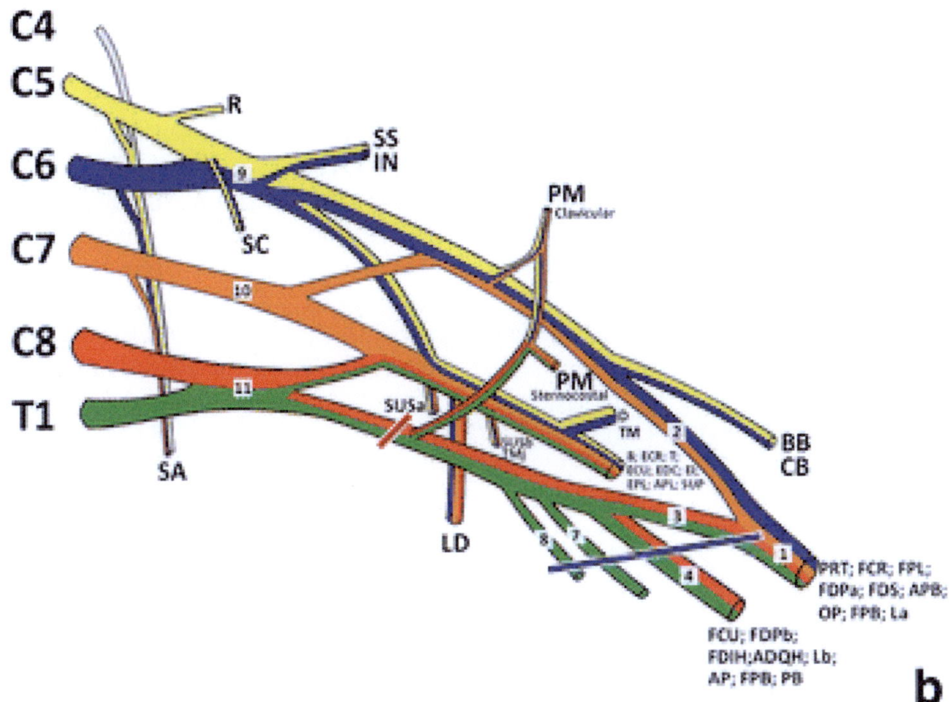

Graphic illustration of the brachial plexus, roots, trunks, divisions, cords, terminal branches, and the muscles (m.) they innervate. 1, median nerve; 2, median nerve root side; 3, medial root of the median nerve; 4, ulnar nerve; 5, axillary artery; 6, axillary vein; 7, medial cutaneous nerve of the arm; 8, medial cutaneous nerve of the forearm; 9, upper trunk of the brachial plexus; 10, middle trunk of the brachial plexus; 11, lower trunk of the brachial plexus. SA serratus anterior m., SC subclavius m., R rhomboids m., SS supraspinatus m., IN infraspinatus m., PM pectoralis major m., SUSa subscapularis m. (upper half), LD latissimus dorsi m., SUSb subscapularis m. (lower half), TMj teres major m., D deltoid m., TM teres minor m., B brachioradialis m., ECR extensor carpi radialis m., T triceps m., ECU extensor carpi ulnaris m., EDC extensor digitorum communis m., EI extensor indicis proprius m., EPL extensor policis longus m., APL abductor pollicis longus m., SUP supinator m., BB biceps brachii m., CB coracobrachialis m., PRT pronator teres m., FCR flexor carpi radialis m., FPL flexor pollicis longus m., FDPa flexor digitorum profundus m. [bellies for the index and middle finger], FDS flexor digitorum superficialis m., APB abductor pollicis brevis m., OP opponens pollicis m., FPB flexor pollicis brevis m., La first and second lumbricals m., FCU flexor carpi ulnaris m., FDPb Flexor digitorum profundus m. [bellies for the ring and small fingers], FDIH first dorsal interosseous m., ADQH abductor digiti quinti m., Lb third and fourth lumbricals m., AP adductor pollicis m., FPB flexor pollicis brevis m. (deep head), PB palmaris brevis m. (Source: Casal et al via Journal of Medical Case Reports. 2017. CC-BY 4.0 (https://creativecommons.org/licenses/by/4.0/). Image has been cropped to show only panel B. Please see full attribution with citation below in references section for this question)

The medial antebrachial cutaneous nerve is a direct branch of the medial cord of the brachial plexus, and its involvement would support medial cord involvement.

The dorsal scapular nerve branches directly off the C4 to C5 nerve roots.

The brachial plexus is a complex series of nerves that originates in the ventral rami from the mixed spinal nerves in the lower cervical to upper thoracic (C5–T1). It is anatomically divided into five sections:

1. *Roots*—sensory (dorsal roots) and motor axons (ventral roots) exiting the spinal fuse within the intervertebral foramina just beyond the dorsal root ganglia to form mixed spinal nerves. Each nerve divides into a posteriorly directed branch (posterior primary ramus) and an anteriorly directed branch (anterior primary ramus). Anatomically, the anterior primary rami from C5 to T1 are typically defined as the brachial plexus roots, although in clinical practice, brachial plexus lesions often include structures proximal to the anterior primary rami)
   - The C5–T1 anterior primary rami give off several motor branches:
     – Some of which will directly innervate muscles (scalene and longus colli muscles [C5–C8])
     – Others join to form nerves
       • Long thoracic (C5–C8)
       • Phrenic (C3–C5)
       • Dorsal scapular (C4–C5)
2. *Trunks*—The roots merge into three trunks:
   • *Upper trunk* (C5–C6 anterior primary rami)
     – The suprascapular nerve and the nerve to the subclavius exit from the trunk
   • *Middle trunk* (C7 anterior primary ramus)
   • *Lower trunk* (C8–T1 anterior primary rami)
3. *Divisions*—Each trunk splits into an *anterior* and *posterior* division.
   • The anterior division primarily innervates flexors and the posterior division primarily supplies extensors
4. *Cords*—The divisions reorganize into three cords which are named for their orientation to the axillary artery:
   • *Lateral cord* (from anterior divisions of upper and middle trunks)
     – The lateral cord gives of the lateral and musculocutaneous nerve before terminating as the lateral head of the median nerve
   • *Posterior cord* (from all three posterior divisions)
     – The posterior cord gives off the upper subscapular, thoracodorsal, and lower subscapular nerves before terminating as the axillary and radial nerves
   • *Medial cord* (from anterior division of lower trunk)
     – The medial cord gives off the medial pectoral, medial brachial cutaneous, medial antebrachial cutaneous, and ulnar nerves before terminating as the medial head of the median nerve

5. *Terminal nerves*—The five terminal nerves are distally situated in the axilla and upon exciting become the peripheral nerves of the upper extremity
   • Musculocutaneous
   • Axillary
   • Median
   • Ulnar
   • Radial

References

Casal D, Cunha T, Pais D, et al. A stab wound to the axilla illustrating the importance of brachial plexus anatomy in an emergency context: a case report. *J Med Case Rep.* 2017;11(1):6. Published 2017 Jan 4. https://doi.org/10.1186/s13256-016-1162-6

Ferrante MA. Brachial plexopathies. Continuum (Minneap Minn). 2014 Oct;20(5 Peripheral Nervous System Disorders):1323–42. https://doi.org/10.1212/01.CON.0000455878.60932.37. PMID: 25299285.

Preston, D. C., & Shapiro, B. E. (2020). *Electromyography and Neuromuscular Disorders: Clinical-Electrophysiologic-Ultrasound Correlations* (4th ed.). Elsevier. ISBN: 978-0-323-66180-5.

91. A 28-year-old female presents with acute onset of right shoulder pain and right arm weakness. On exam you note difficulty with left shoulder abduction and elbow flexion, as well atrophy of the left deltoid and biceps. You also notice dysmorphic facial features including hypotelorism, epicanthal folds, and dysmorphic ears as well as short stature. She reports her father has had similar attacks of symptoms throughout his life. Mutations in which of the following genes would be most likely associated with the disorder she likely has?
    A. *SCN1A*
    B. *SEPT9*
    C. *PNP22*
    D. *DYSF*
    Correct answer: B

Explanation

Hereditary neuralgic amyotrophy is a rare disorder that is characterized by recurrent episodes of brachial plexopathy. Symptoms usually begin in the second or third decade of life, although they can occur even earlier. There can be associated phenotypic features including dysmorphic facies (hypotelorism, cleft palate, widely spaced teeth, dysmorphic ears), and short stature. Attacks are similar to Parsonage-Turner syndrome, but are associated with higher recurrence rates. Greater propensity to affect individual nerves, involvement of lumbosacral nerves and postpartum attacks have been described as more common in hereditary neurologic amyotrophy.

Mutations in the septin gene *SEPT9* on chromosome 17q25 have been identified as causal of hereditary neurologic amyotrophy. However, genetic heterogeneity exists, and not all cases are linked to this locus.

References

Bhatti A, Ravat S, Desai K, Shekhar BR, Menon SR, Kumbhar BV, Kunwar A, Jain N, Das DK. Spectrum of Clinical Variability with SEPT9 Gene Mutation in Hereditary Neuralgic Amyotrophy: Understanding the Pathogenesis Using Molecular Dynamics Simulation Study. Neurol India. 2024 Sep 1;72(5):1021–1026. https://doi.org/10.4103/neurol-india.NI_823_19. Epub 2024 Oct 19. PMID: 39428775.

Laccone F, Hannibal MC, Neesen J, Grisold W, Chance PF, Rehder H. Dysmorphic syndrome of hereditary neuralgic amyotrophy associated with a SEPT9 gene mutation--a family study. Clin Genet. 2008 Sep;74(3):279–83. https://doi.org/10.1111/j.1399-0004.2008.01022.x. Epub 2008 May 19. PMID: 18492087.

Meiling JB, Boon AJ, Niu Z, Howe BM, Hoskote SS, Spinner RJ, Klein CJ. Parsonage-Turner Syndrome and Hereditary Brachial Plexus Neuropathy. Mayo Clin Proc. 2024 Jan;99(1):124–140. https://doi.org/10.1016/j.mayocp.2023.06.011. PMID: 38176820.

Rubin DI. Diseases of The Plexus. Continuum. 2008 June;2008 (Spinal Cord, Root, and Plexus Disorders): 156–179. https://doi.org/10.1212/01.CON.0000324129.85559.74

Linked questions: 92–96

92. A 58-year-old woman with a history of cervical cancer treated with pelvic radiation therapy 5 years ago presents with progressive, painless weakness in her lower legs. She reports difficulty rising from a chair and alteration in her gait. Motor exam is notable for 4/5 right hip flexion strength, 5/5 right knee extension, 3/5 strength in right dorsiflexion and plantarflexion, 3/5 left hip flexion strength, 3/5 left thigh abduction. She has depressed reflexes throughout the legs. You note fasciculations in her left thigh and right calf. Where would her symptoms best localize?

A. Bilateral sciatic nerves
B. Right L5 radiculopathy
C. The lumbosacral plexus
D. Lower thoracic cord
E. Bilateral femoral nerves
Correct answer: C

Explanation

The diffuse asymmetric involvement of the lower extremities with depressed reflexes, and fasciculations on exam is most consistent with a peripheral process that best localized to the lumbosacral plexus (see below for description). Proximal leg muscles (hip flexion) should not be affected in sciatic neuropathy. The lower leg involvement would not be seen with femoral neuropathy. L5 radiculopathy would not explain the extent of her muscle weakness, and she has symptoms bilaterally arguing against unilateral radiculopathy. While diffuse lower extremity weakness could be seen with a thoracic cord lesion, the absence of upper motor neuron signs make lumbosacral plexopathy more likely.

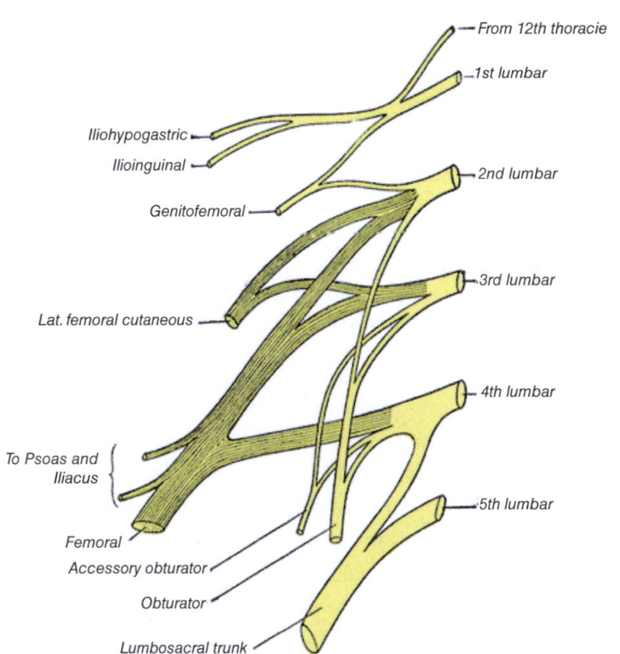

Plan of lumbar plexus. (Source: Henry Gray. *Gray H. Anatomy of the Human Body. 20th ed. Philadelphia, PA: Lea & Febiger; 1918*: Plate 822. Accessed via Bartleby.com. Public Domain. (https://creativecommons.org/publicdomain/zero/1.0/). https://www.bartleby.com/lit-hub/anatomy-of-the-human-body/fig-822)

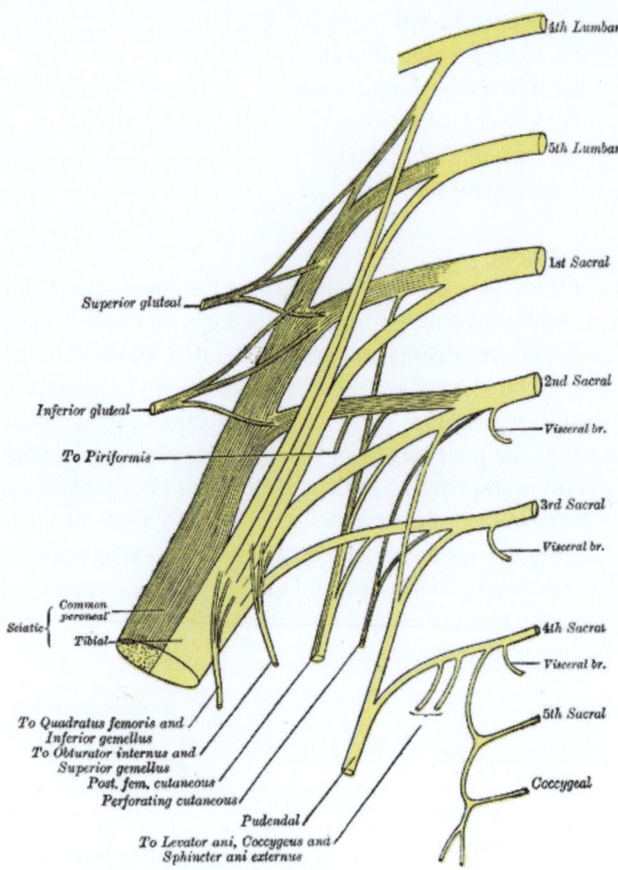

Plan of sacral and pudendal plexuses. (Source: Henry Gray. *Gray H. Anatomy of the Human Body. 20th ed. Philadelphia, PA: Lea & Febiger; 1918*: Plate 828. Accessed via Bartleby.com: Public Domain. (https://creativecommons.org/publicdomain/zero/1.0/). https://www.bartleby.com/lit-hub/anatomy-of-the-human-body/fig-828)

The lumbosacral plexus is a complex network of nerves that arises from the ventral rami of the L1–S4 nerve roots. Anatomically, it is typically thought of as two sections, an upper portion consisting of an upper lumbar plexus, and a lower portion consisting of a lower lumbosacral plexus. The lumbosacral plexus provides sensory and motor innervation to the lower limb and pelvic girdle.

Upper lumbar plexus (L1–L4 nerve roots, with variable contribution from T12). Situated behind the psoas muscles in the retroperitoneum. Several major nerves are derived from the upper portion of the plexus including:

- *Iliohypogastric (T12–L1) and ilioinguinal (L1) nerves*:
  - *Muscular innervation*: to the transverse and internal oblique muscles.
  - *Sensation*:
    - *Iliohypogastric*: to a strip over the lower anterior abdomen
    - *Ilioinguinal*: an area of skin over the inguinal ligament, an area of skin over the rostral medial thigh, upper part of scrotum in males or labia in females

- *The genitofemoral nerve (L1–L2)*: divides into a genital and femoral branch at the level of the medial inguinal ligament
  - *Genital branch*: muscular innervation to the cremasteric muscles in males and sensation to the skin over the lower part of the scrotum in males and labia in females
  - *Femoral branch*: supplies sensation to an area of skin over the femoral triangle
- *Lateral femoral cutaneous nerve of the thigh (L2–L3)*
  - *Sensation*: A pure sensory nerve, also known as the lateral cutaneous nerve of the thigh. It passes under the inguinal ligament and it is here that the nerve is susceptible to injury and compression which can lead to meralgia paresthetica. It supplies a large oval area of skin over the lateral and anterior thigh.
- *The femoral nerve (L2–L4)*: The anterior rami of L2-L3-L4 divide into anterior and posterior divisions, the posterior divisions form the femoral nerve
  - *Muscular innervation*: iliopsoas, pectineus, sartorius, quadriceps
  - *Sensation*: medial calf (*saphenous nerve*), anterior medial thigh (*medial and intermediate cutaneous nerves of the thigh*)
- *The obturator nerve (L2–L4)*: the anterior divisions of L2-L3-L4 form the obturator nerve. This exits the pelvis through the obturator foramen
  - *Muscular innervation*: thigh adductors (adductor, longus, adductor brevis, adductor magnus, and gracilis)
  - *Sensation*: to a small area of skin on the medial thigh

Lower Lumbar PLexus (L4–S4 nerve roots). The L4 contribution joins with the L5 root to form the *lumbosacral trunk* which then descends below the pelvic outlet to join the sacral plexus. The major nerves from the lower lumbosacral plexus include

- *Superior gluteal nerve (L4–S1)*
  - *Muscular innervation*: tensor fasciae latae, gluteus medius, gluteus minimus
- *The inferior gluteal nerve (L5–S2)*
  - *Muscular innervation*: gluteus maximus
- *The sciatic nerve (L4–S3)*: made of the tibial and fibular [peroneal] components.
  - *Muscular innervation*: hamstrings(semimembranosus, semitendinosus, long and short head of the biceps femoris), lateral division of the adductor magnus, all muscles innervated by the peroneal and tibial nerves
  - *Sensation*: entire lower leg below the knee excluding the medial calf which is innervated by the saphenous nerve
- *The posterior femoral cutaneous nerve (S1–S3)*
  - *Sensation*: lower buttock and posterior thigh

- *The pudendal nerve (S1–S4)*
  - *Motor*: urinary and anal sphincters
  - *Sensation:* genital and rectal areas

References

Blumenfeld, H. (2021). *Neuroanatomy through Clinical Cases* (3rd edition). Oxford University Press. ISBN 9781605359265

Dyck PJ, Thaisetthawatkul P. Lumbosacral plexopathy. Continuum (Minneap Minn). 2014 Oct;20(5 Peripheral Nervous System Disorders):1343–58. https://doi.org/10.1212/01.CON.0000455877.60932.d3. PMID: 25299286.

Preston, D. C., & Shapiro, B. E. (2020). *Electromyography and Neuromuscular Disorders: Clinical-Electrophysiologic-Ultrasound Correlations* (4th ed.). Elsevier. ISBN: 978-0-323-66180-5.

Linked question

93. What is the *most likely* diagnosis in this case?
    - A. Cauda equina syndrome due to a herniated disc
    - B. Radiation-induced lumbosacral plexopathy
    - C. Neoplastic lumbosacral plexopathy
    - D. A retroperitoneal hematoma
    - E. Psoas muscle abscess
    - **Correct answer**: B

Explanation

The patient's history of radiation therapy, in combination with a delayed presentation of weakness is most concerning for radiation-induced lumbosacral plexopathy. Radiation can affect peripheral nerves by causing chronic inflammation, organized fibrosis, and microvascular injury. The effects depend on the dose or intensity of the radiation. The effects can be seen both early and late. The lumbosacral plexus can be affected by radiation therapy for neoplasm of the pelvic organs, like prostate or testicular cancer in men, cervical or ovarian cancer in women, and colon cancer in both genders. Typical symptoms of radiation-induced lumbosacral plexopathy are slowly progressive muscle weakness and atrophy in the lower extremities which can be asymmetric or unilateral. There can be stepwise progression with long stable periods. Sensory symptoms are typically absent or minimal. Pain is not commonly seen or is typically mild. Neoplastic lumbosacral plexopathy is an important differential diagnosis to con sider and should be worked up as well. This is typically more painful.

Reference

Dyck PJ, Thaisetthawatkul P. Lumbosacral plexopathy. Continuum (Minneap Minn). 2014 Oct;20(5 Peripheral Nervous System Disorders):1343–58. https://doi.

org/10.1212/01.CON.0000455877.60932.d3. PMID: 25299286.

Linked question

94. What characteristic findings *that are most specific to the patient's suspected diagnosis* would you expect to see on electromyography in this patient?
    - A. Fibrillations and positive sharp waves
    - B. Myotonic discharges
    - C. Large, polyphasic motor unit action potentials
    - D. Complex repetitive discharges
    - E. Myokymia
    - **Correct answer**: E

Explanation

While many of these findings may be seen in several etiologies of lumbosacral plexopathy myokymic discharges are the most specific to radiation induced nerve damage. Myotonic discharges are characteristically seen in myotonic dystrophy, myotonia congenita, and paramyotonia congenita.

References

Dyck PJ, Thaisetthawatkul P. Lumbosacral plexopathy. Continuum (Minneap Minn). 2014 Oct;20(5 Peripheral Nervous System Disorders):1343–58. https://doi.org/10.1212/01.CON.0000455877.60932.d3. PMID: 25299286.

Ko K, Sung DH, Kang MJ, Ko MJ, Do JG, Sunwoo H, Kwon TG, Hwang JM, Park Y. Clinical, Electrophysiological Findings in Adult Patients with Non-traumatic Plexopathies. Ann Rehabil Med. 2011 Dec;35(6):807–15. https://doi.org/10.5535/arm.2011.35.6.807. Epub 2011 Dec 30. PMID: 22506209; PMCID: PMC3309383.

Preston, D. C., & Shapiro, B. E. (2020). *Electromyography and Neuromuscular Disorders: Clinical-Electrophysiologic-Ultrasound Correlations* (4th ed.). Elsevier. ISBN: 978-0-323-66180-5.

Linked question

95. If the patient had reported numbness over the anterolateral thigh, what nerve and root combination below is correct and localizable to her symptoms?
    - A. Saphenous nerve (L5)
    - B. Lateral femoral cutaneous nerve of the thigh (L2–L3)
    - C. Lateral femoral cutaneous nerve of the thigh (L1)
    - D. Intermediate femoral cutaneous nerve of the thigh (L3–L4)
    - E. Obturator nerve (L2–L4)
    - **Correct answer**: B

Explanation

The lateral femoral cutaneous nerve of the thigh is derived from the L2–L3 nerve roots and supplies sensation to the lateral and anterior thigh.

Reference

Preston, D. C., & Shapiro, B. E. (2020). *Electromyography and Neuromuscular Disorders: Clinical-Electrophysiologic-Ultrasound Correlations* (4th ed.). Elsevier. ISBN: 978-0-323-66180-5.

Linked question

96. Which of the following is true about the nerve the patient's thigh adduction weakness best localizes to?
    A. It is derived from the anterior divisions of the L2-L3-L4 nerve roots
    B. It is derived from the posterior divisions of the L2-L3-L4 nerve roots
    C. It supplies sensation to the perineum
    D. It arises from the lumbosacral trunk
    E. It is derived from the L4–L5 nerve roots

    Correct answer: A

Explanation

The anterior rami of L2-L3-L4 divides into anterior and posterior divisions. The anterior divisions form the obturator nerve and the posterior divisions form the femoral nerve. The obturator nerve provides innervation to the thigh adductors (adductor, longus, adductor brevis, adductor magnus, and gracilis) and sensation to a small area of skin on the medial thigh.

Reference

Preston, D. C., & Shapiro, B. E. (2020). *Electromyography and Neuromuscular Disorders: Clinical-Electrophysiologic-Ultrasound Correlations* (4th ed.). Elsevier. ISBN: 978-0-323-66180-5.

97. A 65-year-old male with hypertension, hyperlipidemia, and type 2 diabetes presents with a 6-week history of acute onset severe burning pain in his right hip and thigh followed by progressive weakness in the right leg. He also reports a 10-pound unintentional weight loss over the past two months. Examination reveals asymmetric proximal weakness in the right lower extremity with preserved distal strength and reduced patellar reflex on the right. Electrodiagnostic studies show active denervation in the right femoral-innervated muscles and lumbosacral paraspinals, with no demyelinating features. All of the following features would be supportive of the most likely diagnosis *except*?
    A. Elevated protein on CSF studies
    B. Nerve biopsy with multifocal nerve fiber loss and perivascular mononuclear inflammation.
    C. Normal MRI spine
    D. Retroperitoneal lymph node enlargement on imaging
    E. MRI lumbosacral plexus showing increased T2 signal intensity and thickening of right femoral nerve

    Correct answer: D

Explanation

Diabetic lumbosacral radiculoplexus neuropathy, also known as diabetic amyotrophy or Bruns-Garland syndrome, occurs most commonly in individuals with type 2 diabetes. Patients who experience lumbosacral radiculoplexus neuropathy often have fairly well-controlled diabetes. It often occurs in the setting of weight loss. Typically, patients will experience acute, severe pain in the hip or thigh described as burning, tightness, or allodynia followed by weakness of the limb. Typically, pain improves first and weakness can progress over months. On exam, depending on when patients present, there is asymmetric lower limb weakness, muscle atrophy, and absent or reduced reflexes. Sensory loss is atypical. Patients typically improve over time, although this recovery is slow (often up to 2 years) and frequently incomplete. Typically, this is a monophasic illness. Patients can have subsequent episodes on the opposite leg. The suspected pathogenesis is focal microvasculitis of individual nerves.

Diagnosis is largely clinical. Laboratory studies are generally normal. Biopsy of an involved nerve can show focal or multifocal nerve fiber loss, perivascular mononuclear inflammation and neovascularization in the epineurium, segmental demyelination, and axonal degeneration. CSF studies are notable for elevated protein, reflective of the nerve root involvement in this disorder. Nerve conduction studies will show low amplitude or absent compound muscle action potentials, that is often asymmetric, and needle EMG will show increased insertional activity, fibrillation potentials, and reduced recruitment of large motor unit action potentials. The findings are often patchy. MRI spine is often normal, but MRI of the lumbosacral plexus may show increased T2 signal intensity and nerve thickening.

Currently no treatment has been proven effective although IV steroids can be helpful for pain if the patient presents early enough.

Retroperitoneal lymph node involvement would be consistent with a neoplastic cause of lumbosacral plexopathy. This story is more consistent with diabetic amyotrophy.

Reference

Elafros MA, Callaghan BC. Diabetic Neuropathies. Continuum (Minneap Minn). 2023 Oct 1;29(5):1401–1417. https://doi.org/10.1212/CON.0000000000001291. PMID: 37851036; PMCID: PMC11088946.

Linked questions: 98–102

98. A 45-year-old right-handed woman presents with intermittent pain and paresthesias in her right hand. She describes tingling that awakens her from sleep which she can alleviate by shaking out her wrists. Symptoms are also provoked by driving or holding her phone. She describes symptoms in her thumb, index, and middle finger. What of the following exam findings would be most consistent with the suspected diagnosis?
    A. Weakness in finger abduction
    B. Tapping at the medial elbow causes tingling of the first three digits
    C. When attempting to hold a piece of paper between the thumb and index finger with the thumb held straight and adducted as the examiner pulls out the paper the patient is unable to hold the paper and flexes the thumb
    D. Normal sensation over the thenar eminence
    E. Pressing the wrists together in a flexed posture causes tingling in the dorsum of the hand
    Correct answer: D

Explanation

Median entrapment at the wrist is the most common of the entrapment neuropathies and the usual site of compression occurs in the carpal tunnel resulting in a constellation of signs and symptoms known as carpal tunnel syndrome. Typically, patients will experience wrist and arm pain and paresthesias of the hand. Pain can localize to the wrist but often may radiate into the forearm and arm. Paresthesias are often in the median nerve distribution (medial thumb, index, middle, and lateral ring finger) although patients frequently describe the whole hand being involved. Symptoms are classically provoked by flexing or extending the wrist and nocturnal symptoms are particularly common. Tinel's sign is often present-tapping at the wrist produces paresthesias in the median-innervated fingers. Phalen's maneuver, holding the wrists flexed and pressing them together, can also produce paresthesias in the median-innervated fingers (not the dorsum of the hand). When there are sensory findings from carpal tunnel syndrome the thenar eminence will be spared as it is supplied by a sensory branch from the median nerve before it enters the carpal tunnel. Furthermore, carpal tunnel syndrome is a clinical diagnosis and patients may not have exam findings of sensory change and weakness despite being symptomatic.

Weakness in finger abduction and when attempting to hold a piece of paper between the thumb and index finger with the thumb held straight and adducted as the examiner pulls out the paper the patient is unable to hold the paper and flexes the thumb (Froment's sign) are signs seen in ulnar neuropathy. Tapping at the elbow producing hand paresthesias (positive Tinel's at the elbow) can be seen in ulnar neuropathy at the elbow and would produce symptoms in the fourth and fifth digit.

Reference

Preston, D. C., & Shapiro, B. E. (2020). *Electromyography and Neuromuscular Disorders: Clinical-Electrophysiologic-Ultrasound Correlations* (4th ed.). Elsevier. ISBN: 978-0-323-66180-5.

Linked question

99. On exam tapping at the volar wrist and pressing the backs of the patient's wrists together with the wrists flexed produces tingling in the first three digits of the right hand. There is mild loss of sensation to pinprick over the medial thumb, the index finger, middle finger, and lateral ring finger. There is preserved strength in the hand and no muscle atrophy. What is the next most appropriate step in management?
    A. Splinting of the right wrist at night
    B. Splinting of the right elbow at night
    C. Surgical referral for carpal tunnel release
    D. Prednisone course
    E. MRI cervical spine
    Correct answer: A

Explanation

This clinical scenario is most consistent with carpal tunnel syndrome. Wrist splinting is considered a first-line treatment and can often be very effective in managing symptoms. Splinting of the elbow would not help with carpal tunnel syndrome but rather ulnar neuropathy at the elbow. Surgical referral can be made in more severe cases where wrist splinting has failed. Corticosteroid injections, not oral steroids, can provide short-term relief. MRI cervical spine would be appropriate if she was endorsing symptoms concerning for radiculopathy.

Reference

Wipperman J, Penny ML. Carpal Tunnel Syndrome: Rapid Evidence Review. Am Fam Physician. 2024 Jul;110(1):52–57. PMID: 39028782.

Linked question

100. The patient comes back several months later, symptoms have worsened and she now has weakness despite wrist splinting. You are considering surgical referral but first-order electrodiagnostic testing for further characterization, all of the findings below would be consistent with carpal tunnel syndrome *except*?
    A. Prolonged distal latency from the median nerve compound muscle action potential as recorded over the abductor pollicis brevis
    B. Fibrillations and positive sharp waves seen in the first dorsal interosseous
    C. Absent sensory nerve action potential recorded over the second digit
    D. Fibrillations and positive sharp waves seen in the APB

    Correct answer: B

Explanation

Changes in the first dorsal interossei would be consistent with ulnar neuropathy. The remaining changes could be seen in median neuropathy at the wrist (carpal tunnel syndrome).

Reference

Preston, D. C., & Shapiro, B. E. (2020). *Electromyography and Neuromuscular Disorders: Clinical-Electrophysiologic-Ultrasound Correlations* (4th ed.). Elsevier. ISBN: 978-0-323-66180-5.

Linked question

101. All of the following conditions are associated with carpal tunnel syndrome, except?
    A. Pregnancy
    B. Hypothyroidism
    C. Acromegaly
    D. Rheumatoid arthritis
    E. Hypertension

    Correct answer: E

Explanation

Most cases of carpal tunnel syndrome are idiopathic, but there are several conditions associated with the development of carpal tunnel syndrome.

Reference

Preston, D. C., & Shapiro, B. E. (2020). *Electromyography and Neuromuscular Disorders: Clinical-Electrophysiologic-Ultrasound Correlations* (4th ed.). Elsevier. ISBN: 978-0-323-66180-5.

Linked question

102. If the patient had instead presented with inability to flex the distal phalanx of the thumb, index, and middle finger as well as weakness of pronation without sensory changes, which of the following findings would support your suspected diagnosis?
    A. Fibrillations and positive sharp waves in the flexor pollicis longus
    B. Prolonged distal latency of the median nerve compound muscle action potential as recorded over the abductor pollicis brevis
    C. Absent median sensory nerve action potential as recorded over the second digit
    D. Fibrillations and positive sharp waves in the pronator teres
    E. Reduced median nerve CMAP as recorded over the abductor pollicis brevis.

    Correct answer: A

Explanation

This clinical scenario describes anterior interosseous neuropathy. The flexor pollicis longus is innervated by the anterior interosseous nerve. The remaining findings described above localize to other divisions of the median nerve.

Knowing the anatomy of the median nerve can help differentiate where lesions of the nerve may come from. The median nerve receives contributions from the upper, middle, and lower trunk of the brachial plexus and is formed by combining the medial and lateral cords. It descends the upper arm where it gives off no muscular branches, and as it passes into the forearm the median nerve runs between the two heads of the pronator teres before giving off branches to the pronator teres, flexor carpi radialis, and flexor digitorum superficialis. Next the anterior interosseous nerve branches off in the forearm, a pure motor nerve that innervates the flexor pollicis longus, the flexor digitorum profundus to digits 2 and 3, and the pronator quadratus. The median nerve continues toward the wrist and just proximal to the wrist and carpal tunnel the palmar cutaneous sensory branch arises which supplies sensation to the thenar eminence. The median nerve then enters the wrist through the carpal tunnel and in the palm divides into motor and sensory branches. The motor division travels into the palm where it supplies the first and second lumbricals. The recurrent motor branch is also given off from this division, and turns around to supply many of the thenar eminence muscles including the opponens pollicis, the abductor pollicis brevis, and the superficial head of the flexor pollicis brevis. The sensory division supplies the medial thumb, index finger, middle finger, and lateral half of the ring finger.

Reference

Preston, D. C., & Shapiro, B. E. (2020). *Electromyography and Neuromuscular Disorders: Clinical-*

Electrophysiologic-Ultrasound Correlations (4th ed.). Elsevier. ISBN: 978-0-323-66180-5.

103. A 40-year-old presents numbness and tingling in the fourth and fifth digits of her right hand. She is an avid cyclist and notes that symptoms worsen after long rides. On examination, she has weakness in finger abduction and adduction but preserved wrist flexion strength. You suspect ulnar neuropathy at the wrist.

      Which of the following findings would be most consistent with this diagnosis?
      A. Weakness in the flexor digitorum profundus (digits 4 and 5)
      B. Normal dorsal ulnar cutaneous nerve sensory nerve action potential
      C. Fibrillations and positive sharp waves in the flexor carpi ulnaris
      D. Slowed conduction velocity across the elbow in the ulnar nerve CMAP recorded over the adductor digiti minimi
      E. Neurogenic motor unit action potentials in the abductor pollicis brevis.

      Correct answer: B

Explanation

Understanding the anatomy of the ulnar nerve can assist with appropriately localizing lesions of the ulnar nerve. The ulnar nerve is essentially derived from the C8 and T1 roots and nearly all fibers travel through the lower trunk of the brachial plexus and continue into the medial cord. The ulnar nerve descends the medial arm where it does not give off any branches. The ulnar nerve travels to the elbow where it enters the ulnar groove (formed by the olecranon process and the medial epicondyle). It then travels through the cubital tunnel which is formed by the tendinous arch of the two heads of the flexor carpi ulnaris muscle. This is the common site of entrapment of the ulnar nerve. After this, it provides innervation to the flexor carpi ulnaris and the medial division of the flexor digitorum profundus (FDP) (to digits four and five). It then travels down through the medial forearm. Five to eight cm proximal to the wrist, the dorsal ulnar cutaneous nerves comes off to supply sensation to the dorsal medial hand, dorsal fourth, and medial fifth digits. The nerve than enters the medial wrist, traveling through Guyon's canal to supply sensation to the volar fifth and medial fourth digits, and muscular innervation to the palmar and dorsal interossei, the third and fourth lumbricals, the adductor pollicis, the deep head of the flexor pollicis longus, and the hypothenar muscles including the abductor digiti minimi.

Abnormalities in the flexor digitorum profundus and flexor carpi ulnaris would not be expected with ulnar neuropathy at the wrist. Slowed conduction velocity of the ulnar nerve at the elbow would be seen in ulnar neuropathy at the

elbow. Changes in the abductor pollicis brevis would be seen in median neuropathy, medial cord, lower trunk, or C8–T1 lesions. The dorsal ulnar cutaneous nerve is spared in ulnar neuropathy at the wrist so normal findings would be expected and consistent with ulnar neuropathy at the wrist.

Reference

Preston, D. C., & Shapiro, B. E. (2020). *Electromyography and Neuromuscular Disorders: Clinical-Electrophysiologic-Ultrasound Correlations* (4th ed.). Elsevier. ISBN: 978-0-323-66180-5.

104. A 30-year-old male after a night of drinking falls asleep with his right arm draped over a chair. The next day he notices weakness in raising his wrist and extending his fingers and altered sensation over the dorsum of his hand. All of the following would be consistent with the suspected diagnosis *except*?
      A. Weakness in elbow extension
      B. Mild weakness in elbow flexion
      C. Weakness supination
      D. Reduced sensation to pinprick over the lateral dorsum of the hand, part of the thumb and dorsal proximal index, middle and ring fingers
      E. Weakness in thumb extension

      Correct answer: A

Explanation

The radial nerve receives innervation from the C5–T1 nerve roots and all three trunks of the brachial plexus. It is a branch of the posterior cord. High in the arm it gives off the posterior cutaneous nerve of the arm, the lower lateral cutaneous nerve of the arm, and the posterior cutaneous nerve of the forearm as well as branches to the triceps. The nerve wraps around the posterior humerus, traveling in the spiral groove and travels toward the elbow. In the arm, it pierces the lateral intermuscular septum to enter the anterior compartment of the arm. It gives branches to the brachioradialis and long head of the extensor carpi radialis. Next, it enters the radial tunnel and passes by the elbow and bifurcates into superficial and deep branches. The superficial branch is the superficial radial sensory nerve which travels distally into the forearm, eventually becoming subcutaneous over the radial bone and supplying sensation to the lateral dorsum of the hand, part of the thumb, and dorsal proximal index middle and ring fingers. The deep branch supplies the extensor carpi radialis brevis and supinator muscle before entering the supinator muscle under the Arcade of Frohse, after which it is known as the posterior interosseous nerve. Note, some sources consider the entire deep branch to be the posterior interosseous nerve. The nerve then supplies the remaining extensors of the wrist, thumb, and fingers.

The above scenario describes the characteristic "Saturday night palsy" leading to compression of the radial nerve at the spiral groove. The triceps is spared in this scenario due to the innervation coming from the radial nerve above the spiral groove. The remaining findings are all from the radial nerve below the spiral groove.

Reference

Preston, D. C., & Shapiro, B. E. (2020). *Electromyography and Neuromuscular Disorders: Clinical-Electrophysiologic-Ultrasound Correlations* (4th ed.). Elsevier. ISBN: 978-0-323-66180-5.

105. A 50-year-old woman presents with weakness in right elbow flexion and paresthesias in the lateral forearm on the right. Exam confirms weakness in elbow flexion and absent right biceps reflex, as well as decreased sensation in the lateral forearm on the right. Electrodiagnostic testing demonstrates absent right lateral antebrachial cutaneous nerve sensory response, normal right median and radial nerve sensory responses, fibrillations and positive sharp waves in the right biceps and brachialis muscle, as well as neurogenic motor unit action potentials in those muscles and normal electromyography of the right flexor carpi radialis, pronator teres, deltoid, supraspinatus, infraspinatus, and cervical paraspinal muscles.

     Where would the lesion best localize?
     A. Lateral cord of the brachial plexus
     B. Musculocutaneous nerve
     C. C5 radiculopathy
     D. Upper trunk of the brachial plexus
     E. Medial cord of the brachial plexus
     Correct answer: B

Explanation

The pathology described here best localizes to the musculocutaneous nerve. The musculocutaneous nerve arises from the lateral cord of the brachial plexus, and in the upper arm runs between the biceps and brachialis muscles which it also innervates. It additionally supplies the coracobrachialis. It runs past the elbow where it becomes a pure sensory nerve, the lateral antebrachial cutaneous sensory nerve and supplies sensation to the lateral half of the forearm.

If the lesion was in the lateral cord of the brachial plexus, changes in the pronator teres and flexor carpi radialis would be expected as well as changes in the musculocutaneous innervated muscles. C5 radiculopathy is inconsistent with sparing of other C5 innervated muscles (deltoid, supraspinatus) as well as the cervical paraspinals. With lesions of the upper trunk of the brachial plexus changes in the supraspinatus and infraspinatus would be expected. Lesions in the

medial cord of the brachial plexus would affect sensation in the medial aspect of the arm (medial brachial and antebrachial cutaneous nerves branch from here) as well as ulnar innervated muscles among others.

Reference

Preston, D. C., & Shapiro, B. E. (2020). *Electromyography and Neuromuscular Disorders: Clinical-Electrophysiologic-Ultrasound Correlations* (4th ed.). Elsevier. ISBN: 978-0-323-66180-5.

106. A 32-year-old female develops weakness of her left arm after a shoulder dislocation. Exam is notable for left shoulder abduction weakness as well as more mild weakness in external rotation of the shoulder and a patch of numbness over the left lateral shoulder. Nerve conduction studies are notable for normal left radial nerve and lateral antebrachial cutaneous nerve sensory studies and normal left radial motor responses. Electromyography reveals denervation in the left deltoid and teres minor, and normal findings in the left triceps, biceps, supraspinatus, infraspinatus, brachioradialis, and cervical paraspinals.

     Where would the suspected pathology best localize?
     A. Posterior cord of the brachial plexus
     B. C5 radiculopathy
     C. Upper trunk of the brachial plexus
     D. C6 radiculopathy
     E. Axillary neuropathy
     Correct answer: E

Explanation

The patient's findings and electrodiagnostic testing is consistent with axillary neuropathy. The axillary is a branch off of the posterior cord of the brachial plexus, and largely receives its fibers from C5 and C6 running through the upper trunk of the brachial plexus. It supplies the teres minor (aids in external rotation of the shoulder), the deltoid (shoulder abduction) muscles, and sensation to an oval-shaped area over the lateral shoulder. With a lesion to the posterior cord of the brachial plexus, changes to the radial responses would be expected. Lack of findings in the cervical paraspinals and normal findings in non-axillary limb muscles localizing to C5 and C6 make radiculopathy unlikely. Upper trunk brachial plexopathy is less likely given normal findings in the supraspinatus and infraspinatus (supplied by the suprascapular nerve which branches off the upper trunk).

Reference

Preston, D. C., & Shapiro, B. E. (2020). *Electromyography and Neuromuscular Disorders: Clinical-Electrophysiologic-Ultrasound Correlations* (4th ed.). Elsevier. ISBN: 978-0-323-66180-5.

107. All of the following are true about diabetic neuropathy, except?
    A. Length-dependent axonal polyneuropathy is the most common manifestation of diabetic neuropathy.
    B. The most common diabetic mononeuropathies involve the cranial nerves.
    C. Neuropathy related to type 1 diabetes is less strongly linked to glycemic control than in type 2 diabetes.
    D. Diabetic radiculopathy can lead to bulging of the abdomen
    E. Diabetes increases risk for entrapment neuropathy

Correct answer: C

Explanation

Diabetic neuropathy involves a broad range of conditions that can manifest in a variety of ways. The most common presentation is of length-dependent axonal polyneuropathy. Diabetic neuropathy from type 1 and 2 diabetes are different; type 1 is more directly linked to glycemic control. While in type 2 diabetes, glycemic control is an important risk factor for neuropathy, it is not as tightly linked and evidence indicates that components of the metabolic syndrome including hypertriglyceridemia and hypertension are also important determinants of neuropathy risk and progression. More rarely, diabetes can manifest as mononeuropathies. Cranial mononeuropathy is the most common form of this, and the oculomotor nerve tends to be most commonly affected. Diabetic radiculopathy is a mononeuropathy that involves a single nerve root, typically presenting with rapid onset of unilateral pain in the thorax or abdomen in a single or multiple dermatome distribution. In severe cases, there can be bulging of the abdomen with upright posture due to denervation of the abdominal wall. Peripheral nerves are susceptible to damage from external pressure in diabetes; it is thought that this related to glycosylation of protein leading to cross-linking of collagen which produces a stiffer form of connective tissue, creating more risk for compression due to restricted anatomic channels for nerves that may already be damaged due to diabetes.

References

Bell DSH. Diabetic Mononeuropathies and Diabetic Amyotrophy. *Diabetes Ther*. 2022;13(10):1715–1722. https://doi.org/10.1007/s13300-022-01308-x. PMID: 35969368

Gibbons CH. Diabetes and Metabolic Disorders and the Peripheral Nervous System. Continuum (Minneap Minn). 2020 Oct;26(5):1161–1183. https://doi.org/10.1212/CON.0000000000000906. PMID: 33002997

Linked questions: 108–111

108. A 68-year-old male presents for numbness and weakness in his extremities. Five weeks prior to evaluation, he developed a right foot drop accompanied by pain and paresthesias. A few weeks later, he developed pain, numbness, and tingling in the right hand. A week later, he developed a left foot drop and pain. During this time period, he had a 10 lb unintentional weight loss. Exam is notable for weakness in dorsiflexion and eversion bilaterally, weakness in the right interossei, wrist flexion and finger flexion of digits 4 and 5, and sensory loss in the bilateral feet and right hand. Initial laboratory studies are notable for elevated inflammatory markers. Of the choices below, what is this presentation most consistent with?
    A. Vasculitic neuropathy
    B. Guillain- Barre syndrome
    C. Transverse myelitis
    D. Chronic Inflammatory Demyelinating Polyneuropathy (CIDP)
    E. Diabetic neuropathy

Correct answer: A

Explanation

This describes a presentation of painful mono neuritis multiplex, with the acute development of multiple mononeuropathies. Together with the weight loss and elevated inflammatory markers this is consistent with vasculitic neuropathy. Guillain-Barré syndrome, transverse myelitis, and CIDP do not present with mononeuritis multiplex. Diabetic neuropathy can present as mononeuritis multiplex but this is an uncommon presentation.

The typical presentation of vasculitic neuropathy is of mononeuritis multiplex with sequential painful peripheral neuropathies. Although vasculitis can also be more diffuse leading to painful and less commonly non-painful distal symmetric polyneuropathy or can be limited to the brachial or lumbosacral plexus. Vasculitic neuropathy can occur in the setting of systemic vasculitis, including primary vasculitides (such as ANCA-associated vasculitis) and secondary vasculitis (such as sarcoid, infection, and malignancy). Vasculitic neuropathy can also be classified as non-systemic vasculitic neuropathy. This includes recurrent/chronic conditions like non-systemic skin/nerve vasculitis and Wartenberg migratory sensory neuritis, and self-limiting conditions including diabetic inflammatory plexopathy and post-surgical inflammatory neuropathy.

References

Kapoor M, Reddel SW. Ways to think about vasculitic neuropathy. Curr Opin Neurol. 2024 Oct 1;37(5):478–486. https://doi.org/10.1097/WCO.0000000000001301. Epub 2024 Jul 24. PMID: 39046107.

Karam C. Peripheral Neuropathies Associated With Vasculitis and Autoimmune Connective Tissue Disease. Continuum (Minneap Minn). 2020 Oct;26(5):1257–1279. https://doi.org/10.1212/CON.0000000000000917.   PMID: 33003001.

Linked question

109. The patient undergoes nerve biopsy, you suspect vasculitic neuropathy, all of the following pathologic findings would be consistent with this diagnosis except?
A. Normal findings
B. Multifocal nerve fiber loss
C. Inflammation in the blood vessel well
D. Thrombosed blood vessel with recanalization
E. Focal thickening of the myelin sheath
Correct answer: E

Explanation

Normal findings can be seen because vasculitis is a patchy process and can be missed on biopsy. Multifocal nerve fiber loss is not definitely diagnostic of vasculitis neuropathy but is suggestive of it. Inflammation in the blood vessel wall and vascular wall damage is consistent with definite vasculitis. Definite vasculitis consists of inflammation in the blood vessel wall and vascular wall damage. Thrombosed blood vessels with recanalization is suggestive of chronic or prior vasculitis. Pathology will also depend on the cause of the vasculitis.

Focal thickening of the myelin sheath (tomacula) is seen in HNPP.

References

Kapoor M, Reddel SW. Ways to think about vasculitic neuropathy. Curr Opin Neurol. 2024 Oct 1;37(5):478–486. https://doi.org/10.1097/WCO.0000000000001301. Epub 2024 Jul 24. PMID: 39046107.

Karam C. Peripheral Neuropathies Associated With Vasculitis and Autoimmune Connective Tissue Disease. Continuum (Minneap Minn). 2020 Oct;26(5):1257–1279. https://doi.org/10.1212/CON.0000000000000917.   PMID: 33003001.

Klein CJ. Charcot-Marie-Tooth Disease and Other Hereditary Neuropathies. Continuum (Minneap Minn). 2020 Oct;26(5):1224–1256.   https://doi.org/10.1212/CON.0000000000000927. Erratum in: Continuum (Minneap Minn). 2021 Feb 1;27(1):289. https://doi.org/10.1212/CON.0000000000000990.   PMID: 33003000.

Linked question

110. Vasculitic neuropathy is associated with all of the following rheumatologic disorders *except*?
A. Systemic lupus erythematosus
B. Sjogren syndrome
C. Systemic sclerosis
D. Systemic vasculitides
E. Autoinflammatory disorders
Correct answer: C

Explanation

There can be a range of neurologic manifestations of various rheumatologic disorders, involving both the central and peripheral nervous system. Certain rheumatologic disorders have been shown to be associated with vasculitic neuropathy including systemic lupus erythematosus, sjogren syndrome and rheumatoid arthritis, although they are more commonly associated with other types of neuropathy including length-dependent axonal neuropathy and small fiber neuropathy. Systemic vasculitides and autoinflammatory disorders are strongly associated with vasculitic neuropathy. Systemic sclerosis has not been associated with vasculitic neuropathy, but is known to be associated with myopathy.

Reference

Toledano M. Neurologic Manifestations of Rheumatologic Disease. Continuum (Minneap Minn). 2023 Jun 1;29(3):734–762.   https://doi.org/10.1212/CON.0000000000001263. PMID: 37341329.

Linked question

111. Further workup is notable for negative ANCA antibodies, + hepatitis B virus antigen, and normal chest x ray. The patient develops significant abdominal pain and undergoes abdominal angiography demonstrating small aneurysms in the mesenteric arteries.

Which of the following systemic diseases do you suspect?
A. Polyarteritis nodosa
B. Giant cell arteritis
C. Eosinophilic granulomatosis with polyangiitis (Churg-Strauss syndrome)
D. Essential mixed cryoglobulinemia
E. Granulomatosis with polyangiitis (Wegener granulomatosis)
Correct answer: A

Explanation

Systemic vasculitis is often classified by small, medium, and large vessel vasculitis. Vasculitides of the small or medium blood vessels can involve the vasa nervorum or nerve arterioles, leading to neuropathy. The large vessel vasculitides rarely produce vasculitic neuropathy. Giant cell arteritis is a large vessel vasculitis that affects the aorta and its major branches. Symptoms include headache, jaw claudication, and monocular vision loss. ANCA-associated vasculitis, cryoglobulinemia, and polyarteritis nodosa are the vasculitides most often associated with neuropathy. Anca-associated vasculitis, including microscopic polyangiitis, granulomatosis with polyangiitis, and eosinophilic granulomatosis with polyangiitis, and immune complex vasculitis including cryoglobulinemic vasculitis are small vessel vasculitis. Polyarteritis nodosa is a medium vessel vasculitis.

While there is overlap in these different disorders, there are some features that can be used to distinguish them. Frequently, patients with ANCA-associated vasculitis have constitutional symptoms, such as fever and weight loss, involvement of the kidneys, and respiratory tract. In granulomatosis with polyangiitis, there is inflammation of the respiratory tract leading to sinus and respiratory system involvement. Eosinophilic granulomatosis with polyangiitis is accompanied by peripheral blood eosinophilia and asthma. ANCA can show specificity to either MPO (usually perinuclear ANCA) which is typically seen in microscopic polyangiitis or eosinophilic granulomatosis with polyangiitis or PR3 (usually cytoplasmic ANCA) which is typically seen in granulomatosis with polyangiitis.

Polyarteritis nodosa affects the small and medium vessels and leads to vasculopathy in multiple organ systems. Patients often have constitutional symptoms like fever, weight loss, and myalgia. There can be gastrointestinal, renal, and cardiac involvement. It can be associated with chronic hepatitis B infection. Skin manifestations can include livedo reticularis. Rarely there can be central nervous system involvement including stroke. Angiography of the visceral arteries can characteristically demonstrate arterial saccular or fusiform microaneurysms coexisting with stenotic lesions.

Cryoglobulinemia is caused by serum protein complexes (circulating immunoglobulins) that precipitate at cold temperature. Type I cryoglobulins consist of isolated monoclonal proteins (IgM or IgG) and can be seen in b cell lymphoproliferative diseases like multiple myeloma, Waldenström macroglobulinemia, chronic lymphocytic leukemia, and B-cell non-Hodgkin lymphoma. Type II cryoglobulins are mixed with a monoclonal component as well as polyclonal IgG. Type III cryoglobulins are mixed polyclonal cryoglobulins that are usually immunoglobulin-anti-immunoglobulin immune complexes. Type II and II cryoglobulins can also be associated with lymphoproliferative disorders but are mostly seen in patients with hepatitis C virus infection. Not all patients with cryoglobulins develop vasculitis, and when neuropathy develops it is most commonly a generalized neuropathy (although mononeuritis multiplex can occur). Patients with Sjögren syndrome, SLE, hepatocarcinoma, lymphoma, or hepatitis B virus may also have cryoglobulinemia. A classic triad of symptoms in cryo-

globulinemia includes diffuse joint pain, generalized weakness, and palpable purpura.

References

Karam C. Peripheral Neuropathies Associated With Vasculitis and Autoimmune Connective Tissue Disease. Continuum (Minneap Minn). 2020 Oct;26(5):1257–1279. https://doi.org/10.1212/CON.0000000000000917. PMID: 33003001.

Kapoor M, Reddel SW. Ways to think about vasculitic neuropathy. Curr Opin Neurol. 2024 Oct 1;37(5):478–486. https://doi.org/10.1097/WCO.0000000000001301. Epub 2024 Jul 24. PMID: 39046107.Toledano M. Neurologic Manifestations of Rheumatologic Disease. Continuum (Minneap Minn). 2023 Jun 1;29(3):734–762. https://doi.org/10.1212/CON.0000000000001263. PMID: 37341329.

Linked questions: 112–114

112. A 12 -year-old female presents for evaluation of clumsiness. Since she was young, she has struggled to keep up with her peers in gym class and frequently trips. She particularly has trouble going up hills. Her younger brother has similar symptoms. Her father and paternal uncle have needed braces their whole lives and were told they have a "nerve condition" based on biopsy done in childhood but have not regularly followed with a neurologist since their 20s. On examination, she has pes cavus, hammer toes, and distal muscle atrophy. Strength testing reveals distal lower extremity weakness. Reflexes are absent at the ankles and reduced at the knees. Sensation is decreased in a stocking-glove pattern.

    Which of the following is most likely to yield a precise diagnosis?
    A. Ganglioside antibody panel
    B. Nerve biopsy
    C. Genetic testing
    D. Lumbar spine MRI
    E. Electromyography and nerve conduction study (EMG/NCS)

Correct answer: C

Explanation

The above scenario is consistent with hereditary neuropathy, the most common of which is Charcot-Marie-Tooth disease (CMT), also called hereditary motor and sensory neuropathy (HMSN). Patients with CMT have slowly progressive distal muscle weakness and atrophy. Patients do not have significant pain and may not notice sensory changes so clinical presentation is most often due to weakness. Foot and ankle abnormalities (hammer toes, pes cavus) are common.

Genetic testing would be most helpful in yielding a precise diagnosis. While nerve biopsy and EMG/NCS can help characterize the neuropathy, genetic testing will give a more precise diagnosis and if positive obviates the need for additional expensive and uncomfortable testing. Ganglioside antibodies would be helpful if an immune-mediated neuropathy was suspected but this presentation is more consistent with a genetic condition. Lumbar spine MRI is not necessary as the symptoms do not localize to the lumbar spine.

Reference

Klein CJ. Charcot-Marie-Tooth Disease and Other Hereditary Neuropathies. Continuum (Minneap Minn). 2020 Oct;26(5):1224–1256. https://doi.org/10.1212/CON.0000000000000927. Erratum in: Continuum (Minneap Minn). 2021 Feb 1;27(1):289. https://doi.org/10.1212/CON.0000000000000990. PMID: 33003000.

Linked question

113. The genetic testing results were consistent with CMT1A, what mutation did they show?
    A. *PMP22* duplication
    B. *PMP22* deletion
    C. *GJB1*
    D. *MFN2*
    E. *MPZ*
    Correct answer: A

Explanation

CMT1A, a subtype of CMT 1 (autosomal dominant, demyelinating hereditary neuropathy) is caused by mutations in the peripheral myelin protein 22 gene (PMP22), most often a duplication, although point mutations may cause a similar or more severe phenotype. *PMP22* deletions are seen in hereditary neuropathy with liability to pressure palsies (HNPP) This presents with recurrent mononeuropathies with mild nerve trauma/compression, often with complete recovery between attacks. Mutations in GJB1 are seen in CMTX1, the most common CMTX, or x-linked CMT. CMT2A is the most common subtype of CMT2 (axonal neuropathy) and is caused by mutations in the mitofusin 2 gene (MFN2). Mutations in myelin protein zero (MPZ) are seen in CMT 1B, which is clinically and electrodiagnostically very similar to CMT1A. More rarely, MPZ mutation can also be seen in CMT2J, a late-onset axonal neuropathy.

References

Klein CJ. Charcot-Marie-Tooth Disease and Other Hereditary Neuropathies. Continuum (Minneap Minn). 2020 Oct;26(5):1224–1256. https://doi.org/10.1212/CON.0000000000000927. Erratum in: Continuum (Minneap Minn). 2021 Feb 1;27(1):289. https://doi.org/10.1212/CON.0000000000000990. PMID: 33003000.

Van Paassen, B.W., et al., PMP22 related neuropathies: Charcot-Marie-Tooth disease type 1A and Hereditary Neuropathy with liability to Pressure Palsies. Orphanet J Rare Dis, 2014. 9: p. 38.

Linked question

114. The patient's father remembers that he had EMG/NCS done when he was a child. What findings would you expect his EMG/NCS to have shown?
    A. Uniform conduction velocity slowing in the demyelinating range
    B. Mild slowing with low amplitudes
    C. Partial conduction block and abnormal temporal dispersion
    D. Small motor unit action potentials with early full recruitment
    E. Normal EMG/NCS
    Correct answer: A

Explanation

CMT 1A is an inherited demyelinating neuropathy which causes uniform conduction velocity slowing. Mild slowing with low amplitudes would be consistent with an axonal neuropathy. Acquired demyelinating neuropathies would cause patchy slowing in addition to partial conduction blocks and abnormal temporal dispersion. Small motor unit action potentials with early full recruitment describes a myopathic pattern. Normal EMG/NCS would not be expected in CMT

References

Klein CJ. Charcot-Marie-Tooth Disease and Other Hereditary Neuropathies. Continuum (Minneap Minn). 2020 Oct;26(5):1224–1256. https://doi.org/10.1212/CON.0000000000000927. Erratum in: Continuum (Minneap Minn). 2021 Feb 1;27(1):289. https://doi.org/10.1212/CON.0000000000000990. PMID: 33003000.

Preston, D. C., & Shapiro, B. E. (2020). *Electromyography and Neuromuscular Disorders: Clinical-Electrophysiologic-Ultrasound Correlations* (4th ed.). Elsevier. ISBN: 978-0-323-66180-5.

115. A 22-year-old man presents with progressive vision difficulties, hearing loss, gait instability, and loss of smell. He has had difficulty seeing in dim light since adolescence, and his balance has worsened over the past few years. Neurologic exam notable for absent deep tendon reflexes, distal muscle weakness, and distal sensory loss. He is also noted to have thickened, scaly skin on his palms and soles. Fundoscopic exam shows retinitis pigmentosa.

    Which of the following tests would be the most appropriate next step in confirming the suspected diagnosis?

A. Serum very long-chain fatty acids
B. Serum phytanic acid
C. Arylsulfatase A activity
D. Genetic testing for PMP22 duplication
E. Galactocerebrosidase activity
Correct answer: B

Explanation

The above clinical scenario describes Refsum disease, a peroxisomal disorder caused by a deficiency in the enzyme phytanoyl-CoA hydroxylase due to mutations in the *PHYH* gene. Less commonly it can be associated with pathogenic variants in the *PEX7* gene. This leads to the accumulation of phytanic acid which will be elevated in serum. Age of onset of symptoms can be variable from infancy to late adulthood. Typically patients present with late childhood onset retinitis pigmentosa and a variable combination of anosmia, polyneuropathy (sensory and motor), hearing loss, ataxia, ichthyosis, and cardiac arrhythmias and cardiomyopathy.

Serum very long-chain fatty acids are used in the diagnosis of adrenoleukodystrophy. Arylsulfatase A activity is reduced in metachromatic leukodystrophy. PMP22 duplication is seen in CMT1A. Galactocerebrosidase activity can be used to diagnose Krabbe disease.

References

Adang L. Leukodystrophies. Continuum (Minneap Minn). 2022 Aug 1;28(4):1194–1216. https://doi.org/10.1212/CON.0000000000001130. PMID: 35938662; PMCID: PMC11320896.

Klein CJ. Charcot-Marie-Tooth Disease and Other Hereditary Neuropathies. Continuum (Minneap Minn). 2020 Oct;26(5):1224–1256. https://doi.org/10.1212/CON.0000000000000927. Erratum in: Continuum (Minneap Minn). 2021 Feb 1;27(1):289. https://doi.org/10.1212/CON.0000000000000990. PMID: 33003000.

Waterham HR, Wanders RJA, Leroy BP. Adult Refsum Disease. 2006 Mar 20 [Updated 2021 Sep 30]. In: Adam MP, Feldman J, Mirzaa GM, et al., editors. GeneReviews® [Internet]. Seattle (WA): University of Washington, Seattle; 1993–2025. Available from: https://www.ncbi.nlm.nih.gov/books/NBK1353/

116. A 3-year-old girl is brought to the clinic due to progressive difficulty walking and frequent falls over the past several months. Previously, she had met all developmental milestones. On exam, she was noted to have distal extremity weakness and reduced deep tendon reflexes. EMG was consistent with a demyelinating neuropathy. Over the next several months, she experienced rapid decline and lost the ability to walk independently, and also speak. MRI showed confluent T2-hyperintensities in the periventricular and subcortical white matter. Further testing revealed reduced arylsulfatase A activity and increased urinary sulfatides.

   What is the diagnosis?
   A. Metachromatic leukodystrophy
   B. CMT1a
   C. Refsum disease
   D. CMTX
   E. Alexander disease
   Correct answer: A

Explanation

This scenario describes Metachromatic leukodystrophy. Metachromatic leukodystrophy is a lysosomal storage disorder typically caused by mutations in the ARSA gene which leads to insufficient arylsulfatase A enzymatic activity. The enzyme deficiency causes accumulation of sulfatides in the peripheral and central nervous system as well as the gallbladder. There are late infantile, juvenile, and adult-onset forms.

In the late infantile form, there are symptoms of rapid loss of motor and then cognitive function in the first few years of life. There is both central and peripheral demyelination and peripheral neuropathy can precede the central demyelination. Cranial neuropathies can also occur. In the juvenile form, the clinical decline is slower, but once ambulation is lost, it is rapid. In the adult form, there is a slow progression of neuropsychiatric symptoms.

Metachromatic leukodystrophy can be diagnosed by the combination of low arylsulfatase A enzymatic activity and elevated urinary sulfatides, as well as genetic testing confirming pathogenic variants in the *ARSA* gene.

Reference

Adang L. Leukodystrophies. Continuum (Minneap Minn). 2022 Aug 1;28(4):1194–1216. https://doi.org/10.1212/CON.0000000000001130. PMID: 35938662; PMCID: PMC11320896.

117. A 28-year-old female presents with progressive weakness and difficulty walking. She first noticed symptoms in her late teens with poor balance and mild foot weakness. Symptoms have progressively worsened. She also notes difficulty with fine motor tasks in the hands. Her father and paternal grandfather had similar issues. Exam is notable for mild distal atrophy in the legs, high arched feet, hammertoes, weakness in dorsiflexion, and plantar flexion, as well as the intrinsic foot muscles, absent ankle jerks, and distal sensory loss. EMG is consistent with an axonal neuropathy.

   Of the options below, which diagnosis fits the clinical scenario best?
   A. CMT1

B. CMT 2
C. CMT X
D. CMT 4
E. HNPP
Correct answer: B

Explanation

Charcot-Marie Tooth (CMT) also known as hereditary motor and sensory neuropathy (HMSN) (a term that is often used interchangeably) was classified into seven types as understanding of the genetic patterns, histopathologic findings, and neurophysiologic characteristics evolved. Now, in the era of next-generation sequencing and the discovery of numerous genes leading to overlapping phenotypes, traditional classifications of Charcot-Marie-Tooth (CMT) may fall out of favor. However, these terms remain widely used in clinical practice, helping guide diagnostic evaluation and patient counseling.

CMT1 refers to an autosomal-dominant form of CMT with demyelinating findings on electrodiagnostic testing. CMT2 is autosomal dominant with axonal features. CMT3, also known as Déjérine-Sottas neuropathy, is an early-onset severe form caused by several different mutations and now is no longer considered a separate category. Instead, depending on the mutation, these patients are categorized as CMT 1, CMTX (x-linked CMT), or CMT4 (autosomal recessive CMT). Of note CMT4 is not the same as HMSN4-HMSN4 now refers to Refsum disease and CMT4 is the term for all autosomal recessive demyelinating forms of CMT. CMT 5 (HSMN associated with spastic paraplegia), CMT6 (HMSN associated with optic atrophy), and CMT 7 (HMSN associated with retinitis pigmentosa) are not used in favor of genetic descriptions. For CMT types 1, 2, and 4 there are additional subclassifications by letters (CMT1a, etc.) based on the specific phenotype and causal gene. Although this is complicated by the large number of genes (more than letters in the alphabet), and the fact that the same gene can be both dominant and recessive

Reference

Klein CJ. Charcot-Marie-Tooth Disease and Other Hereditary Neuropathies. Continuum (Minneap Minn). 2020 Oct;26(5):1224–1256. https://doi.org/10.1212/CON.0000000000000927. Erratum in: Continuum (Minneap Minn). 2021 Feb 1;27(1):289. https://doi.org/10.1212/CON.0000000000000990. PMID: 33003000.

118. A 7-year-old boy with no significant past medical history is brought to the clinic due to declining school performance and difficulty walking over the last several months. Family history is notable for his mother having subtle difficulty with ambulation. On examination, he has spasticity in the lower limbs, hyperreflexia, impaired vibration sense, a tan complexion, and difficulty with fine motor skills. Brain MRI reveals symmetric T2 hyperintensities in the periventricular white matter, most prominently in the parieto-occipital regions.

What of the following tests would be consistent with his diagnosis (select all that apply).
A. Insufficient arylsulfatase A enzymatic activity
B. Elevated serum phytanic acid
C. Elevated serum very long chain fatty acids
D. Mutation in *ABCA1* gene
E. Mutation in *ABCD1* gene
Correct answer: C, E

Explanation

The case described here is consistent with adrenoleukodystrophy. Adrenoleukodystrophy is an X-linked peroxisomal disorder caused by mutations in the *ABCD1* gene. This leads to deficiency of the peroxisomal transporter ATP binding cassette transporter subfamily D member 1 (ABCD1) and accumulation of very long chain fatty acids. These very long chain fatty acids accumulate and result in pathology in the brain, spinal cord, and adrenal glands. It can present as three distinct phenotypes: cerebral adrenoleukodystrophy, adreno-myeloneuropathy, and Addison only (adrenal insufficiency). Women can present with an attenuated form of adrenomyeloneuropathy.

Most cases of cerebral adrenoleukodystrophy occur in childhood, although there can be onset in adulthood as well. This is characterized by behavioral change, cognitive decline, and fine motor difficulties. Hematopoietic stem cell transplant is standard of care for pre or minimally symptomatic cerebral adrenoleukodystrophy.

Adults typically present with adrenomyeloneuropathy which is characterized by demyelination and atrophy within the spinal cord, preferentially affecting the corticospinal tracts. Clinically, it manifests as progressive difficulty walking, urinary and sexual dysfunction.

Most affected boys will have some degree of adrenal insufficiency.

References

Adang L. Leukodystrophies. Continuum (Minneap Minn). 2022 Aug 1;28(4):1194–1216. https://doi.org/10.1212/CON.0000000000001130. PMID: 35938662; PMCID: PMC11320896.

Raymond GV, Moser AB, Fatemi A. X-Linked Adrenoleukodystrophy. 1999 Mar 26 [Updated 2023 Apr 6]. In: Adam MP, Feldman J, Mirzaa GM, et al., editors.

GeneReviews® [Internet]. Seattle (WA): University of Washington, Seattle; 1993–2025. Available from: https://www.ncbi.nlm.nih.gov/books/NBK1315/

119. A 55-year-old man presents with 6 months of slowly progressive weakness in the lower extremities and a longer duration of paresthesias and loss of sensation in his feet. He also complains of constipation, dizziness with standing, and sexual dysfunction. Examination is notable for reduced sensation to temperature, pain, and light touch. Additional workup reveals orthostatic hypotension and elevated creatinine.

Of the options below, which gene mutation is most likely to be found in this patient?

A. *GAN*
B. *TTR*
C. *PMP22*
D. *ABCD1*
E. *GFAP*

Correct answer: B

Explanation

This clinical scenario is consistent with hereditary transthyretin amyloidosis with neuropathy (familial amyloid neuropathy). These are a group of autosomal-dominant disorders caused by aggregates of abnormal precursor protein of amyloid. Most commonly, this is transthyretin and is caused by mutations in *TTR*. Clinical manifestations include length-dependent sensorimotor polyneuropathy, autonomic dysfunction, heart failure, cardiac arrhythmias, and nephrotic disease. There are several small oligonucleotide-based gene therapies, approved by the FDA for treatment: including patisiran (small interfering RNA) and inotersen (antisense oligonucleotide).

GAN mutations lead to GAN-related neurodegeneration which can range from severe to milder. The more severe phenotype is called giant axonal neuropathy and typically presents in infancy, starting with severe sensorimotor neuropathy and evolving to have central nervous system involvement. Tightly coiled hair is also characteristic.

PMP22 mutations can be seen in Charcot-Marie-tooth and hereditary neuropathy with liability to pressure palsies. The former is characterized by a progressive sensorimotor neuropathy, and the latter by recurrent mononeuropathies.

ABCD1 mutations are seen in adrenoleukodystrophy, an x-linked peroxisomal disorder, with features of cognitive decline, fine motor difficulties, and adrenal insufficiency.

Pathogenic variants in the *GFAP* gene can lead to Alexander disease, an autosomal-dominant leukodystrophy characterized by neurologic decline, ataxia, and eye movement dysfunction.

References

Adang L. Leukodystrophies. Continuum (Minneap Minn). 2022 Aug 1;28(4):1194–1216. https://doi.org/10.1212/CON.0000000000001130. PMID: 35938662; PMCID: PMC11320896.

Klein CJ. Charcot-Marie-Tooth Disease and Other Hereditary Neuropathies. Continuum (Minneap Minn). 2020 Oct;26(5):1224–1256. https://doi.org/10.1212/CON.0000000000000927. Erratum in: Continuum (Minneap Minn). 2021 Feb 1;27(1):289. https://doi.org/10.1212/CON.0000000000000990. PMID: 33003000.

Opal P. GAN-Related Neurodegeneration. 2003 Jan 9 [Updated 2021 Oct 14]. In: Adam MP, Feldman J, Mirzaa GM, et al., editors. GeneReviews® [Internet]. Seattle (WA): University of Washington, Seattle; 1993–2025. Available from: https://www.ncbi.nlm.nih.gov/books/NBK1136/

120. A 34-year-old woman presents with several days of altered cognition followed by acute-onset of severe abdominal pain, nausea, and vomiting. Following these symptoms, she developed progressive weakness. Her medical history is significant for intermittent episodes of abdominal pain over the past few years, but no clear diagnosis was made. She reports that she started a new sulfa-containing antibiotic last week for a urinary tract infection. She is noted to have dark urine. Neurological exam is notable for proximal > than distal weakness in the extremities as well as reduced deep tendon reflexes.

Which of the following tests would be the *most appropriate next step* in confirming the suspected diagnosis?

A. Urinary levels of δ-aminolevulinic acid and porphobilinogen
B. Arylsulfatase A enzymatic activity
C. Serum phytanic acid level
D. CSF analysis for albuminocytologic dissociation
E. Galactocerebrosidase activity

Correct answer: A

Explanation

The clinical presentation described here is consistent with porphyric neuropathy.

Porphyrias are inherited disorders caused by several different mutations in the genes encoding for enzymes in the heme biosynthetic pathways. They are classified as either hepatic or erythropoietic depending on the site of production of the heme. They can also be categorized as acute neurovisceral or cutaneous porphyrias based on the primary expression of symptoms. The acute hepatic porphyrias (AHP) which present with neurological symptoms predominately include acute intermittent porphyria (AIP), hereditary coproporphyria (HCP), variegate porphyria (VP), and delta-aminolevulinic acid dehydratase (ALAD) deficiency porphyria (ADP).

Clinically the acute hepatic porphyrias can present with acute neurovisceral attacks which can be triggered by different factors including medications. Typically, patients develop neuropsychiatric symptoms followed by severe abdominal pain and vomiting. Patients can also have darkening of the urine. With acute intermittent porphyria, peripheral neuropathy can develop after these symptoms, termed porphyric neuropathy. Onset can be rapid with maximal involvement within 4 weeks and can be severe. Proximal weakness is common, and there tends to be more motor rather than sensory involvement. Autonomic dysfunction can also occur.

During an attack, confirmation of an acute intermittent porphyria relies on elevated urinary levels of δ-aminolevulinic acid and porphobilinogen.

Reference

Gandhi Mehta RK, Caress JB, Rudnick SR, Bonkovsky HL. Porphyric neuropathy. Muscle Nerve. 2021 Aug;64(2):140–152. https://doi.org/10.1002/mus.27232. Epub 2021 Mar 31. PMID: 33786855.

Linked questions: 121–124

121. A four-year-old boy presents to a neuromuscular clinic due to falls and difficulty running and jumping. His parents report that he is unable to run well and also has difficulty with stairs. Family history is notable for a maternal uncle who was in a wheelchair and died in his early 20s due to cardiac complications. Examination is notable for atrophy of the thigh muscles and enlargement of his calves, a waddling gait, diminished reflexes with preserved ankle jerks, and using his hands to push up his legs to stand from sitting. Laboratory evaluation was notable for CK that is 10 times the upper limit of normal.

    Which of the following genes is most likely to be mutated in this patient?
    A. *DMD*
    B. *MYOT*
    C. *COL6*
    D. *LMNA*
    E. *CAV3*

    Correct answer: A

Explanation

The case scenario described here is consistent with Duchenne's muscular dystrophy (DMD), a dystrophinopathy. Dystrophinopathies are x-linked conditions due to mutations in the *DMD* gene which encodes for dystrophin, a skeletal muscle protein that connects the contractile apparatus to the extracellular matrix via the muscle membrane. These include DMD—the most severe form, Becker's muscular dystrophy (BMD) —a milder form, and an intermediate form. Mutations cause limited production of the dystrophin protein, causing loss of myofiber membrane integrity and necrosis and replacement of muscle with fibrous and connective tissue.

Characteristically in boys with DMD, development is normal in the first few years of life, although milestones may be slightly delayed and there may be mild hypotonia. In the first 2–3 years of life, weakness will typically manifest with symptoms like frequent falls and difficulty walking. Weakness is typically most pronounced in the proximal legs. Classic features include calf pseudohypertrophy and a Gower's sign (needing to push up with the arms from sitting). Weakness is progressive. There is also cardiac involvement. Typically, patients become wheelchair bound by around age 12, and affected patients usually die in their 20s from cardiac or respiratory complications. Dilated cardiomyopathy will develop eventually in almost all patients. Mild intellectual disability is common. Serum CK levels are often 10–20 times the upper limit of normal. Muscle biopsy is not typically needed as part of the workup but would demonstrate endomysial connective tissue proliferation, scattered degeneration, and regeneration of myofibers, muscle fiber necrosis with a mononuclear cell infiltrate, and replacement of muscle with adipose tissue and fat.

Mutations in the *MYOT* are seen in limb-girdle muscular dystrophy (LGMD) type 1A (myotilinopathy). LGMDs are a diverse group of genetic disorders generally characterized by weakness of the shoulder and pelvic girdle muscles that can present from childhood through adulthood. By convention, LGMD type 1 are autosomal-dominant and LGMD type 2 are autosomal recessive. LGMD1A has variable onset from the 20s to the 70s. Typically, it will present with first weakness in the legs and then the arms, facial and neck extensor weakness can occur as well. Cardiomyopathy can also occur, typically later in life. CK can be normal or elevated.

Mutations in *COL6* lad to collagen-6-related muscular dystrophy phenotypes, a type of congenital muscular dystrophy. Congenital muscular dystrophies (CMDs) are a group of inherited conditions defined by muscle weakness occurring before the acquisition of ambulation, delayed motor milestones, and characterized by muscle dystrophic pathology. Collagen-VI related muscular dystrophies exist on a spectrum from the more severe Ullrich's congenital muscular dystrophy phenotype to the milder Bethlem myopathy phenotype. Characteristic clinical features include progressive muscle weakness, distal joint laxity and proximal joint contractures, and keloid scars and hyperkeratosis pilaris.

Mutations in the *LMNA* gene which encodes Lamin A/C, a nuclear envelope protein, are seen in LGMD1B. Different phenotypes can be associated with mutations in this gene. LGMD1B generally presents before age 20 with proximal lower extremity weakness, with later involvement of the arms. Cardiac abnormalities are common including cardiomyopathy and rhythm abnormalities. Serum CK can be normal or mildly elevated. Emery-Dreifuss muscular dystrophy is another phenotype which manifests as contractures of the elbows, ankles and posterior cervical muscles, slowly progressive weakness, cardiac abnormalities and a slight elevation in CK levels. Congenital muscular dystrophy phenotypes can be seen as well.

CAV3 mutations are seen in LGMD1C (caveolinopathy and rippling muscle disease). LGMD1C typically can manifest between childhood and adulthood. It involves proximal muscle weakness in the lower extremities and frequently cramps after exercise. It can often have a benign clinical course and life expectancy is not reduced. Caveolin 3 mutations can also result in rippling muscle disease phenotypes. This is characterized by wormlike movements in the muscle surface, muscle mounding, and percussion-related contraction.

References

Iyadurai SJ, Kissel JT. The Limb-Girdle Muscular Dystrophies and the Dystrophinopathies. Continuum (Minneap Minn). 2016 Dec;22(6, Muscle and Neuromuscular Junction Disorders):1954–1977. https://doi.org/10.1212/CON.0000000000000406. PMID: 27922502.

Venugopal V, Pavlakis S. Duchenne Muscular Dystrophy. [Updated 2023 Jul 10]. In: StatPearls [Internet]. Treasure Island (FL): StatPearls Publishing; 2025 Jan-. Available from: https://www.ncbi.nlm.nih.gov/books/NBK482346/

Zambon AA, Muntoni F. Congenital muscular dystrophies: What is new? Neuromuscul Disord. 2021 Oct;31(10):931–942. https://doi.org/10.1016/j.nmd.2021.07.009. Epub 2021 Jul 28. PMID: 34470717.

Linked question

122. The patient undergoes genetic testing which confirms mutation in the dystrophin gene expected to cause Duchenne muscular dystrophy.

    Where is dystrophin expressed? Select all that apply.
    A. Striated muscle
    B. Liver
    C. Cardiac muscle
    D. Brain
    E. Kidney
    Correct answer: A, C, D

Explanation

Dystrophin is expressed in both striated and cardiac muscle which is why there is weakness and cardiomyopathy seen in the dystrophinopathies. To a lesser extent, it is also expressed in the brain and retina which explains some of the central nervous system manifestations of Duchenne's muscular dystrophy.

Reference

Iyadurai SJ, Kissel JT. The Limb-Girdle Muscular Dystrophies and the Dystrophinopathies. Continuum (Minneap Minn). 2016 Dec;22(6, Muscle and Neuromuscular Junction Disorders):1954–1977. https://doi.org/10.1212/CON.0000000000000406. PMID: 27922502.

Linked question

123. Which of the following should the patient's family be counseled about?
    A. The patient's father should have neuromuscular evaluation
    B. The patient's mother should consider genetic testing for *DMD* mutation
    C. Severe intellectual impairment is expected
    D. The patient's sister has a 50% chance of being symptomatic
    Correct answer: B

Explanation

Duchenne's muscular dystrophy (DMD) is due to an x-linked mutation and while spontaneous mutations can lead to DMD, it can be passed from the affected patient's biological mother. It would not be passed on from his biological father. Given the history of an affected uncle, this is most likely the case. While female carriers can be unaffected, they can also have (typically mild) symptoms and are at risk for cardiomyopathy. It is important for carrier females to have a cardiac evaluation.

Mild, not severe, intellectual impairment is common in patients with DMD.

The patient's sister most likely has a 50% chance of being a carrier of a mutated *DMD* gene, but carriers are not necessarily symptomatic.

Reference

Lee BH. The Dystrophinopathies. Continuum (Minneap Minn). 2022 Dec 1;28(6):1678–1697. https://doi.org/10.1212/CON.0000000000001208. PMID: 36537975.

Linked question

124. Regarding management options for Duchenne's muscular dystrophy (DMD), which of the following is true?
    A. All DMD patients are started on exon skipping therapy
    B. Oral corticosteroids are recommended
    C. All exercise should be avoided
    D. B and C
    E. None of the above
    Correct answer: B

Explanation

Exon skipping therapy uses antisense oligonucleotides to restore the reading frame of a mutated dystrophin gene by "skipping" an exon. The patient needs to have a specific mutation in order to be eligible for exon skipping therapy. Eteplirsen is the first exon skipping therapy to be approved by the FDA and is an exon-51-skipping therapy. Approximately 14% of individuals with dystrophinopathy are amenable to mutation-specific exon-51–skipping therapy,

Oral corticosteroids have been shown to prolong the ability to walk, preserve upper extremity strength, have cardiopulmonary benefits, and reduce the risk of scoliosis in patients with Duchenne's muscular dystrophy (DMD). Commonly used corticosteroids include prednisone and deflazacort. There are a variety of regimens that are used and the use may be limited by side effects.

Gentle exercise is recommended to prevent disuse atrophy. If myoglobinuria or significant muscle pain develops, activity should be reduced.

References

Lee BH. The Dystrophinopathies. Continuum (Minneap Minn). 2022 Dec 1;28(6):1678–1697, https://doi.org/10.1212/CON.0000000000001208. PMID: 36537975.

Venugopal V, Pavlakis S. Duchenne Muscular Dystrophy. [Updated 2023 Jul 10]. In: StatPearls [Internet]. Treasure Island (FL): StatPearls Publishing; 2025 Jan-. Available from: https://www.ncbi.nlm.nih.gov/books/NBK482346/

Linked questions: 125–127

125. A 42-year-old male is evaluated in clinic. He reports gradually progressive weakness since his 20s. He also describes difficulty relaxing his hand and jaw, with movements like letting go from a handshake and chewing food. He reports his mother also has difficulty relaxing her grip but no weakness. Exam is notable for ptosis, temporal atrophy, weakness in neck flexion, weakness in the distal limb muscles, and grip and percussion myotonia.

Which of the following is this presentation most consistent with?
    A. Myotonia congenita
    B. Paramyotonia congenita
    C. Myotonic dystrophy type 1
    D. Myotonic dystrophy type 2
    E. Sodium Channel myotonia
    Correct answer: C

Explanation

Of the above choices, this clinical scenario is most consistent with Myotonic dystrophy type 1 (DM1). DM1 is caused by an expanded CTG triplet in the *DMPK* gene on chromosome 19. 50 to more than 1000 CTG repeats can be present, compared to fewer than 37 in people without DM1. Clinically, characteristic patterns of weakness in DM1 include involvement of cranial, oropharyngeal, trunk, and distal limb muscles. Temporal wasting is seen. Myotonia, delayed relaxation of muscles, can be seen characteristically in the hands, tongue, and jaw. Patients may describe difficulty releasing from a handshake or from a doorknob. In the tongue and jaw, it can impact chewing and speaking.

DM2 is caused by an expanded CCTG tetramer in the *CNPB* gene on chromosome 3. Normal repeats range from 11 to 25, while in DM2 the number ranges from 75 to 10,000. The age of onset tends to be later as compared to DM1. Typical clinical symptoms include leg weakness, myalgia, and myotonia. Neck flexors, truncal musculature, and proximal limb muscles are preferentially affected. Later in life distal muscles can be affected as well.

DM1 and DM2 are multisystem disorders and multidisciplinary care is essential. Respiratory involvement is common, particularly in DM1. Cardiac conduction deficits are common in both DM1 and DM2. Cataracts are also seen in DM1 and DM2. They are also associated with increased cholesterol levels, hypertriglyceridemia, and insulin resistance. Diabetes is common, and more common in patients with DM2 as compared to those with DM1

Myotonia congenita, paramyotonia congenita, and sodium channel myotonia are non-dystrophic myotonias. In the non-dystrophic myotonias, symptoms usually occur in the first two decades of life and include muscle stiffness, weakness, fatigue, and pain. In contrast to DM1 and DM2, there is not severe fixed weakness or muscle atrophy. Clinical features are varied and can range from mild muscle stiffness to severe myotonia. Myotonia can be treated with sodium-channel blockers including antiseizure medications, anesthetics, and antiarrhythmics-like mexiletine.

Myotonia congenita is seen in *CLCN1* mutations, which encodes the main skeletal muscle chloride channel ClC-1 and can be autosomal dominant (Thomsen disease) or autosomal recessive (Becker disease- more severe). Patients will have muscular builds due to hypertrophy. Action myotonia is seen- stiffness with rapid movement. The stiffness improves with exercise ("warm-up phenomenon"). More commonly with Becker disease patients can characteristically experience initial weakness with exercise that subsequently improves.

Paramyotonia congenita and sodium-channel myotonias are autosomal-dominant disorders related to *SCN4A* mutations. In paramyotonia congenita, muscle stiffness worsens after sustained exercise ("paradoxical myotonia"). Paramyotonia congenita also more commonly affects the face, and classically there is paradoxical eye closure myotonia (with repetition there is more difficulty with eye closure and opening).

References

Hamel JI. Myotonic Dystrophy. Continuum (Minneap Minn). 2022 Dec 1;28(6):1715–1734. https://doi.org/10.1212/CON.0000000000001184. PMID: 36537977.

Trivedi JR. Muscle Channelopathies. Continuum (Minneap Minn). 2022 Dec 1;28(6):1778–1799. https://doi.org/10.1212/CON.0000000000001183. PMID: 36537980.

Linked question

126. Which of the following gene mutations is paired correctly with the clinical disorder?
    A. Myotonia congenita—*SCN4A*
    B. Paramyotonia congenita—*SCN4A*
    C. Myotonic dystrophy type 1—*CNPB*
    D. Myotonic dystrophy type 22—*DMPK*
    E. None of the above
    Correct answer: B

Explanation

Myotonia congenita is associated with *CLCN1* mutations. Paramyotonia congenita is associated with *SCN4A* mutations. Myotonic dystrophy type 1 is caused by an expanded CTG triplet in the *DMPK* gene on chromosome 19. Myotonic dystrophy type 2 is caused by an expanded CCTG tetramer in the *CNPB* gene on chromosome 3.

Reference

Trivedi JR. Muscle Channelopathies. Continuum (Minneap Minn). 2022 Dec 1;28(6):1778–1799. https://doi.org/10.1212/CON.0000000000001183. PMID: 36537980.

Linked question

127. Regarding myotonic dystrophy type 1 (DM1) and type 2 (DM2), which of the following is true?
    A. DM2 has a congenital form
    B. DM2 characteristically has more facial muscle weakness as compared to DM1
    C. DM1 has more grip myotonia as compared to DM2
    D. Diabetes is more common in DM1 as compared to DM2
    Correct answer: C

Explanation

Congenital myotonic dystrophy can be seen with DM1 and is the most severe form characterized by symptoms within the first month of life. There can be decreased fetal movements prenatally. Symptoms include hypotonia, respiratory weakness, feeding difficulties, and skeletal abnormalities like club feet.

DM2 has more pronounced proximal weakness, including neck flexion, truncal muscles, and proximal leg and arm muscles. DM1 has more facial involvement. In DM1, there is prominent temporal wasting and ptosis as well as weakness of the facial and oropharyngeal muscles, neck flexion, respiratory muscles, truncal muscles, and distal limb muscles. DM1 has more grip and oromandibular myotonia and DM2 has more myotonia in the proximal muscles.

Myotonic dystrophy is associated with increased cholesterol levels, hypertriglyceridemia, and insulin resistance. Diabetes is common, and more common in patients with DM2 as compared to those with DM1.

Reference

Hamel JI. Myotonic Dystrophy. Continuum (Minneap Minn). 2022 Dec 1;28(6):1715–1734. https://doi.org/10.1212/CON.0000000000001184. PMID: 36537977.

128. A 19-year-old man presents to clinic for left-sided shoulder complaints that he noticed after trying a new workout in the gym. He has been having difficulty lifting the arm. He notes that he has always struggled particularly with upper body workouts and feels he has been unable to lift heavier weights despite exercising regularly. On neurological exam, you find the patient has weakness in eye closure, weakness in pursing his lips, and a horizontal smile. You note bilateral scapular winging, more pronounced on the left side. He can only lift the left arm to 120° and has atrophy of the left pectoral major muscle with a horizontal axillary fold.

You suspect that the patient has Facioscapulohumeral Muscular Dystrophy (FSHD) and send genetic testing. What would be consistent with your suspected diagnosis (select all that apply).

A. Mutation in *DYSF* gene
B. D4Z4 repeat contraction
C. Mutation in *FKTN* gene
D. *SMCHD1* (structural maintenance of chromosomes flexible hinge domain containing 1) mutation
E. CGN trinucleotide repeat in *PABN1*

Correct answer: B, D

Explanation

FSHD can be caused by two separate mutations that result in similar clinical presentations. FSHD 1 and FSHD2 have the same downstream mechanism; misexpression of the double homeobox 4 (*DUX4*) gene, which is normally epigenetically silenced in most somatic tissues. In FSHD1, there is a repeat contraction of the D4Z4 on chromosome 4q35.18, which the *DUX4* gene is buried in and this contraction allows for the expression of the *DUX4* gene. FSHD2 is less common, and is most often caused by mutations in the *SMCHD1* (structural maintenance of chromosomes flexible hinge domain containing 1) gene on chromosome 18. Clinically, there is a characteristic pattern of weakness, which often starts in the face, shoulder girdle, and upper arms. Later in the disease, the trunk, pelvic girdle, and leg muscles become involved. Onset is typically in late adolescence through early adulthood although this can vary. Severity of disease is also highly variable even within the same family. Some characteristic findings in FSHD include a transverse smile (due to facial weakness), asymmetric scapular winging (weakness of the serratus anterior and trapezius), and horizontal axillary folds (weakness of the pectoral muscle).

Mutations in the *DYSF* gene are seen in limb girdle muscular dystrophy 2b (LGMD2B), a dysferlinopathy. This can present with different phenotypes including a limb girdle phenotype, Miyoshi myopathy and distal myopathy with anterior tibial onset. Onset is from adolescence to late adulthood, typically beginning with pelvic girdle weakness. Walking can be affected due to involvement of the gastrocnemius. Involvement of the upper extremities develops after the lower extremity weakness. Miyoshi distal myopathy can present with the inability to walk and to get up on the toes. Anterior tibial onset variety presents with steppage gait and foot drop. Muscle biopsy would reveal a reduction or lack of dysferlin staining.

Mutations in the *FKTN* gene are seen in Fukuyama congenital muscular dystrophy. This is a α-dystroglycan–related muscular dystrophy. It is common in Japan due to an ancestral mutation. Clinically patients present with hypotonia, generalized muscle weakness, and CNS migration disturbances including cobblestone lissencephaly. Onset is typi-

cally in early infancy. CK is elevated and muscle biopsy will show findings consistent with muscular dystrophy (interstitial fibrosis) and selective deficiency of α-dystroglycan when this is stained for.

CGN trinucleotide repeat in *PABN1* is seen in oculopharyngeal muscular dystrophy. This tends to have onset in later adult life (late 40s) and is characterized by ptosis and dysphagia. Restricted extraocular movements and limb weakness will also develop. The proximal musculature is the most affected.

References

Iyadurai SJ, Kissel JT. The Limb-Girdle Muscular Dystrophies and the Dystrophinopathies. Continuum (Minneap Minn). 2016 Dec;22(6, Muscle and Neuromuscular Junction Disorders):1954–1977. https://doi.org/10.1212/CON.0000000000000406. PMID: 27922502.

Mul K. Facioscapulohumeral Muscular Dystrophy. Continuum (Minneap Minn). 2022 Dec 1;28(6):1735–1751. https://doi.org/10.1212/CON.0000000000001155. PMID: 36537978.

Saito K. Fukuyama Congenital Muscular Dystrophy. 2006 Jan 26 [Updated 2019 Jul 3]. In: Adam MP, Feldman J, Mirzaa GM, et al., editors. GeneReviews® [Internet]. Seattle (WA): University of Washington, Seattle; 1993–2025. Available from: https://www.ncbi.nlm.nih.gov/books/NBK1206/

Trollet C, Boulinguiez A, Roth F, et al. Oculopharyngeal Muscular Dystrophy. 2001 Mar 8 [Updated 2020 Oct 22]. In: Adam MP, Feldman J, Mirzaa GM, et al., editors. GeneReviews® [Internet]. Seattle (WA): University of Washington, Seattle; 1993–2025. Available from: https://www.ncbi.nlm.nih.gov/books/NBK1126/

129. A 5-year-old girl is brought to the neuromuscular clinic due to generalized hypotonia and delayed motor milestones. She sat independently at 10 months but has never been able to walk. Her parents note that she has significant joint stiffness in her elbows and fingers, but also looseness (hyperlaxity) in her ankles and wrists. On exam, she has proximal muscle weakness, contractures of the elbows, hypermobility of distal joints, and a soft velvety skin texture of the soles of her feet. There is no facial weakness. Muscle biopsy commonly shows dystrophic features (degeneration, regeneration, and replacement of muscle with fat and fibrous connective tissue), and normal merosin staining.

    Which of the following findings would most likely be seen in this patient's workup?

    A. Mutation in *COL6* gene
    B. Mutations in the dystrophin gene
    C. Expanded CTG repeats in the *DMPK* gene

D. Mutation in the *LAMA2* gene

E. CGN trinucleotide repeat in *PABN1*

Correct answer: A

Explanation

The situation described here is consistent with Ullrich's congenital muscular dystrophy, a congenital muscular dystrophy. Congenital muscular dystrophies (CMDs) are a group of inherited conditions defined by muscle weakness occurring before the acquisition of ambulation, delayed motor milestones, and characterized by muscle dystrophic pathology. Collagen-VI related muscular dystrophies exist on a spectrum from the more severe Ullrich's congenital muscular dystrophy phenotype to the milder Bethlem myopathy phenotype. Characteristic clinical features include progressive muscle weakness, distal joint laxity and proximal joint contractures, and skin changes including keloid scars, hyperkeratosis pilaris, and bulbous soft heels.

Mutations in dystrophin cause dystrophinopathies, x-linked conditions due to mutations in the *DMD* gene which encodes for dystrophin, a skeletal muscle protein that connects the contractile apparatus to the extracellular matrix via the muscle membrane. These include DMD—the most severe form, Becker's muscular dystrophy (BMD) —a milder form, and an intermediate form. Mutations cause limited production of the dystrophin protein, causing loss of myofiber membrane integrity, and necrosis and replacement of muscle with fibrous and connective tissue.

An expanded CTG triplet in the *DMPK* gene on chromosome 19 causes myotonic dystrophy type I (DM1). Clinically, characteristic patterns of weakness in DM1 include involvement of cranial, oropharyngeal, trunk, and distal limb muscles. Temporal wasting is seen. Myotonia, delayed relaxation of muscles, can be seen characteristically in the hands, tongue, and jaw. Patients may describe difficulty releasing from a handshake or from a doorknob. In the tongue and jaw, it can impact chewing and speaking.

Mutations in the *LAMA2* gene are seen in LAMA2-related muscular dystrophies. This is another congenital muscular dystrophy, although it also has a limb girdle muscular dystrophy phenotype. Laminin, a heterotrimeric protein composed of α, β, and γ subunits, in skeletal muscle, the laminin-211 isoform (merosin) predominates and mediates attachment of collagens and other extracellular matrix components to the sarcolemmal membrane. Clinically, it is characterized by prominent hypotonia and weakness in infancy, slow progressive weakness and contractures, including facial weakness and respiratory involvement. Muscle biopsy will show lack of merosin staining.

CGN trinucleotide repeat in *PABN1* is seen in oculopharyngeal muscular dystrophy. This tends to have onset in later adult life (late 40s) and is characterized by ptosis and dysphagia. Restricted extraocular movements and limb weakness will also develop. The proximal musculature is the most affected.

References

Hamel JI. Myotonic Dystrophy. Continuum (Minneap Minn). 2022 Dec 1;28(6):1715–1734. https://doi.org/10.1212/CON.0000000000001184. PMID: 36537977.

Iyadurai SJ, Kissel JT. The Limb-Girdle Muscular Dystrophies and the Dystrophinopathies. Continuum (Minneap Minn). 2016 Dec;22(6, Muscle and Neuromuscular Junction Disorders):1954–1977. https://doi.org/10.1212/CON.0000000000000406. PMID: 27922502.

Trollet C, Boulinguiez A, Roth F, et al. Oculopharyngeal Muscular Dystrophy. 2001 Mar 8 [Updated 2020 Oct 22]. In: Adam MP, Feldman J, Mirzaa GM, et al., editors. GeneReviews® [Internet]. Seattle (WA): University of Washington, Seattle; 1993–2025. Available from: https://www.ncbi.nlm.nih.gov/books/NBK1126/

Zambon AA, Muntoni F. Congenital muscular dystrophies: What is new? Neuromuscul Disord. 2021 Oct;31(10):931–942. https://doi.org/10.1016/j.nmd.2021.07.009. Epub 2021 Jul 28. PMID: 34470717.

Linked questions: 130–131

130. A 6-year-old girl is seen in a clinic for weakness. She frequently complains of muscle cramps and has trouble keeping up with the other children in gym class. She was noted to be hypotonic in infancy and also had hip dislocations. Her mother notes that she has also been "unathletic" her whole life and struggles with muscle cramps after exercise. On exam, she is found to have a narrow face, hypotonia, and mild proximal weakness. Comprehensive neuromuscular workup including genetic testing reveals a mutation in the *RYR1* gene, and biopsy which showed absent NADH–tetrazolium reductase (TR)-staining in longitudinal cores in the muscle fibers. This is expected to be consistent with which of the following neuromuscular disorders?

A. Nemaline myopathy

B. Walker-Warburg syndrome

C. Central core myopathy

D. Centronuclear (myotubular) myopathy

E. Muscle-eye brain disease

Correct answer: C

Explanation

Congenital myopathies are inherited disorders with early onset hypotonia that are typically not progressive. Patients can have normal to mildly elevated CK. Differentiating them clinically can be difficult, and they are defined by histopathologic characteristics and increasingly by specific genetic mutations. They are typically caused by abnormalities of the contractile matrix, or structures supporting efficient excitation-contraction coupling, including the T tubules, sarcoplasmic reticulum, and other supporting structures.

Nemaline myopathy is defined by the formation of abnormal rodlike structures (nemaline bodies) that can be seen on muscle biopsy. These tend to cluster under the sarcolemma but can be found in the sarcoplasm and the nucleus. They appear as dark red–blue structures on Gomori one-step trichrome stain. There also tends to be a predominance of type I fibers where the rods tend to predominate. These disrupt the ability of the myofiber to generate adequate force during contraction. Nemaline myopathy is most commonly associated with mutations in NEB (nemaline myopathy type 2 [NEM2]). ACTA1 mutations (nemaline myopathy type 3 [NEM3] are the second most common. Clinically, nemaline myopathy has different phenotypes including severe congenital, intermediate congenital, typical congenital, childhood-onset, and adult-onset forms. Most typically, there is infantile onset hypotonia and weakness which predominates in the proximal muscles including neck flexor and respiratory muscles. Respiratory involvement is common in the more severe forms. Micrognathia, finger contractures, chest deformities, and scoliosis can be seen.

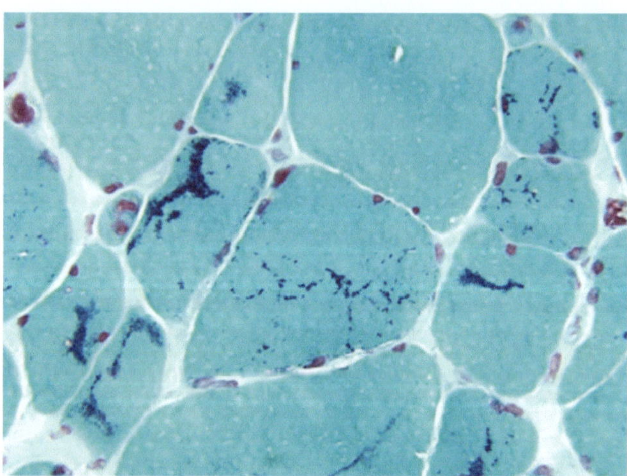

Gomori trichrome staining showing Nemaline Rods. (Source: Sarullo FM, Vitale G, Di Franco A, Sarullo S, Salerno Y, Vassallo L, Baviera EP, Marazia S, Mandalà G, Lanza GA. CC-BY 4.0 (https://creative-commons.org/licenses/by/4.0/) via *BMC cardiovascular disorders (2015)*. No changes were made. Sarullo FM, Vitale G, Di Franco A, et al. Nemaline myopathy and heart failure: role of ivabradine; a case report. *BMC Cardiovasc Disord*. 2015;15:5. Published 2015 Jan 19. https://doi.org/10.1186/1471-2261-15-5)

Core myopathies, including central core disease and multiminicore disease, are defined by findings on muscle biopsy of focally reduced oxidative and glycolytic enzymatic activity with staining. In central core myopathy, these cores are

well demarcated, found centrally and peripherally and extend along the longitudinal axis of the fiber. NADH-tetrazolium reductase staining, succinate dehydrogenase, and cytochrome c oxidase stains are all stains that will demonstrate the absence of oxidative and glycolytic activity in the cores. The cores are most often seen on type 1 fibers, and these fibers may predominate and be hypertrophic. Increased internal nucleation may also be seen. In multiminicore disease, there are "minicores" that appear as areas that do not stain with oxidative enzymes. They are short in length.

Central core myopathy is most commonly caused by mutations in skeletal muscle ryanodine receptor 1 (*RYR1*) gene located in chromosome 19q13.1. *SEPN1* mutations are the second-most common cause. The ryanodine receptor is a calcium channel receptor that releases calcium into the sarcoplasmic reticulum. Mutations in the *RYR1* gene can cause central core myopathy, multiminicore disease, congenital fiber type disproportion, and malignant hyperthermia. Central core myopathy related to *RYR1* mutations is autosomal dominant. Clinically, patients will present with infantile onset weakness (although adult onset disease has also been described) that predominantly affects the central musculature including axial musculature. Most patients will achieve the ability to walk. Bulbar, respiratory, and cardiac involvement is not typical. Exercise induced myalgia is common, and there is risk for malignant hyperthermia (this can also occur without myopathy). *RYR1*-related multiminicore disease is typically autosomal recessive, and clinically characterized by hypotonia and weakness (mostly central, although facial and extraocular weakness can be seen as well) in infancy or childhood.

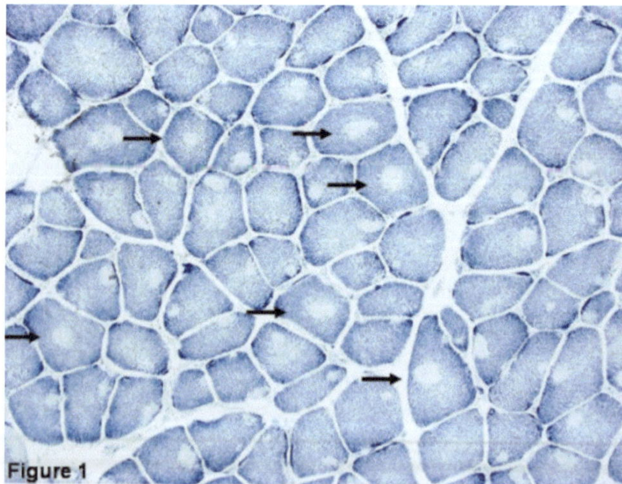

Histopathologic appearance of typical central core disease. (Source: Jungbluth H -Orphanet. CC-BY 2.0 (https://creativecommons.org/licenses/by/2.0/) via *Journal of rare diseases (2007). No changes were made.* Jungbluth H. Central core disease. *Orphanet J Rare Dis*. 2007;2:25. Published 2007 May 15. https://doi.org/10.1186/1750-1172-2-25)

Muscle histology in centronuclear myopathy characteristically shows internal nuclei, sometimes in central longitudinal chains (which is how they appear in embryonic myotubes). There is a predominance of type 1 fibers. There are a variety of modes of inheritance and clinical syndromes associated with centronuclear myopathy.

X-linked, which is caused by mutations in the *MTM1* gene located on chromosome Xq28, is the most common and also the most severe. They will present with hypotonia, proximal and distal weakness, respiratory muscles weakness, facial weakness, ophthalmoplegia. Systemic features include gallstones and hepatic dysfunction among others. Ventilator dependence is common.

Walker-Warburg syndrome is a dystroglycanopathy, a group of disorders caused by abnormal glycosylation of α-dystroglycan. It is autosomal recessive and caused by several different mutations in genes including in *POMT1*, *POMT2*, fukutin (*FKTM*), and *FKRP*. It has a severe phenotype with hypotonia, paralysis at birth, global developmental delay. Brain abnormalities including cobblestone lissencephaly are seen, as well as ocular abnormalities. In the α- dystroglycanopathies, muscle biopsy shows reduced α-dystroglycan when stained for.

Muscle-eye brain disease is another dystroglycanopathy. It is autosomal recessive caused by mutations of *POMGnT1*. Clinically it is characterized by severe hypotonia at birth, progressive weakness, and moderate to severe developmental delay. Brain malformations are seen such as lissencephaly and polymicrogyria. Structural eye abnormalities are also seen.

Reference

Butterfield RJ. Congenital Muscular Dystrophy and Congenital Myopathy. Continuum (Minneap Minn). 2019 Dec;25(6):1640–1661. https://doi.org/10.1212/CON.0000000000000792. PMID: 31794464.

Linked question

131. You diagnose the patient with RYR1 related central core myopathy, what counseling is appropriate?
    A. The patient will likely never be able to walk
    B. There is a high risk of cardiac complications with this condition
    C. There is a risk for malignant hyperthermia with anesthesia
    D. Most cases of this disorder are autosomal recessive, and she likely inherited a pathogenic variant from each parent
    E. Bulbar and respiratory involvement are common
    Correct answer: C

Explanation

Central core myopathy related to *RYR1* mutations is autosomal dominant. Clinically, patients will present with infantile onset weakness (although adult-onset disease has also been described) that predominantly affects the central musculature including axial musculature. Most patients will achieve the ability to walk. Bulbar, respiratory, and cardiac involvement is not typical. Exercise induced myalgia is common, and there is risk for malignant hyperthermia (this can also occur without myopathy).

Reference

Iannaccone ST, Castro D. Congenital muscular dystrophies and congenital myopathies. Continuum (Minneap Minn). 2013 Dec;19(6 Muscle Disease):1509–34. https://doi.org/10.1212/01.CON.0000440658.03557.f1. PMID: 24305446; PMCID: PMC10564049.

132. A 15-year-old boy is brought in for evaluation of generalized weakness, and sensorineural hearing loss. He also has a history of poor vision, and prior ophthalmologic exams have been notable for retinitis pigmentosa. Exam is notable for ptosis, ophthalmoplegia, and mild proximal weakness. Electrocardiogram shows complete heart block. Which of the following is the most likely diagnosis?
    A. Myoclonic epilepsy with ragged red fibers
    B. Mitochondrial encephalopathy, lactic acidosis, and strokes
    C. Kearns-Sayre syndrome
    D. Muscle-eye brain disease
    E. Giant axonal neuropathy
    Correct answer: C

Explanation

This clinical vignette describes a presentation of Kearns-Sayre syndrome, which is characterized by the triad of external ophthalmoplegia, retinitis pigmentosa, and sensorineural hearing loss with symptom onset before age 20. This is a mitochondrial disorder typically caused by a large-scale deletion of a segment of mtDNA, and rarely by duplications. Typically, it is sporadic. Other features that can be seen include myopathy, cardiac conduction defects, renal impairment, dementia, seizure, pancreatic failure, bulbar dysfunction, short stature, parkinsonism, and neuropathy.

Myoclonic epilepsy with ragged red fibers (MERRF) is also a mitochondrial disorder caused by various mutations in mtDNA. Characteristic clinical findings are progressive epilepsy and myoclonus. On muscle biopsy, Gomori trichrome stain will show "ragged red fibers" due to clumps of diseased mitochondria accumulating in the subsarcolemmal region of the muscle fiber. Other clinical features that may be seen include sensorineural hearing loss, myopathy, dementia, neuropathy, short stature, cardiomyopathy, and optic atrophy.

Mitochondrial encephalomyopathy, lactic acidosis, and stroke-like syndrome (MELAS) is a mitochondrial disorder. Most often, it is caused by a few select mutations in the mtDNA *tRNA*^{leu} gene. Symptoms can manifest from infancy into late adulthood. It is characterized by elevated lactate in blood and CSF, stroke and stroke-like events, varying degrees of cognitive impairment, epilepsy, and myopathy. Other clinical features that may be seen include diabetes mellitus, Wolff-Parkinson-White syndrome, and atypical migraine.

Muscle-eye brain disease is a dystroglycanopathy. It is autosomal recessive caused by mutations of *POMGnT1*. Clinically, it is characterized by severe hypotonia at birth, progressive weakness, and moderate to severe developmental delay. Brain malformations are seen such as lissencephaly and polymicrogyria. Structural eye abnormalities are also seen.

Giant axonal neuropathy is due to *GAN* mutations and typically presents in infancy, starting with severe sensorimotor neuropathy and evolving to have central nervous system involvement. Tightly coiled hair is also characteristic.

References

Butterfield RJ. Congenital Muscular Dystrophy and Congenital Myopathy. Continuum (Minneap Minn). 2019 Dec;25(6):1640–1661. https://doi.org/10.1212/CON.0000000000000792. PMID: 31794464.

Cohen BH. Mitochondrial and Metabolic Myopathies. Continuum (Minneap Minn). 2019 Dec;25(6):1732–1766. https://doi.org/10.1212/CON.0000000000000805. PMID: 31794469.

Opal P. GAN-Related Neurodegeneration. 2003 Jan 9 [Updated 2021 Oct 14]. In: Adam MP, Feldman J, Mirzaa GM, et al., editors. GeneReviews® [Internet]. Seattle (WA): University of Washington, Seattle; 1993–2025. Available from: https://www.ncbi.nlm.nih.gov/books/NBK1136/

Linked questions: 133–135

133. A 42-year-old male is seen in clinic due to chronically elevated CK of about 700. Careful questioning reveals that he has avoided exercise since childhood as he always felt that he was bad at sports and unable to keep up with his peers. He would also experience cramps with exercise. He finds that his ability to tolerate physical activity will improve after a short rest from initial activity. He had a prior episode of rhabdomyolysis after participating in a charity 5k race. He has a normal neurologic exam. What diagnosis is this most consistent with?
A. McArdle disease
B. Pompe disease
C. Carnitine palmitoyltransferase 2 deficiency
D. Muscle eye brain disease
E. Kearns-Sayre syndrome
Correct answer: A

Explanation

This is a typical presentation for a patient with McArdle disease (glycogenosis type V). McArdle disease is an autosomal-recessive disorder due to myophosphorylase deficiency. Myophosphorylase is involved in breaking down glycogen into glucose, and its deficiency results in the accumulation of glycogen in the muscles. Clinically, patients will present with exercise induced weakness and muscle cramps and can develop rhabdomyolysis. CK can be chronically elevated. Characteristically, there is a second wind phenomena where exercise intolerance can be alleviated by briefly reducing the intensity of exercise or stopping exercise and then resuming slowly. High carbohydrate meals before exercise and graded exercise can help alleviate symptoms.

Pompe disease (glycogenosis type II) is an autosomal recessive disorder due to acid maltase deficiency (also known as α-glucosidase (GAA)). This leads to impaired glycogen breakdown in lysosomes. There are both early and late onset forms. The early-onset set form is more severe manifesting in infancy with hypotonia, hypertrophic cardiomyopathy, respiratory failure, and developmental delays. The late-onset form can occur in childhood or adulthood with proximal muscle weakness and respiratory insufficiency due to diaphragmatic involvement. Enzyme replacement therapy (ERT) with α-glucosidase alfa is the primary treatment.

Carnitine palmitoyltransferase 2 (CPT2) deficiency is autosomal recessive and due to disordered long chain fatty acid oxidation. It can present as a lethal neonatal form, severe infantile hepatocardiomuscular form, and myopathic form (milder can have symptom onset from infancy to adulthood). The myopathic form is characterized by exercise-induced myalgias and weakness. There can be associated myoglobinuria. Treatment includes a high-carbohydrate diet, carnitine supplementation, and avoidance of triggers.

Muscle-eye brain disease is a dystroglycanopathy. It is autosomal recessive caused by mutations of *POMGnT1*. Clinically, it is characterized by severe hypotonia at birth, progressive weakness, and moderate to severe developmental delay. Brain malformations are seen such as lissencephaly and polymicrogyria. Structural eye abnormalities are also seen.

Kearns-Sayre syndrome is characterized by the triad of external ophthalmoplegia, retinitis pigmentosa, and sensorineural hearing loss with symptom onset before age 20. This is a mitochondrial disorder typically caused by a large-scale deletion of a segment of mtDNA, and rarely by duplications. Typically, it is sporadic. Other features that can be seen include myopathy, cardiac conduction defects, renal impairment, dementia, seizure, pancreatic failure, bulbar dysfunction, short stature, parkinsonism, and neuropathy.

References

Berardo A, DiMauro S, Hirano M. A diagnostic algorithm for metabolic myopathies. Curr Neurol Neurosci Rep. 2010 Mar;10(2):118–26. https://doi.org/10.1007/s11910-010-0096-4. PMID: 20425236; PMCID: PMC2872126.

Cohen BH. Mitochondrial and Metabolic Myopathies. Continuum (Minneap Minn). 2019 Dec;25(6):1732–1766. https://doi.org/10.1212/CON.0000000000000805. PMID: 31794469.

Lam JR, Anastasopoulou C, Khattak ZE, et al. McArdle Disease (Glycogen Storage Disease Type 5) [Updated 2025 Jan 22]. In: StatPearls [Internet]. Treasure Island (FL): StatPearls Publishing; 2025 Jan-. Available from: https://www.ncbi.nlm.nih.gov/books/NBK560785/

Morales A, Siqueira Tavares De Melo MH, Anastasopoulou C, et al. Glycogen Storage Disease Type II. [Updated 2025 Jan 28]. In: StatPearls [Internet]. Treasure Island (FL): StatPearls Publishing; 2025 Jan-. Available from: https://www.ncbi.nlm.nih.gov/books/NBK470558/

Tarnopolsky MA. Metabolic Myopathies. Continuum (Minneap Minn). 2022 Dec 1;28(6):1752–1777. https://doi.org/10.1212/CON.0000000000001182. PMID: 36537979.

Wieser T. Carnitine Palmitoyltransferase II Deficiency. 2004 Aug 27 [Updated 2019 Jan 3]. In: Adam MP, Feldman J, Mirzaa GM, et al., editors. GeneReviews® [Internet]. Seattle (WA): University of Washington, Seattle; 1993–2025. Available from: https://www.ncbi.nlm.nih.gov/books/NBK1253/

Linked question

134. Which of the following metabolic myopathies is correctly paired with the correlating problem?
    A. Pompe disease (glycogenosis type 2)- phosphofructokinase deficiency
    B. McArdle disease (glycogenesis type 5)- myophosphorylase deficiency
    C. Tarui disease (glycogenesis type 7)- anti–3-hydroxy-3-methylglutaryl coenzyme A reductase antibody
    D. Kearns-Sayre syndrome- carnitine palmitoyl transferase 2 deficiency
    E. Mitochondrial encephalopathy, lactic acidosis, and strokes (MELAS)—carnitine deficiency
    F. Myoclonic epilepsy with ragged red fibers (MERRF)—acid maltase deficiency
Correct answer: B

Explanation

Pompe disease (glycogenosis type 2) is due to acid maltase deficiency. McArdle disease (glycogenosis type V) is due to myophosphorylase deficiency. Tarui disease (glycogenesis type VII) is due to phosphofructokinase deficiency. Kearns-Sayre syndrome is caused by a large-scale deletion of a segment of mtDNA, and rarely by duplications. MELAS is caused by a few select mutations in the mtDNA *tRNA*[leu] gene. Myoclonic epilepsy with ragged red fibers (MERRF) is also a mitochondrial disorder caused by various mutations in mtDNA

References

Berardo A, DiMauro S, Hirano M. A diagnostic algorithm for metabolic myopathies. Curr Neurol Neurosci Rep. 2010 Mar;10(2):118–26. https://doi.org/10.1007/s11910-010-0096-4 PMID: 20425236; PMCID: PMC2872126.

Cohen BH. Mitochondrial and Metabolic Myopathies. Continuum (Minneap Minn). 2019 Dec;25(6):1732–1766. https://doi.org/10.1212/CON.0000000000000805. PMID: 31794469.

Linked question

135. Which of the following may mimic metabolic myopathies?
    A. Limb girdle muscular dystrophies
    B. Statin use
    C. Hypothyroidism
    D. Vitamin D deficiency
    E. All of the above
Correct answer: E

Explanation

Metabolic myopathies are genetic disorders that affect the metabolism of glucose and free fatty acids in skeletal muscle. Typical clinical symptoms include exercise-induced cramps or sometimes weakness and a risk for rhabdomyolysis. These includes glycogen storage diseases, fatty acid oxidation defects, and mitochondrial myopathies. Other disorders that are not involved with energy metabolism, and acquired causes can also lead to rhabdomyolysis mimicking metabolic myopathies. Limb girdle muscular dystrophies and Becker muscular dystrophy can present with exercise-induced rhabdomyolysis before weakness develops. This is thought to be related to excessive calcium influx and or sarcolemmal damage induced by calcium. Statins can trigger rhabdomyolysis, and commonly lead to myalgia and a higher CK rise in response to exercise. They can also trigger an autoimmune process mediated by anti–3-hydroxy-3-methylglutaryl coenzyme A reductase antibodies (autoimmune necrotizing myopathy). Vitamin D deficiency can also lead to exercise intolerance, elevated CK, and rhabdomyolysis. Hypothyroidism may be associated with myopathy and elevated CK levels, but will also predispose to exercise-induced rhabdomyolysis.

Reference

Tarnopolsky MA. Metabolic Myopathies. Continuum (Minneap Minn). 2022 Dec 1;28(6):1752–1777. https://doi.org/10.1212/CON.0000000000001182. PMID: 36537979.

136. A 16-year-old girl is referred for evaluation of episodic muscle weakness. Her parents report that since early childhood, she has had intermittent episodes of flaccid paralysis, lasting several hours, often triggered by rest after exercise or carbohydrate-rich meals. Between episodes, her strength is normal.

   She was recently evaluated by cardiology for palpitations and lightheadedness, and her ECG revealed frequent ventricular ectopy and a prolonged QT interval. Holter monitoring captured runs of ventricular tachycardia.

   Examination is notable for low-set ears, hypertelorism, small mandible, and curved pinky fingers.

   What is your suspected diagnosis?

   A. Hypokalemic periodic paralysis

   B. Hyperkalemic periodic paralysis

   C. Andersen-Tawil syndrome

   D. Myotonia congenita

   E. Paramyotonia congenita

   Correct answer: C

Explanation

This case describes Andersen-Tawil syndrome. This is due to a mutation in the *KCNJ2* gene which encodes for an inward rectifier potassium channel that stabilizes the resting membrane potential of skeletal and cardiac myocytes. Classically, there is a triad of episodic weakness, cardiac abnormalities, and distinctive skeletal features. Symptoms usually begin between age 1 and 20 with either episodic weakness or cardiac symptoms like palpitations or syncope. Duration of attacks is variable and potassium can be high, low, or normal during attacks. Cardiac abnormalities include prolonged QT interval and ventricular arrhythmias. Characteristic skeletal features include short stature, scoliosis, low-set ears, hypertelorism, broad nasal bridge, micrognathia, clinodactyly, syndactyly, and toes joined at the base. Treatments include beta blockers, pacemaker/ICD, acetazolamide, and potassium supplementation if potassium is low during attacks.

Hyperkalemic periodic paralysis is associated with mutations in the sodium channel *SCN4a* gene. Most commonly, symptoms begin between 1 and 10 years of age. Patients experience episodic attacks of flaccid paralysis that last 1–4 h. They often occur in the morning. Potassium levels can be normal or elevated during an attack. Triggers include potassium-rich food, rest after exercise, fasting, cold, stress, and pregnancy. Patients can have stiffness from myotonia in between attacks and some patients can develop progressive myopathy. Treatments include thiazide diuretics, glucose or carbohydrate intake, beta agonists, acetazolamide, and avoiding fasting and potassium-rich foods.

Hypokalemic periodic paralysis can be caused by mutations in the calcium channel *CACNA1S* gene and less commonly in the sodium channel *SCN4A* gene. Attacks of weakness can begin between 5 and 35 years of age and will decrease with age. Attacks involve focal or generalized weakness and last hours to days, notably longer than in hyperkalemic periodic paralysis. There will be hypokalemia during attacks. Triggers include carbohydrate-rich meals, alcohol, and rest after strenuous exercise. Patients can develop progressive myopathy. Treatment includes potassium supplementation, acetazolamide, spironolactone, and a low carbohydrate, low salt diet.

Myotonia congenita and paramyotonia congenita and sodium channel myotonia are non-dystrophic myotonias. In the non-dystrophic myotonias, symptoms usually occur in the first two decades of life and include muscle stiffness, weakness, fatigue, and pain. Clinical features are varied and can range from mild muscle stiffness to severe myotonia. Myotonia congenita is seen in *CLCN1* mutations, which encodes the main skeletal muscle chloride channel CIC-1 and can be autosomal dominant (Thomsen disease) or autosomal recessive (Becker disease, more severe). Patients will have muscular builds due to hypertrophy. Action myotonia is seen, stiffness with rapid movement. The stiffness improves with exercise ("warm-up phenomenon"). More commonly with Becker disease, patients can characteristically experience initial weakness with exercise that subsequently improves. Paramyotonia congenita and sodium-channel myotonias are autosomal dominant disorders related to *SCN4A* mutations. In paramyotonia congenita muscle stiffness worsens after sustained exercise ("paradoxical myotonia"). Paramyotonia congenita also more commonly affects the face, and classically there is paradoxical eye closure myotonia (with repetition, there is more difficulty with eye closure and opening).

References

Statland JM, Fontaine B, Hanna MG, Johnson NE, Kissel JT, Sansone VA, Shieh PB, Tawil RN, Trivedi J, Cannon SC, Griggs RC. Review of the Diagnosis and Treatment of Periodic Paralysis. Muscle Nerve. 2018 Apr;57(4):522–530. https://doi.org/10.1002/mus.26009. Epub 2017 Nov 29. PMID: 29125635; PMCID: PMC5867231.

Trivedi JR. Muscle Channelopathies. Continuum (Minneap Minn). 2022 Dec 1;28(6):1778–1799. https://doi.org/10.1212/CON.0000000000001183. PMID: 36537980.

Linked questions: 137–140

137. A 58-year-old female with no significant past medical history presents to clinic due to weakness. She describes difficulty going up stairs as well as doing her hair in the morning. She has also noted a rash on the backs of her hands and on her chest. Exam is notable for proximal muscle weakness, a violaceous rash on the knuckles, and an erythematous rash on her anterior chest, back, and shoulders. CK is 3580. Antinuclear antibodies and double-stranded DNA antibodies are not present. Complement levels are normal.

What condition is this consistent with?
A. Dermatomyositis
B. Polymyositis
C. Necrotizing autoimmune myositis
D. Inclusion-body myositis
E. Overlap myositis

Correct answer: A

Explanation

This case scenario describes a common presentation of dermatomyositis, an idiopathic inflammatory myopathy. In addition to proximal muscle weakness, patients present with distinct skin findings that can co-occur with the muscle weakness or precede it. The skin findings include a periorbital heliotrope rash with edema, Gottron's papule (violaceous eruption on the knuckles), erythematous rash on the knees, elbows, neck, anterior chest ("v-sign"), and back and shoulders ("shawl sign"). Lesions are photosensitive. Other findings include nail changes including dilated capillary loops at the base of the fingernails, irregular and thickened cuticles, and cracked palmar fingertips ("mechanic's hands"). Skin findings can occur without weakness (amyopathic dermatomyositis). There is an increased risk of malignancy, necessitating a thorough annual workup in the first three years after disease onset.

The other conditions are also idiopathic inflammatory myopathies that are less consistent with the clinical picture described above.

Polymyositis is rare, and there is some debate as to whether it is a discrete disorder or poorly defined disease which includes connective tissue disease associated myositis, overlap myositis, and necrotizing autoimmune myopathy. It is a diagnosis of exclusion (exclude rash, family history indicating genetic disorder, exposure to myotoxic drugs, inclusion-body myositis phenotype) in patients with subacute proximal myopathy.

Necrotizing autoimmune myositis can develop acutely or sub acutely and lead to severe weakness and very elevated creatine kinase levels (over 50 times the upper limit of normal). It can occur alone, in association with cancer, in patients with connective-tissue disorders, and in patients taking statins. In patients taking statins, it can continue to worsen after statin withdrawal (if it resolves with statin withdrawal, it was probably due to toxic effects of the statin on the muscle rather than immune myopathy). Most patients with necrotizing autoimmune myositis have antibodies against signal recognition particle (SRP) or against 3-hydroxy-3-methylglutaryl–coenzyme A reductase (HMGCR).

Inclusion-body myositis is the most common acquired myopathy over age 50. It can develop slowly over a period of years. Weakness may be asymmetric, and there is characteristic early involvement of the distal muscles, including the finger flexors and foot extensors and quadriceps. There may be atrophy of the forearms as well as the quadriceps muscles. Axial musculature may also be involved which can result in camptocormia (bending forward of the spine).

Overlap myositis includes patients with myositis associated with an underlying connective tissue disorder such as rheumatoid arthritis or systemic lupus erythematosus. Muscle biopsy may show nonspecific features consistent with myositis or features of necrotizing autoimmune myopathy or dermatomyositis but the patient should have a clinical picture of a multi-system connective tissue disease. Antisynthetase syndrome, which is associated with aminoacyl tRNA synthetase (ARS) antibodies (the most common being Jo-1), has recently been classified as an overlap myositis (previously, it was grouped with dermatomyositis and polymyositis). This is associated with a clinical constellation of myositis, arthritis, Raynaud phenomenon, hyperkeratosis and fissuring of the palmar skin, and interstitial lung disease.

In regards to treatment, corticosteroids are first line for the majority of patients with idiopathic inflammatory myopathies. Further immunosuppression (such as steroid sparing agents like azathioprine or in more aggressive cases IVIG) may be required to prevent disease recurrence after steroid weaning. There are currently no treatments with proven benefit in inclusion body myositis and treatment revolves around non-pharmacologic interventions to maintain independence.

Also of note, there are a variety of solid and hematologic malignancies that can occur in the idiopathic inflammatory myopathies. Dermatomyositis has a particularly strong association with cancer, and screening should be performed in all patients over 40 with dermatomyositis. HMG-CoA reductase

IgG antibody-positive immune-mediated necrotizing myopathy is also associated with malignancy, and cancer can occur regardless of prior statin exposure. Antisynthetase syndrome, anti-SRP antibody immune-mediated necrotizing myopathy, and overlap myositis have low incidence of cancer, and routine screening is not recommended.

References

Ashton C, Paramalingam S, Stevenson B, Brusch A, Needham M. Idiopathic inflammatory myopathies: a review. Intern Med J. 2021 Jun;51(6):845–852. https://doi.org/10.1111/imj.15358. PMID: 34155760.

Dalakas MC. Inflammatory muscle diseases. N Engl J Med. 2015 Apr 30;372(18):1734–47. https://doi.org/10.1056/NEJMra1402225. PMID: 25923553.

Manousakis G. Inflammatory Myopathies. Continuum (Minneap Minn). 2022 Dec 1;28(6):1643–1662. https://doi.org/10.1212/CON.0000000000001179. PMID: 36537973.

Linked question

138. What autoantibodies might be expected with this condition?
    A. Anti-3-hydroxy-3-methylglutaryl–coenzyme A reductase (anti-HMGCR)
    B. Anti-signal recognition particle (anti-SRP)
    C. Anti-cytosolic 5′-nucleotidase 1A (anti-cN1A, or anti-NT5C1A)
    D. Anti-Mi-2
    Correct answer: D

Explanation

Here is a list of common autoantibodies seen in inflammatory myopathies:

- Inclusion body myositis: Anti cytosolic 5′-nucleotidase 1A (anti-cN1A, or anti-NT5C1A)
- Antisynthetase syndrome (historically grouped with dermatomyositis and polymyositis but more recently is considered an overlap myositis): Anti-histidyl–transfer RNA synthetase (anti-Jo-1)
- Necrotizing autoimmune myositis: Anti-3-hydroxy-3-methylglutaryl–coenzyme A reductase (anti-HMGCR) and Anti-signal recognition particle (anti-SRP)
- Dermatomyositis
    - Amyopathic dermatomyositis or rapidly progressive interstitial lung disease: Anti-melanoma differentiation-associated protein-5 (anti-MDA-5)
    - Typical skin lesions of dermatomyositis: Anti-Mi-2
    - Cancer-associated dermatomyositis: Anti-transcriptional intermediary factor 1 γ (anti-TIF-1γ) and anti-nuclear matrix protein 2 (anti-NXP-2)

References

Ashton C, Paramalingam S, Stevenson B, Brusch A, Needham M. Idiopathic inflammatory myopathies: a review. Intern Med J. 2021 Jun;51(6):845–852. https://doi.org/10.1111/imj.15358. PMID: 34155760.

Dalakas MC. Inflammatory muscle diseases. N Engl J Med. 2015 Apr 30;372(18):1734–47. https://doi.org/10.1056/NEJMra1402225. PMID: 25923553.

Linked question

139. The patient was found to have anti-Mi-2 autoantibodies. What pathology findings would be most consistent with the suspected diagnosis
    A. Necrotic and regenerating fibers
    B. Sarcoplasmic rimmed vacuoles
    C. Perifascicular atrophy
    D. Amyloid deposits
    E. Ragged red fibers
    Correct answer: C

Explanation

Here is a list of typical pathology seen in inflammatory myopathies:

- Dermatomyositis: perifascicular atrophy; perivascular/perimysial; reduced capillary density; MAC deposition on small blood vessels

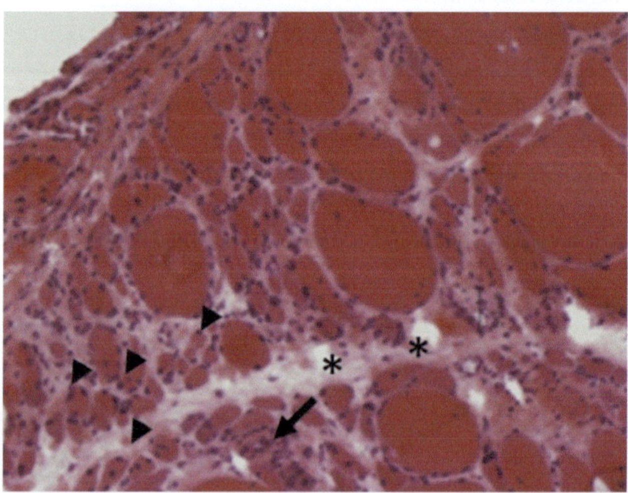

Perifascicular atrophy (arrowheads) with increased endomysial connective tissue (asterisks) and inflammatory infiltrates (arrows) are characteristics of dermatomyositis. (Source: Malik A, Hayat G, Kalia JS, Guzman MA. CC-BY 4.0 (https://creativecommons.org/licenses/by/4.0/) via *Frontiers in neurology (2016)*. No changes were made. Malik A, Hayat G, Kalia JS, Guzman MA. Idiopathic Inflammatory Myopathies: Clinical Approach and Management. *Front Neurol.* 2016;7:64. Published 2016 May 20. https://doi.org/10.3389/fneur.2016.00064)

- Polymyositis: CD8+ cells invading healthy fibers; widespread expression of MHC class I antigen; no vacuoles
- Necrotizing autoimmune myositis: Scattered necrotic fibers with macrophages; regenerating fibers; minimal cellular infiltrate

- Inclusion body myositis: sarcoplasmic rimmed vacuoles; inflammatory infiltrate, CD8+ cells invading healthy fibers; congophilic amyloid deposits; 15–18 nm tubulo-filament inclusion bodies in the sarcoplasm and myonuclei; ragged red fibers

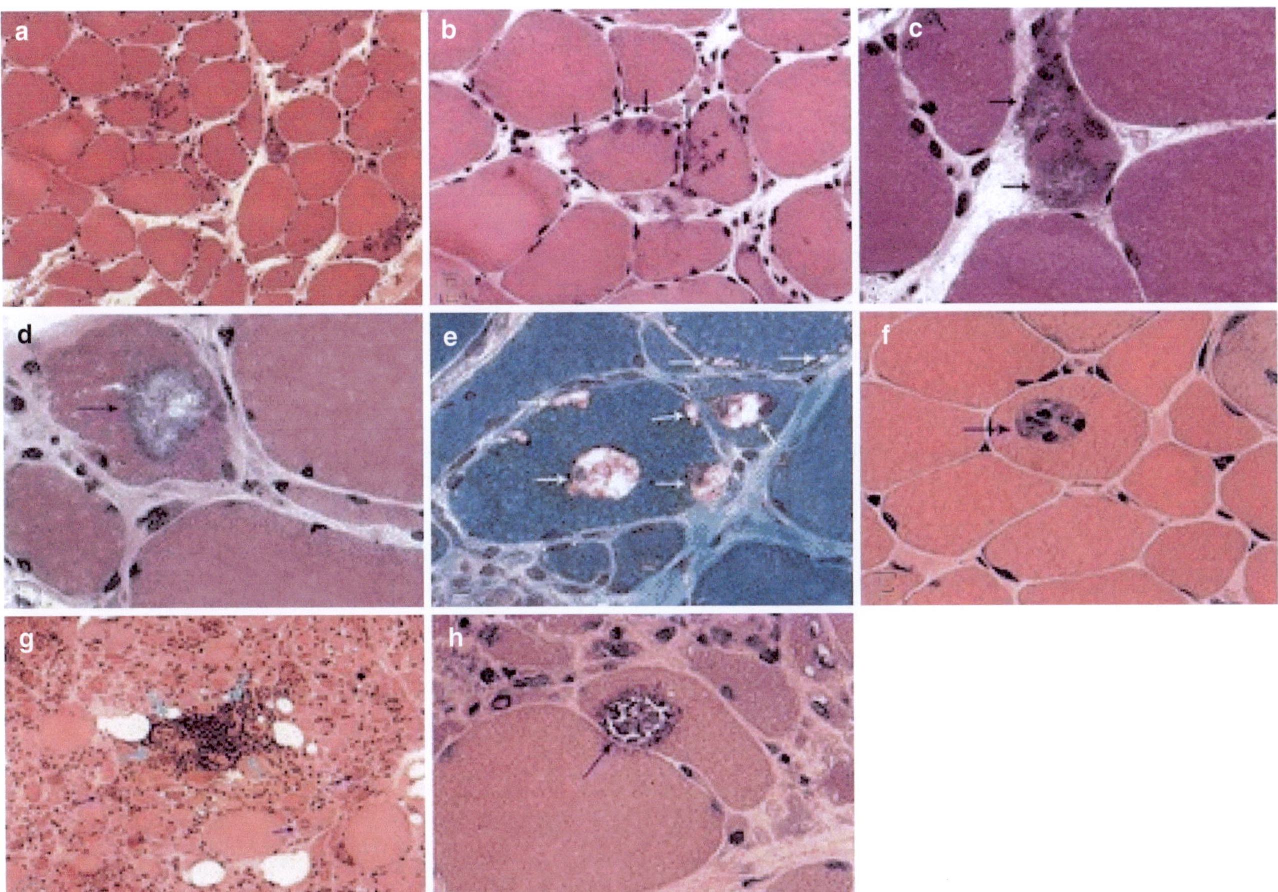

Pathological characteristics of sporadic inclusion body myositis (s-IBM). (**a**) Atrophic muscle fibers were angular, irregular, and round, with muscle fiber hypertrophy, HE staining; (**b**) Fimbriated cavity and inclusion bodies (blue arrows), HE staining; (**c**) Sand-like particles (inclusion bodies) (blue arrows), HE staining; (**d**) round Fimbriated cavities in the atrophic muscle fibers, with sand-like inclusion bodies in which (blue arrows), HE staining; (**e**) Red particles of inclusion bodies in fimbriated cavities (yellow arrows), Gomori staining; (**f**) Non-ecrotic muscle fibers infiltrated by monocytes (blue arrows), HE staining; (**g**) Focal inflammatory infiltration (green arrows) and fimbriated cavities showed in several muscle fibers (blue arrows), HE staining; (**h**) Round fimbriated cavities in atrophic muscle fibers, with gross particles of inclusion bodies in which (blue arrows), HE staining. (Source: Li K, Pu C, Huang X, Liu J, Mao Y, Lu X. CC-BY 4.0 (https://creativecommons. org/licenses/by/4.0/) via *Proteome science (2014). No changes were made.* No changes were made. Li K, Pu C, Huang X, Liu J, Mao Y, Lu X. Proteomic study of sporadic inclusion body myositis. Proteome Sci. 2014;12(1):45. Published 2014 Sep 12. https://doi.org/10.1186/ s12953-014-0045-2)

References

Ashton C, Paramalingam S, Stevenson B, Brusch A, Needham M. Idiopathic inflammatory myopathies: a review. Intern Med J. 2021 Jun;51(6):845–852. https://doi.org/10.1111/imj.15358. PMID: 34155760.

Dalakas MC. Inflammatory muscle diseases. N Engl J Med. 2015 Apr 30;372(18):1734–47. https://doi.org/10.1056/NEJMra1402225. PMID: 25923553.

Linked question

140. What electromyography and nerve conduction study (EMG and NCS) findings would be consistent with the suspected diagnosis (select all that apply)?
    A. Small motor unit action potentials on EMG
    B. Reduced amplitude of sensory nerve action potentials on NCS
    C. Reduced recruitment on EMG
    D. Early full recruitment on EMG
    E. Prolonged distal motor latency of the median nerve compound muscle action potential on NCS

Correct answer: A, D

Explanation

The clinical case describes dermatomyositis. On EMG/NCS, myopathic findings would be expected. Of the findings listed above, small motor unit action potentials and early full recruitment are consistent with myopathy. Reduced amplitude of sensory nerve action potentials would be seen in sensory neuropathy. Reduced recruitment is a neuropathic finding. Prolonged distal motor latency of the median nerve compound muscle action potentials may be seen in median neuropathy at the wrist.

References

Dalakas MC. Inflammatory muscle diseases. N Engl J Med. 2015 Apr 30;372(18):1734–47. https://doi.org/10.1056/NEJMra1402225. PMID: 25923553.

Preston, D. C., & Shapiro, B. E. (2020). *Electromyography and Neuromuscular Disorders: Clinical-Electrophysiologic-Ultrasound Correlations* (4th ed.). Elsevier. ISBN: 978-0-323-66180-5.

141. Which of the following is *not* true about HIV-associated myopathy?
    A. Increased immunosuppression is associated with myopathy
    B. Typically, it presents with slowly progressive proximal limb weakness
    C. One possible mechanism includes direct toxicity of HIV infection
    D. Another possible mechanism includes an aberrant immune response which results in an inflammatory myopathy
    E. ART toxicity can cause myopathy

Correct answer: A

Explanation

Myopathy can occur at any time during the course of HIV infection. It does not appear to be influenced by the degree of immunosuppression. Typically, it presents with slowly progressive proximal weakness. Possible mechanisms include direct toxicity of HIV infection, ART toxicity (especially with zidovune), vasculitis, infection, and an aberrant immune response resulting in an inflammatory myopathy. Serum CK can be elevated. EMG demonstrates myopathic features. Muscle biopsy can show a variety of findings, most commonly nonspecific myofiber degeneration.

References

Saylor D. Neurologic Complications of Human Immunodeficiency Virus Infection. Continuum (Minneap Minn). 2018 Oct;24(5, Neuroinfectious Disease):1397–1421. https://doi.org/10.1212/CON.0000000000000647. PMID: 30273245; PMCID: PMC8006925.

Verma S, Micsa E, Estanislao L, Simpson D. Neuromuscular complications in HIV. Curr Neurol Neurosci Rep. 2004 Jan;4(1):62–7. https://doi.org/10.1007/s11910-004--0014-8. PMID: 14683631.

142. Which of the following is true about sarcoid myopathy?
    A. Clinical myopathy is a common presentation of sarcoid
    B. Acute myositis is the most common way for sarcoid myopathy to present
    C. Granulomas are typically present on muscle biopsy
    D. CK levels are always normal
    E. Steroids should not be used in sarcoid myopathy

Correct answer: C

Explanation

Symptomatic myopathy in sarcoid is uncommon, occurring in only about 1.4–2.3% of patients with sarcoid. Subclinical muscle involvement is more common, and imaging studies or autopsy have showed involvement in 50–80% of patients. There are a variety of ways that sarcoid myopathy can present; most commonly, it is with progressive muscle weakness primarily affecting the proximal muscles. Other patterns reported include a distal predominant pattern, the nodular type with stiffness, pain and palpable nodules, and rarely acute myositis. Non-caseating granulomas are typically present on muscle pathology. Other findings on biopsy can include perimysial connective tissue with histiocyte-associated, and diffuse muscle changes or changes anatomically related to the granulomas. CK levels can be normal or high depending on the myopathy subtype. Treatment options for sarcoid myopathies commonly include steroids.

References

Garret M, Pestronk A. Sarcoidosis, granulomas and myopathy syndromes: A clinical-pathology review. J Neuroimmunol. 2022 Dec 15;373:577975. https://doi.org/10.1016/j.jneuroim.2022.577975. Epub 2022 Oct 3. PMID: 36228383.

Pawate S. Sarcoidosis and the Nervous System. Continuum (Minneap Minn). 2020 Jun;26(3):695–715. https://doi.org/10.1212/CON.0000000000000855. PMID: 32487903.

143. A 65-year-old male patient has been in the ICU for 3 weeks due to severe sepsis and acute respiratory distress syndrome (ARDS). He has been on mechanical ventilation and received high-dose corticosteroids. Over the past week, he has been difficult to wean from the ventilator and a neuromuscular disorder is suspected. Which of the following findings would be supportive of critical illness myopathy as the cause of his weakness?
    A. Asymmetric distal weakness
    B. Increased tone
    C. Extraocular muscle involvement
    D. Nerve conduction studies showing compound muscle action potentials with reduced amplitude and increased duration
    E. Nerve conduction studies showing absent sensory nerve action potentials

Correct answer: D

Explanation

A variety of neuromuscular disorders can complicate an ICU stay including disorders like myasthenia gravis and Guillain-Barre syndrome as well as ICU-acquired weakness which describes weakness in patients that are critically ill that is not caused by an alternative etiology other than the critical illness itself. Three categories of ICU acquired weakness are critical illness neuropathy, critical illness myopathy, and a combination of the two called critical illness neuromyopathy. Both critical illness myopathy and neuropathy present with symmetric proximal weakness. Facial weakness can occur but extraocular muscle involvement would be atypical and should suggest an alternate diagnosis. Tone and reflexes are decreased. Serum CK can be normal or elevated in critical illness myopathy. Electromyography can assist with diagnosis; in critical illness, myopathy compound muscle action potentials (CMAPs) show reduced amplitude and increased duration. In critical illness, polyneuropathy CMAPs and sensory nerve action potentials (SNAPs) are reduced or absent. Muscle biopsy can show selective loss of thick filaments and muscle necrosis in critical illness neuropathy. Patients with critical illness myopathy have a better chance of recovery than patients with critical illness polyneuropathy. Treatment is supportive.

Reference

Birch TB. Neuromuscular Disorders in the Intensive Care Unit. Continuum (Minneap Minn). 2021 Oct 1;27(5):1344–1364. https://doi.org/10.1212/CON.0000000000001004. PMID: 34618763.

Movement Disorders

Nestor Beltre, Kyra Floyd, Xavier Guell, and Betsy Thomas

Chorea

1. Which of the following is FALSE regarding the natural history of Sydenham's chorea?
   A. Pregnancy may induce recurrence of chorea
   B. Psychiatric symptoms frequently persist beyond the acute phase
   C. Patients in remission may display parkinsonism
   D. Most cases develop a chronic course of chorea
   E. Motor symptoms are often preceded by psychiatric symptoms, including obsessive compulsive disorder (OCD) and major depression.
   Correct answer: D

Explanation

Sydenham's chorea is an autoimmune condition which develops as a sequela of group A beta-hemolytic streptococcal infection. One study showed that Sydenham's chorea developed in about 26% of patients with rheumatic fever. The usual onset is at 8–9 years of age, with a greater prevalence in females. Symptoms typically develop 4–8 weeks after pharyngitis infection, but symptoms may develop in a delayed fashion, after 6 months or longer. Neurobehavioral manifestations including irritability, depression, and obsessive-compulsive symptoms may precede the onset of chorea and can persist after remission of motor symptoms. In the acute phase, patients with Sydenham's chorea may exhibit other motor symptoms such as tics, dysarthria, and hypotonia. Treatment is in a tiered approach, first with antibiotics (penicillin) for streptococcal eradication and prophylaxis, symptomatic control (valproic acid, risperidone), and then immunomodulation for refractory cases. In 80% of cases, there is complete remission by 6 months. Pregnancy or oral contraceptives may induce recurrence of chorea.

References

Teixeira AL, Vasconcelos LP, Nunes M, Singer H. Sydenham's chorea: from pathophysiology to therapeutics. Expert Rev Neurother. 2021;21(8):913–22. https://doi.org/10.1080/14737175.2021.1965883.

The Differential Diagnosis of Chorea. Oxford University Press; 2010.

Linked questions: 2–3

2. A 44-year-old man presents with several months of progressive involuntary jerking movements of his limbs, irritability, and difficulty concentrating. His father died of a neurodegenerative condition in his 50s. MRI reveals atrophy of the caudate nuclei. Genetic testing shows a CAG trinucleotide repeat expansion. Which of the following is the most likely diagnosis?
   A. Wilson's disease
   B. Huntington's disease
   C. Parkinson's disease
   D. Essential tremor
   E. Creutzfeldt-Jakob disease
   Correct answer: B

Explanation

Huntington's disease is caused by a CAG trinucleotide repeat expansion in the huntingtin (HTT) gene on chromosome 4, in an autosomal dominant inheritance pattern. Key features include choreiform movements, psychiatric symptoms such as irritability and depression, cognitive decline, and atrophy of the caudate nucleus on imaging.

Incorrect Answers

A. Wilson's disease: While patients with Wilson's disease can present with chorea, it is due to a genetic mutation in

N. Beltre · K. Floyd · X. Guell · B. Thomas (✉)
Department of Neurology, NYU Langone Health,
New York, NY, USA
e-mail: nestor.beltre@nyulangone.org; kyra.floyd@nyulangone.org; xavier.guellparadis@nyulangone.org;
betsy.thomas@nyulangone.org

the ATP7B gene rather than a CAG trinucleotide repeat expansion.

C. Parkinson's disease: Parkinson's disease is characterized by bradykinesia, rigidity, and resting tremor, not chorea or caudate atrophy.

D. Essential tremor: Essential tremor is characterized by bilateral action tremor, without cognitive decline or imaging abnormalities in the caudate.

E. Creutzfeldt-Jakob disease: Creutzfeldt-Jakob disease symptoms include rapidly progressive dementia with myoclonus and characteristic EEG/MRI findings. Inherited forms of prion diseases are responsible for 10–15% of the incidence of human prion disease and are caused by a mutation in the prion protein gene (PRNP) rather than a CAG trinucleotide repeat expansion (seen in Huntington's disease).

References

Członkowska A, Litwin T, Chabik G. Wilson disease: neurologic features. Handb Clin Neurol. 2017;142:101–19. https://doi.org/10.1016/b978-0-444-63625-6.00010-0.

Haubenberger D, Hallett M. Essential Tremor. N Engl J Med. 2018;378(19):1802–10. https://doi.org/10.1056/NEJMcp1707928.

Iwasaki Y. Creutzfeldt-Jakob disease. Neuropathology. 2017;37(2):174–88. https://doi.org/10.1111/neup.12355.

Jankovic J. Parkinson's disease: clinical features and diagnosis. J Neurol Neurosurg Psychiatry. 2008;79(4):368–76. https://doi.org/10.1136/jnnp.2007.131045.

McColgan P, Tabrizi SJ. Huntington's disease: a clinical review. Eur J Neurol. 2018;25(1):24–34. https://doi.org/10.1111/ene.13413.

Linked question

3. For the patient in the last question, which of the following statements is TRUE regarding his likely diagnosis?
   A. The disorder is inherited in an autosomal recessive pattern
   B. The underlying genetic defect involves a trinucleotide (CAG) repeat expansion in the HTT gene
   C. The most common initial symptoms are muscle rigidity and bradykinesia
   D. Anticipation is more common when the mutated gene is passed from mother to child
   E. The number of CAG repeats does not affect age of onset

Correct answer: B

Explanation

Huntington's disease is caused by a CAG trinucleotide repeat expansion in the huntingtin (HTT) gene on chromosome 4, in an autosomal dominant inheritance pattern. Key features

include choreiform movements, psychiatric symptoms (e.g., irritability, depression), cognitive decline, and caudate nucleus atrophy on imaging.

Incorrect Answers
A. The disorder is inherited in an autosomal dominant pattern.
C. Adult-onset Huntington's disease typically manifests first with chorea, whereas juvenile-onset Huntington's disease (with symptom onset less than 20 years old) typically manifests with parkinsonism and rigidity.
D. Anticipation is more common when the mutated gene is passed from father to child, due to the instability of the repeats during spermatogenesis.
E. There is an inverse correlation between repeat length and age of onset. Typically, if there are greater than 60 repeats, the patient will have juvenile-onset Huntington's disease, and chromosomes with 40 or more repeats are 100% penetrant.

Reference

McColgan P, Tabrizi SJ. Huntington's disease: a clinical review. Eur J Neurol. 2018;25(1):24–34. https://doi.org/10.1111/ene.13413.

4. A 27-year-old pregnant female in her first trimester with a past medical history of systemic lupus erythematosus presents with abrupt, involuntary, non-rhythmic movements affecting her face and upper limbs. Neurological examination reveals milkmaid's grip and facial grimacing. Which of the following statements about her condition is FALSE?
   A. Symptoms typically worsen and can persist after delivery
   B. Psychiatric symptoms such as personality changes, depression, or hallucinations may accompany the involuntary movements
   C. The condition is strongly associated with a history of Sydenham's chorea or rheumatic fever
   D. One of the main theories on the pathophysiology of this condition relates to the action of estrogen on dopamine receptors at the striatal level
   E. Treatment relies primarily on dopamine receptor antagonists and dopamine-depleting agents

Correct answer: A

Explanation

In chorea gravidarum, symptoms of chorea usually begin in the first or early second trimester and typically resolve by the third trimester or abate within hours of delivery. The other answers are true.

Reference

Robottom BJ, Weiner WJ. Chorea gravidarum. Handb Clin Neurol. 2011;100:231–5. https://doi.org/10.1016/b978-0-444-52014-2.00015-x.

5. A 38-year-old man with a history of epilepsy presents with progressive involuntary movements of the face and a "rubber man" appearance, obsessive-compulsive behaviors, and peripheral neuropathy. Blood smear reveals acanthocytes and serum creatine kinase (CK) is elevated. Brain MRI reveals caudate atrophy with dilatation of the anterior horns. Which condition is most likely?
   A. Huntington's disease
   B. Wilson's disease
   C. Sydenham's chorea
   D. Chorea-acanthocytosis
   E. Tardive dyskinesia
   Correct answer: D

Explanation

Chorea-acanthocytosis is an autosomal recessive disorder that is a member of the broader group of neuroacanthocytosis syndromes. It is characterized by chorea, psychiatric symptoms (e.g., obsessive-compulsive behaviors), acanthocytes on blood smear, elevated CK, and peripheral neuropathy. Axonal sensorimotor neuropathy and self-injurious tongue/lip biting are hallmark features.

Incorrect Answers

A. Huntington's disease: While chorea, psychiatric symptoms, and caudate atrophy can also be seen in Huntington's disease, acanthocytes and elevated CK are absent.
B. Wilson's disease: Wilson's disease presents with chorea and psychiatric symptoms but is distinguished by Kayser-Fleischer rings, low serum ceruloplasmin, and hepatic involvement.
C. Sydenham's chorea: Sydenham's chorea is an autoimmune condition following group A beta-hemolytic streptococcal infection and lacks acanthocytes or neuropathy.
E. Tardive dyskinesia: Tardive dyskinesia is caused by prolonged antipsychotic use and predominantly manifests as stereotyped oro-buccal-lingual movements.

Reference

Walker RH, Jung HH, Danek A. Neuroacanthocytosis. Handb Clin Neurol. 2011;100.141–51. https.//doi.org/10.1016/b978-0-444-52014-2.00007-0.

6. A 68-year-old man with advanced Parkinson's disease dementia develops worsening involuntary, writhing movements of his limbs and face 1 hour after each dose of his medication. His symptoms improve during "off" periods. MRI of the brain is unremarkable, and serum glucose is slightly elevated. Which medication is most likely responsible for these movements?
   A. Quetiapine
   B. Levodopa-carbidopa
   C. Sertraline
   D. Cocaine
   E. Metformin
   Correct answer: B

Explanation

Levodopa-induced dyskinesia is the most common cause of drug-induced chorea in Parkinson's disease, with around 80% of patients developing levodopa-induced dyskinesias. Peak-dose choreiform movements occur due to pulsatile dopamine receptor stimulation in the basal ganglia, typically 1–2 hours after medication administration. The temporal relationship to dosing and improvement during "off" periods are classic features.

Incorrect Answers

A. Quetiapine: While antipsychotics like quetiapine cause tardive dyskinesia, these movements are typically orobuccolingual and persist beyond drug cessation. They do not fluctuate with dosing schedules. Additionally, quetiapine has a lower risk of developing tardive dyskinesia compared to other antipsychotics.
C. Sertraline: SSRIs, such as sertraline, are more commonly associated with tremor or akathisia. Chorea is rare and typically occurs in the context of serotonin syndrome, which includes additional features (e.g., hyperthermia, clonus).
D. Cocaine: Cocaine-induced chorea ("crack dancing") presents acutely with recreational use, not in a chronic medication regimen. Symptoms typically resolve with drug clearance.
E. Metformin: This medication is not associated with movement disorders.

References

Daras M, Koppel BS, Atos-Radzion E. Cocaine-induced choreoathetoid movements ('crack dancing'). Neurology. 1994;44(4):751–2. https://doi.org/10.1212/wnl.44.4.751.

Hauser RA, Meyer JM, Factor SA, Comella CL, Tanner CM, Xavier RM, et al. Differentiating tardive dyskinesia: a video-based review of antipsychotic-induced movement disorders in clinical practice. CNS Spectr. 2022;27(2):208–17. https://doi.org/10.1017/s109285292000200x.

Kwon DK, Kwatra M, Wang J, Ko HS. Levodopa-Induced Dyskinesia in Parkinson's Disease: Pathogenesis and Emerging Treatment Strategies. Cells. 2022;11(23). https://doi.org/10.3390/cells11233736.

7. A 10-year-old girl with Sydenham's chorea continues to have severe, disabling chorea despite 4 weeks of valproic acid and secondary penicillin prophylaxis. Her parents report no improvement in her involuntary movements or emotional lability. Which intervention is the MOST appropriate next step?
   A. Increase valproic acid dose and add haloperidol
   B. Initiate intravenous immunoglobulin (IVIG)
   C. Switch to carbamazepine
   D. Continue current regimen for 1 more month
   E. Start carbidopa-levodopa
   Correct answer: B

Explanation

For refractory Sydenham's chorea, immunomodulatory therapy (e.g., IVIG, steroids, or plasma exchange) is recommended when symptomatic treatments fail. IVIG (2 g/kg administered over 2–5 days) modulates autoimmune mechanisms by neutralizing pathogenic antibodies and reducing basal ganglia inflammation. Studies show rapid symptom improvement in resistant cases, often within days. Treatment is in a tiered approach, first with antibiotics (penicillin) for streptococcal eradication and prophylaxis, symptomatic control (valproic acid, risperidone), and then immunomodulation for refractory cases.

Incorrect Answers

A. Increase valproic acid and add haloperidol: While valproic acid and dopamine antagonists (e.g., haloperidol) are first-line symptomatic therapies, escalating doses in non responders risks side effects (e.g., sedation, tardive dyskinesia) without addressing the autoimmune etiology.
C. Switch to carbamazepine: Limited evidence supports carbamazepine for Sydenham's chorea. It is less effective than valproic acid or immunomodulators in refractory cases.
D. Continue current regimen: Persisting severe symptoms after 4 weeks warrant escalation to immunomodulation rather than observation.
E. Carbidopa-levodopa: carbidopa-levodopa is contraindicated in Sydenham's chorea, as dopaminergic agents may exacerbate chorea.

Reference

Jummani R, Okun M. Sydenham chorea. Arch Neurol. 2001;58(2):311–3. https://doi.org/10.1001/archneur.58.2.311.

8. A 61-year-old man with a past medical history of schizophrenia presents with rapidly progressive dementia, myoclonus, and gait ataxia over 2 months. He recently developed involuntary, asymmetric jerky movements of the limbs. Brain MRI shows hyperintensity in the basal ganglia on diffusion-weighted imaging. Which diagnosis is MOST likely?
   A. Huntington's disease
   B. Wilson's disease
   C. Sydenham's chorea
   D. Creutzfeldt-Jakob disease (CJD)
   E. Tardive dyskinesia
   Correct answer: D

Explanation

The symptoms of rapidly progressive dementia, myoclonus, and ataxia, combined with MRI findings of basal ganglia hyperintensity on DWI is highly specific for Creutzfeldt-Jakob disease (CJD). Chorea in CJD, though rare in sporadic cases, is more frequently observed in variant CJD and forms part of the diagnostic criteria. Sporadic CJD, which is likely due to spontaneous misfolding of prion protein, is more common and rapidly progressive than variant CJD which is caused primarily by consuming beef infected with bovine spongiform encephalopathy. Chorea has been described as a later-stage manifestation of CJD but can occur at all stages of the disease. Often chorea coexists with other movement disorders like dystonia or myoclonus in CJD.

Incorrect Answers

A. Huntington's disease: Huntington's disease presents with chorea and dementia but progresses over years rather than months. MRI shows caudate atrophy rather than basal ganglia hyperintensity.
B. Wilson's disease: Wilson's disease features chorea and psychiatric symptoms, but also typically includes Kayser-Fleischer rings, low ceruloplasmin, and hepatic involvement.
C. Sydenham's chorea: Sydenham's chorea is an autoimmune condition following group A beta-hemolytic streptococcal infection, occurring in children aged 5–15 years old.
E. Tardive dyskinesia: Tardive dyskinesia is caused by prolonged dopamine antagonist use, with stereotyped orolingual movements (e.g., tongue protrusion), and is not associated with rapidly progressive dementia.

Reference

The Differential Diagnosis of Chorea. Oxford University Press; 2010.

Ballism and Athetosis

Linked questions: 9–10

9. A 74-year-old woman of East Asian descent with poorly controlled type 2 diabetes mellitus presents with sudden-onset involuntary, jerky, high amplitude movements in her right arm and leg. Her serum glucose is 326 mg/dL, hemoglobin A1C is 11.1%, and no ketones are detected. Brain MRI reveals a hyperintense area in the left putamen on T1-weighted imaging. What is the most likely diagnosis?
    A. Huntington's disease
    B. Acute ischemic stroke
    C. Nonketotic hyperglycemic hemichorea and hemiballismus
    D. Methamphetamine-induced chorea
    E. Wilson's disease
    Correct answer: C

Explanation

Nonketotic hyperglycemic hemichorea-hemiballismus is characterized by unilateral choreiform or ballistic movements associated with nonketotic hyperglycemia and imaging abnormalities, typically in the contralateral basal ganglia (putamen or caudate). The patient's clinical presentation, elevated glucose levels, absence of ketones, and MRI findings strongly support this diagnosis. Glycemic control often resolves symptoms.

Incorrect Answers

A. Huntington's disease: While chorea is a hallmark of Huntington's disease, it typically presents with progressive cognitive decline and psychiatric symptoms over years, rather than acute onset chorea. Imaging findings in Huntington's disease show caudate atrophy rather than hyperintensities in the putamen.

B. Acute ischemic stroke: Stroke can cause sudden-onset focal neurological deficits but rarely presents as isolated hemichorea without other signs (e.g., weakness or sensory loss), and imaging would show ischemic changes rather than hyperintensities in the basal ganglia.

D. Methamphetamine-induced chorea: Methamphetamine use can cause chorea but is associated with substance abuse history and systemic toxicity signs, which are absent here.

E. Wilson's disease: Wilson's disease causes basal ganglia dysfunction and a wide spectrum of neurologic manifestations such as chorea, dystonia, bradykinesia, tremor, and rigidity, but typically presents earlier in life with additional features such as hepatic dysfunction and Kayser-Fleischer rings on slit-lamp examination.

References

Aylward EH, Codori AM, Rosenblatt A, Sherr M, Brandt J, Stine OC, et al. Rate of caudate atrophy in presymptomatic and symptomatic stages of Huntington's disease. Mov Disord. 2000;15(3):552–60. https://doi.org/10.1002/1531-8257(200005)15:3<552::Aid-mds1020>3.0.Co;2-p.

Carrion DM, Carrion AF. Non-ketotic hyperglycaemia hemichorea-hemiballismus and acute ischaemic stroke. BMJ Case Rep. 2013;2013. https://doi.org/10.1136/bcr-2012-008359.

Członkowska A, Litwin T, Chabik G. Wilson disease: neurologic features. Handb Clin Neurol. 2017;142:101–19. https://doi.org/10.1016/b978-0-444-63625-6.00010-0.

Danve A, Kulkarni S, Bhoite G. Non-ketotic hyperglycemia unmasks hemichorea. J Community Hosp Intern Med Perspect. 2015;5(4):27825. https://doi.org/10.3402/jchimp.v5.27825.

Everett S, Dalo AM, Ananth D, Alejo AL, Durdella H, Niehaus M. Non-ketotic Hyperglycemia Hemichorea-Hemiballismus Syndrome: A Case Report. Cureus. 2023;15(5):e38434. https://doi.org/10.7759/cureus.38434.

Sperling LS, Horowitz JL. Methamphetamine-induced choreoathetosis and rhabdomyolysis. Ann Intern Med. 1994;121(12):986. https://doi.org/10.7326/0003-4819-121-12-199412150-00019.

Linked question

10. Which intervention is MOST appropriate for initial management?
    A. Administer risperidone
    B. Initiate aggressive insulin therapy
    C. Perform deep brain stimulation (DBS) of the globus pallidus interna
    D. Administer tetrabenazine
    E. Start haloperidol
    Correct answer: B

Explanation

The cornerstone of managing nonketotic hyperglycemic hemichorea-hemiballismus is rapid glycemic control with insulin. The exact pathophysiology is unknown, but it is thought that the symptoms are due to ischemia secondary to hyperviscosity. Hyperglycemia correction often leads to symptom resolution and normalization of imaging findings over days to weeks.

Incorrect Answers

A. Risperidone/D. Tetrabenazine/E. Haloperidol: Dopamine blockers (risperidone, haloperidol) or vesicular mono-amine transporter inhibitors (tetrabenazine) are adjunctive therapies for refractory cases but are not first line. Over 80% of nonketotic hyperglycemic hemichorea-hemiballismus cases improve with insulin alone. These medications carry risks of tardive dyskinesia or sedation and should only follow glycemic control.

C. Deep brain stimulation (DBS): DBS is reserved for severe, medication-refractory cases (e.g., chronic poststroke hemiballismus). Nonketotic hyperglycemic hemichorea-hemiballismus typically resolves with glucose management.

Reference

Danve A, Kulkarni S, Bhoite G. Non-ketotic hyperglycemia unmasks hemichorea. J Community Hosp Intern Med Perspect. 2015;5(4):27825. https://doi.org/10.3402/jchimp.v5.27825.

11. A 4-year-old girl presents with involuntary, jerky movements of the limbs and slow, writhing motions of the hands. Her mother reports that she had severe neonatal jaundice requiring phototherapy. Brain MRI shows T1 hyperintensity in the globus pallidus. Which condition is most likely?
    A. Lesch-Nyhan syndrome
    B. Huntington's disease
    C. Wilson's disease
    D. Dopa-responsive dystonia
    E. Choreoathetoid cerebral palsy
    Correct answer: E

Explanation

Choreoathetoid cerebral palsy, a subtype of dyskinetic cerebral palsy, is characterized by chorea (rapid, irregular movements) and athetosis (slow, writhing motions). The history of severe neonatal jaundice (kernicterus) and brain MRI findings of globus pallidus hyperintensities are pathognomonic. Brain MRI may appear normal or have subtle T1 hyperintensities in the globus pallidus interna, but over time scarring is common and may be visualized with volume loss and increased T2 signal.

Incorrect Answers

A. Lesch-Nyhan syndrome: Lesch-Nyhan syndrome is caused by a deficiency of hypoxanthine-guanine phosphoribosyltransferase (HPRT) activity due to inborn error of purine metabolism and is associated with uric acid overproduction. Its inheritance is X-linked recessive; thus males are typically affected. There is no history of kernicterus, and typically brain MRI shows nonspecific atrophic changes.

B. Huntington's disease: A genetic neurodegenerative disorder with adult-onset chorea, cognitive decline, and caudate atrophy on MRI, which is not linked to neonatal jaundice.

D. Dopa-responsive dystonia: This condition improves dramatically with levodopa and typically presents with dystonia rather than choreoathetosis.

E. Wilson's disease: While one of the common neurologic manifestations of Wilson's disease is chorea, key features of this disease are hepatic dysfunction, Kayser-Fleischer rings, and low serum ceruloplasmin.

References

Li X, Arya K. Athetoid Cerebral Palsy. StatPearls. Treasure Island (FL): StatPearls Publishing Copyright © 2025, StatPearls Publishing LLC.; 2025.

Torres RJ, Puig JG. Hypoxanthine-guanine phosophoribosyltransferase (HPRT) deficiency: Lesch-Nyhan syndrome. Orphanet J Rare Dis. 2007;2:48. https://doi.org/10.1186/1750-1172-2-48.

Dystonia

Linked questions: 12–14

12. A 50-year-old woman with a history of hypothyroidism and hypertension presents for evaluation of neck pain. She states that for the past 3 months, she has been having pain at the back of her neck, on the left side. She also feels that her neck is involuntarily turning to the right side. On examination, the patient is noted to have tilting of her neck to the left side, with turning of the neck to the right side. With effort, she can temporarily straighten her neck, but upon relaxing it immediately reverts to the previously described position. The examination of her cranial nerves, strength, sensation, and reflexes are all normal. Her current medications are levothyroxine and losartan, and she denies any other medication use in the past. What is the correct diagnosis?
    A. Tardive dystonia
    B. Cervical radiculopathy
    C. Cervical osteoarthritis
    D. Cervical dystonia
    E. Cervical myelopathy
    Correct answer: D

Explanation

Dystonia is a syndrome of sustained muscle contraction causing sustained or intermittent abnormal posturing. As this can cause unusual postures of body parts, dystonia can often be misdiagnosed or misinterpreted as a functional disorder. This patient has dystonia affecting the neck muscles, called cervical dystonia. This is often accompanied by pain in the neck.

Incorrect Answers

A. Tardive dystonia: Patients who are exposed to antipsychotic medications or antidopaminergic nausea medications such as metoclopramide can develop tardive dystonia, which is dystonic posturing related to the use or withdrawal of dopaminergic receptor antagonists. Therefore, it is important to do a thorough medication review prior to diagnosing a patient with idiopathic cervical dystonia. As this patient has no current or history of dopaminergic receptor antagonist use, her presentation is not consistent with tardive dystonia.

B. Cervical radiculopathy: Typical symptoms of cervical radiculopathy include pain radiating down the arm, which may be accompanied by paresthesias, numbness, or weakness. This condition would not cause abnormal posturing of the neck.

C. Cervical osteoarthritis can cause neck pain leading to radiculopathy, stenosis, and spondylosis, but would not cause abnormal posturing of the neck.

E. A patient with cervical myelopathy may experience neck pain radiating down one or both arms, along with paresthesias, numbness, and/or weakness. The exam may reveal weakness accompanied by sensory changes and brisk reflexes. These are not seen in this patient, and myelopathy would not cause abnormal posturing of the neck.

Reference

Chan J, Brin MF, Fahn S. Idiopathic cervical dystonia: clinical characteristics. Mov Disord. 1991;6(2):119–26. https://doi.org/10.1002/mds.870060206.

Linked question

13. Which of the following symptoms or exam findings would NOT be expected in this patient?
    A. Alleviation of posturing by touching the chin or back of the head
    B. Jerky irregular shaking of the head and neck
    C. Weakness in extensor muscles of the neck
    D. Improvement in neck posturing with walking backwards
    E. Limited range of motion of the neck
    Correct answer: C

Explanation

When evaluating a patient to determine if they have idiopathic cervical dystonia, it is important to do a thorough examination to exclude other conditions that can mimic cervical dystonia. This includes neck extensor myopathy, a myopathy that causes isolated weakness of neck extensor muscles, leading to a dropped head posture which can be misinterpreted as dystonic posturing. Patients with cervical dystonia should have full strength in their neck muscles, which should be examined prior to making the diagnosis.

Incorrect Answers

A. Patients with cervical dystonia often have a "sensory trick"—which refers to a maneuver that the patient can perform themselves to improve or alleviate the neck posturing. Common sensory tricks include touching the chin with a hand, or touching the back of the head. In some series, 84% of patients with cervical dystonia reported a sensory trick, and the presence of a sensory trick is helpful in confirming the diagnosis. The mechanism of the sensory trick remains poorly understood.

B. Patients with cervical dystonia may experience a jerky and irregular shaking of the neck, often worsened by turning the head in one direction. This is often referred to as a dystonic tremor, though the term tremor is not necessarily an accurate term for this shaking, as it is typically very irregular in nature. It is important to differentiate this from the head tremor of essential tremor, which should be a very regular, oscillatory tremor.

D. Dystonia is often very task-specific, often referred to as "state function behavior"—the tendency of dystonia symptoms to be more prominent during certain activities or when the body is in a particular state. Many patients with various forms of dystonia note that their symptoms worsen upon walking forwards and improve upon walking backwards.

E. Many patients with cervical dystonia have limited range of motion of the neck, and this should be assessed on the examination.

References

LeDoux MS. Dystonia: phenomenology. Parkinsonism Relat Disord. 2012;18 Suppl 1(Suppl 1):S162–4. https://doi.org/10.1016/s1353-8020(11)70050-5.

Martino D, Liuzzi D, Macerollo A, Aniello MS, Livrea P, Defazio G. The phenomenology of the geste antagoniste in primary blepharospasm and cervical dystonia. Mov Disord. 2010;25(4):407–12. https://doi.org/10.1002/mds.23011.

Raju S, Ravi A, Prashanth LK. Cervical Dystonia Mimics: A Case Series and Review of the Literature. Tremor Other

Hyperkinet Mov (N Y). 2019;9. https://doi.org/10.7916/tohm.v0.707.

Linked question

14. Which of the following treatments is NOT likely to improve the patient's symptoms?
    A. Clonazepam
    B. Valproic acid
    C. Baclofen
    D. Botulinum toxin injections
    E. Trihexyphenidyl

Correct answer: B

Explanation

Clonazepam (a benzodiazepine), baclofen (antispasmodic agent), and trihexyphenidyl (an anticholinergic) are all medications that have been used in dystonia with success. However, botulinum toxin injections are the mainstay of treatment for cervical dystonia and are typically necessary in addition to use of oral medications. Valproic acid has not been validated for use in dystonia.

Reference

Velickovic M, Benabou R, Brin MF. Cervical dystonia pathophysiology and treatment options. Drugs. 2001;61(13):1921–43. https://doi.org/10.2165/00003495-200161130-00004.

15. A 12-year-old boy with no prior medical history presents with difficulty writing. He complains of tightness in his arm that develops as soon as he starts writing. This does not affect any other activity. The patient is examined, and it is noted that he develops posturing of the arm only when writing, characterized by involuntary flexion of the wrist. He is diagnosed with writer's cramp. However, about a year after this he starts to develop difficulty walking. Upon examining the patient, it is noted that his right foot inverts when he walks. He then begins to develop foot inversion even at rest. What test is likely to reveal the cause of the patient's symptoms?
    A. MRI of the brain
    B. Genetic testing
    C. Head CT
    D. Nerve conduction velocity
    E. Basic metabolic panel

Correct answer: B

Explanation

This patient initially presented with writer's cramp, a focal dystonia. His dystonia then spreads to other body regions, representing a generalized dystonia. Given the young age of onset and development of a generalized dystonia, this raises suspicion for a genetic cause of dystonia. The family history would also be a useful part of the evaluation. DYT1 dystonia would be a compelling consideration for this case, though DYT6, DYT25, and dopa-responsive dystonia may also mimic this.

Incorrect Answers

A, C. Standard CT or MRI scans of the brain will be normal in most patients with dystonia and do not assist in confirming the diagnosis.

D. An EMG may reveal increased activity in the muscles involved in the patient's dystonia, but a nerve conduction velocity test should be normal, or at most show mild nonspecific slowing.

E. A BMP would be normal in a patient with dystonia.

Reference

Ozelius L, Lubarr N. DYT1 Early-Onset Isolated Dystonia. In: Adam MP, Feldman J, Mirzaa GM, Pagon RA, Wallace SE, Amemiya A, editors. GeneReviews(®). Seattle (WA): University of Washington, Seattle Copyright © 1993–2025, University of Washington, Seattle. GeneReviews is a registered trademark of the University of Washington, Seattle. All rights reserved.; 1993.

16. A 6-year-old girl with no prior medical history presents for evaluation of difficulty walking for the past year. On examination, the patient has mild bilateral foot plantarflexion and inversion at rest, which becomes severe when walking, with posturing of the right arm. Brisk reflexes in the bilateral lower extremities are noted, with clonus at the bilateral ankles. Her parents describe that she often appears to walk normally early in the day, but by late afternoon/evening develops more significant symptoms. Her paternal uncle also had similar symptoms. What medication would be most helpful in this case?
    A. Levodopa
    B. Methocarbamol
    C. Sertraline
    D. Gabapentin
    E. Amantadine

Correct answer: A

Explanation

This patient presents with dystonic posturing, with significant diurnal variation (symptoms are worse later in the day) and lower extremity hyperreflexia, a constellation of symptoms consistent with dopa-responsive dystonia (DRD). Patients with this condition respond robustly to levodopa, and this response is helpful in confirming the diagnosis. Genetic testing should also be pursued, looking for an autosomal dominant heterozygous mutation in the GTP cyclohydrolase I gene

(GCH-1). The other listed options—methocarbamol, sertraline, gabapentin and amantadine—are unlikely to produce significant benefit. Other medication options used for dystonia, such as benzodiazepines, trihexyphenidyl, and baclofen, can all be helpful in this condition, but the most effective treatment is typically levodopa.

References

Lee WW, Jeon BS. Clinical spectrum of dopa-responsive dystonia and related disorders. Curr Neurol Neurosci Rep. 2014;14(7):461. https://doi.org/10.1007/s11910-014-0461-9.

Wijemanne S, Jankovic J. Dopa-responsive dystonia–clinical and genetic heterogeneity. Nat Rev Neurol. 2015;11(7):414–24. https://doi.org/10.1038/nrneurol.2015.86.

17. A 65-year-old man, diagnosed with Parkinson's disease 1 year ago, presents for follow-up. His main symptom has been mild right-sided slowness and stiffness. As his symptoms have not been functionally impairing, he has remained unmedicated for his Parkinson's disease thus far. Today he presents with a new complaint of right foot pain, which waxes and wanes throughout the day. On examination, he has mild facial masking, no hypophonia, no tremor, and mild bradykinesia and cogwheel rigidity in the right arm and leg. On his right foot, he appears to have mild toe curling in digits 2–5, with mild extension of the big toe. With walking, this becomes slightly more pronounced. There is no weakness or sensory deficit, and his reflexes are normal. What is the diagnosis?
    A. Idiopathic primary dystonia
    B. Charcot Marie Tooth disease
    C. Secondary dystonia
    D. Dopa-responsive dystonia with GCH-1 mutation
    E. Hammer toes

Correct answer: C

Explanation

This patient with Parkinson's disease has developed secondary dystonia related to his condition. This is characterized by posturing causing toe curling and big toe extension in his foot, on the same side of his body that is affected by his Parkinson's disease. Dystonia is seen in 30% or more of patients with Parkinson's disease and can even be the first presentation of the disease. Therefore, when patients with Parkinson's disease complain of pain or other discomfort, it is important to do a thorough examination to evaluate for dystonic posturing. The response of dystonia to levodopa can be variable, but this would be a good first option for treating these symptoms. Medications that are used for any form of dystonia, including benzodiazepines, trihexyphenidyl, and baclofen, can be helpful as well, and botulinum toxin injections are an excellent treatment option as well. Deep brain stimulation for Parkinson's disease can help with dystonia as well.

Incorrect Answers

A. Though idiopathic primary dystonia is a possibility in this case, given that this patient has a condition known to cause secondary dystonia (Parkinson's disease), and the symptoms are on the same side where the patient experiences his Parkinson's disease symptoms, this is more likely to be a secondary dystonia.

B. Charcot Marie Tooth is a hereditary peripheral neuropathy, causing a constellation of symptoms including weakness, hammer toes, paresthesias and sensory loss, loss of reflexes, and gait issues. The patient's age would be atypical for a first presentation of CMT, though there are late-onset forms. The normal strength, sensation, and reflexes make CMT less likely in this case.

D. Dopa-responsive dystonia is a condition characterized by dystonic posturing, often accompanied by lower extremity hyperreflexia and significant diurnal variation, with symptoms often worsening later in the day. This condition most typically begins in childhood, though late-onset cases have been described as well. In this case, the later age of onset, the lack of diurnal variation or hyperreflexia, and the fact that the symptoms are only on the right side which is affected more by Parkinson's disease make dopa-responsive dystonia less likely.

E. Hammer toes are an orthopedic deformity where the proximal interphalangeal joint assumes a bent position. This is a consideration for this patient's toe curling, but a hammer toe is a fixed deformity and should not vary with activities. The variation in symptom severity with different activities, which is called state function behavior, a classic finding in dystonia, makes hammer toes a less likely etiology of the patient's symptoms.

Reference

Shetty AS, Bhatia KP, Lang AE. Dystonia and Parkinson's disease: What is the relationship? Neurobiol Dis. 2019;132:104462. https://doi.org/10.1016/j.nbd.2019.05.001.

18. A 51-year-old woman with a history of hypertension and hyperlipidemia presents with involuntary movements of the lower face. Six months prior to the evaluation, she began to experience involuntary closing of the jaw, making it difficult to speak and chew food. One month prior to the evaluation, she began to notice involuntary eye closure. On examination, the patient is noted to have frequent involuntary closing of the eyes, occasionally lasting for several seconds at a time, posturing of the lips in

a pursed manner, and involuntary jaw closing interfering with her ability to speak and provide the history. She notes that there are other members of her family with involuntary eye closure. She is taking losartan and rosuvastatin and denies any other medication exposure in the past. What is the diagnosis?

A. Tardive dyskinesia
B. Meige syndrome
C. Functional movement disorder
D. Hemifacial spasm
E. Chronic motor tics

Correct answer: B

Explanation

Meige syndrome is a dystonic movement disorder characterized by blepharospasm (involuntary bilateral eye closure) and oromandibular dystonia (in this patient's case, lip pursing and jaw closing). Hereditary factors may be involved in this syndrome, as a positive family history is found in some patients with Meige syndrome. Medications for dystonia treatment, such as clonazepam, baclofen, or trihexyphenidyl, may be used. OnabotulinumtoxinA injections can also be helpful in managing symptoms.

Incorrect Answers

A. Tardive dyskinesia and dystonia can mimic a primary dystonic process, and it is important to do a thorough medication review. Given the lack of exposure to dopamine receptor blocking agents, this is not consistent with a tardive movement disorder.
C. There are no specific features in this case to suggest a functional movement disorder.
D. As the patient has bilateral movements, and they are not myoclonic in nature, this is not consistent with hemifacial spasm.
E. As the patient has not endorsed any urge to perform her movements or relief with performing them, this is unlikely to represent tics. This would also be a somewhat unusual age to present with new tics.

Reference

Pandey S, Sharma S. Meige's syndrome: History, epidemiology, clinical features, pathogenesis and treatment. J Neurol Sci. 2017;372:162–70. https://doi.org/10.1016/j.jns.2016.11.053.

Linked questions: 19–20

19. A 35-year-old man of Filipino descent presents for evaluation regarding involuntary movements. Seven years prior he developed involuntary bilateral eye closure. He was diagnosed with blepharospasm and was treated with OnabotulinumtoxinA injections with good effect. Four years later, he developed torticollis and writer's cramp. As of 6 months ago, he has developed posturing in all four of his limbs, which is making it challenging for him to perform his activities of daily living or walk stably. He has also developed involuntary tongue protrusion and mild symmetric bilateral bradykinesia and cogwheel rigidity. He has been taking clonazepam and trihexyphenidyl, which help somewhat with his symptoms. He continues to get OnabotulinumtoxinA injections, but he has developed symptoms in so many different parts of his body that the OnabotulinumtoxinA can no longer effectively manage his issues. What is the most likely diagnosis?

A. Parkinson's disease
B. Huntington's disease
C. X-linked dystonia parkinsonism
D. Tardive dystonia
E. Motor neuron disease

Correct answer: C

Explanation

X-linked dystonia parkinsonism, also known as Lubag disease, is a condition that causes progressive dystonia, with or without parkinsonism. This is seen in Filipino males and can present with a wide spectrum of movement disorders including dystonia, parkinsonism, myoclonus, and chorea. Patients may present with a focal dystonia, which then progresses to a multifocal or generalized dystonia. Involuntary tongue protrusion and a characteristic gait with phasic knee bending may be seen as well.

Reference

Evidente VG, Advincula J, Esteban R, Pasco P, Alfon JA, Natividad FF, et al. Phenomenology of "Lubag" or X-linked dystonia-parkinsonism. Mov Disord. 2002;17(6):1271–7. https://doi.org/10.1002/mds.10271.

Linked question

20. What is the next best step in the management for this patient?

A. Levodopa
B. Deep brain stimulation
C. High-intensity focused ultrasound
D. Quetiapine
E. Amantadine

Correct answer: B

Explanation

This patient has refractory dystonic symptoms despite being on multiple oral anti-dystonia drugs and receiving

OnabotulinumtoxinA injections, and he is having difficulty with his activities of daily living including walking. This is an appropriate time to explore deep brain stimulation for the patient, and this has been described as an effective treatment for patients with X-linked dystonia parkinsonism.

Incorrect Answers

A. Levodopa has not been found to be helpful in this disease. The patient does have mild parkinsonism, but his main issue is dystonia.

C. High-intensity focused ultrasound is a procedure that can be used to address tremor in patients with essential tremor and Parkinson's disease. It would not have a role for this patient's dystonia.

D, E. Quetiapine is an antipsychotic and amantadine is used in Parkinson's disease, these medications would not have a role for this patient.

Reference

Evidente VG, Advincula J, Esteban R, Pasco P, Alfon JA, Natividad FF, et al. Phenomenology of "Lubag" or X-linked dystonia-parkinsonism. Mov Disord. 2002;17(6):1271–7. https://doi.org/10.1002/mds.10271.

Functional Movement Disorders

Linked questions: 21–23

21. A 50-year-old woman presents for evaluation due to pain and stiffness in her neck. She is concerned about cervical dystonia, as one of her friends was recently diagnosed with this. On examination, her head is fully turned to the left, and she cannot voluntarily move her head in any other direction. She does not have a sensory trick (a maneuver that can help her straighten her head, such as touching her chin or the back of her head), and her neck posture does not demonstrate any variability with different activities. When you test the range of motion in her neck, at times you are able to obtain a degree of horizontal movement, at other times you are unable to move her neck. You obtain an MRI and CT scan of the patient's neck, which are unremarkable. What is the likely diagnosis?
    A. Cervical dystonia
    B. Atlantoaxial subluxation
    C. Congenital torticollis
    D. Functional dystonia
    E. Osteoarthritis
    Correct answer: D

Explanation

This patient's presentation is suggestive of a functional disorder. Clues that suggest this are the absence of typical features of cervical dystonia, including a sensory trick, or state-function behavior, the variability of dystonic posturing, and movements with different activities. While patients with cervical dystonia can have some limitation of range of motion of the neck, total inability to move the neck at all is not expected. The variable resistance to passive movement of the neck—at times the range of motion is completely absent, other times it can be obtained to a degree—is also a feature of a functional disorder. When a patient presents with fixed posturing of the neck, it is always important to rule out an orthopedic issue, which is why the MRI and CT scan were obtained.

References

Espay AJ, Aybek S, Carson A, Edwards MJ, Goldstein LH, Hallett M, et al. Current Concepts in Diagnosis and Treatment of Functional Neurological Disorders. JAMA Neurol. 2018;75(9):1132–41. https://doi.org/10.1001/jamaneurol.2018.1264.

Hallett M. Functional Neurologic Disorder, La Lésion Dynamique: 2024 Wartenberg Lecture. Neurology. 2024;103(11):e210051. https://doi.org/10.1212/wnl.0000000000210051.

Linked question

22. A diagnosis of functional dystonia is suspected. Which of the following would NOT be consistent with this diagnosis?
    A. Variable resistance to passive movement of the neck
    B. Resolution of neck posturing with distraction
    C. Further history that onset of neck posturing occurred at the time of a stressful life event
    D. Improvement of neck posturing when walking backwards
    E. Spontaneous resolution of neck posturing for two weeks, followed by recurrence
    Correct answer: D

Explanation

Functional neurologic disorders are a constellation of motor and sensory signs and symptoms that are inconsistent with a known neurologic disease. This is involuntary, in contrast to malingering, where the patient is knowingly producing symptoms with the goal of secondary gain. Naturally, a thorough evaluation for any known neurologic disease should be done in a patient with a suspected functional disorder. However, in addition to this, there should be an evaluation done for the features that help rule in a functional disorder. A feature that is often seen in functional disorders is variability of performance, with the patient often demonstrating resolution of symptoms when distracted. Though idiopathic cervical dystonia can certainly have variability in its severity depending on the activity that the patient is doing, features like total resolution of neck posturing with distraction and spontaneous resolution of the dystonia for multiple weeks (answers B and E) are suggestive of a functional disorder and would not be seen in cervical dystonia. Variable resistance to passive movement of the neck can be seen in functional dystonia (answer A), as is described in the previous question. It is also prudent to assess for any underlying medical or psychological stressor that occurred at the time of symptom onset, which may have provoked a functional disorder. However, this cannot always be identified. Improvement of neck posturing when walking backwards is a feature that can be seen in many forms of organic dystonia (answer D) and therefore would not confirm a diagnosis of a functional disorder.

References

Espay AJ, Aybek S, Carson A, Edwards MJ, Goldstein LH, Hallett M, et al. Current Concepts in Diagnosis and Treatment of Functional Neurological Disorders. JAMA Neurol. 2018;75(9):1132–41. https://doi.org/10.1001/jamaneurol.2018.1264.

Hallett M. Functional Neurologic Disorder, La Lésion Dynamique: 2024 Wartenberg Lecture. Neurology. 2024;103(11):e210051. https://doi.org/10.1212/wnl.0000000000210051.

Linked question

23. What is the most appropriate next step for treating this patient?
    A. Discussion of the diagnosis and referral to cognitive behavioral and physical therapy
    B. Psychiatry referral for discussion of the diagnosis
    C. OnabotulinumtoxinA injections
    D. Discharge from the clinic, as this is not an organic neurological disorder
    E. Referral for massage therapy

    Correct answer: A

Explanation

Discussion of the diagnosis and referral to cognitive behavioral and physical therapy. When a diagnosis of a functional disorder has been confirmed, this should be discussed with the patient to help them understand what is happening to their body. This should ideally be done once the provider has established a trusting relationship with the patient. The patient should then be referred for cognitive behavioral therapy and physical therapy focused on functional disorders.

Incorrect Answers

B. While psychiatric issues such as depression and anxiety can be one of the underlying causes that precipitate a functional disorder, and a psychiatry referral can be helpful in this case, the diagnosis should be discussed with the patient first. Referring the patient straight to a psychiatrist without discussing the diagnosis is inappropriate, as the diagnosis should come from a trusted provider. Additionally, a psychiatrist may not be comfortable explaining why this is not an organic cervical dystonia, that is, a discussion that is most appropriate for a neurologist.

C. OnabotulinumtoxinA injections are not appropriate for functional disorders.

D. A supportive approach to a functional diagnosis is most likely to produce improvement in the patient, and patients can significantly improve with good support and therapeutic interventions. It would be most appropriate to schedule a follow-up for this patient, to continue to answer questions and assess the efficacy of the planned interventions.

E. While massage therapy may be helpful for neck comfort, it would not address the underlying functional disorder.

References

Espay AJ, Aybek S, Carson A, Edwards MJ, Goldstein LH, Hallett M, et al. Current Concepts in Diagnosis and Treatment of Functional Neurological Disorders. JAMA Neurol. 2018;75(9):1132–41. https://doi.org/10.1001/jamaneurol.2018.1264.

Hallett M. Functional Neurologic Disorder, La Lésion Dynamique: 2024 Wartenberg Lecture. Neurology. 2024;103(11):e210051. https://doi.org/10.1212/wnl.0000000000210051.

24. A 50-year-old man presents for evaluation of tremor. He reports that this started suddenly 1 month ago. He is noticing tremor both at rest and with action, interfering with all of his ADLs. On examination, the patient does not have any abnormal movements during the history-taking portion of the visit aside from when he is talking about the tremor, but upon beginning the examination develops prominent large amplitude shaking movements in both arms. The movements appear non-rhythmic and are not oscillatory. They vary in their severity. When he is distracted with cognitive tasks such as recalling three words, these movements cease. Additionally, when the patient is asked to tap his fingers or do tasks with his right arm, the left arm tremor ceases. His exam is otherwise normal. When asked about whether anything changed at the time of symptom onset, he reports that he was fired from his job around that time, though he

reports that he did not find this to be particularly stressful and he is now looking for a new job. What is the likely diagnosis?

A. Parkinson's disease
B. Holmes tremor
C. Functional tremor
D. Essential tremor
E. Enhanced physiological tremor

Correct answer: C

Explanation

Tremor is defined as an involuntary, rhythmic, oscillatory movement. This patient's movements do not follow these characteristics, which rules out the other organic tremor disorders that are listed as options here. Additionally, several features of a functional disorder are present here, such as variability in severity and symptoms fully resolving with distraction. Often, an inciting event or medical issue can be uncovered as the trigger for a functional disorder, though this is not always the case, and even if an event is described, the patient may not describe the event as having been stressful.

References

Espay AJ, Aybek S, Carson A, Edwards MJ, Goldstein LH, Hallett M, et al. Current Concepts in Diagnosis and Treatment of Functional Neurological Disorders. JAMA Neurol. 2018;75(9):1132–41. https://doi.org/10.1001/jamaneurol.2018 1264.

Hallett M. Functional Neurologic Disorder, La Lésion Dynamique: 2024 Wartenberg Lecture. Neurology. 2024;103(11):e210051. https://doi.org/10.1212/wnl.0000000000210051.

Paroxysmal Movement Disorders

Linked questions: 25–27

25. A 50-year-old woman with a history of well-controlled hypertension presents for evaluation of right facial movements. She reports that about 3 months ago, she started to notice involuntary twitching involving her right eye and right upper lip. She denies any history of trauma or any other inciting event. On examination, you noted quick jerking movements of the right eye and right cheek, causing the patient's right eye to close and the right cheek to pull upwards. She denies any urge to perform these movements, or any relief with performing them. The exam is otherwise normal. What is the correct diagnosis?

    A. Tardive dyskinesia
    B. Facial dystonia
    C. Hemifacial spasm

    D. Motor tic disorder
    E. Benign fasciculations

    Correct answer: C

Explanation

This is an involuntary paroxysmal movement disorder involving myoclonic movements in muscles innervated by the facial nerve. This is seen on the examination as small myoclonic jerks, often involving the orbicularis oculi, but can involve many other muscles innervated by the facial nerve. Patients described painless involuntary twitching. It can be provoked on examination by having the patient activate muscles and then relax, for example, by having them close their eyes very tightly and then relax.

Incorrect Answers

A. Tardive dyskinesia would not commonly affect only one side of the face, but regardless the patient does not have a history of using dopamine receptor blocking agents, which is what causes tardive movements.

B. Facial dystonia can cause a variety of movements, but would be less common to affect only one side of the face, and typically causes more slow and sustained posturing movements, rather than the quick jerking movements that are described, which are classic for myoclonus.

D. As the patient describes completely involuntary movements without any preceding urge or relief after performing the movement, this is less consistent with motor tics.

E. Benign fasciculations can commonly present in the eyelids, especially when patients are sleep deprived, but this degree of movement causing upwards pulling of the cheek is not likely to represent a fasciculation.

Reference

Abbruzzese G, Berardelli A, Defazio G. Hemifacial spasm. Handb Clin Neurol. 2011;100:675–80. https://doi.org/10.1016/b978-0-444-52014-2.00048-3.

Linked question

26. What is the best next step in workup?

    A. MRI/MRA of the brain
    B. Genetic testing
    C. EMG/NCV
    D. Routine EEG
    E. Venous sinus imaging

    Correct answer: A

Explanation

Hemifacial spasm can be caused by irritation of the facial nerve by ectatic blood vessels, so every patient should undergo imaging to investigate for this. Genetic testing, routine EEG, and venous sinus imaging would be expected to be normal in a patient with hemifacial spasm. While surface EMG can detect myoclonus, a routine EMG/NCV would be low yield.

Reference

Abbruzzese G, Berardelli A, Defazio G. Hemifacial spasm. Handb Clin Neurol. 2011;100:675–80. https://doi.org/10.1016/b978-0-444-52014-2.00048-3.

Linked question

27. What is the best treatment option for this patient?
    A. Carbamazepine
    B. Gabapentin
    C. Levetiracetam
    D. OnabotulinumtoxinA injections
    E. Focused ultrasound therapy
    Correct answer: D

Explanation

Though several oral medications (answers A, B, C) have been studied for hemifacial spasm, few have demonstrated consistent benefit, and it is now standard of care to start treatment with OnabotulinumtoxinA toxin injections, which are generally well tolerated and sustain efficacy over years. For patients who are found to have neurovascular contact between the facial nerve and an ectatic blood vessel, surgical management with microvascular decompression can be considered.

Reference

Abbruzzese G, Berardelli A, Defazio G. Hemifacial spasm. Handb Clin Neurol. 2011;100:675–80. https://doi.org/10.1016/b978-0-444-52014-2.00048-3.

Linked questions: 28–30

28. A 55-year-old woman with a history of depression, hyperlipidemia, hypertension, and well-controlled diabetes presents for evaluation of leg discomfort. She reports that once or twice a month, around 9 PM, when she gets into bed she feels an intense discomfort and need to move her legs. She moves them around in the bed, or sits up and swings her legs at the edge of the bed, and this helps—however, as soon as she relaxes back in bed, the discomfort builds up again. She often needs to get up and walk around to relieve this sensation. This does not occur during the daytime and only affects her legs. Her exam is normal. What is the most likely diagnosis?
    A. Tardive akathisia
    B. Motor tic disorder
    C. Peripheral neuropathy
    D. Peripheral vascular disease
    E. Restless legs syndrome
    Correct answer: E

Explanation

Restless legs syndrome is a chronic movement disorder where patient develops restlessness in their legs at night, improved with movement. There is a diurnal pattern, where symptoms occur mainly at night, though they can occur earlier in the day as the disease progresses.

Incorrect Answers

A. Tardive akathisia can present with restlessness and a need to move, similar to restless legs syndrome, but would be expected to be present to a degree throughout the day, and no history of antipsychotic use has been uncovered here.

B. Though motor tics are in some ways described similarly—an urge to perform a movement, followed by relief—again the fact that this occurs mainly at night time points more towards restless legs syndrome, as does the fact that it is only occurring in the legs.

C, D. Findings of these conditions are not evident from the examination.

Reference

Gossard TR, Trotti LM, Videnovic A, St Louis EK. Restless Legs Syndrome: Contemporary Diagnosis and Treatment. Neurotherapeutics. 2021;18(1):140–55. https://doi.org/10.1007/s13311-021-01019-4.

Linked question

29. The patient is wondering if one of her medications could be causing her symptoms. She is currently on amlodipine, lisinopril, escitalopram, melatonin, empagliflozin, and rosuvastatin. What would you tell her?
    A. None of these medications are contributing
    B. Melatonin may be contributing
    C. Escitalopram may be contributing
    D. Empagliflozin may be contributing
    E. Rosuvastatin may be contributing
    Correct answer: C

Explanation

Escitalopram may be contributing. Medications can exacerbate or even cause restless legs syndrome. These medications include neuroleptics, SSRIs (such as escitalopram), tricyclic antidepressants, SNRIs, lithium, and diphenhydramine. The other listed medications are less likely to cause this.

Linked question

30. What are your next steps for this patient?
    A. MRI of the brain
    B. MRI of the lumbar spine
    C. Check iron lab work and supplement as needed
    D. Start tramadol
    E. Start pramipexole TID
    Correct answer: C

Explanation

This patient has infrequent restless legs syndrome, occurring only once to twice a month, and therefore may not need pharmacologic intervention, but this should be discussed in a shared decision-making process. Low iron levels can precipitate or worsen restless legs syndrome; therefore, every patient with this condition should have lab work done to investigate their iron levels. The ferritin levels are the best way to measure iron levels over an extended time, and all RLS patients with a level below 50–75 ng/mL should receive iron supplementation. For a patient with mild RLS, this may be adequate to control their symptoms. MRIs are unlikely to be helpful in this patient with classic RLS symptoms and a normal exam (answers A, B); tramadol is an opiate and would not be an appropriate initial treatment for this patient (answer D). Pramipexole is a medication that can be used for RLS, but starting it three times a day would not be needed in a patient who only has symptoms at nighttime. Additionally, based on the patient's description of the symptoms (mild), pharmacologic treatment may not be needed at this time (Answer E).

Reference

Gossard TR, Trotti LM, Videnovic A, St Louis EK. Restless Legs Syndrome: Contemporary Diagnosis and Treatment. Neurotherapeutics. 2021;18(1):140–55. https://doi.org/10.1007/s13311-021-01019-4.

31. A 35-year-old man with restless legs syndrome (RLS) returns for follow-up. He is not on any medications that worsen RLS. His iron levels were checked, and he was found to have an adequate ferritin level of 125. He tried gabapentin but even at low doses found it difficult to tolerate due to GI upset. You have decided to use a low-dose dopamine agonist for his RLS. Which of the following is a side effect seen with dopamine agonists?
    A. Impulse control disorder
    B. Augmentation of RLS
    C. Sleep attacks
    D. A and B
    E. A, B, and C
    Correct answer: E

Explanation

Impulse control disorder, which can manifest in a variety of ways including gambling, overspending, compulsive shopping, hypersexuality, and others, is an important side effect that should be discussed with every patient prior to starting them on a dopamine agonist. Augmentation of RLS refers to the concept that use of dopamine agonists can cause RLS symptoms to paradoxically become worse with time—this may present as worsening in severity of symptoms, spread of symptoms to other limbs, or presentation of symptoms earlier in the day. The use of dopamine agonists is clearly necessary in some patients who do not achieve adequate symptomatic control with iron supplementation, minimization of RLS-provoking drugs, and gabapentin, but the risk of augmentation should be discussed with the patient prior to starting a dopamine agonist, and the dose should be minimized as much as possible. Additionally, sleep attacks, an uncommon side effect of dopamine agonists where the patient suddenly falls asleep without warning, should also be discussed.

32. A 16-year-old boy with no prior medical issues presents for evaluation of involuntary movements. He notes that when he is at rest, he does not develop any involuntary movements. When he is initiating a movement, such as when he is getting out of bed or starting to run in gym class, he may suddenly develop an involuntary movement. This is typically characterized by writhing or flinging movements of his right arm and leg, lasting for about 20 s, and occurring a few times per day. Often, he gets a sense of discomfort or anticipation prior to the movement occurring, which served as a warning that the movement was going to occur. His neurological examination in the office is normal. An MRI of the brain and an EEG are normal, and routine lab work including thyroid function testing and calcium levels are normal. What is the diagnosis?
    A. Surface negative seizure
    B. Chorea
    C. Episodic ataxia
    D. Paroxysmal kinesigenic dyskinesia
    E. A functional movement disorder
    Correct answer: D

Explanation

Paroxysmal kinesigenic dyskinesia (PKD) is a rare condition characterized by involuntary movements that are precipitated by initiating a movement. These movements can be choreoathetotic in nature, or ballistic or dystonic. Patients may have a type of aura before the movements, described as a premonitory sensation that the movement is coming. Movements can be unilateral or bilateral, and attack frequency can be as high as more than 20 attacks per day.

PRRT2 is a gene that has been associated with PKD. Carbamazepine, even at low doses, is often a very effective medication for these patients and completely controls the movements.

Reference

Lotze T, Jankovic J. Paroxysmal kinesigenic dyskinesias. Semin Pediatr Neurol. 2003;10(1):68–79. https://doi.org/10.1016/s1071-9091(02)00012-8.

33. A 12-year-old boy with autism spectrum disorder presents for evaluation of abnormal movements. His parents have noticed that when he is excited, he tends to flap his hands, sometimes for up to 30 s at a time. If they distract him during these episodes, the flapping will stop, but sometimes it is difficult to distract him. He retains awareness and motor function during these episodes, and if he is spoken to he will respond normally. They have been noticing these movements for many years, but lately they have been happening much more often. They note that he got a new train set that he is very excited about recently, and the movement tends to occur most while he is using it, but can also happen with other activities that he enjoys. The patient states that he is somewhat aware of the movements but is not able to explain why he does them. He denies that the movements bother him. Outside of poor eye contact, the neurological examination in the office is normal. What is the likely diagnosis?
    A. Automatisms
    B. Stereotypies
    C. Chronic motor tics
    D. Seizure
    E. Chorea
    Correct answer: B

Explanation

Motor stereotypies are repetitive movements with a fixed pattern. Common stereotypies include hand flapping, nail biting, hair twisting, etc. These movements can be stopped by distraction and usually occur when the patient is experiencing excitement, boredom, or stress. These are more common in children but occur in adults as well. Many patients with autism spectrum disorder do experience stereotypies. This patient has a movement that is typical for a stereotypy (hand flapping), which is distractible, and occurs mainly when he is excited.

Incorrect Answers

A. Automatisms are involuntary, repetitive motor activities that can occur during seizure activity. These may include rubbing the hands together, smacking lips or chewing, and other movements. Given that this patient's movements are bilateral but are also distractible and he is alert and verbal during the movements, it is much less likely that these movements represent seizure activity.

C. Tics can often be seen in patients with autism spectrum disorder, and it can be challenging to distinguish these from stereotypies given that the patient may not be aware of or able to express a clear description of what prompts them to perform the movement, or whether they are getting relief from performing the movement. However, given that this patient's movements seem to occur only in circumstances where he is excited, and not in other circumstances, a stereotypy is more likely.

D. This patient's movements are distractible and occur only in the setting of excitement, and he is awake and alert during the movements, so these are less likely to represent seizure events.

E. Chorea is a fluid, dance-like movement that flows from one body part to the next. The description of the patient's movements is not consistent with chorea.

Reference

Péter Z, Oliphant ME, Fernandez TV. Motor Stereotypies: A Pathophysiological Review. Front Neurosci. 2017;11:171. https://doi.org/10.3389/fnins.2017.00171.

Myoclonus

34. A 63-year-old man with a history of hypertension, hyperlipidemia, and poorly controlled diabetes is admitted to the hospital for decompensated cirrhosis. While admitted, the inpatient team notes shaking movements and consults neurology regarding concern for a tremor. On your examination, the patient is mildly drowsy, but fully oriented and conversant, and has no abnormal movements at rest. When his arms are held outstretched, he develops quick jerking movements of the arms, with loss of tone. What test will help reveal the cause of this patient's symptoms?
    A. Ammonia level
    B. MRI of the brain
    C. EMG/NCV
    D. Lumbar puncture
    E. EEG
    Correct answer: A

Explanation

This patient's examination is suggestive of myoclonus, quick, lightning-like irregular nonrhythmic jerky movements. Myoclonus can be positive (due to sudden muscle contractions) or negative (due to loss of muscle tone). Negative myoclonus, especially in the context of cirrhosis and hyperammonemia, is often referred to as asterixis.

Myoclonus can be induced by medications and a variety of toxic-metabolic etiologies, and therefore, consultation for "tremor" in the hospital will often represent myoclonus in the setting of a medical illness. However, rhythmic myoclonus, especially when present at rest, can represent seizure activity, so there should also be a low threshold for obtaining EEG data in a patient who is spontaneously having myoclonic activity, especially if mental status is impaired. In this patient with asterixis, an MRI, EMG/NCV, lumbar puncture, or EEG will not yield additional information about his movements.

35. A 31-year-old woman with a history of obsessive-compulsive disorder (OCD) on fluoxetine 80 mg daily, and hair loss on minoxidil, presents for evaluation of shaking in her hands. She reports that for about 1 year, she has noted mild shaking in her hands when she is holding her arms out straight. The movements do not interfere with her daily activities. On examination, the patient has no movements at rest. When her arms are held outstretched, there are mild, low amplitude, irregular, quick jerking movements seen in her arms. When she performs finger-nose-finger testing, there is no shaking as she approaches her target. Her exam is otherwise normal. She reports that her OCD is well-controlled with fluoxetine, which she started a year ago. What should the next step be?
    A. No further testing
    B. Start propranolol for enhanced physiologic tremor
    C. EMG of the upper limbs
    D. Start primidone for essential tremor
    E. Start clonazepam for anxiety
    Correct answer: A

Explanation

The description of the patient's examination—quick, jerky movements that are irregular—is consistent with mild myoclonus. This is likely induced by fluoxetine, which she has been taking for the same amount of time that she has been noticing the myoclonus. A thorough examination should be done in every patient with myoclonus, to ensure that there are no other abnormalities such as dystonia, epilepsy, cognitive impairment, or parkinsonism, which have not been found here. As the patient is not bothered by her symptoms, fluoxetine can be continued without changes and her examination can be monitored.

Incorrect Answers

B. The patient's examination is not consistent with tremor. Tremor is a regular, rhythmic, oscillatory movement. This patient has irregular, jerky movements which are consistent with myoclonus.

C. EMG will not provide additional information here.

D. The patient's examination is not consistent with tremor, as explained above, and she does not have any intention tremor, which suggests that this is not essential tremor.

E. There is no description that the patient has uncontrolled anxiety, and while clonazepam can aid in controlling myoclonus, the patient's movements are not bothering her, so addition of further medication is not warranted at this time.

Reference

Rissardo JP, Fornari Caprara AL, Bhal N, Repudi R, Zlatin L, Walker IM. Drug-Induced Myoclonus: A Systematic Review. Medicina (Kaunas). 2025;61(1). https://doi.org/10.3390/medicina61010131.

Linked questions: 36–37

36. A 55-year-old man with a history of hypertension, hyperlipidemia, and diabetes collapses suddenly while at work. On EMS arrival 5 min later, he is found to be pulseless and CPR is initiated. After 5 min of CPR, he is successfully resuscitated and taken to the hospital. He remains on a ventilator for the next 7 days due to cardiac complications and is then weaned from sedation and from the ventilator. As sedation is weaned, the patient wakes up and can answer basic questions and follow simple commands. However, when he tries to lift his arms to follow commands, he develops severe irregular jerking movements of his arms and legs. He does not have these movements at rest. What is the likely diagnosis?
    A. Myoclonic epilepsy
    B. Acute stroke
    C. Dystonia
    D. Chorea
    E. Lance-Adams syndrome
    Correct answer: E

Explanation

This patient has suffered hypoxic injury to the brain as a result of hypoperfusion during his cardiac arrest and has developed post-hypoxic myoclonus, also known as Lance-Adams syndrome. This type of myoclonus is typically initiated by movement, startle response, and tactile stimuli and resolves at rest.

Incorrect Answers

A. As the patient only has myoclonus with action, and is awake and alert during the movements, and they are non-rhythmic, this is not likely to represent epilepsy.

B. Acute stroke would not be expected to present with isolated bilateral action myoclonus.

C, D. The description of the movements is not consistent with dystonia (involuntary posturing) or chorea (fluid, dance-like movements flowing from one body part to the next)

Reference

Shin JH, Park JM, Kim AR, Shin HS, Lee ES, Oh MK, et al. Lance-adams syndrome. Ann Rehabil Med. 2012;36(4):561–4. https://doi.org/10.5535/arm.2012.36.4.561.

Linked question

37. Which of the following is an appropriate first choice for treatment of the patient's movements?
    A. Levodopa
    B. Valproic acid
    C. Propranolol
    D. Zoloft
    E. Trihexyphenidyl
    Correct answer: B

Explanation

Clonazepam, valproic acid, and levetiracetam have all been identified as good primary drug Lance-Adams syndrome and can be combined together in treatment as well. The myoclonic movements in this disorder can sometimes be highly refractory to treatments and may require multiple medications for partial control.

Reference

Shin JH, Park JM, Kim AR, Shin HS, Lee ES, Oh MK, et al. Lance-adams syndrome. Ann Rehabil Med. 2012;36(4):561–4. https://doi.org/10.5535/arm.2012.36.4.561.

38. A 21-year-old woman presents for evaluation of shaking movements. She has been noticing involuntary jerking in her arms more than her legs, for as long as she can remember. You examine the patient and notice that she has action myoclonus, as well as dystonic posturing. You obtain genetic testing, which shows a pathogenic variant in the SGCE gene. Which of the following features are NOT likely to be seen in this patient?
    A. Improvement in jerking movements with alcohol
    B. A sibling with the same symptoms
    C. A history of OCD
    D. Choreiform movements
    E. A parent with the same symptoms
    Correct answer: D

Explanation

SGCE myoclonus-dystonia is a movement disorder combining irregular rapid brief muscle jerking movements (myoclonus) and sustained posturing movements (dystonia). Symptom onset is variable, but typically by age 10–20. Non-motor features of this condition can include OCD, anxiety, and the finding that alcohol helps control the movements. This disorder is inherited in an autosomal dominant fashion, and penetrance is determined by whether the altered SGCE allele is inherited from the patient's father (results in disease) or mother (typically does not result in disease). Therefore, each child of an individual with SGCE myoclonus-dystonia has a 50% chance of inheriting the pathogenic variant, so it is easily possible that our patient would have a sibling and parent with the condition as well. Choreiform movements are not a feature of SGCE myoclonus-dystonia. SCGE encodes the protein epsilon-sarcoglycan.

Reference

Raymond D, Saunders-Pullman R, Ozelius L. SGCE Myoclonus-Dystonia. In: Adam MP, Feldman J, Mirzaa GM, Pagon RA, Wallace SE, Amemiya A, editors. GeneReviews(®). Seattle (WA): University of Washington, Seattle Copyright © 1993–2025, University of Washington, Seattle. GeneReviews is a registered trademark of the University of Washington, Seattle. All rights reserved.; 1993.

Critical Care

39. A 28-year-old man with a past psychiatric history of schizophrenia develops a fever of 39.5 °C (103.1 °F), generalized "lead-pipe" rigidity, and confusion 10 days after starting haloperidol. Laboratory tests reveal leukocytosis (WBC 18,000/µL) and creatine kinase (CK) of 12,000 U/L. Which diagnosis is most likely?
    A. Neuroleptic malignant syndrome
    B. Serotonin syndrome
    C. Malignant hyperthermia
    D. Bacterial meningitis
    E. Sepsis
    Correct answer: A

Explanation

Neuroleptic malignant syndrome (NMS) is a life-threatening reaction to dopamine antagonists like haloperidol. Key features include hyperthermia (>38 °C), severe muscle rigidity, autonomic instability, and altered mental status, typically emerging within days to weeks of starting the drug. Elevated CK (due to rhabdomyolysis) and leukocytosis further support this diagnosis.

Incorrect Answers

B. Serotonin syndrome: While also a drug-induced hyperthermic disorder, serotonin syndrome is caused by serotonergic agents (e.g., SSRIs) and features hyperreflexia, clonus, and diarrhea, not lead-pipe rigidity.
C. Malignant hyperthermia: Malignant hyperthermia is triggered by volatile anesthetics or succinylcholine during surgery, not antipsychotics. Genetic testing for RYR1 mutations can help support diagnosis.
D. Bacterial meningitis: Bacterial meningitis presents with fever and altered mental status, but lacks muscle rigidity. CSF analysis would show elevated white blood cells (typically neutrophilic predominance) and elevated protein.
E. Sepsis: Systemic infection causes fever and leukocytosis, but does not explain severe rigidity or CK elevation without a primary infectious source.

Reference

Tormoehlen LM, Rusyniak DE. Neuroleptic malignant syndrome and serotonin syndrome. Handb Clin Neurol. 2018;157:663–75. https://doi.org/10.1016/b978-0-444-64074-1.00039-2.

Linked questions: 40–41

40. A 27-year-old woman with past medical history of depression presents to the emergency department with agitation, diaphoresis, and generalized tremors. Her husband reports that she started taking sertraline 2 weeks ago and began using dextromethorphan for a cough yesterday. On examination, she has ocular clonus, hyperreflexia in the lower extremities, and a temperature of 38.9 °C (102 °F). Which diagnosis is most likely?
    A. Neuroleptic malignant syndrome
    B. Serotonin syndrome
    C. Anticholinergic toxicity
    D. Malignant hyperthermia
    E. Meningitis
    Correct answer: B

Explanation

The clinical triad of serotonin syndrome is altered mentation, autonomic instability (hyperthermia, tachycardia, hypertension), and motor hyperactivity (clonus, hyperreflexia, tremor, and rigidity). This patient's recent use of two serotonergic agents (sertraline and dextromethorphan) and findings of ocular clonus, hyperreflexia, and fever meet diagnostic criteria. Symptoms typically emerge within hours of medication changes.

Incorrect Answers

A. Neuroleptic malignant syndrome (NMS): Neuroleptic malignant syndrome is associated with dopamine antagonists (e.g., antipsychotics), not SSRIs. NMS presents with "lead-pipe" rigidity, hyporeflexia, and slower symptom onset (days to weeks).
B. Anticholinergic toxicity: Anticholinergic toxicity causes dry skin, absent bowel sounds, and mydriasis—not clonus or hyperreflexia.
D. Malignant hyperthermia: Malignant hyperthermia is triggered by anesthetic agents (e.g., succinylcholine), and features include severe rigidity, hyporeflexia, and metabolic acidosis.
E. Meningitis: Meningitis presents with neck stiffness, photophobia, and CSF pleocytosis, and there is no link to serotonergic drugs.

Reference

Tormoehlen LM, Rusyniak DE. Neuroleptic malignant syndrome and serotonin syndrome. Handb Clin Neurol. 2018;157:663–75. https://doi.org/10.1016/b978-0-444-64074-1.00039-2.

Linked question

41. Which intervention is MOST critical in her initial management?
    A. Administer acetaminophen for fever
    B. Initiate haloperidol for agitation
    C. Discontinue sertraline and provide IV benzodiazepines
    D. Apply physical restraints to prevent self-injury
    E. Continue sertraline at the original dose and add cyproheptadine
    Correct answer: C

Explanation

First-line management of serotonin syndrome requires immediate discontinuation of the offending serotonergic agent (sertraline and dextromethorphan) and administration of benzodiazepines (e.g., lorazepam) to reduce agitation, neuromuscular hyperactivity, and autonomic instability. Benzodiazepines also mitigate the risk of hyperthermia, a key driver of mortality. Many cases of serotonin syndrome resolve within 24 h of discontinuing the offending agent and initiating supportive treatment. For moderate to severe cases, cyproheptadine can be added to block serotonin receptors, and severe hyperthermia requires sedation, paralysis, and mechanical ventilation.

Incorrect Answers

A. Acetaminophen: Acetaminophen is ineffective for serotonin syndrome-related hyperthermia, as the fever stems from muscle hyperactivity, not hypothalamic dysregulation.

B. Haloperidol: Antipsychotics risk exacerbating symptoms by affecting dopamine pathways and may precipitate neuroleptic malignant syndrome.

D. Physical restraints: Physical restraints are relatively contraindicated as they can enforce isometric muscle contractions which worsen hyperthermia and rhabdomyolysis.

E. Continue sertraline: Continuing the causative agent perpetuates serotonin toxicity. Cyproheptadine (a serotonin antagonist) is adjunctive but does not replace stopping the drug.

Reference

Boyer EW, Shannon M. The serotonin syndrome. N Engl J Med. 2005;352(11):1112–20. https://doi.org/10.1056/NEJMra041867.

42. A 17-year-old boy with a history of Tourette syndrome and obsessive-compulsive disorder presents with continuous, nonrhythmic jerking of his face, arms, and legs for 6 h. His parents report no recent medication changes. Vital signs are normal, and creatine kinase (CK) is mildly elevated at 450 U/L. EEG shows no epileptiform activity. Which diagnosis is most likely?
    A. Tic status
    B. Neuroleptic malignant syndrome
    C. Serotonin syndrome
    D. Epilepsia partialis continua
    E. Acute dystonic reaction
    Correct answer: A

Explanation

Tic status is characterized by severe, continuous tics lasting hours to days without resolution, often occurring in patients with preexisting tic disorders like Tourette syndrome. The absence of hyperthermia, normal consciousness, and lack of epileptiform activity on EEG distinguish it from other hyperkinetic emergencies.

Incorrect Answers

B. Neuroleptic malignant syndrome (NMS): Neuroleptic malignant syndrome presents with hyperthermia, "lead-pipe" rigidity, and autonomic instability, typically triggered by dopamine antagonists. Normal vital signs and lack of rigidity rule this out.

C. Serotonin syndrome: Serotonin syndrome features hyperreflexia, clonus, and hyperthermia due to serotonergic agents. This patient lacks clonus or autonomic instability.

D. Epilepsia partialis continua: While epilepsia partialis continua can present with preserved consciousness and a normal EEG (as the focus of the seizures may be subcortical), the movements would be rhythmic and unilateral.

E. Acute dystonic reaction: Acute dystonic reaction causes sustained muscle contractions (e.g., torticollis, oculogyric crisis) typically after dopamine antagonist use. The continuous, jerky movements here are consistent with tics, not dystonia.

Reference

Parmera JB, Yamamoto JYS, Cury RG. Tic Status in Tourette Syndrome Due to Depletion of the Deep Brain Stimulation Battery. JAMA Neurol. 2023;80(3):320–1. https://doi.org/10.1001/jamaneurol.2022.4774.

43. A 15-year-old boy with dystonic cerebral palsy secondary to bilirubin encephalopathy presents with continuous, painful twisting movements of all limbs, arching of the back (opisthotonos), and tachycardia (HR 140 bpm). He was previously managed on risperidone for agitation but recently discontinued it due to weight gain. His parents report he had a febrile illness 2 days prior. Labs show creatine kinase (CK) of 25,000 U/L and myoglobinuria. Which diagnosis is most likely?
    A. Serotonin syndrome
    B. Neuroleptic malignant syndrome
    C. Dystonic storm
    D. Malignant hyperthermia
    E. Generalized tonic-clonic seizure
    Correct answer: C

Explanation

Dystonic storm (status dystonicus) is a life-threatening exacerbation of dystonia characterized by severe, continuous muscle contractions, autonomic instability (e.g., tachycardia), and complications like rhabdomyolysis (elevated CK) and myoglobinuria. Triggers include infection, fever, or medication changes such as discontinuation of dopamine receptor blockers (such as risperidone). This patient's history of dystonic cerebral palsy, recent febrile illness, discontinuation of risperidone, and lab findings are consistent with this diagnosis.

Incorrect Answers

A. Serotonin syndrome: Serotonin syndrome typically presents with clonus and tremor rather than dystonia, and this patient was not exposed to any serotonergic agents.

B. Neuroleptic malignant syndrome (NMS): Neuroleptic malignant syndrome is caused by exposure to dopamine antagonists rather than withdrawal, and symptoms include "lead-pipe" rigidity rather than dystonic movements. Another less common but important cause of NMS is abrupt withdrawal of dopamine agonists and can be seen when patients are not slowly tapered off of dopamine agonists, such as ropinirole or pramipexole, that are used in the treatment of Parkinson's disease or restless legs syndrome.

D. Malignant hyperthermia: Malignant hyperthermia is triggered by anesthesia agents, not infection, and presents with metabolic acidosis and hyporeflexia during surgery.

E. Generalized tonic-clonic seizure: Generalized tonic-clonic seizures involve loss of consciousness and postictal states, not sustained dystonic posturing.

Reference

Termsarasab P, Frucht SJ. Dystonic storm: a practical clinical and video review. J Clin Mov Disord. 2017;4:10. https://doi.org/10.1186/s40734-017-0057-z.

44. A 26-year-old man develops sudden, involuntary upward deviation of the eyes, neck hyperextension, and agitation 48 hours after starting metoclopramide for nausea. Vital signs are stable. Which intervention is MOST appropriate for acute management?
    A. Administer haloperidol for agitation
    B. Discontinue metoclopramide and give intravenous benztropine
    C. Continue metoclopramide and add sertraline
    D. Provide supportive care only
    E. Initiate levetiracetam
    Correct answer: B

Explanation

Oculogyric crisis (OGC) is a drug-induced dystonic reaction, often caused by dopamine receptor antagonists like metoclopramide. Immediate management requires discontinuing the offending agent and administering anticholinergic drugs (e.g., benztropine) or antihistamines (e.g., diphenhydramine) to counteract relative cholinergic excess. Symptoms typically resolve within minutes of treatment.

Incorrect Answers

A. Haloperidol: Antipsychotics exacerbate OGC by further blocking dopamine receptors.

C. Continue metoclopramide and add sertraline: Continuing the causative agent perpetuates symptoms. SSRIs like sertraline have no role in acute OGC management.

D. Supportive care only: While supportive care is important, it is critical to remove the offending agent and administer anticholinergic medication or antihistamines for rapid symptom resolution.

E. Levetiracetam: Oculogyric crises are non-epileptic and should be distinguished through history and examination from epileptic seizures.

Reference

Barow E, Schneider SA, Bhatia KP, Ganos C. Oculogyric crises: Etiology, pathophysiology and therapeutic approaches. Parkinsonism Relat Disord. 2017;36:3–9. https://doi.org/10.1016/j.parkreldis.2016.11.012.

Ataxia

Linked questions: 45–46

45. A 17-year-old boy is referred to the neurology clinic for evaluation of progressive difficulty walking over the past 3 years. His parents report that he began to appear clumsy around age 14, frequently tripping and struggling with balance, especially in low light. Over time, his gait has become increasingly unsteady. He also reports difficulty with handwriting and occasional slurring of speech. There is no history of head trauma, alcohol use, or recent illness. On neurologic examination, he has a wide-based, unsteady gait, dysmetria on finger-to-nose testing, and dysdiadochokinesia. Muscle strength is preserved, but he has absent deep tendon reflexes in the ankles and bilateral Babinski signs. Vibration and position sense are impaired in the feet. He has pes cavus and mild scoliosis. Cardiovascular exam reveals a soft systolic murmur. His older brother has similar symptoms. Which is the most likely diagnosis?
    A. Cerebellar Ataxia with Neuropathy and Vestibular Areflexia Syndrome (CANVAS)
    B. Spinocerebellar ataxia type 3 (SCA3)
    C. Friedreich's ataxia
    D. Postinfectious cerebellitis
    E. Spinocerebellar ataxia type 27B (SCA27B)
    Correct answer: C

Explanation

A. The patient's young age of onset and lack of vestibular areflexia are not suggestive of CANVAS.

B. SCA3 is the most common inherited cause of autosomal dominant cerebellar ataxia worldwide and most commonly starts in adulthood. The patient's young onset of presentation, associated myelopathic signs, and lack of family history in parents or grandparents are not suggestive of SCA3.

C. This is correct. Friedreich's ataxia is the most common autosomal recessive cause of cerebellar ataxia, caused by an expanded GAA trinucleotide repeat in the FXN gene, and is classically associated with myeloneuropathic signs, explaining the patient's absent ankle reflexes (a sign of neuropathy) combined with bilateral Babinski signs (a sign of myelopathy). Pes cavus is a reflection of chronic neuropathy. Scoliosis is also frequently observed in Friedreich's ataxia, as well as cardiomyopathy.

D. The prolonged time course of slowly worsening over multiple years is not suggestive of postinfectious cerebellitis.

E. SCA27B is an autosomal dominant cause of cerebellar ataxia that typically starts in adulthood and is often associated with downbeat nystagmus. The patient's presentation is not suggestive of SCA27B.

References

Cook A, Giunti P. Friedreich's ataxia: clinical features, pathogenesis and management. Br Med Bull. 2017;124(1):19–30. https://doi.org/10.1093/bmb/ldx034.

Rosenthal LS. Neurodegenerative Cerebellar Ataxia. Continuum (Minneap Minn). 2022;28(5):1409–34. https://doi.org/10.1212/con.0000000000001180.

Linked question

46. Which of the following is true regarding the patient in the prior case?

    A. The examination is suggestive of pure cerebellar ataxia

    B. The examination is suggestive of pure sensory ataxia

    C. The examination is suggestive of a frontal gait disorder

    D. The examination is suggestive of mixed cerebellar and sensory ataxia

    E. The examination is suggestive of mixed cerebellar ataxia and frontal gait disorder

    Correct answer: D

Explanation

The patient's exam shows decreased ankle reflexes and Babinski signs, which indicate a myeloneuropathy that is common in Friedreich's ataxia. Pes cavus indicates chronic neuropathy. Proprioceptive loss from both neuropathic and myelopathic pathology contributes to the patient's lack of balance and explains the increased difficulty walking in low-light situations, because patients with proprioceptive loss rely more strongly on visual input to modulate their balance. In addition, finger-to-nose abnormalities, dysdiadochokinesia, and slurred speech are indicative of cerebellar ataxia. There are no signs of executive dysfunction or other frontal signs on exam to suggest that the patient has a frontal gait disorder. For this reason, only (D) is correct.

References

Cook A, Giunti P. Friedreich's ataxia: clinical features, pathogenesis and management. Br Med Bull. 2017;124(1):19–30. https://doi.org/10.1093/bmb/ldx034.

Rosenthal LS. Neurodegenerative Cerebellar Ataxia. Continuum (Minneap Minn). 2022;28(5):1409–34. https://doi.org/10.1212/con.0000000000001180.

47. Which of the following findings would most strongly suggest a diagnosis of ataxia-telangiectasia (AT)?

    A. Gait ataxia and bilateral abnormal head-impulse test in a 60-year-olds

    B. Early-onset ataxia with conjunctival telangiectasias and elevated alpha-fetoprotein

    C. Intermittent ataxia triggered by exertion in a teenage athlete

    D. Progressive ataxia and vertical gaze palsy in a middle-aged adult

    E. Progressive ataxia manifesting in adulthood with a family history of ataxia in the patient's father and paternal grandmother

    Correct answer: B

Explanation

A. A bilateral abnormal head-impulse test in a patient with progressive cerebellar ataxia is most suggestive of Cerebellar Ataxia with Neuropathy and Vestibular Areflexia Syndrome (CANVAS), not AT

B. Correct. AT is a recessively inherited cerebellar ataxia most commonly presenting in early childhood. Classic features include progressive gait ataxia, oculocutaneous telangiectasias, immunodeficiency, and elevated serum alpha-fetoprotein. It is caused by mutations in the *ATM* gene.

C. Episodic features are not typical of ataxia-telangiectasia.

D. Vertical gaze palsy is not observed in AT and suggests an alternative diagnosis. A not-to-miss etiology of progressive cerebellar ataxia with supranuclear gaze palsy is Niemann-Pick type C.

E. A dominant family history is not suggestive of AT. AT is an autosomal recessive condition.

Reference

Rosenthal LS. Neurodegenerative Cerebellar Ataxia. Continuum (Minneap Minn). 2022;28(5):1409–34. https://doi.org/10.1212/con.0000000000001180.

48. Which is FALSE regarding cerebellar ataxia of autoimmune etiology?

    A. Most patients who lose their ability to walk subsequently recover their ability to walk after treatment

    B. Anti-Yo (also known as anti-PCA1) antibodies are a common cause of autoimmune cerebellar ataxia

    C. Screening for neoplasms is an essential feature of the diagnostic work-up of cerebellar ataxia of autoimmune etiology

    D. GAD65 antibodies are associated with cerebellar ataxia

    E. A normal MRI does not exclude cerebellar ataxia of autoimmune etiology

    Correct answer: A

Explanation

A. This statement is false. Most patients who lose their ability to walk as a result of cerebellar ataxia of autoimmune etiology unfortunately do not recover their ability despite immunomodulatory treatment.

B. This is correct. Anti-Yo is the most common antibody accounting for immune-mediated pure cerebellar ataxia. Other causes of pure cerebellar ataxia of autoimmune origin are anti-Tr and anti-mGluR1.

C. This is correct. Screening for neoplasms is an essential feature of the diagnostic work-up of cerebellar ataxia of autoimmune etiology, which can be of paraneoplastic origin.

D. This is correct. GAD65 is most commonly associated with stiff person syndrome, but it is also associated with cerebellar ataxia.

E. This is correct. Normal MRI imaging does not exclude cerebellar ataxia of autoimmune etiology.

References

Abbatemarco JR, Vedeler CA, Greenlee JE. Paraneoplastic cerebellar and brainstem disorders. Handb Clin Neurol. 2024;200:173–91. https://doi.org/10.1016/b978-0-12-823912-4.00030-x.

Shams'ili S, Grefkens J, de Leeuw B, van den Bent M, Hooijkaas H, van der Holt B, et al. Paraneoplastic cerebellar degeneration associated with antineuronal antibodies: analysis of 50 patients. Brain. 2003;126(Pt 6):1409–18. https://doi.org/10.1093/brain/awg133.

49. Which of the following clinical characteristics would be most suggestive of multiple systems atrophy, cerebellar type (MSA-C), in a patient presenting with 3 years of worsening cerebellar ataxia?
    A. Age of onset younger than 30 years old
    B. Family history of cerebellar ataxia
    C. Pontine atrophy
    D. Lack of a history of REM-sleep behavior disorder (RSBD)
    E. Improvement of cerebellar ataxia with carbidopa-levodopa

    Correct answer: C

Explanation

A. A young age of onset would be unusual for MSA-C

B. Family history is not expected for MSA-C. This is considered a sporadic disease, without monogenic inheritance

C. This is correct. Pontine atrophy is commonly seen in MSA-C. However, it is important to note that other forms of ataxia can present with pontine atrophy. A key differentiating imaging feature of MSA-C compared to other forms of ataxia is the rapid loss of pontine size; a study suggests that a loss of pontine anterior-posterior diameter of more than 0.8 mm per year is specific for MSA-C

D. REM-sleep behavior disorder is commonly found in MSA-C

E. Carbidopa-levodopa does not improve cerebellar ataxia

Reference

Stephen CD, Vangel M, Gupta AS, MacMore JP, Schmahmann JD. Rates of change of pons and middle cerebellar peduncle diameters are diagnostic of multiple system atrophy of the cerebellar type. Brain Commun. 2024;6(1):fcae019. https://doi.org/10.1093/braincomms/fcae019.

50. Which of the following clinical characteristics would be most suggestive of spinocerebellar ataxia type 3 (also known as Machado-Joseph disease), in a patient presenting with five years of worsening cerebellar ataxia?
    A. Multiple siblings affected but no parents or grandparents affected
    B. Loss of pontine size at a rate higher than 1 mm per year
    C. Deterioration to wheelchair dependence from symptom onset in 6 months
    D. Portuguese ancestry
    E. History of chronic cough

    Correct answer: D

Explanation

A. SCA3 is an autosomal dominant disorder. Multiple siblings affected, but no parents or grandparents affected, would suggest an autosomal recessive pattern of inheritance, rather than an autosomal dominant pattern of inheritance.

B. Loss of pontine size at a rate higher than 1 mm per year in a patient with progressive cerebellar ataxia is suggestive of multiple systems atrophy cerebellar type.

C. A rapidly progressive course is not expected in inherited forms of cerebellar ataxia and should trigger work-up of alternative causes including immune-mediated cerebellar ataxia.

D. This is correct. SCA3 is the most common cause of inherited ataxia worldwide, and its prevalence is higher in patients with Portuguese ancestry.

E. Chronic cough is not associated with SCA3. Chronic cough is associated with a different form of inherited ataxia called Cerebellar Ataxia with Neuropathy and Vestibular Areflexia Syndrome (CANVAS).

Reference

Rosenthal LS. Neurodegenerative Cerebellar Ataxia. Continuum (Minneap Minn). 2022;28(5):1409–34. https://doi.org/10.1212/con.0000000000001180.

51. Which of the following clinical characteristics would be most suggestive of spinocerebellar ataxia type 27B, in a patient presenting with 5 years of worsening cerebellar ataxia?
    A. Prominent downbeat nystagmus
    B. Lack of improvement with dalfampridine
    C. Ataxia combined with parkinsonism
    D. Ataxia combined with prominent cognitive impairment
    E. Wheelchair dependence developing five years after symptom onset

Correct answer: A

Explanation

A. SCA27B is an autosomal dominant inherited form of cerebellar ataxia. A large portion of patients show downbeat nystagmus.
B. SCA27B imbalance improves with dalfampridine in a large portion of patients.
C. Parkinsonism is not expected in SCA27B. Parkinsonism can be found in some forms of SCA including most commonly SCA2 and SCA3, as well as in later stages of multiple systems atrophy cerebellar type (MSA-C)
D. Prominent cognitive impairment is not expected in SCA27B. Prominent cognitive changes can be seen in other forms of SCA, most notably SCA17 and SCA48.
E. Only a minority of SCA27B require the use of a wheelchair, even after more than 10 years of symptom onset.

References

Jummani R, Okun M. Sydenham chorea. Arch Neurol. 2001;58(2):311–3. https://doi.org/10.1001/archneur.58.2.311.

Wilke C, Pellerin D, Mengel D, Traschütz A, Danzi MC, Dicaire MJ, et al. GAA-FGF14 ataxia (SCA27B): phenotypic profile, natural history progression and 4-aminopyridine treatment response. Brain. 2023;146(10):4144–57. https://doi.org/10.1093/brain/awad157.

Tics

52. Which of the following is true regarding Tourette's syndrome?
    A. Neuropsychological problems are unusual in Tourette's syndrome and should make the physician think of an alternative diagnosis
    B. A family history is unusual in Tourette's syndrome
    C. Variations in the repertoire of tics over years are unusual in Tourette's syndrome and should make the physician consider an alternative diagnosis
    D. Both motor and vocal tics should be present for a diagnosis of Tourette's syndrome according to current diagnostic criteria
    E. Deep brain stimulation is not used for the treatment of Tourette's syndrome

Correct answer: D

Explanation

A. Neuropsychological problems are commonly comorbid in Tourette's, including ADHD, OCD, and anxiety disorders.
B. Family history is common in Tourette's syndrome; there is a 15-fold increased risk of developing Tourette syndrome or chronic motor or vocal tic disorder in siblings of individuals with Tourette syndrome, and a positive family history for tics is seen in about one-half of patients.
C. Variations in tic repertoire over time are common in Tourette's syndrome; for example, patients may report a prior tendency to imitate animal sounds, but tell the examiner that this has not happened for the last five years.
D. This is correct, both motor and vocal tics should be present for a diagnosis of Tourette's syndrome according to current diagnostic criteria.
E. Deep brain stimulation is sometimes used for the treatment of Tourette's syndrome.

References

Robertson MM, Eapen V, Singer HS, Martino D, Scharf JM, Paschou P, et al. Gilles de la Tourette syndrome. Nat Rev Dis Primers. 2017;3:16097. https://doi.org/10.1038/nrdp.2016.97.

Singer HS. Tics and Tourette Syndrome. Continuum (Minneap Minn). 2019;25(4):936–58. https://doi.org/10.1212/con.0000000000000752.

53. Which of the following is not used for the pharmacological treatment of tics?
    A. Clonazepam
    B. Risperidone
    C. Lithium
    D. Topiramate
    E. Clonidine

Correct answer: C

Explanation

Medications commonly used to treat tics include clonazepam, clonidine and guanfacine (alpha-adrenergic agonists), and antipsychotics such as risperidone and pimozide. Other classes that are sometimes used include anticonvulsants such as topiramate and vesicular monoamine transporter-2 inhibitors such as tetrabenazine and deutetrabenazine. Lithium is not used for the treatment of tics.

References

Robertson MM, Eapen V, Singer HS, Martino D, Scharf JM, Paschou P, et al. Gilles de la Tourette syndrome. Nat Rev Dis Primers. 2017;3:16097. https://doi.org/10.1038/nrdp.2016.97.

Singer HS. Tics and Tourette Syndrome. Continuum (Minneap Minn). 2019;25(4):936–58. https://doi.org/10.1212/con.0000000000000752.

54. Which of the medications from the prior question are associated with a risk of developing tardive dyskinesia?
    A. Clonazepam
    B. Risperidone
    C. Lithium
    D. Topiramate
    E. Clonidine
    Correct answer: B

Explanation

Dopamine-receptor blocking agents, such as risperidone, are associated with a risk of developing tardive dyskinesia. The other medications listed are not dopamine-receptor blocking agents. There are many features that can be helpful to differentiate tardive dyskinesia from tics: tics often start in early life; many patients have a family history of tics or anxiety or OCD-like features and include a premonitory urge. Tardive dyskinesia happens only in the context of exposure to agents known to cause tardive dyskinesia and often includes stereotyped oral-lingual movements (see tardive dyskinesia section for more details on this).

Reference

Singer HS. Tics and Tourette Syndrome. Continuum (Minneap Minn). 2019;25(4):936–58. https://doi.org/10.1212/con.0000000000000752.

55. Which of the medications from the prior question would be considered second-line rather than first-line for the treatment of tics?
    A. Clonazepam
    B. Risperidone
    C. Guanfacine
    D. Topiramate
    E. Clonidine
    Correct answer: B

Explanation

Dopamine-receptor blocking agents are considered second-line options of treatment due to their risk of tardive dyskine-sia. The other options would be commonly considered first-line of treatment before considering the use of dopamine-receptor blocking agents.

Reference

Singer HS. Tics and Tourette Syndrome. Continuum (Minneap Minn). 2019;25(4):936–58. https://doi.org/10.1212/con.0000000000000752.

56. Which of the following is most UNCOMMON in the phenomenology of tics?
    A. Premonitory feelings or sensations that happen before the execution of the tic
    B. Increase in discomfort immediately following the execution of the tic
    C. Worsening in periods of increased anxiety
    D. Worsening in periods of increased fatigue
    E. Ability to partially suppress tics
    Correct answer: B

Explanation

A. Premonitory feelings or sensations that happen before the execution of the tic are common. They may include an abnormal sensation (sometimes described as an itch, or pressure sensation) in a specific part of the body, or a more complex urge to perform a specific action.
B. Execution of a tic most commonly leads to a resolution or improvement of the premonitory feeling or sensation, rather than a worsening of it.
C. Patients with tics often report increased tic severity in periods of increased anxiety.
D. Patients with tics often reported increased tic severity in periods of increased fatigue.
E. Patients with tics often have at least partial control over their tics and are often able to reduce or suppress them for brief periods of time.

Reference

Singer HS. Tics and Tourette Syndrome. Continuum (Minneap Minn). 2019;25(4):936–58. https://doi.org/10.1212/con.0000000000000752.

57. Which of the following would be considered a complex rather than simple motor tic?
    A. Shoulder shrugging
    B. Head jerking
    C. Eye blinking
    D. Touching objects
    E. Facial grimacing
    Correct answer: D

Explanation

Complex motor tics involve multiple steps or a cluster of simple actions. Of the options listed, all are simple actions except for touching objects.

Reference

Singer HS. Tics and Tourette Syndrome. Continuum (Minneap Minn). 2019;25(4):936–58. https://doi.org/10.1212/con.0000000000000752.

58. Which of the following is true regarding clonidine for the treatment of tic disorders?
    A. It is in the same pharmacological class as baclofen.
    B. It is in the same pharmacological class as pimozide.
    C. It is in the same pharmacological class as risperidone.
    D. It is associated with a risk of developing tardive dyskinesia.
    E. It is used for the treatment of tics in addition to impulsivity associated with attention-deficit/hyperactivity disorder (ADHD).
    Correct answer: E

Explanation

A. Baclofen is a GABA-B receptor agonist, while clonidine is an alpha-adrenergic agonist.
B. Pimozide is a dopamine receptor antagonist, while clonidine is an alpha-adrenergic agonist.
C. Risperidone is a dopamine receptor antagonist, while clonidine is an alpha-adrenergic agonist.
D. Clonidine is not a dopamine-receptor blocking agent, and it is therefore not associated with the risk of developing tardive dyskinesia.
E. Clonidine may be helpful for the treatment of impulsivity associated with ADHD, which is often comorbid in patients with tic disorders. The same is true for guanfacine.

Reference

Singer HS. Tics and Tourette Syndrome. Continuum (Minneap Minn). 2019;25(4):936–58. https://doi.org/10.1212/con.0000000000000752.

Tardive Syndromes

59. Which of the following presentations is NOT compatible with tardive dyskinesia?
    A. Repetitive oral and lingual movements
    B. Stereotyped movements of the arms and legs
    C. Oral pain
    D. An internal sensation of intense restlessness
    E. Rigidity and rest tremor
    Correct answer: E

Explanation

A. Buccal and lingual movements are very commonly present in patients with tardive dyskinesia.
B. Stereotyped movements of the arms or legs may be present in patients with tardive dyskinesia, such as repetitively adjusting their position in the chair while sitting following a fixed repetitive motor sequence.
C. Tardive pain, most commonly buccal, is sometimes observed in patients with tardive dyskinesia.
D. Akathisia, defined as an internal sensation of restlessness that improves when moving, is commonly observed in patients with tardive dyskinesia.
E. Rigidity and rest tremor are suggestive of parkinsonism, which is not a tardive syndrome. Of note, dopamine receptor antagonists may cause parkinsonism including rigidity and rest tremor, but drug-induced parkinsonism, by definition, resolves after discontinuing the offending drug, while tardive syndromes tend to persist and sometimes worsen after discontinuing the offending drug.

Reference

Friedman JH. Tardive Syndromes. Continuum (Minneap Minn). 2019;25(4):1081–98. https://doi.org/10.1212/con.0000000000000754.

60. Which of the following medications is NOT associated with a risk of developing tardive dyskinesia?
    A. Haloperidol
    B. Pimozide
    C. Aripiprazole
    D. Metoclopramide
    E. Clozapine
    Correct answer: E

Explanation

Dopamine receptor antagonists (such as haloperidol, pimozide, metoclopramide) or dopamine receptor partial agonists (such as aripiprazole) are all associated with a risk of developing tardive dyskinesia. However, clozapine has shown no convincing risk of tardive dyskinesia, theoretically due to its relatively less D2 and relatively more D1 blockade. For this reason, clozapine is used when patients with tardive dyskinesia continue to require the use of an antipsychotic (such as in patients with schizophrenia who continue to require the use of an antipsychotic) because clozapine will not result in a risk of long-term worsening of their tardive dyskinesia. Clozapine can also be used to treat tardive dyskinesia, most commonly in patients that have not responded to more conventional pharmacological strategies to treat tardive dyskinesia.

Reference

Friedman JH. Tardive Syndromes. Continuum (Minneap Minn). 2019;25(4):1081–98. https://doi.org/10.1212/con.0000000000000754.

61. A 64-year-old woman presents to a neurology clinic with a chief complaint of involuntary tongue movements, manifesting 1 year ago. Examination reveals stereotyped lip and tongue movements and a tendency to invert and evert her ankle joints while sitting. She does not have a diagnosis of psychiatric illness, and she is not aware of any medications taken for this reason. Her primary care physician prescribes medication for blood pressure, and she also follows with a gastroenterologist and has taken medication to treat nausea of unclear etiology in the past. Which of the following is true regarding the likelihood that her presentation is a manifestation of tardive dyskinesia?
    A. Her gender does not influence the likelihood of tardive dyskinesia
    B. Her history of prescriptions for blood pressure control supports the possibility of tardive dyskinesia
    C. Her history of prescriptions for nausea control supports the possibility of tardive dyskinesia
    D. The fact that her feet are involved argues against the possibility of tardive dyskinesia
    E. Her age of presentation argues against the possibility of tardive dyskinesia

Correct answer: C

Explanation
A. Female gender is associated with a higher risk of tardive dyskinesia.
B. Blood pressure medication agents are not associated with a risk of tardive dyskinesia.
C. Metoclopramide and prochlorperazine are sometimes prescribed as medications to treat nausea and are associated with a risk of tardive dyskinesia given their dopamine receptor antagonist properties.
D. Foot involvement does not argue against the possibility of tardive dyskinesia. The phenomenology of tardive dyskinesia can include virtually any part of the body.
E. Her age of presentation does not argue against the possibility of tardive dyskinesia. In fact, older age is a risk factor for the development of tardive dyskinesia

Reference

Friedman JH. Tardive Syndromes. Continuum (Minneap Minn). 2019;25(4):1081–98. https://doi.org/10.1212/con.0000000000000754.

Linked questions: 62–63

62. A 32-year-old woman with a diagnosis of schizophrenia, with a longstanding history of haloperidol use, presents with retrocollic dystonic movements. Her neurologist diagnosed her with tardive dyskinesia. Which of the following is true?
    A. The dose of the causative medication is independent of the risk of developing tardive dyskinesia
    B. The duration of exposure to the causative medication is independent of the risk of developing tardive dyskinesia
    C. Deep brain stimulation treatment of her case would most likely target the GPi (globus pallidus, internal segment)
    D. Anticholinergics are not indicated for the treatment of this case
    E. Botox is not indicated for the treatment of this case

Correct answer: C

Explanation
A. Higher doses of antipsychotics are associated with a higher risk of tardive dyskinesia.
B. Higher duration of treatment with antipsychotics is associated with a higher risk of tardive dyskinesia.
C. Deep brain stimulation can be considered for the treatment of tardive dyskinesia in patients that do not respond to other forms of treatment; in the case of dystonia, the most common target for deep brain stimulation is the Gpi.
D. Anticholinergics such as trihexyphenidyl can be useful for the treatment of the dystonic elements of tardive dyskinesia.
E. OnabotulinumtoxinA can be used for the treatment of the dystonic elements of tardive dyskinesia.

Reference

Friedman JH. Tardive Syndromes. Continuum (Minneap Minn). 2019;25(4):1081–98. https://doi.org/10.1212/con.0000000000000754.

Linked question

63. The patient from the prior case is treated with tetrabenazine. Which of the following is FALSE about tetrabenazine?
    A. Tetrabenazine can cause parkinsonism
    B. Tetrabenazine can cause akathisia
    C. Tetrabenazine can cause dystonia
    D. Tetrabenazine can decrease the likelihood of recovery from tardive dyskinesia
    E. Tetrabenazine can cause somnolence

Correct answer: D

Explanation

Tetrabenazine is a VMAT2 inhibitor that decreases the release of dopamine, and because of this it can cause parkinsonism (A), akathisia (B), and dystonic crises such as oculogyric crises (C). This risk is shared with other VMAT2 inhibitors (valbenazine, deutetrabenazine) and with many antipsychotics that act as dopamine receptor antagonists. Tetrabenazine can also cause somnolence, and the risk of this is likely lower with the newer VMAT2 inhibitor formulations (valbenazine and deutetrabenazine). Tetrabenazine and the other VMAT2 inhibitor formulations (valbenazine and deutetrabenazine) do not decrease the likelihood of recovery from tardive dyskinesia. Dopamine receptor antagonists such as haloperidol or risperidone would decrease the likelihood of recovery from tardive dyskinesia.

References

Friedman JH. Tardive Syndromes. Continuum (Minneap Minn). 2019;25(4):1081–98. https://doi.org/10.1212/con.0000000000000754.

Makhoul K, Jankovic J. Real-world experience with VMAT2 inhibitors in Tourette syndrome. J Neurol. 2023;270(9):4518–22. https://doi.org/10.1007/s00415-023-11769-0.

64. Which of the following situations best matches the description of "masked tardive dyskinesia"?
    A. Tardive dyskinesia treated with tetrabenazine
    B. Acute dystonia in patients on antipsychotics
    C. Dyskinesia that emerges when antipsychotic dose is reduced
    D. Parkinsonism masking symptoms of tardive dyskinesia
    E. Choreiform movements due to trihexyphenidyl
    Correct answer: C

Explanation

A. Tetrabenazine, as well as the newer formulations of VMAT2 inhibitors (valbenazine and deutetrabenazine), can treat tardive dyskinesia, but this does not correspond to the concept of "masked tardive dyskinesia."

B. Antipsychotics can cause acute dystonia, but this does not correspond to the concept of "masked tardive dyskinesia."

C. This is correct. Antipsychotics can cause tardive dyskinesia, but also paradoxically treat tardive dyskinesia.

When the offending medication is reduced or discontinued, the symptoms may "unmask" and become more apparent.

D. Drug-induced parkinsonism can coexist with tardive dyskinesia, but this does not correspond to the concept of "masked tardive dyskinesia."

E. Trihexyphenidyl can induce choreiform movements. These movements disappear when trihexyphenidyl is discontinued, and for this reason this would be considered a drug-induced movement disorder and not tardive dyskinesia. This does also not correspond to the concept of "masked tardive dyskinesia."

Reference

Friedman JH. Tardive Syndromes. Continuum (Minneap Minn). 2019;25(4):1081–98. https://doi.org/10.1212/con.0000000000000754.

65. Which of the following clinical features best describes tardive akathisia?
    A. Involuntary lip movements without inner distress
    B. Rocking movements with a subjective feeling of restlessness
    C. Repetitive hand clapping without discomfort
    D. Sudden myoclonic jerks
    E. Sustained upward eye deviation
    Correct answer: B

Explanation

A. These movements are common in tardive dyskinesia, but do not correspond to akathisia.

B. This is correct. Patients with tardive akathisia often show pelvic rocking movements, and the condition includes a subjective inner feeling of restlessness and an urge to move.

C. These movements, without associated inner feeling of restlessness or urge to move, are not compatible with tardive akathisia.

D. This is not compatible with tardive akathisia.

E. Sustained upward gaze is more consistent with oculogyric crisis, a form of acute dystonia that is most commonly induced by dopamine-receptor antagonists.

Reference

Friedman JH. Tardive Syndromes. Continuum (Minneap Minn). 2019;25(4):1081–98. https://doi.org/10.1212/con.0000000000000754.

Parkinsonism

Linked questions: 66–68

66. A 63-year-old right-handed female presents to the office to the neurology clinic with complaints of a 2-year history of difficulty with fine motor tasks such as typing and stiffness. She also notices that she is taking longer to get dressed in the morning and her voice is softer. She has had no falls, but she feels less agile when playing tennis. Her symptoms have been slowly progressing over time, and she denies stepwise decline. She is working full time without difficulty and is independent in her activities of daily living. She has a history of depression, well-controlled on monotherapy with escitalopram 10 mg daily. On examination there is mild facial masking with decreased blink rate and mild increased rigidity on her right arm and leg, and on finger tapping there is slight asymmetric slowness on her right hand with amplitude of movements decreasing with repeated tapping. She walks with an erect posture, narrow base, appropriate stride, and reduced arm swing on the right. She has no tremor, no cranial nerve deficits, and no motor weakness or sensory loss. What clinical features, if present, should raise a concern for atypical parkinsonism?
    A. Lack of rest tremor 5 years into diagnosis
    B. Cerebellar dysmetria on finger to nose testing
    C. Exposure to neuroleptic agents 6 years ago for severe depression with psychotic features
    D. Subcortical white matter disease on magnetic resonance imaging

    Correct Answer: B

Explanation

The Movement Disorder Society (MDS) Clinical Diagnostic Criteria for Parkinson's Disease (PD) establishes both the clinical features in Parkinson's disease and delineates red flags and absolute exclusion criteria that may suggest an atypical form of parkinsonism or alternative diagnosis. The MDS establishes criteria for both clinically established PD and clinically probable PD. To be diagnosed with PD, a patient must have clinical syndrome of parkinsonism, which requires bradykinesia to be present alongside either tremor, rigidity, or both. Additionally, to meet the criteria for a clinically established criteria for PD, patients must have at least two supportive criteria, which include a clinical response to levodopa therapy, the presence of levodopa-induced dyskinesia, rest tremor, or the presence of olfactory loss. Patients with red flag criteria may still meet the criteria for clinically probable PD depending on the presence of supportive criteria.

This patient meets clinical criteria for clinically probably PD on the basis of her parkinsonism and lack of exclusion criteria. The presence of red flag symptoms may raise the concern for an alternative diagnosis. Answer choice B, cerebellar dysmetria on finger to nose testing, would be concerning for multiple-system atrophy, an alpha-synucleinopathy which can present with parkinsonism and cerebellar findings.

Incorrect Answers

A. Rest tremor is not necessary for a diagnosis of PD, and patients can have parkinsonism with both rigidity and bradykinesia without tremor.
C. Treatment with a dopamine receptor blocker or dopamine-depleting agent in a dose and time-course consistent with drug-induced parkinsonism is an exclusion criterion for PD. However, exposure 6 years ago, with symptom onset 2 years ago, makes this diagnosis unlikely.
D. Subcortical white matter changes in magnetic resonance imaging are not a red flag or exclusion criteria for PD. Although it can be seen in cases of vascular parkinsonism, it is a nonspecific finding. Parkinsonism restricted to the lower extremities for 3 years, in conjunction with white matter changes on MRI, would be consistent with vascular parkinsonism.

Reference

Postuma RB, Berg D, Stern M, Poewe W, Olanow CW, Oertel W, et al. MDS clinical diagnostic criteria for Parkinson's disease. Mov Disord. 2015;30(12):1591–601. https://doi.org/10.1002/mds.26424.

Linked question

67. Continuing from Question 66, you discuss the diagnosis of clinically probable PD with this patient, and the shared decision is made to monitor clinically without pharmacotherapy. You prescribe physical therapy and occupational therapy and encourage aerobic exercise, which has been shown to slow disease progression.

    Six months later, the patient returns to the clinic, having completed therapy and having started an exercise routine. However, her symptoms have progressed, and she is now having trouble meeting deadlines at work and doing chores at home. On examination, she has moderate rigidity and bradykinesia on her right side and now has mild findings of parkinsonism on the left side of her body. Her gait exam shows slight forward flexion at the waist, a narrow base, and some shuffling in stride with reduced arm swing on the left and mild rest tremor.

    She is interested in starting pharmacologic therapy. Which of the following agents is not indicated as monotherapy in Parkinson's disease?
    A. Entacapone
    B. Carbidopa/Levodopa
    C. Rasagiline

D. Amantadine
E. Ropinirole
Correct Answer: A

Explanation

The decision of which agent to start as monotherapy in Parkinson's disease (PD) should be a shared decision made with the patient, taking into account severity of symptoms, risk of side effects, and medication adherence. Carbidopa/levodopa is considered the gold standard therapy, as it replaces dopamine, which is the primary neurotransmitter deficiency in PD. Levodopa has significant benefit in motor symptoms with a favorable side effect profile, with the most common side effects being gastrointestinal upset and orthostatic blood pressure fluctuations. However, patients may be concerned about developing levodopa-induced dyskinesias, although the evidence suggests that levodopa-induced dyskinesias are associated most with disease duration rather than early initiation of the drug.

Entacapone, which is a catechol-O-methyltransferase inhibitor, is approved as an adjective agent to levodopa therapy by reducing the breakdown of dopamine to 3-O-methyldopa. It is not approved for monotherapy.

Incorrect Answers

B. Carbidopa/levodopa is the gold standard oral medication for PD.
C. Rasagiline is a monoamine oxidase (MAO) B inhibitor which is approved as monotherapy for Parkinson's disease. It has a modest effect and is best reserved as monotherapy for patients with mild symptoms and who desire once a day dosing. Similarly to entacapone, it is also used as an adjunct to levodopa therapy by reducing the breakdown of monoamines including dopamine, serotonin, and norepinephrine.
D. Amantadine is an NMDA receptor antagonist that can be used as monotherapy for PD, although it is more commonly used for its effect on reducing levodopa-induced dyskinesias in PD.

Reference

Tanner CM, Ostrem JL. Parkinson's Disease. N Engl J Med. 2024;391(5):442–52. https://doi.org/10.1056/NEJMra2401857.

Linked question

68. Three years later, you continue to manage the patient's Parkinson's disease, which has had a clinical course complicated by motor fluctuations, dyskinesias, and non-motor symptoms of fatigue and constipation. She is now on a medical regimen that contains carbidopa/levodopa, amantadine, and entacapone, and she is receiving regular physical therapy. However, she remains impaired by her condition and is interested in advanced therapies for Parkinson's disease. You discuss deep brain stimulation, and she is interested in having a formal evaluation for these symptoms. She has a detailed physical examination both on and off medication, a formal neuropsychological evaluation, and a magnetic resonance imaging study. The presence of which of these symptoms would be a contraindication for deep brain stimulation for this patient?
A. The lack of a clinical response to levodopa
B. The presence of subjective cognitive impairment on neuropsychological evaluation
C. Lower limb dystonia impacting gait
D. Severe motor fluctuations with freezing of gait when off medication
Correct answer: A

Explanation

Deep brain stimulation (DBS) is a neuromodulation therapy for Parkinson's disease (PD) that alters basal ganglia circuitry to improve the motor symptoms of Parkinson's disease. Following initial approval for Advanced PD in 2002, in 2016 the approval was expanded to earlier forms of PD (4-year duration) with early motor complications based on the EARLYSTIM clinical trial, which showed improvement in motor symptoms and quality of life with DBS. In practice, patients with severe motor fluctuations and/or dyskinesias, or medication refractory tremor, are candidates for deep brain stimulation. The two most common anatomical targets for DBS for PD are the subthalamic nucleus and the globus pallidus interna.

The lack of a clinical response to levodopa therapy is a contraindication to deep brain stimulation. In clinical evaluation for deep brain stimulation, a levodopa-challenge is often performed, where patients are evaluated off medications and then reevaluated after administration of their oral medications to assess for clinical response. Lack of clinical response is considered a contraindication for deep brain stimulation and may raise concern for an alternative diagnosis such as multiple-system atrophy.

Incorrect Answers

B. The presence of dementia is a contraindication for deep brain stimulation, which has been implicated in worsening neurocognitive dysfunction. Due to this concern, formal neuropsychological evaluation is often done as part of the preoperative workup to screen for a neurocognitive dysfunction. Subjective cognitive impairment on a formal neuropsychological evaluation is not a contraindication to DBS, although possible worsening of these symptoms should be discussed with the patient.

C. Patients with PD may develop dystonia, which is not a contraindication for deep brain stimulation. In fact, deep brain stimulation of the globus pallidus is used in generalized dystonia, and the presence of dystonia in patient with PD may be a factor in considering globus pallidus stimulation as opposed to subthalamic nucleus stimulation.

D. Severe motor fluctuations are one of the indications for DBS in PD. Freezing of gait when the patient is off medication is not a contraindication, particularly if the symptom improves after taking medication. If the patient continues to have freezing of gait when on medication, they should be counseled that DBS has less consistent impact on gait and that they may remain impaired by this symptom postoperatively.

References

Katz M, Kilbane C, Rosengard J, Alterman RL, Tagliati M. Referring patients for deep brain stimulation: an improving practice. Arch Neurol. 2011;68(8):1027–32. https://doi.org/10.1001/archneurol.2011.151.

Schuepbach WM, Rau J, Knudsen K, Volkmann J, Krack P, Timmermann L, et al. Neurostimulation for Parkinson's disease with early motor complications. N Engl J Med. 2013;368(7):610–22. https://doi.org/10.1056/NEJMoa1205158.

69. A 52-year-old male with a history of hypertension and remote history of alcohol use disorder in remission presents to your clinic for follow-up of his idiopathic Parkinson's disease accompanied by his spouse. During the last clinic assessment, he had left greater than right rigidity and bradykinesia and was experiencing gait festination, for which a new medication was added. Today the patient reports that his motor symptoms have had moderate improvement, which you confirm on examination. However, the spouse is concerned that he has recently been spending his retirement savings on lottery tickets, which is causing both financial and marital issues. The patient endorses that he has an irresistible urge to gamble, which he had before, and admits to buying lottery tickets in secret despite feelings of guilt and attempts to stop. Which of the following medications is most likely to have led to these symptoms and should be reduced?
    A. Amantadine
    B. Carbidopa/levodopa
    C. Pramipexole
    D. Rasagiline

    Correct answer: C

Explanation

This patient is experiencing symptoms concerning for impulse control disorder (ICD), which is an inability to resist impulses that may be harmful to oneself or others, including pathological gambling, compulsive shopping, binge eating, and related behaviors. Patients with Parkinson's disease on dopaminergic therapy are at increased risk for developing ICDs, and it has been well-demonstrated in the medical literature that risk is highest with dopamine agonists, including pramipexole. The pathophysiology is thought to involve the mesolimbic system and, in particular, the dopamine transmission from the ventral tegmental area to the nucleus accumbens. Risk factors for developing ICDs include younger age at Parkinson's disease onset, male gender, a history of substance abuse or psychiatric disorders, and certain personality traits such as impulsivity.

Dopamine agonists with high affinity for D3 receptors, in particular, pramipexole and ropinirole, are thought to pose a higher risk of developing ICDs, although it has also been described with levodopa therapy. Patients with Parkinson's disease started on dopamine agonists should be counseled on the risk for developing ICDs before initiation of therapy, and the offending agent should have a dose reduction or discontinuation. Dopamine agonists at higher dosages often require a gradual weaning to avoid withdrawal side effects.

Incorrect Answers

A. Amantadine—Amantadine can be associated with increased risk for sedation, insomnia, and neuropsychiatric side effects including confusion, agitation, and psychosis. However, it is not commonly associated with impulse control disorder.

B. Carbidopa/levodopa—Although there are reports in the medical literature of levodopa-induced impulse control disorder, dopamine agonists (and pramipexole in particular) are a much more common offenders and should be addressed first.

D. Rasagiline—Rasagiline is a monoamine oxidase (MAO) B inhibitor which is approved as monotherapy for Parkinson's disease and also used as adjunctive therapy with carbidopa/levodopa to reduce the breakdown of dopamine in the CNS. Common side effects include headache and dyspepsia, and there is a risk of serotonin syndrome in patients taking supratherapeutic doses of serotonergic agents, although the risk is lower than nonselective MAO inhibitors (e.g., phenelzine) due to selectivity of both rasagiline and selegiline for MAO-B receptor.

References

Moore TJ, Glenmullen J, Mattison DR. Reports of pathological gambling, hypersexuality, and compulsive shopping associated with dopamine receptor agonist drugs. JAMA Intern Med. 2014;174(12):1930–3. https://doi.org/10.1001/jamainternmed.2014.5262.

Probst CC, van Eimeren T. The functional anatomy of impulse control disorders. Curr Neurol Neurosci Rep. 2013;13(10):386. https://doi.org/10.1007/s11910-013-0386-8.

Speiser Z, Fine T, Litinetsky L, Eliash S, Blaugrund E, Cohen S. Differential behavioral syndrome evoked in the rats after multiple doses of SSRI fluoxetine with selective MAO inhibitors rasagiline or selegiline. J Neural Transm (Vienna). 2008;115(1):107–16. https://doi.org/10.1007/s00702-007-0811-8.

70. A 67-year-old man followed in a neurologic clinic for a progressive neurodegenerative condition dies from pneumonia. On autopsy, histologic examination revealed intracellular aggregates of misfolded α-synuclein. This finding is most consistent with which of the following conditions?
    A. Multiple system atrophy
    B. Alzheimer's disease
    C. Idiopathic Parkinson's disease
    D. Corticobasal degeneration
    E. Progressive supranuclear palsy
    Correct answer: C

Explanation

The two abnormal protein aggregates most relevant for movement disorders are alpha-synuclein and tau protein.

α-Synucleinopathies include Parkinson's disease, multiple system atrophy, pure autonomic failure, and dementia with Lewy bodies, all characterized by intracellular aggregates of misfolded α-synuclein. They share certain clinical characteristics that help differentiate them among similar conditions, including autonomic failure and REM sleep behavior disorders. Tauopathies encompass Alzheimer's disease, progressive supranuclear palsy, and corticobasal degeneration; all these conditions are associated with significant cognitive or cortical deficits.

Lewy bodies are spherical eosinophilic intracellular aggregations with a clear surrounding (described as a halo), composed mostly of insoluble fibrils of alpha-synuclein. These findings are most commonly associated with idiopathic Parkinson's disease and dementia with Lewy bodies. The Braak hypothesis proposes that Parkinson's disease (PD) and dementia with Lewy bodies (DLB) share a common neuropathological substrate—α-synuclein aggregates—but differ in the pattern and timing of pathological spread. In PD, pathology begins in the lower brainstem and olfactory regions, ascending over time to affect cortical areas. In contrast, DLB shows earlier and more prominent cortical involvement, explaining its earlier cognitive symptoms despite similar underlying pathology.

Incorrect Answer

A. Multiple system atrophy (MSA) is also an alpha-synucleinopathy and shares clinical features with Parkinson's disease and dementia with Lewy bodies, including shared prodromal features of autonomic dysfunction and REM behavior disorder. However, the key neuropathological findings in MSA are glial cytoplasmic inclusions, which are more prominent in glial tissue as opposed to neurons. Morphologically, they appear as triangular, sickle, or conical forms, suggesting compositional and organizational differences. It is proposed that the different neuropathology of MSA as opposed to PD and DLB explains the difference in both clinical features and prognosis.

B. Alzheimer's disease has two hallmark neuropathological findings: neurofibrillary tangles and amyloid-beta (Aβ) plaques. Neurofibrillary tangles are intracellular aggregates of hyperphosphorylated tau protein. Amyloid plaques are extracellular deposits of misfolded Aβ peptides, derived from abnormal cleavage of the amyloid precursor protein.

C & D. Both corticobasal degeneration (CBD) and progressive supranuclear palsy (PSP) are tauopathies and are therefore not associated with Lewy bodies. They share clinical features of parkinsonism with no or limited response to levodopa replacement therapy. They also have distinct neuropathological findings, which may explain their distinguishing clinical features. In PSP, there is significant midbrain atrophy as well as *tufted astrocytes*; the midbrain involvement is thought to explain the supranuclear gaze deficit. CBD is characterized by prominent cortical deficits, such as ideomotor apraxia and higher-sensory deficits (e.g., stereognosis), which is reflected in the neuropathological findings of cortical atrophy and the presence of *astrocytic plaques*.

References

Braak H, Del Tredici K, Rüb U, de Vos RA, Jansen Steur EN, Braak E. Staging of brain pathology related to sporadic Parkinson's disease. Neurobiol Aging. 2003;24(2):197–211. https://doi.org/10.1016/s0197-4580(02)00065-9.

Graves NJ, Gambin Y, Sierecki E. α-Synuclein Strains and Their Relevance to Parkinson's Disease, Multiple System Atrophy, and Dementia with Lewy Bodies. Int J Mol Sci. 2023;24(15). https://doi.org/10.3390/ijms241512134.

Menšíková K, Matěj R, Colosimo C, Rosales R, Tučková L, Ehrmann J, et al. Lewy body disease or diseases with

Lewy bodies? NPJ Parkinsons Dis. 2022;8(1):3. https://doi.org/10.1038/s41531-021-00273-9.

Mimuro M, Yoshida M. Chameleons and mimics: Progressive supranuclear palsy and corticobasal degeneration. Neuropathology. 2020;40(1):57–67. https://doi.org/10.1111/neup.12590.

Trejo-Lopez JA, Yachnis AT, Prokop S. Neuropathology of Alzheimer's Disease. Neurotherapeutics. 2022;19(1):173–85. https://doi.org/10.1007/s13311-021-01146-y.

Wakabayashi K, Takahashi H. Cellular pathology in multiple system atrophy. Neuropathology. 2006;26(4):338–45. https://doi.org/10.1111/j.1440-1789.2006.00713.x.

For questions 71–76, choose the imaging finding most consistent with the clinical presentation.

A.

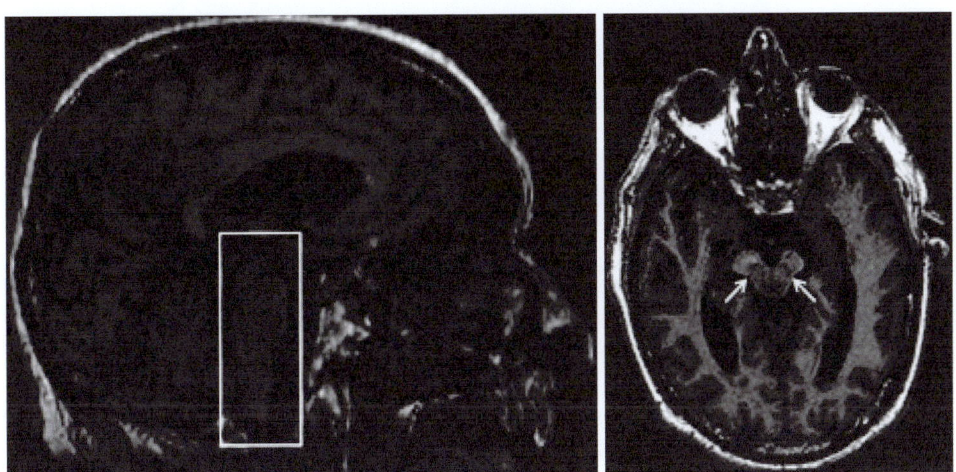

Sagittal and axial MRI brain. (Source: Saeed, U., Compagnone, J., Aviv, R., Strafella, A., Black, S., Lang, A., Masellis, M. CC-BY 4.0 (https://creativecommons.org/licenses/by/4.0/) via *Translational Neurodegeneration*. Image has not been modified from source Please see full attribution with citation below in references section for this question.)

B.

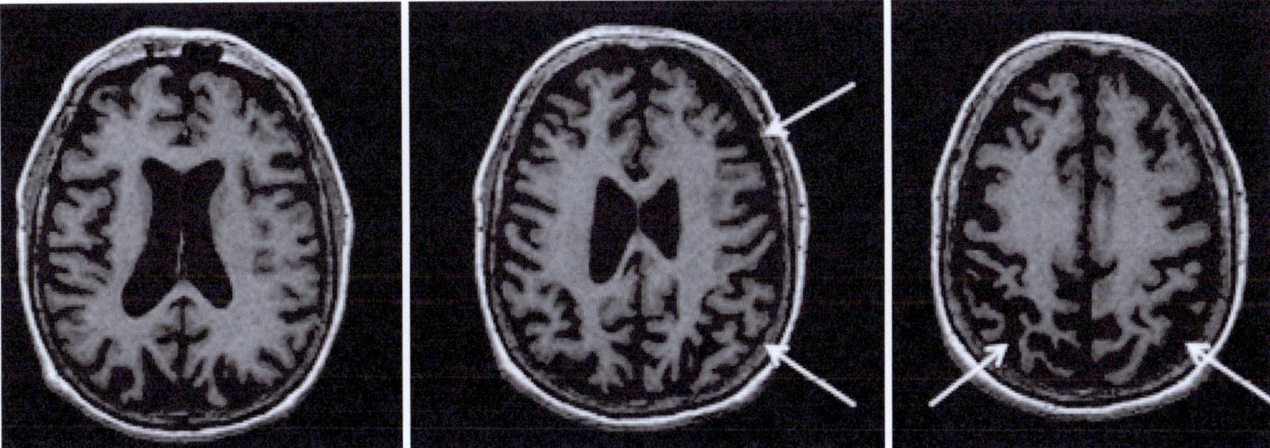

Axial MRI brain—three sections. (Source: Saeed, U., Compagnone, J., Aviv, R., Strafella, A., Black, S., Lang, A., Masellis, M. CC-BY 4.0 (https://creativecommons.org/licenses/by/4.0/) via Translational Neurodegeneration. Image has not been modified from source Please see full attribution with citation below in references section for this question.)

C.

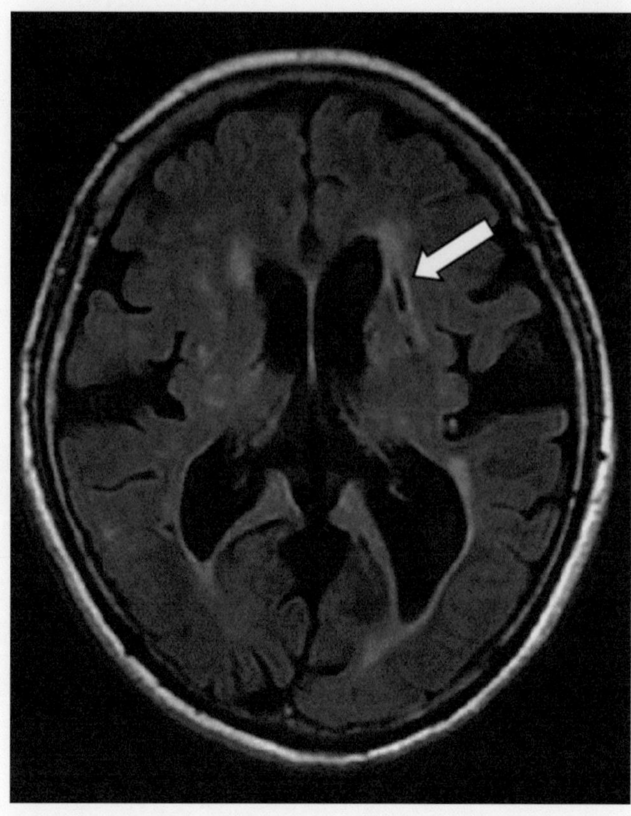

Axial MRI brain. (Source: Shan, Y., Lin, J., Xu, P., Zeng, M., Lin, H., Yan, H. CC-BY 4.0 (https://creativecommons.org/licenses/by/4.0/) via *BioMed Research International*. Image has not been modified from source Please see full attribution with citation below in references section for this question.)

D.

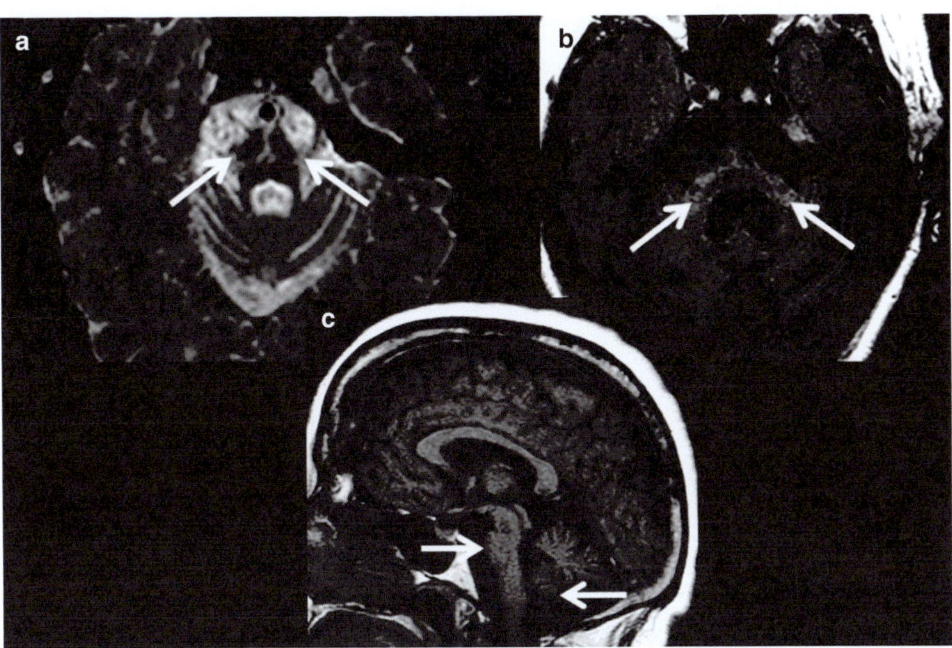

Axial MRI brain (**a** and **b**), sagittal MRI brain (**c**). (Source: Saeed, U., Compagnone, J., Aviv, R., Strafella, A., Black, S., Lang, A., Masellis, M. CC-BY 4.0 (https://creativecommons.org/licenses/by/4.0/) via Translational Neurodegeneration. Image has not been modified from source Please see full attribution with citation below in references section for this question.)

E.

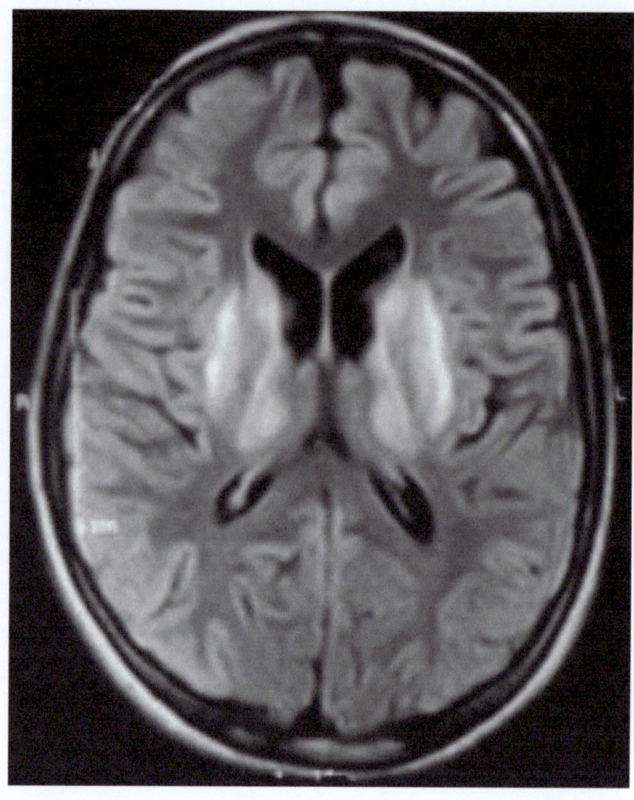

Axial MRI brain. (Source: Karimzadeh, P., Jafari, N., Biglari, H. N., Jabbehdari, S., Zadeh, S. K., Abadi, F. A., Lotfi, A. CC-BY 3.0 (https://creativecommons.org/licenses/by/3.0/) via *Iranian Journal of Child Neurology*. Image has not been modified from source Please see full attribution with citation below in references section for this question.)

F.

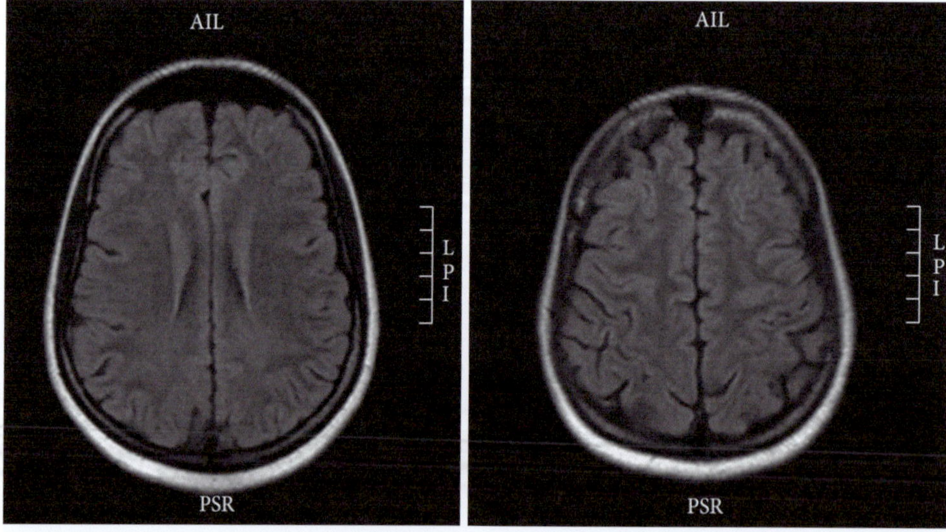

Axial MRI brain sections. (Source: Al-Hashel, J. Y., Ahmed, S. F., Alexnader, K. J., Ahmed, W. CC-BY 3.0 (https://creativecommons.org/licenses/by/3.0/) via *Case Reports in Neurological Medicine*. Image has not been modified from source Please see full attribution with citation below in references section for this question.)

71. An 84-year-old female with poorly controlled hypertension and prior tobacco use presents with a short-stepped gait and frequent falls. On examination, there is rigidity in the bilateral lower extremities with minimal involvement of the upper extremities, slowness in movements in lower extremities, and no tremor. Levodopa is started without response.

72. A 63-year-old male with obstructive sleep apnea presents for evaluation of personality changes and frequent falls. He began having falls within the past year, with one fall resulting in a hip fracture. He also has become increasingly emotionally labile, easily becoming tearful or agitated. On examination, there is prominent neck and truncal rigidity, dysarthria, impaired voluntary downgaze with preserved oculocephalic reflex, and positive snout sign and glabellar reflex.

73. A 52-year-old male with urinary retention presents with frequent falls. On examination, there are hypometric saccades on extraocular movements, cerebellar dysmetria, symmetric bradykinesia, and rigidity. There was a partial response to levodopa therapy, which was discontinued due to severe orthostatic hypotension.

74. A 59-year-old right-handed female complains of progressive impairment of dexterity of the left arm, accompanied by pain and stiffness. The symptoms began 12 months ago, and recently the affected arm began to extend on its own without her volition. Her right arm is minimally impacted. On examination, extraocular movements are intact, and there is significant impairment in fine motor movements of the left hand, with moderate rigidity but normal functioning of her right arm. She is unable to recognize objects placed in her left hand, but quickly identifies them in her right hand.

75. A 74-year-old female presents with a 3-year history of right arm rest tremor and difficulty with handwriting. On examination, there is a right-hand rest tremor, asymmetric appendicular rigidity, and bradykinesia on finger tapping on the right. Levodopa is started, and she has improvement in tremor, but now is experiencing dyskinesias.

76. A 19-year-old man presents with a 6-month history of progressive tremor, slurred speech, and difficulty walking. His parents report behavioral changes including irritability and declining academic performance. On examination, he has a wing-beating tremor, dysarthria, and mild rigidity. Ocular slit-lamp examination reveals golden-brown rings at the corneal margins. Liver enzymes are mildly elevated.

Correct answers: 71. C, 72. A, 73. D, 74. B, 75. F, 76. E

Explanations

71. C

The presence of vascular risk factors in a patient with lower limb parkinsonism, gait disturbance, and without improvement on levodopa replacement therapy is consistent with vascular parkinsonism. Characteristic imaging findings are subcortical white matter lesions in periventricular regions and/or basal ganglia.

72. A

Midbrain atrophy, also known as the hummingbird sign, is a characteristic finding of progressive supranuclear palsy (PSP). The examination findings of impaired vertical gaze with intact oculocephalic reflexes in a patient with parkinsonism, is consistent with PSP. Other features include early falls, cognitive symptoms, and dysarthria.

73. D

Cruciform hyperintensity on axial T2-weighted MRI of the pons, often described at the "hot cross bun sign," is consistent with multiple system atrophy. Other MRI findings include cerebellar atrophy and the "putaminal rim sign," which is a hyperintense rim along the lateral putamen on T2-weighted MRI. This patient has significant autonomic dysfunction (orthostatic hypotension and urinary retention), cerebellar dysfunction, and parkinsonism consistent with multiple system atrophy.

74. B

This patient has exam findings of alien-limb phenomena and stereognosis in one affected limb, corresponding to the contralateral parietal lobe. Corticobasal degeneration often presents with marked asymmetric findings, in contrast with other atypical parkinsonism syndromes such as multiple system atrophy and progressive supranuclear palsy. MRI imaging often demonstrates markedly asymmetric cortical atrophy, most prominently in the parietal lobes and dorsolateral prefrontal cortex.

75. F

This patient has clinically established Parkinson's disease, given the exam findings of parkinsonism without red flags and with appropriate response to levodopa replacement therapy and presence of levodopa-induced dyskinesias. MRI findings in patients with idiopathic Parkinson's disease are often normal, and MRI is not a necessary part of the diagnostic evaluation in a patient with no red flag clinical features.

76. E

A teenage or young adult patient with progressive tremor, dysarthria, and rigidity is concerned for a genetic movement disorder and warrants MRI imaging and targeted laboratory testing. Characteristic MRI findings include symmetric, bilateral hyperintensities of the basal ganglia. The patient in this question stem also has Kayser-Fleischer rings and hepatic dysfunction, consistent with Wilson's disease, a genetic syndrome caused by impaired copper metabolism due to an autosomal recessive mutation in the ATP7B gene.

References

Al-Hashel JY, Ahmed SF, Alexnader KJ, Ahmed W. Cerebral venous thrombosis in a patient with clinically isolated spinal cord syndrome. Case Rep Neurol Med. 2013;2013:364869. https://doi.org/10.1155/2013/364869.

Boxer AL, Yu JT, Golbe LI, Litvan I, Lang AE, Höglinger GU. Advances in progressive supranuclear palsy: new diagnostic criteria, biomarkers, and therapeutic approaches. Lancet Neurol. 2017;16(7):552–63. https://doi.org/10.1016/s1474-4422(17)30157-6.

Karimzadeh P, Jafari N, Nejad Biglari H, Jabbehdari S, Khayat Zadeh S, Ahmad Abadi F, et al. Neurometabolic Diagnosis in Children who referred as Neurodevelopmental Delay (A Practical Criteria, in Iranian Pediatric Patients). Iran J Child Neurol. 2016;10(3):73–81.

Ling H, O'Sullivan SS, Holton JL, Revesz T, Massey LA, Williams DR, et al. Does corticobasal degeneration exist? A clinicopathological re-evaluation. Brain. 2010;133(Pt 7):2045–57. https://doi.org/10.1093/brain/awq123.

Maiti B, Perlmutter JS. Imaging in Movement Disorders. Continuum (Minneap Minn). 2023;29(1):194–218. https://doi.org/10.1212/con.0000000000001210.

Parekh JR, Agrawal PR. Wilson's disease: 'face of giant panda' and 'trident' signs together. Oxf Med Case Reports. 2014;2014(1):16–7. https://doi.org/10.1093/omcr/omu005.

Saeed U, Compagnone J, Aviv RI, Strafella AP, Black SE, Lang AE, et al. Imaging biomarkers in Parkinson's disease and Parkinsonian syndromes: current and emerging concepts. Transl Neurodegener. 2017;6:8. https://doi.org/10.1186/s40035-017-0076-6.

Shan Y, Lin J, Xu P, Zeng M, Lin H, Yan H. Association of Aortic Compliance and Brachial Endothelial Function with Cerebral Small Vessel Disease in Type 2 Diabetes Mellitus Patients: Assessment with High-Resolution MRI. Biomed Res Int. 2016;2016:1609317. https://doi.org/10.1155/2016/1609317.

Tokumaru AM, Saito Y, Murayama S, Kazutomi K, Sakiyama Y, Toyoda M, et al. Imaging-pathologic correlation in corticobasal degeneration. AJNR Am J Neuroradiol. 2009;30(10):1884–92. https://doi.org/10.3174/ajnr.A1721.

77. A neurologist orders a DaTscan, a striatal dopamine visualization study using single photon emission computed tomography (SPECT), to assist in the evaluation of a patient. In what scenario is this imaging study most helpful?

- A. A patient with parkinsonism and features of both progressive supranuclear palsy and corticobasal degeneration
- B. For prognostication of development of motor symptoms in a patient with idiopathic Parkinson's disease
- C. Presurgical evaluation for a patient undergoing deep brain stimulation
- D. To differentiate between essential tremor and tremor due to parkinsonian syndromes

Correct answer: D

Explanation

The DaTscan is a SPECT imaging study that assesses the integrity of nigral dopaminergic neurons using the radiotracer [123I]-ioflupane ([123I]-fluoropropyl βCIT), which targets the dopamine transporter (DAT), a presynaptic membrane-bound protein essential for the reuptake of dopamine from the synaptic cleft into the presynaptic nerve terminal. It was approved by the FDA in 2011 to aid clinicians in differentiating between essential tremor and tremor due to parkinsonian syndromes. Of note, clinical diagnosis without imaging studies has a sensitivity of 90% with a positive predictive value of 98.6%. Therefore, DaTscans are not a routine part of the diagnostic work up in Parkinson's disease and are reserved for patients with early symptoms who wish to have more diagnostic clarity and are not amenable to or cannot tolerate a levodopa challenge (600 mg per day over 2 weeks).

In early Parkinson's disease, posterior putaminal loss is most characteristic and reflects loss of cell bodies in the substantia nigra.

- DaTscans are not able to reliably differentiate between atypical parkinsonism syndromes. FDG-PET scan imaging does show promise, although pathologic diagnosis remains the gold standard.
- DaTscans are not approved for and do not correlate with severity or prognosis of symptoms in patients with Parkinson's disease.
- DaTscans are not part of the presurgical evaluation for deep brain stimulation. Standard parts of the evaluation in Parkinson's disease include ON–OFF assessments to gauge levodopa responsiveness, a neuropsychological

evaluation, and magnetic resonance imaging for presurgical planning.

References

GE Healthcare. DaTscan (Ioflupane I-123 Injection) for Intravenous Use, CII. Package insert. Revised January 2011. Accessed April 8, 2025.

Katz M, Kilbane C, Rosengard J, Alterman RL, Tagliati M. Referring patients for deep brain stimulation: an improving practice. Arch Neurol. 2011;68(8):1027–32. https://doi.org/10.1001/archneurol.2011.151.

Maiti B, Perlmutter JS. Imaging in Movement Disorders. Continuum (Minneap Minn). 2023;29(1):194–218. https://doi.org/10.1212/con.0000000000001210.

Linked questions: 78–79

78. A 68-year-old male with a 7-year history of Parkinson's disease presents to the clinic with increasing cognitive difficulties, including memory loss, difficulty concentrating, and occasional confusion. He denies any episodes of visual hallucinations and confusion. These symptoms have gradually worsened over the past few months. He remains fully independent in performing ADLs and iADLs. His tremor and bradykinesia are stable, although he has postural instability and freezing of gait. He is currently on carbidopa-levodopa, trihexyphenidyl, and entacapone. Which of the following is the most appropriate next step in management?
    A. Start low-dose quetiapine at night to address cognitive symptoms
    B. Start donepezil to address cognitive complaints
    C. Discontinue trihexyphenidyl
    D. Reduce his dose of carbidopa/levodopa
    Correct answer: C

Explanation

Cognitive symptoms in patients with Parkinson's disease are common, with 10–20% of newly diagnosed PD patients having cognitive deficits and 30% of patients progressing to Parkinson's disease dementia (PDD). However, a careful assessment of other causes of cognitive symptoms, including co-pathology with Alzheimer's disease and other causes of dementia, pseudodementia from depression, sleep dysfunction, and medication effects, should be considered.

Anticholinergic agents such as trihexyphenidyl are common causes of cognitive deficits, and studies have shown that anticholinergic use is associated with increased risk of developing dementia in patients with Parkinson's disease. Additionally, this medication class has a modest effect on the motor symptoms of Parkinson's disease and should be weaned or discontinued.

Incorrect Answers

A. Quetiapine is an atypical antipsychotic with dopamine D2 and serotonin type 2A receptor antagonism. It is often used off-label for Parkinson's disease psychosis, partially because it does not significantly worsen parkinsonism. However, it would not be helpful in a patient with cognitive symptoms without psychosis.

B. Donepezil is not an FDA-approved medication for cognitive symptoms in Parkinson's disease. Additionally, other causes of cognitive complaints should be addressed prior to adding a medication for cognitive symptoms. Rivastigmine, another cholinesterase inhibitor, is FDA approved for use in Parkinson's disease on the basis of a positive randomized controlled trial which showed a modest benefit in Parkinson's disease-associated dementia.

D. Reduction of the dose of carbidopa/levodopa would be a reasonable option in a patient with cognitive symptoms. However, in this patient with gait instability and freezing of gait, reduction of trihexyphenidyl would be a more prudent first step, as reduction of levodopa may increase risk of falls.

References

Sheu JJ, Tsai MT, Erickson SR, Wu CH. Association between Anticholinergic Medication Use and Risk of Dementia among Patients with Parkinson's Disease. Pharmacotherapy. 2019;39(8):798–808. https://doi.org/10.1002/phar.2305.

Weintraub D, Irwin D. Diagnosis and Treatment of Cognitive and Neuropsychiatric Symptoms in Parkinson Disease and Dementia With Lewy Bodies. Continuum (Minneap Minn). 2022;28(5):1314–32. https://doi.org/10.1212/con.0000000000001151.

Linked question

79. You reduce the trihexyphenidyl dosage and his cognitive symptoms improve. You continue to manage his care, and in 2 years he presents with his spouse, who endorses that he has recently developed delusions of persecution, as well as formed visual hallucinations of people in his home. Last week he fell in an attempt to interact with these visions. What is the mechanism of action of the FDA-approved medication for Parkinson's disease psychosis?
    A. Cholinesterase inhibitor
    B. Dopamine D2 receptor antagonism and antagonist of serotonin 5-HT2A receptors
    C. Inverse agonist and antagonist at the serotonin 5-HT2A receptors
    D. NMDA receptor antagonist
    Correct answer: C

Explanation

Pimavanserin is the only FDA-approved medication for Parkinson's disease dementia and is an inverse agonist and antagonist at the serotonin 5-HT2A receptors. It does not have activity at the dopamine receptors, which makes it an appropriate choice in avoiding drug-induced worsening of parkinsonism. It shares many of the same side effects associated with dopamine-blocking neuroleptics, including prolongation of the QTC interval with risk for arrhythmia, and a black box warning for increased mortality in patients with dementia. It is not approved to manage psychosis due to other forms of dementia.

Incorrect Answers

A. Rivastigmine can be used for cognitive symptoms, but evidence is mixed for its use in psychosis, and a recent large trial did not show benefit in using rivastigmine for prophylaxis of psychosis. Also, it is not FDA approved for this indication.

B. Quetiapine is an atypical antipsychotic with dopamine D2 and serotonin type 2A receptor antagonism and is not an FDA-approved medication for the treatment of Parkinson's disease psychosis, although it is often used clinically. Additionally, quetiapine acts as an antagonist on adrenergic alpha-1 receptors and histamine H1 receptors, which can worsen non-motor PD symptoms of orthostasis and fatigue, respectively.

D. NMDA antagonism is a feature of multiple neurologic agents, including amantadine and memantine. These agents are not used in Parkinson's disease psychosis.

References

Hawkins T, Berman BD. Pimavanserin: A novel therapeutic option for Parkinson disease psychosis. Neurol Clin Pract. 2017;7(2):157–62. https://doi.org/10.1212/cpj.0000000000000342.

Weintraub D, Irwin D. Diagnosis and Treatment of Cognitive and Neuropsychiatric Symptoms in Parkinson Disease and Dementia With Lewy Bodies. Continuum (Minneap Minn). 2022;28(5):1314–32. https://doi.org/10.1212/con.0000000000001151.

80. A 58-year-old right-handed man presented with a 3-year history of progressive neurologic symptoms that began with impotence, urinary incontinence followed by urinary retention, and loss of balance leading to multiple falls. He then developed curling of the toes on his right foot, rigidity, and generalized slowing. He had no rest or action tremor. He had been diagnosed with Parkinson disease, but developed severe orthostasis when given carbidopa/levodopa. Attempts to control orthostasis with fludrocortisone and then midodrine led to episodes of hypertension. His exam showed occasional square-wave jerks and bilateral sustained end-gaze nystagmus, moderate hypomimia, and mild hypophonia with tachyphemia. Mild cogwheel rigidity was seen bilaterally, worse on the left, and his gait was broad based. Which of the following clinical features would not be expected in this patient?

A. Unexplained anosmia on olfactory testing
B. Development of inappropriate laughter or crying
C. Cold discolored hands and feet
D. Inspiratory sighs
E. Abnormal dopamine nuclear imaging study (DaTscan)
F. Presence of REM sleep behavior disorder

Correct answer: A

Explanation

Multiple system atrophy (MSA) is a progressive neurodegenerative disease that clinically presents with autonomic failure, parkinsonism, and a cerebellar syndrome. It is associated with abnormal aggregation of alpha synuclein, with deposition in glial tissue. However, it is not associated with anosmia, and a study with formal olfactory testing demonstrated specificity of 95.7% for distinguishing Parkinson's disease (PD) from MSA. According to the movement disorders society criteria, unexplained anosmia is an exclusion criterion for a diagnosis of MSA, and its presence is instead supportive of a diagnosis of Parkinson's disease.

Incorrect Answers

B, C, and D. Pseudobulbar affect, cold discolored hands and feet, and inspiratory sighs can be seen in multiple system atrophy and have a >90% specificity in contrast to PD and Lewy Body dementia.

E. A dopamine nuclear imaging study (DaTscan) can be abnormal in multiple types of parkinsonian syndromes (PD, MSA, CBD, and PSP among others). There have been reported cases of pathologically confirmed MSA with a normal DaTscan image.

F. The presence of REM sleep behavior disorder is a shared clinical feature that is seen in alpha-synucleinopathies (Parkinson's disease, dementia with Lewy bodies, and multiple system atrophy).

References

Bu LL, Liu FT, Jiang CF, Guo SS, Yu H, Zuo CT, et al. Patterns of dopamine transporter imaging in subtypes of multiple system atrophy. Acta Neurol Scand. 2018;138(2):170–6. https://doi.org/10.1111/ane.12932.

Krismer F, Pinter B, Mueller C, Mahlknecht P, Nocker M, Reiter E, et al. Sniffing the diagnosis: Olfactory testing in neurodegenerative parkinsonism. Parkinsonism Relat

Disord. 2017;35:36–41. https://doi.org/10.1016/j. parkreldis.2016.11.010.

Wenning GK, Stankovic I, Vignatelli L, Fanciulli A, Calandra-Buonaura G, Seppi K, et al. The Movement Disorder Society Criteria for the Diagnosis of Multiple System Atrophy. Mov Disord. 2022;37(6):1131–48. https://doi.org/10.1002/mds.29005.

81. A 53-year-old male with a history of depression with psychotic features (now in remission) presents with new-onset parkinsonism. He has been taking escitalopram and aripiprazole for the past 5 months with good control of his mood disorder under the care of his psychiatrist. His symptoms include marked bradykinesia, rigidity, and a resting tremor in both arms. There is no significant family history of movement disorders. Which of the following is the next best step in evaluating whether his parkinsonism is drug-induced or due to idiopathic Parkinson's disease?
   A. Perform a dopamine transporter (DAT) scan
   B. Discuss discontinuation of aripiprazole with the patient's psychiatrist
   C. Start a trial of levodopa to assess symptom response
   D. Obtain an MRI of the brain to evaluate for structural lesions
   E. Start benztropine for treatment of parkinsonism

Correct answer: B

Explanation

Drug-induced parkinsonism (DIP) is a common iatrogenic movement disorder most commonly caused by dopamine receptor blockers, although other medication classes include vesicular monoamine transporter 2 (VMAT2) inhibitors, certain antiemetics, and gastrointestinal prokinetics. Drug-induced parkinsonism has clinical features of rigidity, bradykinesia, gait impairment, and resting tremor that can be challenging to distinguish from idiopathic Parkinson's disease (PD), although progression over time and presence of prominent non-motor symptoms are suggestive of underlying idiopathic PD.

The best next step in management is either a discontinuation of the offending agent or transition to a similar drug with lower risk for causing drug-induced parkinsonism (e.g., quetiapine or clozapine). The expected course of drug-induced parkinsonism is resolution or marked improvement of the symptoms within weeks to months of drug cessation, in contrast to tardive dyskinesia which can frequently continue after cessation. Consultation with the prescribing physician, in this case the patient's psychiatrist, is recommended to ensure a safe transition to alternative agents as regards to his mood disorder.

Incorrect Answers

A. A dopamine transporter scan (DaTscan) has high sensitivity and specificity in differentiating drug-induced from idiopathic Parkinson's disease. However, the best next step is to reduce offending agents regardless of underlying diagnosis of DIP or PD and could also provide diagnostic clarity.

   In the case that the patient is unable to have the offending agent reduced due to unstable psychiatric disease, a DaTscan or similar fluorodopa (F-DOPA) PET scan would be the next best step to clarify the diagnosis.

C. Levodopa therapy can induce psychosis and should be used cautiously in patients with a history of psychosis. Although low-dose levodopa can be used judiciously in this patient population, it would not be the safest next step.

D. Magnetic resonance imaging has limited utility in evaluating parkinsonism without atypical features or clinical suspicion for an alternative diagnosis (e.g., Wilson's disease, neurodegeneration with brain iron accumulation (NBIA) syndromes). A normal MRI brain would not help differentiate DIP from PD.

E. Benztropine is an anticholinergic agent commonly used for side effects of neuroleptic agents, including acute dystonia and akathisia. It is also used in DIP, although it has limited clinical benefit, and would not aid in clarifying the diagnosis.

References

Brigo F, Matinella A, Erro R, Tinazzi M. [^{123}I]FP-CIT SPECT (DaTSCAN) may be a useful tool to differentiate between Parkinson's disease and vascular or drug-induced parkinsonisms: a meta-analysis. Eur J Neurol. 2014;21(11):1369–e90. https://doi.org/10.1111/ene.12444.

Conn H, Jankovic J. Drug-induced parkinsonism: diagnosis and treatment. Expert Opin Drug Saf. 2024;23(12):1503–13. https://doi.org/10.1080/14740338.2024.2418950.

82. A 41-year-old female presents to a neurologic clinic with a 4-year history of progressive parkinsonism with symmetric rigidity and bradykinesia, with minimal tremor and recent development of right leg dystonia. She wakes up every morning with minimal symptoms, which worsen throughout the day with significant dysfunction in the evening. A fundoscopic exam is normal, as is a cognitive screen done in the office. Laboratory testing, including hepatic enzymes and ceruloplasmin revealed no abnormalities, and a brain MRI is read as normal. She has no family history of Parkinson's disease.

She is started on low-dose levodopa with marked improvement in parkinsonism, but develops levodopa-induced dyskinesias with residual wearing off dystonia. You discuss genetic testing for young-onset Parkinson's disease. Which is the most likely genetic mutation in this case?

A. Leucine rich repeat kinase 2 (LRRK2)
B. Glucocerebrosidase (GBA)
C. Parkin
D. GTP-cyclohydrolase I (DYT5)
E. ATP7B

Correct answer: C

Explanation

There are several monogenic causes of Parkinson's disease that have been identified in the last several decades and can be tested for in routine clinical practice with the increasing availability of gene panels. 2–3% of idiopathic PD can be attributed to a single gene factor (monogenic parkinsonism); however, in select patient populations, this proportion can be much higher, including 40% in patients of North African Arab descent and 20% in patients of Ashkenazi Jewish descent.

This patient has young-onset Parkinson's disease (<50 years of age), with symmetric parkinsonism, dystonia, and diurnal pattern (less symptoms in the morning with progression throughout the day) with low threshold for both clinical benefit and side effects from levodopa therapy. This is consistent with a mutation in the *PARK2* gene, which encodes Parkin. This produces an autosomal recessive form of genetic parkinsonism with age of onset in 30–40s. Additional features include lower incidence of cognitive decline and very gradual progression of motor symptoms.

Incorrect Answers

A. For the practicing neurologist, it is important to be familiar with the most common cause of monogenic parkinsonism. Mutations in leucine-rich repeat kinase 2 (LRRK2) are the most common autosomal dominant cause of PD. These cases often are late in onset, with incomplete penetrance. This patient's young onset and lack of family history makes this unlikely.

B. Homozygous mutations in glucocerebrosidase leads to Gaucher's disease, a debilitating lysosomal storage disorder with onset in infancy; heterozygous mutations lead to an increased risk of late-onset Parkinson's disease with higher risk of cognitive and psychiatric symptoms. In this patient with no family history, lack of cognitive symptoms, and early onset, this mutation is unlikely.

D. GTP-cyclohydrolase I is the gene responsible for tetrahydrobiopterin (BH4), which is crucial for dopamine synthesis, and leads to dopamine-responsive dystonia

(DRD). This syndrome classically presents as limb dystonia in childhood with a marked response to levodopa replacement therapy at low dosages. The phenotype of *PARK2* mutation shares features of DRD including dystonia and levodopa responsiveness, but *PARK2* presents later in life with predominantly parkinsonism, and DRD presents in childhood predominantly with dystonia and minimal to no parkinsonism

E. ATP7B is the gene responsible for Wilson's disease, an autosomal recessive condition of impaired copper metabolism. It is on the differential for patients with young-onset parkinsonism, although it generally presents earlier in life (20–30s), and would be unlikely in a patient with a normal brain MRI, lack of Kayser-Fleischer rings, and normal ceruloplasmin and hepatic enzymes.

Reference

Klein C. Genetics of Parkinson's Disease – An Overview. In: *Movement Disorders 4*. 1st ed. Blue books of neurology; 34. Saunders Elsevier; 2010:15-39.

83. A 66-year-old woman with a history of 2 years of gradually progressive gait disturbance and urinary incontinence presents to the neurology clinic with mild cognitive complaints. Family members are concerned that in addition to her gait issues requiring use of a walker, she now is disinhibited and increasingly irritable.

    Examination reveals an oriented and cooperative patient with intact recall but difficulty with the Luria sequence and serial 7's. She has no evidence of weakness, and she has mild rigidity in her lower extremities. On gait assessment, she has a mildly wide base, shuffling stride with difficulty lifting the feet off the floor, and hesitancy in doorways and on turning. Her MRI brain revealed enlarged ventricles out of proportion to cortical atrophy with periventricular T2 hyperintensities.

    The patient has a lumbar puncture with a large volume of cerebrospinal fluid removed, which results in significant although brief improvements in gait and subjective improvements in urinary control. Which of the following clinical features is supportive evidence of the suspected diagnosis?

    A. The presence of Alzheimer's pathology on cerebrospinal fluid testing
    B. Ratio of the maximal width of the frontal horns to the maximum inner skull diameter of 0.25
    C. Enlarged temporal horns of the lateral ventricles with hippocampal atrophy
    D. Absence of macroscopic obstruction to CSF flow
    E. Elevated CSF pressure on lumbar puncture

    Correct answer: D

Explanation

The patient in this question has progressive gait dysfunction, urinary dysfunction, and cognitive complaints. MRI imaging revealed enlarged ventricles and periventricular T2 hyperintensities, consistent with hydrocephalus. The improvement after large volume lumbar puncture is consistent with idiopathic normal pressure hydrocephalus (iNPH).

iNPH is a syndrome characterized by a clinical triad of gait disturbance, urinary incontinence, and memory impairment, with normal CSF pressure on lumbar puncture and radiologic findings of enlarged cerebral ventricles. The etiology of iNPH remains unclear, and this is a distinct entity from obstructive hydrocephalus due to a macroscopic obstruction to CSF flow. Hence, the absence of macroscopic obstruction is necessary for the diagnosis of iNPH.

The clinical evaluation of suspected normal pressure hydrocephalus most commonly involves a trial of CSF removal, in which gait is assessed before and after a large volume lumbar puncture to gauge clinical benefit. If there is a positive response to a large volume lumbar puncture, this increases the chance of response to ventricular shunting. Other features that can predict response to shunting include improvements in gait after external lumbar drainage, MRI-measured high CSF velocity through the aqueduct, and abnormal intracranial CSF hydrodynamics.

However, response to shunting is highly variable, and fewer than half of patients showed improvement in all presenting iNPH symptoms after 18 months. The American Academy of Neurology clinical practice guidelines recommend that the risks and benefits of the procedure should be carefully weighed against adverse outcomes, which include risk of shunt failure, ventriculitis, and shunt infections.

Incorrect Answers

A. The presence of Alzheimer's pathology on cerebrospinal fluid testing is a clinical marker of poor response to ventricular shunting and may be concerning for Alzheimer's disease, which can also lead to "hydrocephalus ex vacuo," which can provide the appearance of enlarged ventricles in the presence of cortical atrophy.

B. The ratio of the maximal width of the frontal horns to the maximum inner skull diameter is called the Evans index, and a value >0.30 is supportive of normal pressure hydrocephalus.

C. Enlarged temporal horns of the lateral ventricles *without* hippocampal atrophy are consistent with disproportionately enlarged subarachnoid-space hydrocephalus (DESH), an imaging feature in a subset of patients with iNPH, which correlates with higher probability of benefit from shunting.

E. Elevated pressure on lumbar puncture is inconsistent with iNPH. Furthermore, if elevated CSF pressure is present, then a large volume tap should not be performed due to risk of precipitating herniation.

References

Greenberg BM, Williams MA. Infectious complications of temporary spinal catheter insertion for diagnosis of adult hydrocephalus and idiopathic intracranial hypertension. Neurosurgery. 2008;62(2):431–5; discussion 5–6. https://doi.org/10.1227/01.neu.0000316010.19012.35.

Halperin JJ, Kurlan R, Schwalb JM, Cusimano MD, Gronseth G, Gloss D. Practice guideline: Idiopathic normal pressure hydrocephalus: Response to shunting and predictors of response: Report of the Guideline Development, Dissemination, and Implementation Subcommittee of the American Academy of Neurology. Neurology. 2015;85(23):2063–71. https://doi.org/10.1212/wnl.0000000000002193.

Nakajima M, Yamada S, Miyajima M, Ishii K, Kuriyama N, Kazui H, et al. Guidelines for Management of Idiopathic Normal Pressure Hydrocephalus (Third Edition): Endorsed by the Japanese Society of Normal Pressure Hydrocephalus. Neurol Med Chir (Tokyo). 2021;61(2):63–97. https://doi.org/10.2176/nmc.st.2020-0292.

Tremor

84. Enhanced physiologic tremor can be exacerbated by all of the following, except:
    A. Anxiety
    B. Caffeine
    C. Hyperthyroidism
    D. Alcohol use
    E. β-adrenergic agonists
    Correct answer: D

Explanation

Enhanced physiological tremor is a high-frequency (typically 8–12 Hz), low-amplitude postural tremor that is present in all individuals, but usually subclinical. It can become clinically noticeable or exaggerated (i.e., "enhanced") in response to various factors that increase adrenergic tone or excitability of peripheral motor units.

Alcohol usually reduces tremor amplitude in both essential tremor and enhanced physiologic tremor, due to depressant effects on the central nervous system. Multiple stimulant medications (e.g., caffeine, β-adrenergic agonists), endocrine abnormalities (e.g., hyperthyroidism), and emotional states such as anxiety can enhance tremor.

Reference

Deuschl G, Bain P, Brin M. Consensus statement of the Movement Disorder Society on Tremor. Ad Hoc Scientific Committee. Mov Disord. 1998;13 Suppl 3:2–23. https://doi.org/10.1002/mds.870131303.

85. A 68-year-old man presents with a several-year history of progressive hand tremor that is most noticeable when reaching for objects, as well as increasing unsteadiness while walking. He reports frequent near-falls and requires a cane for ambulation. His family history is notable for a grandson with intellectual disability. On examination, he has an intention tremor of the upper extremities and a wide-based, unsteady gait. Brain MRI reveals white matter changes in the middle cerebellar peduncles. What is the most likely diagnosis?
    A. Spinocerebellar ataxia
    B. Essential tremor
    C. Normal pressure hydrocephalus
    D. Fragile X-associated tremor/ataxia syndrome
    E. Parkinson's disease
    Correct answer: D

Explanation

Fragile X-associated tremor/ataxia syndrome (FXTAS) is distinguished by the combination of late-onset intention tremor, cerebellar ataxia, and characteristic MRI findings of hyperintensities in the middle cerebellar peduncles. FXTAS is caused by a premutation expansion (55–200 CGG repeats) in the 5′ untranslated region of the FMR1 gene on the X chromosome. This premutation leads to elevated levels of FMR1 mRNA, which is thought to cause neurotoxicity. The full mutation (>200 CGG repeats) leads to fragile X syndrome with intellectual disability (as seen in the grandson in the family history). The condition is inherited in a X-linked dominant pattern. Males are therefore at higher risk and may develop more severe symptoms.

Incorrect Answers

A. Spinocerebellar ataxia can cause gait instability and appendicular ataxia, but a family history of intellectual disability and the MRI findings are more consistent with FXTAS.

B. Essential tremor is an isolated tremor syndrome with an autosomal dominant pattern of inheritance. There are no abnormal MRI findings associated with essential tremor.

C. Normal pressure hydrocephalus does not have tremor as a clinical feature.

E. Parkinson's disease classically has a rest tremor and rigidity, with a shuffling gait with a narrow base. MRI findings of cerebellar hyperintensities would be inconsistent with this diagnosis.

References

Brunberg JA, Jacquemont S, Hagerman RJ, Berry-Kravis EM, Grigsby J, Leehey MA, et al. Fragile X premutation carriers: characteristic MR imaging findings of adult male patients with progressive cerebellar and cognitive dysfunction. AJNR Am J Neuroradiol. 2002;23(10):1757–66.

Jacquemont S, Hagerman RJ, Leehey M, Grigsby J, Zhang L, Brunberg JA, et al. Fragile X premutation tremor/ataxia syndrome: molecular, clinical, and neuroimaging correlates. Am J Hum Genet. 2003;72(4):869–78. https://doi.org/10.1086/374321.

86. A 71-year-old female with asthma presents to a neurology clinic for management of bilateral arm tremor that affects her handwriting and ability to drink liquids. She has a family history of tremor in her brother and mother, and alcohol improves her tremor. Examination is notable for tremor in both hands in action and in posture, but no tremor at rest. The rest of the exam is unremarkable. Which of the following medications should be offered for tremor relief?
    A. Propranolol
    B. Levodopa
    C. Amantadine
    D. Gabapentin
    E. Primidone
    Correct answer: E

Explanation

This patient with an isolated bilateral upper limb action tremor, with positive family history and alcohol responsiveness, has essential tremor. The first-line pharmacologic agents are propranolol, a beta-blocker, and primidone, an antiepileptic agent. A second-line option is topiramate, although higher dosages (>200 mg/day) and side effects of weight loss, cognitive impairment, paresthesia, and renal stones limit use. In this patient with asthma, propranolol is contraindicated due to risk of bronchospasm, making primidone the preferred agent.

Incorrect Answers

Levodopa and amantadine can be used to treat tremor associated with Parkinson's disease, but are not recommended agents for essential tremor. Gabapentin is sometimes used for tremor control in essential tremor, but evidence has been inconclusive and this should be considered a third-line option.

Reference

Ferreira JJ, Mestre TA, Lyons KE, Benito-León J, Tan EK, Abbruzzese G, et al. MDS evidence-based review of treatments for essential tremor. Mov Disord. 2019;34(7):950–8. https://doi.org/10.1002/mds.27700.

87. A patient with medication refractory essential tremor is being referred for deep brain stimulation for management. Which of the following surgical targets is most established for this indication?
    A. Ventral intermediate nucleus of the thalamus
    B. Globus pallidus
    C. Subthalamic nucleus
    D. Cerebellar deep nuclei
    E. Anterior nucleus of the thalamus
    Correct answer: A

Explanation

Deep brain stimulation is an FDA-approved treatment for management of medication refractory essential tremor since 1997, on the basis of clinical trials demonstrating efficacy in tremor control and improvements in quality of life metrics. DBS targeting the ventral intermediate nucleus (VIM) of the thalamus has been studied most extensively for essential tremor. Bilateral DBS is more effective in tremor reduction than unilateral, but has a higher rate of adverse events such as dysarthria, gait impairment, and incoordination. Long-term studies over a 10-year postoperative period have demonstrated continued tremor benefit. Serious complications were rare, but include infection and intracranial hemorrhage.

Incorrect Answers

The globus pallidus and subthalamic nucleus are targets for DBS in Parkinson's disease. The anterior nucleus of the thalamus is a DBS target for medication refractory epilepsy. Cerebellar deep nuclei are investigational and are not currently used in clinical practice.

References

Baizabal-Carvallo JF, Kagnoff MN, Jimenez-Shahed J, Fekete R, Jankovic J. The safety and efficacy of thalamic deep brain stimulation in essential tremor: 10 years and beyond. J Neurol Neurosurg Psychiatry. 2014;85(5):567–72. https://doi.org/10.1136/jnnp-2013-304943.

Wharen RE, Jr., Okun MS, Guthrie BL, Uitti RJ, Larson P, Foote K, et al. Thalamic DBS with a constant-current device in essential tremor: A controlled clinical trial. Parkinsonism Relat Disord. 2017;40:18–26. https://doi.org/10.1016/j.parkreldis.2017.03.017.

88. A 48-year-old man with bipolar disorder presents with a several-week history of fine, bilateral hand tremor that is most noticeable when holding objects or performing tasks such as writing. His medication regimen includes fluoxetine, risperidone, and lithium. Laboratory findings reveal normal electrolyte levels and thyroid function and a lithium serum level of 1.4 mmol/L. On examination, he has a low amplitude, high-frequency postural tremor in his bilateral hands, no tremor at rest, and no evidence of bradykinesia or rigidity. What is the next best step?
    A. Reduction or discontinuation of risperidone
    B. Reduction or discontinuation of lithium
    C. Start propranolol for tremor control
    D. Obtain MRI brain imaging
    Correct answer: B

Explanation

Lithium is a monovalent cation, most commonly used as a mood stabilizer in bipolar disorder. It is effective for management of both acute mania and depressive episodes. Unfortunately, lithium toxicity can lead to multiorgan dysfunction, and neurologic toxicity can range from acute toxicity with coma and seizures to chronic toxicity ranging from action tremor to chronic cerebellar toxicity (Irreversible Lithium-Effectuated Neurotoxicity). Older patients on chronic lithium therapy are more susceptible and lithium toxicity can occur with normal serum values due to variability in correlation of serum to CNS concentrations of lithium.

Reduction of the lithium dose or discontinuation of lithium is the mainstay of treatment. In acute toxicity, hemodialysis is used as an emergent therapy.

Incorrect Answers

Risperidone can lead to drug-induced parkinsonism, which would include a rest tremor without features of parkinsonism. Propranolol could be used if, after coordinating with the patient's treating psychiatrist and adjusting the lithium regimen, tremors continue. MRI of the brain would be unlikely to change management and is not the best next step in a patient on lithium with elevated lithium levels.

References

Baek JH, Kinrys G, Nierenberg AA. Lithium tremor revisited: pathophysiology and treatment. Acta Psychiatr Scand. 2014;129(1):17–23. https://doi.org/10.1111/acps.12171.

Chan BS, Cheng S, Isoardi KZ, Chiew A, Siu W, Shulruf B, et al. Effect of age on the severity of chronic lithium poisoning. Clin Toxicol (Phila). 2020;58(11):1023–7. https://doi.org/10.1080/15563650.2020.1726376.

Marmol S, Beltre N, Margolesky J. Syndrome of Irreversible Lithium-Effectuated Neurotoxicity (SILENT): A Preventable Cerebellar Disorder.

89. A 61-year-old female with hypertension present to a neurologic clinic with frequent falls upon standing. When she rises to a standing position, she has bilateral leg tremors that can lead to her collapsing on the floor, and the symptoms improve when she is walking. When examined in a chair, she has a normal neurological exam, but upon standing her bilateral quadriceps muscles develop a high-frequency tremor. She walks with a wide base and reduced step length. What is the diagnosis?
    A. Vascular parkinsonism
    B. Orthostatic tremor
    C. Essential tremor
    D. Cerebellar ataxia
    E. Peripheral neuropathy
    Correct answer: B

Explanation
Orthostatic tremor is characterized by a high-frequency (13–18 Hz) tremor of the legs and trunk upon standing, leading to unsteadiness that resolves with sitting. Pathophysiological studies implicate abnormal oscillatory activity within the ponto-cerebello-thalamo-cortical network, with functional imaging and neurophysiological data supporting a central generator involving the cerebellum, thalamus, and brainstem, as well as altered connectivity with the supplementary motor area. There is limited evidence to guide treatment, although clonazepam is the most often used.

Incorrect Answers
Vascular parkinsonism can affect the lower extremities, but is characterized by rigidity, slowness, and a shuffling gait possibly with freezing of gait; high-frequency leg tremor is not a feature. Essential tremor rarely affects the legs, and isolated leg involvement in particular would be highly uncharacteristic. Cerebellar ataxia and peripheral neuropathy can both cause a wide-based gait, which is also seen in orthostatic tremor, likely as a compensatory mechanism.

Reference
Whitney D, Bhatti D, Torres-Russotto D. Orthostatic Tremor: Pathophysiology Guiding Treatment. Curr Treat Options Neurol. 2018;20(9):35. https://doi.org/10.1007/s11940-018-0524-3.

Questions 90–94
Match the description of each tremor type with the clinical description of the tremor:

    A. Essential tremor
    B. Parkinsonian tremor
    C. Dystonic tremor
    D. Holmes tremor
    E. Enhanced physiologic tremor

90. A 45-year-old female has an irregular tremor of the neck, with abnormal posturing that improves when she lightly touches her chin.
91. A 70-year-old female reports a resting tremor in her right hand, which abates immediately upon assuming a posture, but appears after a latency of a few seconds.
92. A 65-year-old male with a bilateral hand and vocal tremor, which worsens with stress and improves after consuming alcohol.
93. A 56-year-old female with a renal transplant with high-frequency tremor of both hands present in action and posture and no family history of tremor.
94. A 62-year-old male with a right arm proximal tremor present in rest, action, and posture, worsened in wing beating position.
    Correct answers: 90. C, 91. B, 92. A, 93. E, 94. D

Explanations
90. C – Dystonic tremor is a jerky, irregular tremulous movement that accompanies dystonia, a syndrome of sustained muscle contraction causing sustained or intermittent abnormal posturing. Unlike other tremors, dystonic tremors do not oscillate around a point and are asymmetric, are associated with a *geste antagoniste* or sensory trick (e.g., improvement with touching the chin), and can be relieved by allowing the abnormal posture to develop (e.g., a null point).
91. B – A parkinsonian tremor is characterized by a 4–7 Hz rest tremor of the hand, lower limb, jaw, tongue, or foot. A classic and specific feature of a parkinsonian tremor is the *postural re-emergent* tremor, which is when tremor abates when assuming a posture but then resumes when the posture is sustained.
92. A – Essential tremor is an isolated tremor syndrome that most commonly affects the bilateral upper extremities but can also involve other body parts. The second most commonly affected areas are head and voice, with leg and truncal involvement being less common. Vocal tremor is much more common in ET than in enhanced physiologic tremor and not seen in Parkinson's disease. Relief with alcohol is also common.
93. E – Enhanced physiologic tremor should be suspected in a patient with a kidney transplant, as they are commonly prescribed tacrolimus, which is a common offender in causing tremor.

94. D – Holmes tremor is a syndrome of rest, postural, and intention tremor that usually emerges from a lesion in the brainstem near the red nucleus. Given the structural etiology, it is usually unilateral and accompanied by other neurological findings. Other names for this tremor include rubral or midbrain tremor.

Reference

Bhatia KP, Bain P, Bajaj N, Elble RJ, Hallett M, Louis ED, et al. Consensus Statement on the classification of tremors. from the task force on tremor of the International Parkinson and Movement Disorder Society. Mov Disord. 2018;33(1):75–87. https://doi.org/10.1002/mds.27121.

95. A 41-year-old male presents with a 6-month history of right-hand tremor. The tremor began abruptly and is described as variable in both frequency and amplitude. On examination, the tremor is present at rest and with action, but markedly diminishes when she is asked to perform a cognitive task such as serial sevens. When asked to tap rhythmically with her left hand, the tremor in the right-hand changes to match the tapping frequency. There is no family history of tremor, and the neurological examination is otherwise normal. Which of the following clinical features is most characteristic of functional tremor?
   A. Tremor that is present in rest and action
   B. Tremor that is suppressed with distraction and shows changes to match the tapping frequency
   C. Tremor with variable amplitude
   D. Present of variability throughout the clinical examination
   E. Abrupt onset of tremor
   Correct answer: B

Explanation

A functional neurological disorder (FND) is a condition that can be identified by the positive clinical features that are specific to FND. These features include inconsistency (symptoms changing over time and with distraction), incongruence with a known neuroanatomical pathway or disease pattern, and positive physical signs.

Functional tremor is the most common functional movement disorder. Eliciting the features of functional tremor requires a clinical understanding of the features of tremor syndromes to ascertain incongruence, as well as positive physical signs. Among the positive physical signs is entrainment, in which the tremor adopts the frequency of a repetitive task elsewhere, and the suppression of tremor with distraction, known as distractibility.

Incorrect Answers

Multiple forms of tremor can be present in rest and action, including Holmes tremor, tremor associated with Wilson's disease, and others. Variability in tremor amplitude throughout the examination is common in many types of tremor. Of note, amplitude can change depending on stress levels in multiple tremor conditions, but change in frequency is more consistent with functional tremor. A common example is a patient with Parkinson's disease tremor who has no tremor in the beginning of a clinical encounter, but subsequently develops tremor when discussing a stressful topic. Finally, an abrupt onset of tremor can be seen in multiple etiologies, including stroke and demyelinating disease.

References

Espay AJ, Aybek S, Carson A, Edwards MJ, Goldstein LH, Hallett M, et al. Current Concepts in Diagnosis and Treatment of Functional Neurological Disorders. JAMA Neurol. 2018;75(9):1132–41. https://doi.org/10.1001/jamaneurol.2018.1264.

Schwingenschuh P, Espay AJ. Functional tremor. J Neurol Sci. 2022;435:120208. https://doi.org/10.1016/j.jns.2022.120208.

96. A patient presents for follow-up for management of medically refractory essential tremor and is interested in high-intensity focused ultrasound (HIFU) lesioning therapy. All of the following are true regarding this therapy, except for which of the following?
   A. HIFU is not typically performed bilaterally on the same date, due to the risk of adverse effects with bilateral procedures
   B. A low skull density ratio can be a contraindication for the procedure
   C. The most common persistent adverse effects are paresthesia/numbness and gait disturbance
   D. HIFU is associated with a higher rate of severe intracranial hemorrhage compared to deep brain stimulation
   E. HIFU is an incisionless, MRI-guided procedure targeting the ventral intermediate nucleus of the thalamus
   Correct answer: D

Explanation

High-intensity focused ultrasound (HIFU) is an incisionless, MRI-guided procedure that creates a lesion in the ventral intermediate nucleus of the thalamus. It provides significant improvement in contralateral hand tremor and quality of life, although there are side effects of paresthesia and gait disturbance. It is most commonly performed unilaterally due to the risk of irreversible adverse effects with bilateral lesioning and is now FDA approved to be performed on the second side after a 9-month interval. The risk of severe intracranial hemorrhage is considered lower than with invasive surgical procedures such as deep brain stimulation. One of the inclusion criteria for the clinical trial that led to the approval of HIFU was an adequate skull density ratio (the ratio of cortical to cancellous bone) to ensure adequate transmission of ultrasound energy through the skull.

References

Elias WJ, Lipsman N, Ondo WG, Ghanouni P, Kim YG, Lee W, et al. A Randomized Trial of Focused Ultrasound Thalamotomy for Essential Tremor. N Engl J Med. 2016;375(8):730–9. https://doi.org/10.1056/NEJMoa1600159.

Mortezaei A, Essibayi MA, Mirahmadi Eraghi M, Alizadeh M, Taghlabi KM, Eskandar EN, et al. Magnetic resonance-guided focused ultrasound in the treatment of refractory essential tremor: a systematic review and meta-analysis. Neurosurg Focus. 2024;57(3):E2. https://doi.org/10.3171/2024.6.Focus24326.

97. A 68-year-old man with essential tremor is started on primidone. Within hours of his first dose, he develops dizziness, ataxia, and nausea. Which of the following statements regarding the side effects of primidone in essential tremor is *incorrect*?
    A. Acute neurotoxic symptoms such as dizziness, ataxia, and nausea are common at treatment initiation and typically resolved within several days with continued therapy or dose reduction.
    B. Slow titration and starting at low doses (e.g., 25–62.5 mg) can help minimize acute intolerance to primidone.
    C. Persistent or severe hematologic abnormalities, such as agranulocytosis or megaloblastic anemia, are common and usually require permanent discontinuation of primidone.
    D. Fatigue, malaise, and somnolence are among the most frequently reported early side effects of primidone.
    E. Most patients who experience early side effects are able to continue therapy after the initial period.

Correct answer: C

Explanation

Primidone is an enzyme-inducing drug that can cause acute neurotoxic symptoms (dizziness, ataxia, nausea, fatigue, malaise, somnolence). These are typically mild and resolved within 1–4 days, and most patients are able to continue therapy. Slow titration and low starting doses reduce acute intolerance.

Hematologic abnormalities such as agranulocytosis and megaloblastic anemia are rare, not common, and secondary to impairment of folic acid metabolism. The rare megaloblastic anemia often responds to folic acid without requiring discontinuation. Additionally, as an enzyme-inducing drug, a careful medication review is critical to avoid medication interactions.

References

Food and Drug Administration. *Mysoline [prescribing information]*. Silver Spring, MD: US Department of Health and Human Services; Updated July 6, 2020. Accessed [insert date]. https://www.accessdata.fda.gov

Haubenberger D, Hallett M. Essential Tremor. N Engl J Med. 2018;378(19):1802–10. https://doi.org/10.1056/NEJMcp1707928.

Hesdorffer CS, Longo DL. Drug-Induced Megaloblastic Anemia. N Engl J Med. 2015;373(17):1649–58. https://doi.org/10.1056/NEJMra1508861.

Zesiewicz TA, Elble RJ, Louis ED, Gronseth GS, Ondo WG, Dewey RB, Jr., et al. Evidence-based guideline update: treatment of essential tremor: report of the Quality Standards subcommittee of the American Academy of Neurology. Neurology. 2011;77(19):1752–5. https://doi.org/10.1212/WNL.0b013e318236f0fd.

98. A 38-year-old right-handed woman presents with a 3-year history of fine, irregular, jerky movements in her hands, most noticeable when holding objects or performing precise tasks such as writing. She reports occasional brief, involuntary muscle jerks in her fingers and forearms, which sometimes cause her to drop objects. There is a family history of similar symptoms in her mother and a maternal uncle with epilepsy. She has never experienced loss of consciousness, but describes rare, brief episodes of limb "shaking" without clear triggers. Neurologic examination reveals a high-frequency (9–18 Hz), low-amplitude, irregular tremor in both hands during posture and action.

    Which of the following findings would most strongly support the most likely diagnosis in this patient?
    A. Symmetric, 4–12 Hz postural and kinetic tremor of the upper limbs, responsive to propranolol
    B. High-frequency (9–18 Hz) postural and action tremor with superimposed myoclonic jerks, giant somatosensory evoked potentials, and cortical spikes on EEG
    C. Unilateral, 4–7 Hz resting tremor with bradykinesia and rigidity
    D. Low-frequency (2–5 Hz) intention tremor with dysmetria and nystagmus
    E. High-frequency (13–18 Hz) tremor of the legs present only when standing, relieved by walking

Correct answer: B

Explanation

This patient is experiencing cortical tremor, which is a high-frequency, low amplitude, irregular postural and action tremor. It can be distinguished from essential tremor by the presence of myoclonic jerks and cortical hyperexcitability on neurophysiologic testing such as giant somatosensory evoked potential and cortical spikes on EEG.

Cortical tremor with a family history and comorbid epilepsy is suggestive of autosomal dominant cortical tremor, myoclonus, and epilepsy syndromes (ADCME).

Incorrect Answers

A. Unlike essential tremor, cortical tremor is refractory to standard tremor treatments, although antiepileptic agents such as levetiracetam can be used.

C. These features are suggestive of Parkinson's disease.

D. This is more consistent of a cerebellar syndrome, which is less commonly associated with either myoclonus or epilepsy.

E. High-frequency tremor in the legs is more consistent with orthostatic tremor.

References

Haubenberger D, Hallett M. Essential Tremor. N Engl J Med. 2018;378(19):1802–10. https://doi.org/10.1056/NEJMcp1707928.

Latorre A, Rocchi L, Magrinelli F, Mulroy E, Berardelli A, Rothwell JC, ct al. Unravelling the enigma of cortical tremor and other forms of cortical myoclonus. Brain. 2020;143(9):2653–63. https://doi.org/10.1093/brain/awaa129.

Terada K, Ikeda A, Mima T, Kimura M, Nagahama Y, Kamioka Y, et al. Familial cortical myoclonic tremor as a unique form of cortical reflex myoclonus. Mov Disord. 1997;12(3):370–7. https://doi.org/10.1002/mds.870120316.

Wilson's Disease

99. A 17-year-old boy presents with a 6-month history of progressive hand tremor, difficulty with speech, and declining school performance. Examination reveals dysarthria, a wing-beating tremor, and mild jaundice. Slit-lamp examination identifies brownish rings at the corneal margin. Laboratory studies show elevated liver enzymes, low serum ceruloplasmin, and increased 24-h urinary copper excretion. There is no family history of liver disease. What is the most likely diagnosis?

A. Juvenile Parkinson's disease
B. Wilson's disease
C. Niemann-Pick disease type C
D. Urea cycle disorders

Correct answer: B

Explanation

This presentation is characteristic of Wilson's disease, which typically involves hepatic dysfunction, neurologic manifestations (including tremor and dysarthria), psychiatric disturbances, and Kayser–Fleischer rings. The condition follows an autosomal recessive inheritance pattern due to pathogenic variants in the ATP7B gene located on chromosome 13q14. ATP7B encodes a copper-transporting P-type ATPase primarily expressed in hepatocytes. Mutations impair copper excretion into bile and its incorporation into ceruloplasmin, resulting in copper accumulation in the liver and subsequent deposition in extrahepatic tissues such as the brain.

Wilson's disease has a highly variable disease presentation, and the diagnosis should be excluded in any patient <40 years of age with unexplained progressive movement disorder. Patients with Wilson's disease can have isolated neurologic symptoms, with the most common symptoms being dysarthria followed by dystonia, gait abnormalities, and tremor. Laboratory findings include low serum ceruloplasmin and increased 24-h urinary copper excretion. Making a diagnosis is critical as Wilson's disease progression can be halted with appropriate treatment.

Incorrect Answer

A. Juvenile Parkinson's disease can lead to tremor in a young patient, but will have symptoms classically associated with Parkinson's disease without hepatic dysfunction or cognitive symptoms.

C. Niemann–Pick disease type C is a lysosomal storage disorder that often presents in juveniles with hepatosplenomegaly, progressive neuropsychiatric symptoms (cognitive impairment, psychiatric changes), and movement disorders such as ataxia and dystonia. It is not associated with Kayser–Fleischer rings or changes in ceruloplasmin and urine copper levels.

D. Urea cycle disorders can lead to acute or chronic hepatic dysfunction, hyperammonemia, and neuropsychiatric symptoms, including movement disorders. Diagnosis is based on plasma ammonia, amino acid analysis, and urine orotic acid. However, this would not be associated with Kayser–Fleischer rings or changes in ceruloplasmin and urine copper levels.

References

Bolton SC, Soran V, Marfa MP, Imrie J, Gissen P, Jahnova H, et al. Clinical disease characteristics of patients with Niemann-Pick Disease Type C: findings from the International Niemann-Pick Disease Registry (INPDR). Orphanet J Rare Dis. 2022;17(1):51. https://doi.org/10.1186/s13023-022-02200-4.

Lorincz MT. Neurologic Wilson's disease. Ann N Y Acad Sci. 2010;1184:173–87. https://doi.org/10.1111/j.1749-6632.2009.05109.x.

Roberts EA, Schilsky ML. Current and Emerging Issues in Wilson's Disease. N Engl J Med. 2023;389(10):922–38. https://doi.org/10.1056/NEJMra1903585.

Simpson KL, MacLeod EL, Kakajiwala A, Gropman AL, Ah Mew N. Urea Cycle Disorders Overview. In: Adam MP, Feldman J, Mirzaa GM, Pagon RA, Wallace SE, Amemiya A, editors. GeneReviews(®). Seattle (WA): University of Washington, Seattle. Copyright © 1993–2025, University of Washington, Seattle. GeneReviews is a registered trademark of the University of Washington, Seattle. All rights reserved.; 1993.

100. A 24-year-old patient with dysarthria and generalized dystonia was recently diagnosed with Wilson's disease. Which of the following is true regarding pharmacologic treatment of Wison's disease?
    A. Initial treatment includes high dosages of D-penicillamine to normalize copper metabolism
    B. Trientine can lead to drug-induced lupus, limiting its use
    C. Zinc oral therapy cannot be used as monotherapy for maintenance therapy
    D. Recommended initial treatment is a low-dose trientine
    E. Monitoring for maintenance therapy is based on serial magnetic resonance imaging changes

    Correct answer: B

Explanation

Prior to the treatment era, the median survival for patients with Wilson's disease after the development of neurologic symptoms was ~5 years. It is critical to establish treatment quickly after diagnosis to prevent significant morbidity and mortality. The American Association for the Study of Liver Diseases recommends starting with a copper chelating agent—either D-penicillamine or trientine. Trientine is preferred in most situations due to the side effect profile of penicillamine, which includes drug-induced lupus. Either medication is started at a low dose to prevent paradoxical worsening with overly aggressive treatment, with serial monitoring relying on clinical symptoms and laboratory monitoring of urinary copper excretion, ceruloplasmin levels, and liver biochemistries. MRI imaging does not have an established role in monitoring for therapy. Zinc is another pharmacologic option that limits copper absorption and promotes fecal excretion of copper and can be used as monotherapy during the maintenance phase.

References

Lorincz MT. Neurologic Wilson's disease. Ann N Y Acad Sci. 2010;1184:173–87. https://doi.org/10.1111/j.1749-6632.2009.05109.x.

Roberts EA, Schilsky ML. Current and Emerging Issues in Wilson's Disease. N Engl J Med. 2023;389(10):922–38. https://doi.org/10.1056/NEJMra1903585.

101. A 19-year-old woman with Wilson's disease is being treated with D-penicillamine. She presents with new-onset numbness and weakness in her lower extremities, along with pallor and mild gait instability. Laboratory evaluation reveals anemia, leukopenia, low serum copper, and a 24-h urinary copper excretion of 60 µg/24 h (target: 200–500 µg/24 h for chelation therapy). What is the most appropriate next step in management?
    A. Reduce or temporarily discontinue chelation therapy, with close monitoring and consideration of copper supplementation if symptoms are severe
    B. Switch to zinc maintenance therapy at the current time
    C. Initiate copper supplementation and continue current chelation therapy
    D. Continue current chelation therapy without changes
    E. Increase the dose of chelation therapy

    Correct answer: A

Explanation

These findings are consistent with copper deficiency secondary to overtreatment of Wilson's disease. Overtreatment with copper chelators can lead to copper deficiency, manifesting as cytopenias and neurologic complications such as myelopathy or neuropathy. When these symptoms develop, the most appropriate next step is prompt reduction or interruption of chelation therapy, with careful monitoring of clinical and laboratory parameters to prevent irreversible neurologic damage. Due to these concerns, treatment of Wilson's disease requires careful serial monitoring of urinary copper levels, ceruloplasmin levels, and serial neurological examination, as well as co-management with hepatology colleagues.

Incorrect Answers

B. This may be an appropriate next step after discontinuation of chelation therapy and normalization of copper levels.

C. It would not be appropriate to both supplement copper and continue the chelation therapy.

D and E would both lead to worsening of the copper deficiency and the patient's symptoms.

References

Lorincz MT. Neurologic Wilson's disease. Ann N Y Acad Sci. 2010;1184:173–87. https://doi.org/10.1111/j.1749-6632.2009.05109.x.

Roberts EA, Schilsky ML. Current and Emerging Issues in Wilson's Disease. N Engl J Med. 2023;389(10):922–38. https://doi.org/10.1056/NEJMra1903585.

102. Which of the following is not an MRI finding commonly associated with Wilson's disease?
    A. T2-weighted hyperintense signal in the bilateral thalami and putamen
    B. Gyriform cortical restriction diffusion on DWI imaging sequence
    C. T2-weighted axial MRI with hyperintensity in the tegmentum, with normal signal of the red nucleus
    D. T2-weighted axial MRI of the pons with hypointensity of central tegmental tracts, with hyperintensity of aqueductal opening to the fourth ventricle

Correct answer: B

Explanation

Changes in magnetic resonance imaging studies are common in patients with neurological symptoms in Wilson's disease. Commonly described findings in the literature include T2 hyperintensities in bilateral thalami and putamina, T2 hyperintensities in the tegmentum with normal signal in the red nucleus (face of the giant panda), and T2 hypointensity in the central tegmental tract with hyperintensities in the aqueductal opening of the fourth ventricle (face of the miniature panda). Cortical ribboning, described as gyriform cortical restriction diffusion on DWI imaging sequences, is not commonly associated with Wilson's disease, but rather cortical ribboning is seen in Creutzfeldt-Jakob disease (CJD).

Reference

Singh P, Ahluwalia A, Saggar K, Grewal CS. Wilson's disease: MRI features. J Pediatr Neurosci. 2011;6(1):27–8. https://doi.org/10.4103/1817-1745.84402.

Demyelinating Diseases

6

Thomas Flagiello, Vito Arena, and Tyler Ellis Smith

1. A 37-year-old male artist with a history of MS on dimethyl fumarate presents to clinic reporting worsened right arm and leg weakness for 2 weeks. MRI reveals a new enhancing right-sided cervical cord lesion. You prescribe 5 days of IV methylprednisolone 2 days after symptom onset, but the patient does not notice any improvement and has significant impairment in dominant limb function and gait. Clinical evidence best supports which of the following as a second-line treatment?
   A. A steroid taper over 2 weeks
   B. IVIG
   C. Therapeutic plasma exchange
   D. Cyclophosphamide
   E. No further intervention and monitor for resolution

   Correct answer: C

Explanation

Multiple sclerosis (MS) relapses can be severe, and while some degree of natural recovery is expected even in the absence of treatment, it can be variable and often incomplete. While high-dose steroids are the first-line treatment for MS relapses, severe relapses can be refractory. In such cases, various options may be considered, but evidence best supports the use of therapeutic plasma exchange (TPE) as the second-line therapy. TPE is considered an overall safe and well-tolerated therapy with evidence for recovery in steroid-refractory relapses supported by various retrospective studies and randomized clinical trials. Some retrospective studies even suggest a decrease in long-term disability in patients with steroid-refractory relapses.

References

Marrodan M, Crema S, Rubstein A, Alessandro L, Fernandez J, Correale J, et al. Therapeutic plasma exchange in MS refractory relapses: Long-term outcome. Mult Scler Relat Disord. 2021;55:103168. https://doi.org/10.1016/j.msard.2021.103168.

Weinshenker BG, O'Brien PC, Petterson TM, Noseworthy JH, Lucchinetti CF, Dodick DW, et al. A randomized trial of plasma exchange in acute central nervous system inflammatory demyelinating disease. Ann Neurol. 1999;46(6):878–86. https://doi.org/10.1002/1531-8249(199912)46:6<878::aid-ana10>3.0.co;2-q.

2. A 27-year-old woman comes to your office for evaluation. She reports that 1 year ago she developed numbness and tingling in the toes of her right foot that spread up the right leg over the course of 5 days. She assumed she pinched a nerve after having helped her friend move out of her apartment the weekend before. Symptoms lasted for 3 weeks before resolving. She presents for evaluation at the urging of her colleague whose mother has multiple sclerosis (MS). Exam is notable for normal cranial nerve function, intact strength, symmetric reflexes, and normal sensation with the exception of reduced vibratory sense in the distal right lower extremity. A brain MRI reveals multiple T2/FLAIR hyperintense periventricular and juxtacortical lesions and a spine MRI showsa right-sided dorsal spinal cord lesion at the T8 level. None of the lesions enhance. You explain that based on the 2017 McDonald Criteria, the patient currently meets dissemination in space criteria, but not dissemination in time for multiple sclerosis. Which of the following would *not* qualify to satisfy dissemination in time criteria under the 2017 McDonald Criteria?

T. Flagiello (✉) · V. Arena · T. E. Smith
Department of Neurology—Multiple Sclerosis, New York University Langone Medical Center, New York, NY, USA
e-mail: Thomas.Flagiello@nyulangone.org;
Vito.Arena@nyulangone.org; Tyler.Smith@nyulangone.org

T. E. Smith, V. Arena (eds.), *Essential Neurology Board Review Q & A*, https://doi.org/10.1007/978-3-032-17213-6_6

A. MRI brain/spinal cord with both enhancing and non-enhancing lesions on the same scan.

B. Cerebrospinal fluid (CSF) demonstrating four or more CSF-specific oligoclonal bands.

C. Serial MRI showing new T2/FLAIR non-enhancing lesions.

D. An additional clinical attack implicating a different CNS site with objective clinical evidence.

E. MRI scan with some lesions with associated T1 hypointensity.

Correct answer: E

Explanation

The 2017 revision to the McDonald Criteria was built on earlier iterations in an attempt to further enhance the sensitivity without sacrificing specificity. Consideration of prior symptoms alone can sometimes be helpful when description is compatible with a syndrome typical for MS, though it is recommended this be supported by evidence of a CNS lesion either by neurological exam or paraclinical testing. The criteria above were established to aid in objective demonstration of dissemination in time, including addition of CSF-specific oligoclonal bands in patients with one clinical attack and MRI only demonstrating dissemination in space. This allows for earlier diagnosis of MS.

Reference

Thompson AJ, Banwell BL, Barkhof F, Carroll WM, Coetzee T, Comi G, et al. Diagnosis of multiple sclerosis: 2017 revisions of the McDonald criteria. Lancet Neurol. 2018;17(2):162–73. https://doi.org/10.1016/s1474-4422(17)30470-2

Linked questions: 3–5

3. A 29-year-old woman presents to the ER with new neurological symptoms. She notes she woke up with numbness in her right hand extending halfway up her arm as well as mild numbness in her right foot up to the shin. Symptoms persisted and severity intensified and progressed to include the right side of her face over the course of the day. An MRI is obtained and key images are shown. Which of the following lesion locations is not part of the diagnostic criteria for dissemination in space for MS according to the 2017 McDonald Criteria?

A. Juxtacortical

B. Deep gray nuclei

C. Brain stem

D. Cerebellum

E. Spinal cord

Correct answer: B

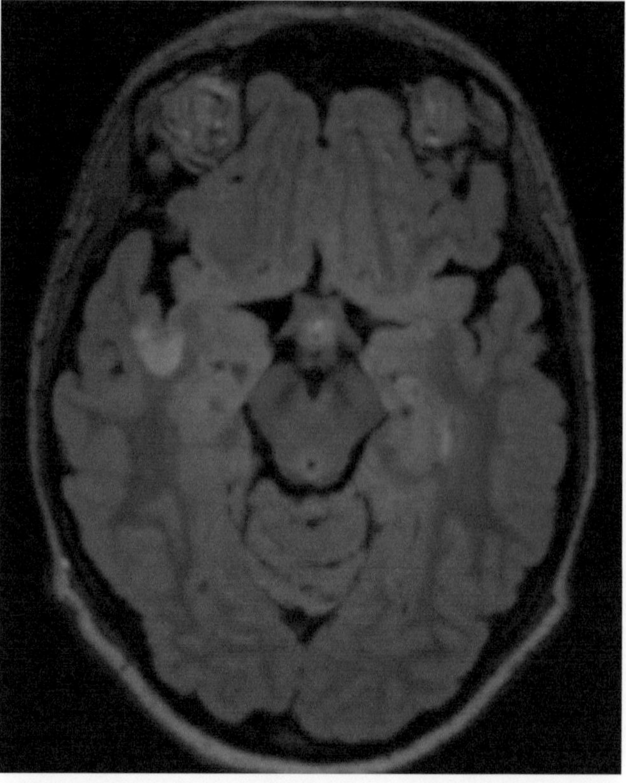

Axial FLAIR MRI brain. (Images courtesy of Dr. Vito Arena)

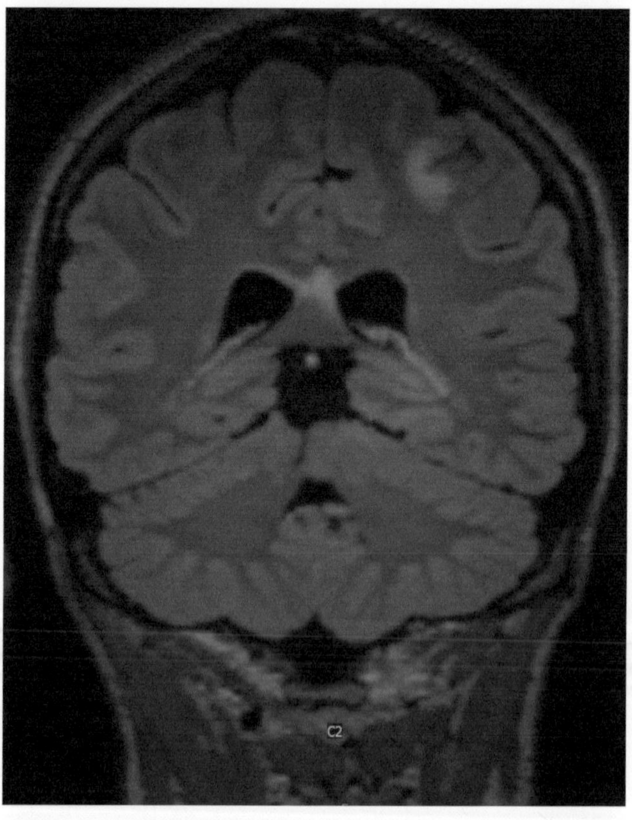

Coronal FLAIR MRI brain. (Images courtesy of Dr. Vito Arena)

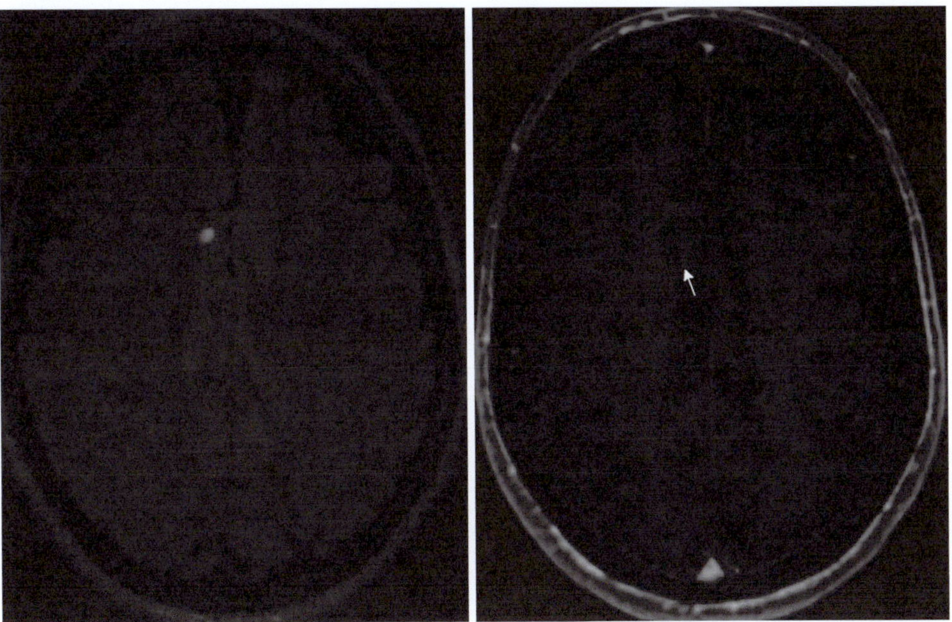

Left: Axial FLAIR MRI brain; Right: Axial post-contrast MRI brain. (Images courtesy of Dr. Vito Arena)

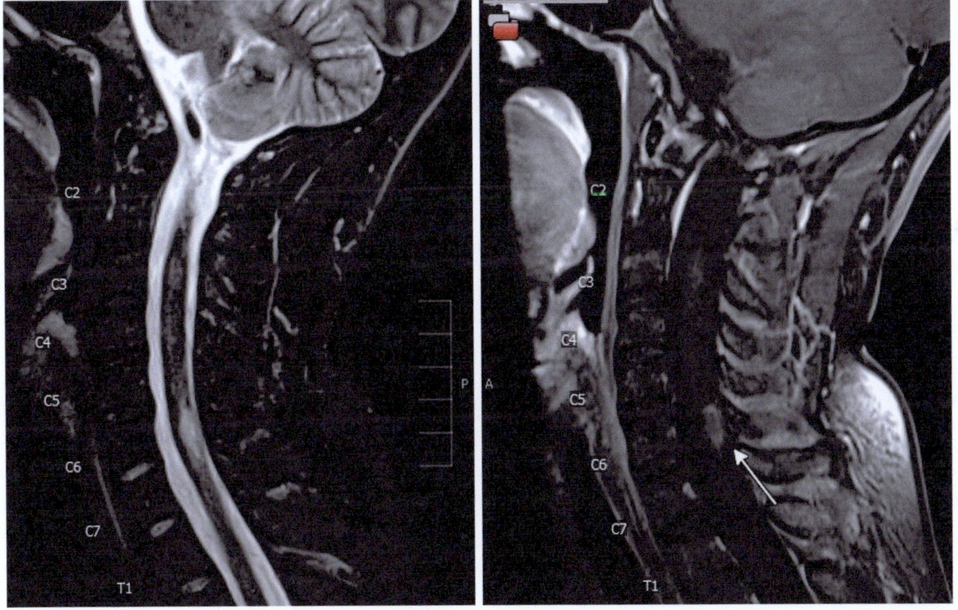

Left: Sagittal STIR MRI cervical spine; Right: Sagittal post-contrast MRI cervical spine. (Courtesy of Dr. Vito Arena)

Explanation

The four cardinal lesion locations designated in the 2017 McDonald Criteria include juxtacortical (no intervening white matter between the cortex and the lesion), periventricular (touching the ventricular surface and radiating perpendicularly, as often seen with Dawnson's fingers), infratentorial lesions (i.e., brainstem, middle cerebellar peduncle, cerebellum), and spinal cord. The optic nerve will be included as a lesion site in the 2024 McDonald Criteria.

Reference

Thompson AJ, Banwell BL, Barkhof F, Carroll WM, Coetzee T, Comi G, et al. Diagnosis of multiple sclerosis: 2017 revisions of the McDonald criteria. Lancet Neurol. 2018;17(2):162–73. https://doi.org/10.1016/s1474-4422(17)30470-2

Linked question

4. The patient notes that 2 months earlier while on vacation she felt very off balance for 3 days. She denies any history of abnormal rashes, joint pains, oral or genital ulcers, or other systemic symptoms. She has no other relevant past medical history. Based on her history and your review of the MRI, is further testing necessary to make a diagnosis and if so which testing?
   A. Yes, a lumbar puncture must be performed for oligoclonal bands.
   B. Yes, serum testing to check for aquaporin-4 antibody is necessary.
   C. No, the patient presented with a typical syndrome and the MRI findings above satisfy diagnostic criteria.
   D. Yes, an MRI of the spine must be completed.
   Correct answer: C

Explanation

This patient presented with a typical syndrome of MS. She has a brain MRI demonstrating periventricular and infratentorial regions, satisfying dissemination in space. She has lesions that are enhancing and lesions that are non-enhancing, satisfying dissemination in time. Her history does not suggest other red flags, making other diagnostic considerations less likely.

Reference

Thompson AJ, Banwell BL, Barkhof F, et al. Diagnosis of multiple sclerosis: 2017 revisions of the McDonald criteria.

Lancet Neurol. 2018;17(2):162–173. https://doi.org/10.1016/S1474-4422(17)30470-2

Linked question

5. You make a diagnosis of relapsing remitting multiple sclerosis (RRMS). The patient asks you about the prognosis. Which of the following carries higher risk of poor prognosis?
   A. Optic neuritis at onset
   B. Monosymptomatic onset
   C. Short inter-attack interval
   D. Poor recovery from initial relapse
   E. Both C and D
   Correct answer: E

Explanation

Prognostication in multiple sclerosis is challenging and imperfect. A host of variables may influence disease course. Disease-related clinical factors that may portend worse prognosis include higher number of relapses early in the disease; brief inter-attack intervals; poor recovery from first relapse; pyramidal, cerebellar, sphincteric, and cognitive symptoms at onset; multifocal presentation at onset; and progression at onset.

Reference

Amato MP, Ponziani G, Bartolozzi ML, Siracusa G. A prospective study on the natural history of multiple sclerosis: clues to the conduct and interpretation of clinical trials. J Neurol Sci. 1999;168(2):96–106. https://doi.org/10.1016/s0022-510x(99)00143-4

6. A 47-year-old man with a history of hyperlipidemia and current tobacco use presents to your clinic for evaluation. He developed numbness and weakness in the left hand several months ago. It worsened over the course of a week and persisted for 4 weeks. It has improved but has not fully resolved back to baseline. He notes he has had significant fatigue over the last 6 months and a history of insomnia. He reports numbness and tingling in the legs that started 2–3 years ago. An outside neurologist had performed a nerve conduction study which was unrevealing, and further evaluation was not pursued at that time. Numbness and tingling did not fully resolve. You order an MRI (see below).

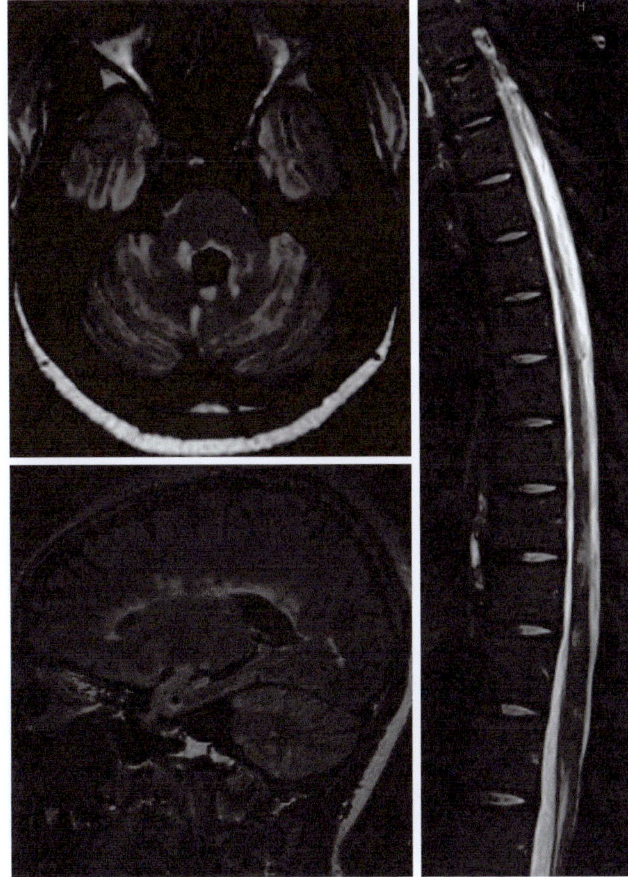

Top Left: Axial FLAIR MRI brain; Bottom Left: Sagittal FLAIR MRI brain; Right: Sagittal STIR MRI thoracic spine. (Images Courtesy of Dr. Vito Arena)

Of the following patient demographics, which has *not* been found to be a factor carrying worse prognosis at the time of MS diagnosis?

A. Older age at onset
B. Male sex
C. Smoking
D. White race and northern European ancestry
E. Comorbidities including hypertension

Correct answer: D

Explanation

Demographic features that may carry a worse prognosis at the time of MS diagnosis include older age at onset, male sex, smoking, psychiatric comorbidities (depression, anxiety, bipolar disorder), cardiovascular comorbidities, and social construct of race/ethnicity (Black, Hispanic/Latinx, middle eastern, north African, or Asian ancestry compared to white or Northern European ancestry).

References

Marrie RA, Rudick R, Horwitz R, Cutter G, Tyry T, Campagnolo D, et al. Vascular comorbidity is associated with more rapid disability progression in multiple sclerosis. Neurology. 2010;74(13):1041–7. https://doi.org/10.1212/WNL.0b013e3181d6b125.

Mowry EM, Pesic M, Grimes B, Deen SR, Bacchetti P, Waubant E. Clinical predictors of early second event in patients with clinically isolated syndrome. J Neurol. 2009;256(7):1061–6. https://doi.org/10.1007/s00415-009-5063-0.

7. Which of the following MRI features seen in multiple sclerosis is *not* associated with worse prognosis?
   A. Gadolinium-enhancing lesions within 6 to 9 months of starting a disease-modifying therapy (DMT)
   B. Infratentorial lesions
   C. Spinal cord lesions and atrophy
   D. Higher number of T2 lesion at baseline
   E. Paramagnetic rim lesions
   F. Periventricular predominance

Correct answer: F

Explanation

Various MRI features seen in MS have been studied for their prognostic value. A longitudinal study demonstrated a positive relationship between higher lesion load and proportion of patients reaching Expanded Disability Status Scale (EDSS) of 6.0 20 years later, where higher numbers indicate greater disability. Infratentorial lesions at baseline have been associated with higher risk of reaching EDSS of 3.0 and higher risk of conversion from clinically isolated syndrome (CIS) or radiographically isolated syndrome (RIS) to MS. Spinal cord lesions have been associated with higher rates of relapse, conversion from RIS to MS and CIS to MS. Spinal cord lesions and atrophy have been associated with disability progression in various studies. Having new gadolinium-enhancing lesions at 6 to 9 months after treatment initiation was associated with future relapse risk. Another study showed that two or more gadolinium-enhancing lesions on baseline MRI of CIS patients independently increased the risk of secondary progressive MS by a factor of 3.2 after 15 years of follow-up. Paramagnetic rim lesions have been associated with progression independent of relapse activity. Many other MRI measures have also been studied and may be associated with disability progression and worse clinical outcomes including various brain volume measures (whole brain, cortical, thalamic).

References

Cordonnier C, de Seze J, Breteau G, Ferriby D, Michelin E, Stojkovic T, et al. Prospective study of patients presenting with acute partial transverse myelopathy. J Neurol. 2003;250(12):1447–52. https://doi.org/10.1007/s00415-003-0242-x.

Fisniku LK, Brex PA, Altmann DR, Miszkiel KA, Benton CE, Lanyon R, et al. Disability and T2 MRI lesions: a 20-year follow-up of patients with relapse onset of multiple sclerosis. Brain. 2008;131(Pt 3):808–17. https://doi.org/10.1093/brain/awm329.

Sormani MP, Bruzzi P. MRI lesions as a surrogate for relapses in multiple sclerosis: a meta-analysis of randomised trials. Lancet Neurol. 2013;12(7):669–76. https://doi.org/10.1016/s1474-4422(13)70103-0

Tintore M, Rovira A, Arrambide G, Mitjana R, Río J, Auger C, et al. Brainstem lesions in clinically isolated syndromes. Neurology. 2010;75(21):1933–8. https://doi.org/10.1212/WNL.0b013e3181feb26f.

Linked questions: 8–10

8. A 28-year-old woman presents to her primary care doctor with several years of migraine with aura. An MRI is ordered and is shown below. She is referred to your office. On history, she describes typical scintillating scotoma preceding her migraines. She denies any other transient or episodic neurological symptoms. Your neurological exam is normal. This would best be described as follows:

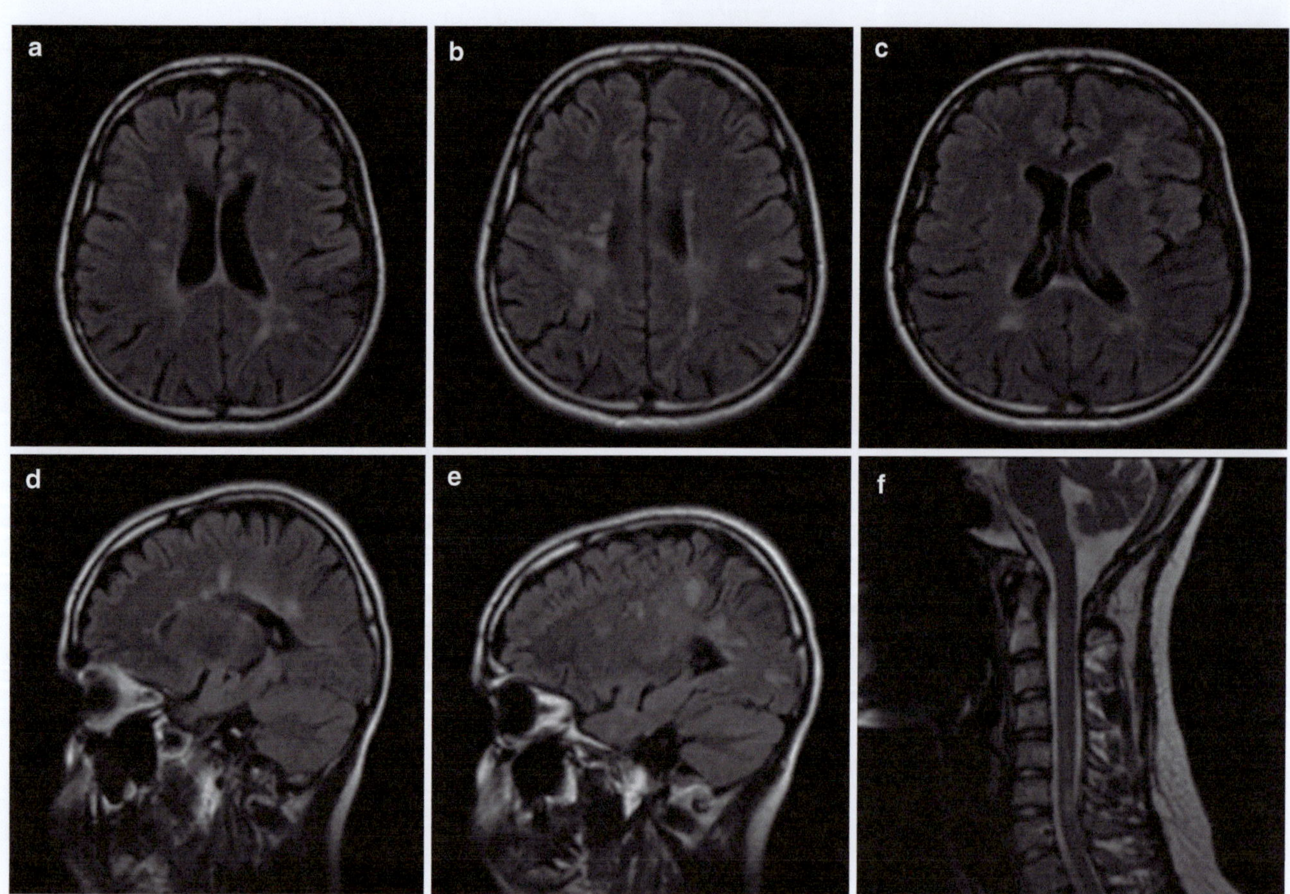

Axial MRI brain (**a–e**) and sagittal MRI cervical spine. (Image source: Alroughani, R., Ahmed, S., Khan, R., and Al-Hashel, J. CC-BY 4.0 (https://creativecommons.org/licenses/by/4.0/) via *SpringerPlus*. Image has not been modified from source. Please see full attribution with citation below in references section for this question.)

A. Relapsing remitting multiple sclerosis
B. Benign white matter abnormality associated with migraines
C. Radiologically isolated syndrome
D. Early onset microvascular ischemic changes
Correct answer: C

Explanation

The MRI demonstrates features that are typical of multiple sclerosis; however, she has no history suggestive of prior typical demyelinating syndromes and has a normal neurological exam. Radiologically isolated syndrome is defined as the presence of asymptomatic, incidentally identified demyelinating-appearing white matter lesions in the CNS within individuals lacking symptoms typical of MS in the 2017 McDonald Criteria. Note that the criteria for RIS will be modified under the 2024 McDonald Criteria (these individuals may be simply diagnosed as multiple sclerosis in the future).

References

Alroughani R, Ahmed SF, Khan R, Al-Hashel J. Status migrainosus as an initial presentation of multiple sclerosis. Springerplus. 2015;4:28. https://doi.org/10.1186/s40064-015-0818-9.

Lebrun-Frénay C, Okuda DT, Siva A, Landes-Chateau C, Azevedo CJ, Mondot L, et al. The radiologically isolated syndrome: revised diagnostic criteria. Brain. 2023;146(8):3431–43. https://doi.org/10.1093/brain/awad073.

Linked question

9. What further testing can help you stratify risk for this patient for conversion to clinically definite multiple sclerosis?
   A. MRI spinal cord
   B. Myelin basic protein levels
   C. CSF testing for oligoclonal bands
   D. Serum testing for ESR/CRP, ANA, MOG antibody
   E. MR angiogram of the head
   F. A and C
   Correct answer: F

Linked question

10. Which is not a factor that has been shown to increase the risk for conversion to clinically definite MS?
    A. Age greater than 37
    B. Infratentorial lesions
    C. Spinal cord lesions
    D. Oligoclonal bands
    E. Gadolinium enhancing lesions on follow up scan
    Correct answer: A

Explanation (Questions 9 and 10)

Studies suggest that about 50% of people with RIS will develop relapsing or progressive symptoms of multiple sclerosis within 10 years. Age (younger), positive cerebrospinal fluid for CSF-specific oligoclonal bands, and infratentorial lesions and spinal cord lesions on MRI were baseline independent predictors associated with a subsequent clinical event at 5 and 10 years. The presence of gadolinium-enhanced lesions during follow-up was also associated with the risk of a seminal event at 10 years. Note that the criteria for RIS will be modified under the 2024 McDonald Criteria (these individuals may be simply diagnosed as multiple sclerosis in the future).

Reference

Lebrun-Frenay C, Kantarci O, Siva A, Sormani MP, Pelletier D, Okuda DT. Radiologically Isolated Syndrome: 10-Year Risk Estimate of a Clinical Event. Ann Neurol. 2020;88(2):407–17. https://doi.org/10.1002/ana.25799.

11. What virus has been most implicated in the pathogenesis of multiple sclerosis?
    A. Cytomegalovirus (CMV)
    B. Epstein-Barr virus (EBV)
    C. Human papillomavirus (HPV)
    D. Influenza A virus
    E. Varicella-zoster virus (VZV)
    Correct answer: B

Explanation

Epstein-Barr virus has been identified as a likely immune system stimulus in the development of MS. Nearly 100% of patients with MS have antibodies to EBV in their blood, suggesting the virus serves as a stimulus of the immune system and may be necessary but not sufficient for the development of MS. Of the other viruses listed, CMV and VZV have also been linked to MS, but with less robust evidence.

Reference

Abrahamyan S, Eberspächer B, Hoshi MM, Aly L, Luessi F, Groppa S, et al. Complete Epstein-Barr virus seropositivity in a large cohort of patients with early multiple sclerosis. J Neurol Neurosurg Psychiatry. 2020;91(7):681–6. https://doi.org/10.1136/jnnp-2020-322941.

12. What environmental factor has *not* been positively associated with an increased prevalence of MS?
    A. Increased distance from the equator
    B. Obesity in childhood and adolescence
    C. Tobacco smoking
    D. Increased sunlight exposure
    Correct answer: D

Explanation

Higher latitude, particularly prior to puberty, is linked to a higher prevalence of MS. One proposed explanation for this is that sunlight exposure may be protective, owing to either a direct effect of ultraviolet radiation or higher levels of serum vitamin D. Other modifiable risk factors that are linked to increased risk of developing MS include obesity during childhood and adolescence and tobacco smoking.

References

Jacobs BM, Noyce AJ, Giovannoni G, Dobson R. BMI and low vitamin D are causal factors for multiple sclerosis: A Mendelian Randomization study. Neurol Neuroimmunol Neuroinflamm. 2020;7(2). https://doi.org/10.1212/NXI.0000000000000662.

Riise T, Nortvedt MW, Ascherio A. Smoking is a risk factor for multiple sclerosis. Neurology. 2003;61(8):1122–4. https://doi.org/10.1212/01.wnl.0000081305.66687.d2.

Simpson S, Jr., Wang W, Otahal P, Blizzard L, van der Mei IAF, Taylor BV. Latitude continues to be significantly associated with the prevalence of multiple sclerosis: an updated meta-analysis. J Neurol Neurosurg Psychiatry. 2019;90(11):1193–200. https://doi.org/10.1136/jnnp-2018-320189.

13. Which of the following is considered an uncommon symptom of MS?
    A. Fatigue
    B. Depression
    C. Bladder dysfunction
    D. Seizure
    E. Cognitive dysfunction
    Correct answer: D

Explanation

All of these symptoms can be seen in patients with MS. Fatigue is one of the most commonly reported symptoms manifesting as a physical exhaustion that worsens as the day progresses. This can be worsened by other MS-related symptoms including sleep disturbances and depression, the latter which is seen in more than half of patients with MS. Neurogenic bladder in patients with MS can be characterized by difficulty storing urine or incomplete emptying, and more than one type can exist in the same patient. Common symptoms are urinary frequency, urgency, nocturia, and weak urinary stream. Cognitive dysfunction manifests most often as deficits in attention, processing speed, executive function, and short-term memory loss and has been correlated with cerebral disease burden and cortical atrophy. Seizures are a rare symptom of MS (<5% of patients); however, studies have demonstrated a three to six times higher prevalence in patients with MS compared to the general population.

Reference

Schorner A, Weissert R. Patients with Epileptic Seizures and Multiple Sclerosis in a Multiple Sclerosis Center in Southern Germany Between 2003–2015. Front Neurol. 2019;10:613. https://doi.org/10.3389/fneur.2019.00613.

14. You are consulted on a 27-year-old male patient with a history of sensory myelitis followed 2 years later by diplopia secondary to an internuclear ophthalmoplegia. MRI of the brain and spine shows lesions meeting MS diagnostic criteria. The pathology of MS lesions includes all of the following except:
    A. Pathologic heterogeneity of early active MS plaques with four distinct immunopatterns.
    B. Chronic plaques may be inactive or active/smoldering.
    C. Remyelinated plaques, aka shadow plaques.
    D. Meningeal inflammatory infiltrates characterized by lymphoid follicle-like structures.
    E. Astrocyte loss, dystrophic astrocytic profiles, and GFAP-laden macrophages suggesting phagocytosis of lytic astrocytes by macrophages.
    Correct answer: E

Explanation

The pathology of MS lesions is complex and varies by lesion type and location. Various immunopatterns of active lesions have been described by Luchinetti and colleagues which may suggest inter-patient differences in the targets of injury and mechanisms of demyelination. Astrocytopathy, as alluded to in choice E, is a hallmark of NMOSD.

References

Lucchinetti CF, Guo Y, Popescu BF, Fujihara K, Itoyama Y, Misu T. The pathology of an autoimmune astrocytopathy: lessons learned from neuromyelitis optica. Brain Pathol. 2014;24(1):83–97. https://doi.org/10.1111/bpa.12099.

Popescu BF, Pirko I, Lucchinetti CF. Pathology of multiple sclerosis: where do we stand? Continuum (Minneap Minn). 2013;19(4 Multiple Sclerosis):901–21. https://doi.org/10.1212/01.CON.0000433291.23091.65.

Linked questions: 15–16

15. A 32-year-old man with newly diagnosed MS presents to the emergency room with 1 week of painful spasms in his right arm and leg. He shows you a video of an episode where his right elbow, wrist, and ankle are force-

fully contracted for 1–2 minutes with preserved awareness. These episodes are very painful and have occurred in clusters for the past week. Electroencephalogram (EEG) capturing an episode is normal, and MRI brain and spine do not reveal new lesions. What is the most likely diagnosis?

A. Focal motor seizure
B. Psychogenic movement disorder
C. Paroxysmal dystonia
D. Basal ganglia infarct
E. Tics

Correct answer: C

Linked question

16. What medication can be offered to alleviate these movements described in the question above?

A. Levodopa
B. Venlafaxine
C. Ondansetron
D. Carbamazepine
E. Propranolol

Correct answer: D

Explanation (Questions 15 and 16)

This patient presents with paroxysmal dystonia (PD), which are characterized by sudden, brief, and stereotyped episodes that typically involve unilateral upper and lower extremities and can spread to involve the face. They can be the initial manifestation of MS or occur throughout the disease course. PD belongs to a larger group of paroxysmal symptoms seen in MS, and other examples include trigeminal neuralgia and ataxia/dysarthria. The unrevealing EEG and MRI make choice (a) and (d) unlikely. Treatment options include pulse steroid therapy and antiseizure medications, particularly carbamazepine and oxcarbazepine.

Reference

Freiha J, Riachi N, Chalah MA, Zoghaib R, Ayache SS, Ahdab R. Paroxysmal Symptoms in Multiple Sclerosis-A Review of the Literature. J Clin Med. 2020;9(10). https://doi.org/10.3390/jcm9103100.

17. Which acute demyelinating disorder is characterized by white matter lesions with alternative hyperintense and isointense rings on T1-weighted MRI imaging?

A. Marburg variant of MS
B. ADEM
C. Acute hemorrhagic leukoencephalopathy (AHLE)
D. Baló disease
E. Progressive multifocal leukoencephalopathy (PML)

Correct answer: D

Explanation

Baló disease (also known as Baló concentric sclerosis) is considered a variant of MS. It has a classic "bullseye" or "onion bulb" appearance on MRI due to alternating bands of demyelination and preserved white matter. The Marburg variant of MS is characterized by fulminant demyelination with an aggressive course that often causes death within months of onset. Radiographically, acute disseminated encephalomyelitis (ADEM) appears as multifocal ill-defined lesions throughout the brain and spinal cord, and acute hemorrhagic leukoencephalitis (AHLE) is considered a severe form with associated hemorrhage and extensive mass effect and edema. Progressive multifocal leukoencephalopathy (PML) is an infection caused by the John Cunningham virus and on MRI will appear as multifocal, asymmetric white matter lesions with preferential involvement of the parieto-occipital regions and the subcortical U-fibers.

References

Czeisler BM. Emergent Management of Central Nervous System Demyelinating Disorders. Continuum (Minneap Minn). 2024;30(3):781–817. https://doi.org/10.1212/CON.0000000000001436.

Gavra M, Boviatsis E, Stavrinou LC, Sakas D. Pitfalls in the diagnosis of a tumefactive demyelinating lesion: A case report. J Med Case Rep. 2011;5:217. https://doi.org/10.1186/1752-1947-5-217.

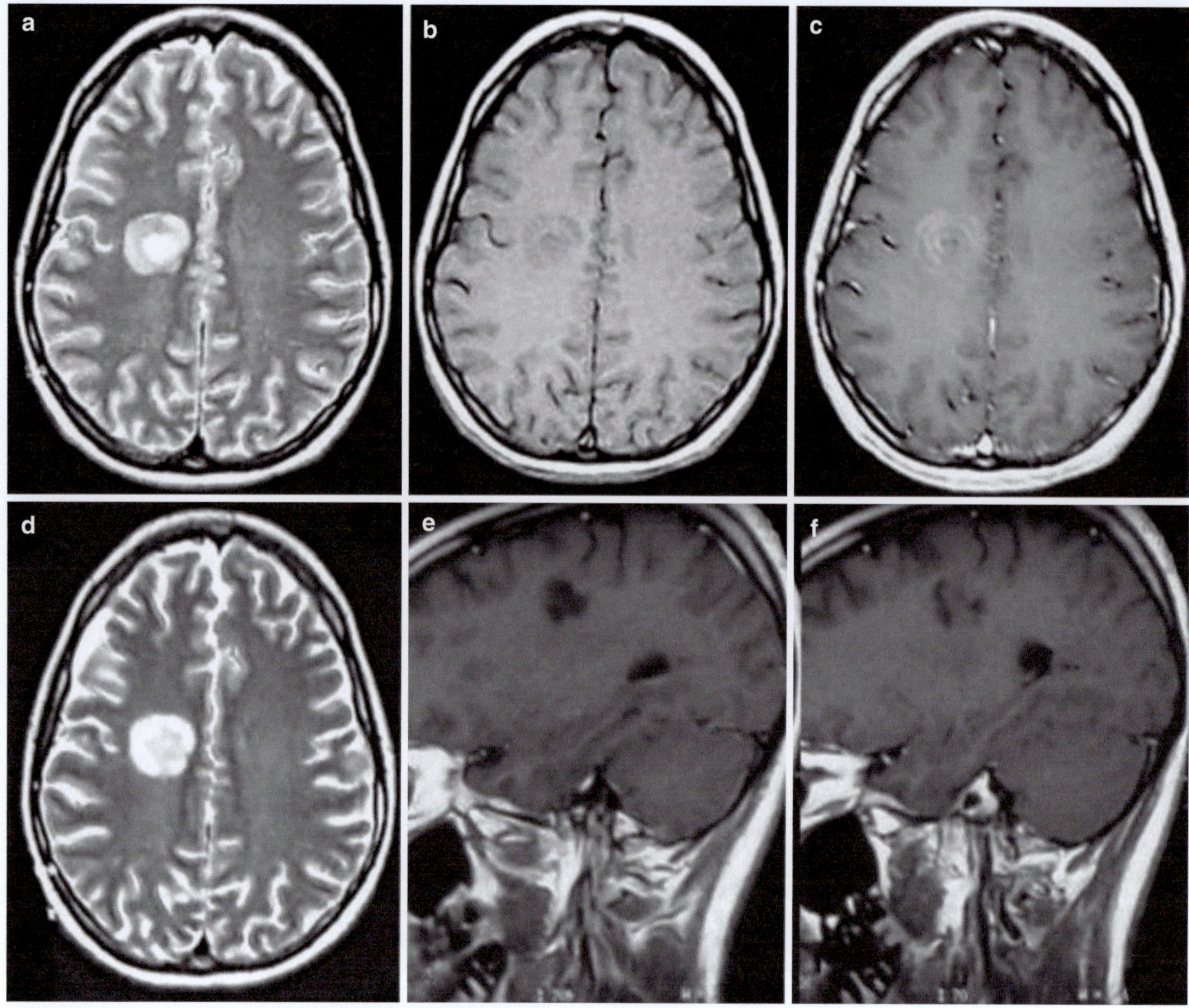

MRI brain of an individual with Baló concentric sclerosis. Note the concentric patterns of signal change, particular in images (**a–c**). Image (**d**) shows 1 month follow-up after therapy. Images (**e** and **f**) are post-contrast T1-weighted images. (Image source: Gavra, M., Boviatsis, E., Stavrinou, L., Sakas, D. CC-BY 2.0. (https://creativecommons.org/licenses/by/2.0/) via Journal of Medical Case Reports. Image has not been modified from source. Please see full attribution with citation below in references section for this question.)

18. Which of the following magnetic resonance imaging findings is *most* suggestive of a tumefactive demyelinating lesion compared to a high-grade glioma?
    A. Significant mass effect
    B. Incomplete ring of enhancement with gadolinium
    C. High cerebral blood volume on perfusion imaging
    D. Involvement of the cortex
    E. Internal susceptibility artifact on susceptibility-weighted imaging

Correct answer: B

Explanation

Tumefactive demyelinating lesions (TDL) are defined as greater than two centimeters in diameter and mimic neoplasm (e.g., lymphoma, glioma) on imaging. They may demonstrate an open ring of enhancement on post-gadolinium sequences with the incomplete portion facing the gray matter. Other characteristics that favor TDL include lack of cortical Involvement, less mass effect than expected for size, and low relative cerebral blood volume on perfusion MRI, although there is significant variability in all of these imaging findings, and caution should be used when relying on them to differentiate between demyelinating and neoplastic lesions.

References

Gavra M, Boviatsis E, Stavrinou LC, Sakas D. Pitfalls in the diagnosis of a tumefactive demyelinating lesion: A case report. J Med Case Rep. 2011;5:217. https://doi.org/10.1186/1752-1947-5-217.

Kim DS, Na DG, Kim KH, Kim JH, Kim E, Yun BL, Chang KH. Distinguishing tumefactive demyelinating lesions from glioma or central nervous system lymphoma: added value of unenhanced CT compared with conventional contrast-enhanced MR imaging. Radiology. 2009;251(2):467–75. https://doi.org/10.1148/radiol.2512072071.

Masdeu JC, Quinto C, Olivera C, Tenner M, Leslie D, Visintainer P. Open-ring imaging sign: highly specific for atypical brain demyelination. Neurology. 2000;54(7):1427–33. https://doi.org/10.1212/wnl.54.7.1427.

19. Which of the following disease-modifying therapies (DMTs) is associated with the highest rate of progressive multifocal leukoencephalopathy (PML)?
    A. Natalizumab
    B. Ocrelizumab
    C. Teriflunomide
    D. Dimethyl fumarate
    E. Glatiramer acetate

Correct answer: A

Explanation

Natalizumab is associated with the highest rate of PML among the DMTs used in the treatment of multiple sclerosis, with a total of 839 cases of PML among 213,000 patients exposed to natalizumab as of August 2020.

Reference

Smith TE, Kister I. Infection Mitigation Strategies for Multiple Sclerosis Patients on Oral and Monoclonal Disease-Modifying Therapies. Curr Neurol Neurosci Rep. 2021;21(7):36. https://doi.org/10.1007/s11910-021-01117-y.

20. A 32-year-old female has been recently diagnosed with RRMS. She is actively trying to conceive, which of the following DMTs would be most important to avoid?
    A. Dimethyl fumarate
    B. Glatiramer acetate
    C. Teriflunomide
    D. Ocrelizumab
    E. Fingolimod

Correct answer: C

Explanation

Of the DMTs listed, teriflunomide has the highest risk of fetotoxicity. Pregnancy should be excluded prior to starting teriflunomide, and effective contraception should be advised while taking teriflunomide. Additionally, if the patient becomes pregnant or is imminently considering pregnancy, teriflunomide should be discontinued and charcoal or cholestyramine should be administered as part of an accelerated-elimination protocol.

Reference

Bove RM, Houtchens MK. Pregnancy Management in Multiple Sclerosis and Other Demyelinating Diseases. Continuum (Minneap Minn). 2022;28(1):12–33. https://doi.org/10.1212/con.0000000000001108.

21. Which of the following DMTs is associated with a risk of macular edema?
    A. Fingolimod
    B. Glatiramer acetate
    C. Cladribine
    D. Ocrelizumab
    E. Ofatumumab

Correct answer: A

Explanation

Fingolimod is a sphingosine-1 phosphate (S1P) receptor modulator, and this class of DMT is associated with a risk of macular edema. Patients should have an ophthalmologic exam to confirm the absence of macular edema prior to starting an S1P modulator and then periodically while on therapy.

Reference

Coyle PK, Freedman MS, Cohen BA, Cree BAC, Markowitz CE. Sphingosine 1-phosphate receptor modulators in multiple sclerosis treatment: A practical review. Ann Clin Transl Neurol. 2024;11(4):842–55. https://doi.org/10.1002/acn3.52017.

22. Which of the following DMTs should not be used in the treatment of multiple sclerosis in a patient with inflammatory bowel disease (IBD)?
    A. Natalizumab
    B. Ocrelizumab
    C. Ozanimod
    D. Teriflunomide
    E. Dimethyl fumarate
    Correct answer: B

Explanation

Anti-CD20 therapies (such as ocrelizumab, and potentially ofatumumab, rituximab, and ublituximab as well) have been associated with an increased risk of developing immune-mediated colitis and should be avoided in those who have a pre-existing diagnosis of IBD.

References

Kim T, Brinker A, Croteau D, Lee PR, Baldassari LE, Stevens J, et al. Immune-mediated colitis associated with ocrelizumab: A new safety risk. Mult Scler. 2023;29(10):1275–81. https://doi org/10.1177/13524585231195854.

Tolaymat S, Sharma K, Kagzi Y, Sriwastava S. Anti-CD20 monoclonal antibody (mAb) therapy and colitis: A case series and review. Mult Scler Relat Disord. 2023;75:104763. https://doi.org/10.1016/j.msard.2023.104763.

23. A 44-year-old female with multiple sclerosis has been treated with natalizumab for 8 months. During this time, she has been clinically stable up until 2 weeks ago, when she developed new right hemiparesis. Her serum JC virus antibody level is negative. Her MRI shows multiple enhancing lesions. Which of the following is the best next step in the workup of these new lesions?
    A. Check anti-natalizumab antibodies in the serum
    B. Check John Cunningham (JC) virus PCR in the serum
    C. Perform a lumbar puncture to check for malignancy
    D. Check a panel of autoimmune encephalitis antibodies in the serum
    Correct answer: A

Explanation

While rare, individuals can develop anti-natalizumab antibodies that lower the efficacy of natalizumab. She is unlikely to have progressive multifocal leukoencephalopathy (PML) with a negative serum JC virus level. While a malignancy could be considered, the less invasive and better next step would be to rule out anti-natalizumab antibodies.

Reference

Calabresi PA, Giovannoni G, Confavreux C, Galetta SL, Havrdova E, Hutchinson M, et al. The incidence and significance of anti-natalizumab antibodies: results from AFFIRM and SENTINEL. Neurology. 2007;69(14):1391–403. https://doi.org/10.1212/01.wnl.0000277457.17420.b5.

24. A 42-year-old female with MS has been treated with natalizumab for 5 years, with no new relapses nor progression. She asks what factors contribute to her risk of PML. What would you counsel her?
    A. Patients with progressive forms of MS are at higher risk of PML.
    B. Higher titers of JC virus antibody are associated with a higher risk of PML.
    C. Pregnancy lowers the risk of developing PML.
    D. Initial JC virus infections are associated with a rash.
    Correct answer: B

Explanation

Higher serum titers of JC virus antibody are associated with a higher risk of PML. The JC virus PCR is best tested in the CSF when there is concern for PML, but is not used for regular monitoring. The type of MS is not associated with a different risk of PML. JC virus infections appear to be asymptomatic.

Reference

Ho PR, Koendgen H, Campbell N, Haddock B, Richman S, Chang I. Risk of natalizumab-associated progressive multifocal leukoencephalopathy in patients with multiple sclerosis: a retrospective analysis of data from four clinical studies. Lancet Neurol. 2017;16(11):925–33. https://doi.org/10.1016/s1474-4422(17)30282-x

25. A 45-year-old male has had a progressively worsening decline in gait over the last 3 years. His MRI demonstrates T2 hyperintensities in periventricular and infratentorial regions, as well as multiple short segment T2 hyperintensities in the cervical and thoracic spine.

He undergoes a lumbar puncture, which reveals eight oligoclonal bands unique to the CSF. Which of the following is the best treatment for him?

A. Siponimod
B. Natalizumab
C. Glatiramer acetate
D. Ocrelizumab
E. Cladribine

Correct answer: D

Explanation

Once alternative etiologies have been reasonably ruled out, this patient meets diagnostic criteria for primary progressive multiple sclerosis. As of publication, ocrelizumab is the only DMT on this list to demonstrate benefit in limiting progression in primary progressive multiple sclerosis.

Reference

Montalban X, Hauser SL, Kappos L, Arnold DL, Bar-Or A, Comi G, et al. Ocrelizumab versus Placebo in Primary Progressive Multiple Sclerosis. N Engl J Med. 2017;376(3):209–20. https://doi.org/10.1056/NEJMoa1606468.

26. A 42-year-old female comes to your clinic for a second opinion. She was diagnosed with multiple sclerosis after she developed cervical myelitis when she was 20 years old. She was started on interferon beta-1a, which she continues to take. Over the years, she had multiple relapses, which responded well to intravenous steroids. Over the last 4 years she has had a progressive decline in strength of her right leg and has not improved with steroid administration. Offering which of the following DMTs would be the best next step?

    A. Siponimod
    B. Natalizumab
    C. Teriflunomide
    D. Cladribine
    E. Satralizumab

    Correct answer: A

Explanation

Her clinical course suggests progression to secondary progressive multiple sclerosis (SPMS). As of publication, siponimod is the only DMT on this list to demonstrate efficacy in reducing the risk of disability progression in SPMS.

Reference

Kappos L, Bar-Or A, Cree BAC, Fox RJ, Giovannoni G, Gold R, et al. Siponimod versus placebo in secondary progressive multiple sclerosis (EXPAND): a double-blind, randomised, phase 3 study. Lancet. 2018;391(10127):1263–73. https://doi.org/10.1016/S0140-6736(18)30475-6

27. Which of the following is the mechanism of action of natalizumab?

    A. Integrin agonist
    B. Binds directly to VCAM-1 on leukocytes
    C. Binds to α4-subunit of α4β1 and α4β7 integrins
    D. Blocks sphingosine-1 phosphate receptor
    E. Binds to CD20 marker on B lymphocytes

    Correct answer: C

Explanation

Natalizumab bands to the α4-subunit of α4β1 (which comprises VLA-4) and α4β7 integrins present on many leukocytes. These integrins allow leukocytes to bind to vascular cell adhesion molecule-1 (VCAM-1) expressed on vascular endothelial cells, to allow transmigration of leukocytes across the blood brain barrier. The oral medications fingolimod, siponimod, ozanimod, and ponesimod target sphingosine-1 phosphate receptors. Ocrelizumab, ofatumumab, and ublituximab bind to the CD20 marker on B lymphocytes.

References

Engelhardt B, Kappos L. Natalizumab: targeting alpha4-integrins in multiple sclerosis. Neurodegener Dis. 2008;5(1):16–22. https://doi.org/10.1159/000109933.

Rice GP, Hartung HP, Calabresi PA. Anti-alpha4 integrin therapy for multiple sclerosis: mechanisms and rationale. Neurology. 2005;64(8):1336–42. https://doi.org/10.1212/01.Wnl.0000158329.30470.D0.

28. Which of the following adverse effects is correctly paired with the disease-modifying therapy used in the treatment of multiple sclerosis?

    A. Teriflunomide; transaminitis
    B. Interferon beta; flushing
    C. Dimethyl fumarate; flu-like symptoms
    D. Ocrelizumab; lipoatrophy
    E. Glatiramer acetate; hypogammaglobulinemia

    Correct answer: A

Explanation

Teriflunomide is associated with transaminitis. As such, hepatic function labs are recommended monthly for the first 6 months of therapy. Interferons are associated with flu-like symptoms, dimethyl fumarate is associated with flushing, ocrelizumab is associated with hypogammaglobulincmia, and glatiramer acetate is associated with lipoatrophy.

References

Confavreux C, O'Connor P, Comi G, Freedman MS, Miller AE, Olsson TP, et al. Oral teriflunomide for patients with relapsing multiple sclerosis (TOWER): a randomised, double-blind, placebo-controlled, phase 3 trial. Lancet

Neurol. 2014;13(3):247–56. https://doi.org/10.1016/s1474-4422(13)70308-9.

Cross A, Riley C. Treatment of Multiple Sclerosis. Continuum (Minneap Minn). 2022;28(4):1025–51. https://doi.org/10.1212/con.0000000000001170.

29. Which of the following vaccinations should be avoided in an individual who is currently being treated with ocrelizumab?
    A. Hepatitis B
    B. Yellow fever
    C. Zoster
    D. Varicella
    E. Influenza
    F. A and B
    G. B and D
    H. C and E
    Correct answer: G

Explanation

Yellow fever and varicella vaccinations are both live vaccines and are not recommended during ocrelizumab treatment. Live vaccines should be administered prior to starting treatment with ocrelizumab. The other options listed are not live vaccines so they can be safely administered, although there is ongoing research into the optimal timing of vaccine administration during the every 6 month ocrelizumab infusion cycle.

Reference

Otero-Romero S, Lebrun-Frénay C, Reyes S, Amato MP, Campins M, Farez M, et al. ECTRIMS/EAN consensus on vaccination in people with multiple sclerosis: Improving immunization strategies in the era of highly active immunotherapeutic drugs. Mult Scler. 2023;29(8):904–25. https://doi.org/10.1177/13524585231168043.

30. A 29-year-old woman with RRMS presents with acute onset right arm weakness and difficulty walking. MRI brain reveals multiple juxtacortical and periventricular lesions with associated enhancement, not present on an MRI from 2 months prior. She tells you that she discontinued her DMT in preparation for pregnancy 4 weeks ago. Of the following options, which medication was she most likely previously taking?
    A. Dimethyl fumarate
    B. Fingolimod
    C. Ublituximab
    D. Glatiramer acetate
    E. Teriflunomide
    Correct answer: B

Explanation

This clinical scenario is most consistent with the "rebound phenomenon," which is characterized by clinical deterioration and/or evidence of new disease activity on MRI. after stopping DMTs. Drugs used in the treatment of MS that are associated with a higher risk of rebound include natalizumab and the sphingosine 1-phosphate modulators (e.g., fingolimod). This should be taken into account when prescribing these medications to people of child-bearing potential. Treatment strategies that have been implemented in rebound activity after fingolimod or natalizumab cessation include corticosteroids, plasma exchange, and anti-CD20 therapies (e.g., ocrelizumab).

Reference

Barry B, Erwin AA, Stevens J, Tornatore C. Fingolimod Rebound: - Review of the Clinical Experience and Management Considerations. Neurol Ther. 2019;8(2):241–50. https://doi.org/10.1007/s40120-019-00160-9.

Linked questions: 31–32

31. A 30-year-old female presents to clinic with a new diagnosis of RRMS. She is not interested in having children in the future. After an extensive discussion of different disease DMTs and a shared decision-making process, you prescribe dimethyl fumarate. After 2 years of disease stability, she experiences a severe relapse in which she loses significant strength in her legs. You recommend switching to a higher-efficacy DMT. Her labs are below. Which of the following disease-modifying therapies (DMT) would be the most appropriate next step?
    CBC unremarkable
    CMP unremarkable
    Hepatitis B core antibody positive
    Hepatitis C antibody negative
    Quantiferon negative
    JC virus antibody negative
    A. Glatiramer acetate
    B. Interferon beta
    C. Ocrelizumab
    D. Natalizumab
    E. Ofatumumab
    Correct answer: D

Explanation

Interferon beta and glatiramer acetate are unlikely to offer a significantly reduced risk of relapse relative to dimethyl fumarate. While anti-CD20 agents such as ocrelizumab and ofatumumab have higher efficacy than dimethyl fumarate, they increase the risk of hepatitis B virus reactivation, and this patient has a history of hepatitis B infection as evidence by the positive hepatitis B core antibody. It is possible to prescribe an antiviral to reduce the risk of hepatitis B reactivation in an individual receiving treatment with an anti-CD20 agent, but the best choice is likely to avoid this additional infectious risk and begin with natalizumab. One of the paramount risks associated with natalizumab is developing PML caused by JC virus, for which this individual has tested negative.

References

Cross A, Riley C. Treatment of Multiple Sclerosis. Continuum (Minneap Minn). 2022;28(4):1025–51. https://doi.org/10.1212/con.0000000000001170.

Terrault NA, Lok ASF, McMahon BJ, Chang KM, Hwang JP, Jonas MM, et al. Update on prevention, diagnosis, and treatment of chronic hepatitis B: AASLD 2018 hepatitis B guidance. Hepatology. 2018;67(4):1560–99. https://doi.org/10.1002/hep.29800

Linked question

32. The patient from the prior question continues on natalizumab for 4 more years with no further relapses. At this time, she develops a positive JC virus antibody. Her MRI shows no changes and she has no new symptoms. Repeat labs demonstrate negative hepatitis B surface antigen, positive hepatitis B core antibody, and negative hepatitis B surface antigen. You discuss a switch to ofatumumab. Which of the following would be needed to safely switch to ofatumumab?
    A. Plasma exchange prior to starting ofatumumab
    B. Regular hepatic panel monitoring while on ofatumumab
    C. Hepatitis B vaccination
    D. None, switching to ofatumumab is not recommended due to history of hepatitis B
    E. Consult hepatology to discuss treatment with an antiviral while on ofatumumab

    Correct answer: E

Explanation

The anti-CD20 agents lead to increased risk hepatitis B virus reactivation. This risk can be mitigated through the use of ongoing antiviral treatment. As such, it is prudent to involve a hepatologist to manage antivirals to limit the risk of hepatitis B virus reactivation if treatment with ofatumumab is being considered.

Reference

Terrault NA, Lok ASF, McMahon BJ, Chang KM, Hwang JP, Jonas MM, et al. Update on prevention, diagnosis, and treatment of chronic hepatitis B: AASLD 2018 hepatitis B

guidance. Hepatology. 2018;67(4):1560–99. https://doi.org/10.1002/hep.29800

33. Which of the following disease-modifying therapies (DMTs) are correctly paired with their mechanism of action?
    A. Ublituximab; impairs DNA synthesis, cytotoxic to T and B lymphocytes.
    B. Cladribine; targets lymphocytes by binding to CD52 and effecting cytolysis.
    C. Alemtuzumab; binds CD20 on B cells and effects cytolysis.
    D. Teriflunomide; targets VLA-4 to impair lymphocyte transmigration.
    E. Ozanimod; targets sphingosine-1-phosphate receptor to impair lymphocyte migration from lymphoid tissues.

    Correct answer: E

Explanation

- Ozanimod is a sphingosine-1-phosphate receptor inhibitor that impairs lymphocyte migration from lymphoid tissues.
- Ublituximab binds to CD20 on B lymphocytes leading to their depletion.
- Cladribine is a nucleoside analogue of deoxyadenosine and is cytotoxic to T and B lymphocytes.
- Alemtuzumab binds to CD52 leading to lymphocyte depletion.
- Natalizumab targets the alpha-4 integrin subunit of VLA-4 to impair lymphocyte transmigration.
- Teriflunomide impairs lymphocyte proliferation through inhibition of dihydroorotate dehydrogenase.

Reference

Cross A, Riley C. Treatment of Multiple Sclerosis. Continuum (Minneap Minn). 2022;28(4):1025–51. https://doi.org/10.1212/con.0000000000001170.

Linked questions: 34–35

34. A 59-year-old man with MS, on natalizumab for 7 years, clinically stable for the last 5 years, presents discoordination over a 3 week period. He does not get regular laboratory tests. On exam, you also identify impaired visual fields. You obtain an MRI, seen below. What is the next step?

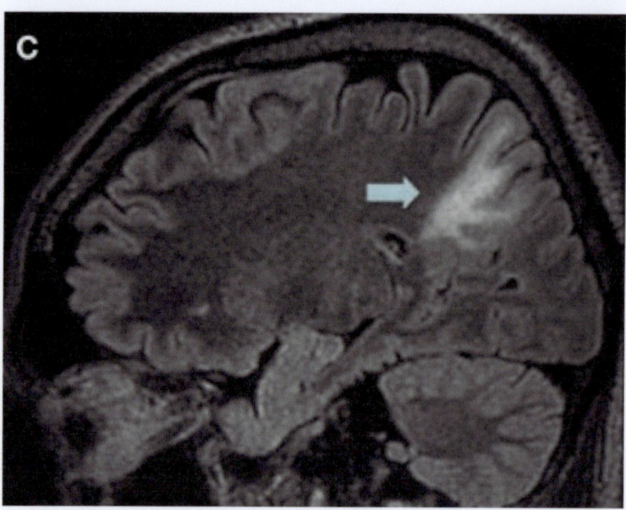

Sagittal MRI brain. (Image source: Lindå, H., von Heijne, A. CC-BY 3.0 (https://creativecommons.org/licenses/by/3.0/), via Frontiers in Neurology. Image has been cropped from the original source. Please see full attribution with citation below in references section for this question.)

A. Steroids to treat an MS relapse
B. Switch to rituximab
C. Repeat MRI in 3–6 months
D. Lumbar puncture
E. Switch to siponimod for secondary progressive MS

Correct answer: D

Linked question

35. For the patient in the prior question, you pursue a lumbar puncture. Which of the following CSF tests is most likely to reveal the underlying cause of this MRI finding?

A. Cell count
B. IgG index
C. JC virus PCR
D. Oligoclonal bands
E. hematopathology/flow cytometry
F. HSV PCR
G. EBV PCR

Correct answer: C

Explanation (Questions 34 and 35)

This MRI finding, in a patient on natalizumab, is most consistent with progressive multifocal leukoencephalopathy (PML). Because natalizumab is such a highly effective therapy, new MRI lesions should be closely evaluated for the possibility of PML (in addition to considering if a new lesion is a multiple sclerosis lesion). PML is a CNS infection caused by the JC virus. Of the multiple sclerosis DMTs, natalizumab confers the highest risk for developing PML. This risk is associated with the amount of time one has been on natalizumab, as well as the JC virus antibody titer. As a result, the serum JC virus antibody titer should be regularly monitored while on natalizumab therapy to identify when an individual becomes infected (often asymptomatic) and estimate the risks of infection based on the antibody titer. The MRI findings of PML can be quite varied and depend in part on the underlying risk factor for the development of PML (e.g., natalizumab-associated vs HIV-associated).

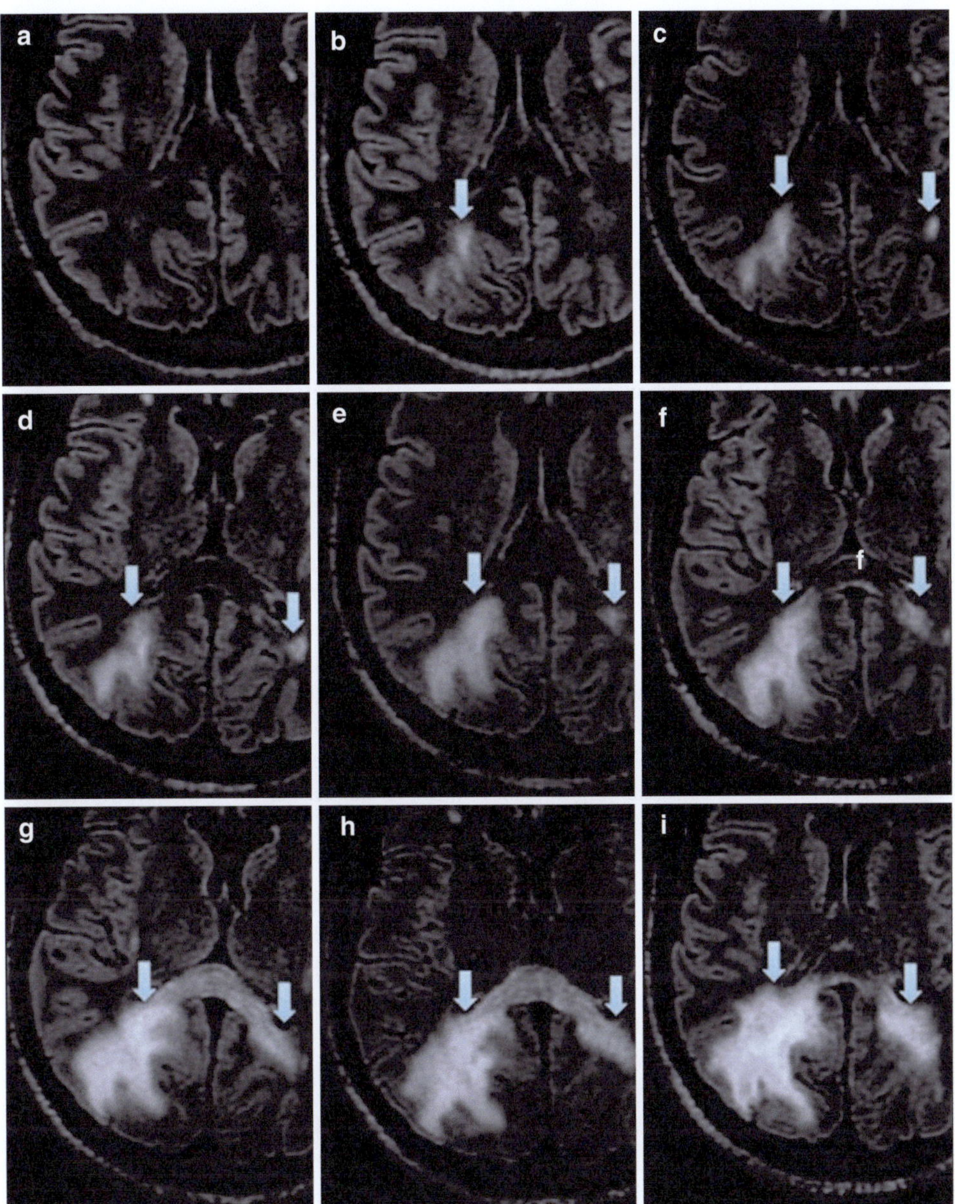

Axial MRI brain. (**a**) shows baseline MRI 1 year prior to the diagnosis of PML. (**b**) shows the findings when PML was diagnosed. Images (**c–i**) show the progression of PML over the course of 2.5 months. (Image source: Lindå, H., von Heijne, A. CC-BY 3.0 (https://creativecommons.org/licenses/by/3.0/), via Frontiers in Neurology. Image has not been modified from the original source. Lindå H, von Heijne A. Presymptomatic diagnosis with MRI and adequate treatment ameliorate the outcome after natalizumab-associated progressive multifocal leukoencephalopathy. Front Neurol. 2013;4:11. Published 2013 Feb 18. https://doi.org/10.3389/fneur.2013.00011)

References

Lindå H, von Heijne A. Presymptomatic diagnosis with MRI and adequate treatment ameliorate the outcome after natalizumab-associated progressive multifocal leukoencephalopathy. Front Neurol. 2013;4:11. https://doi.org/10.3389/fneur.2013.00011.

Wattjes MP, Barkhof F. Diagnosis of natalizumab-associated progressive multifocal leukoencephalopathy using MRI. Curr Opin Neurol. 2014;27(3):260–70. https://doi.org/10.1097/wco.0000000000000099.

36. A 44-year-old woman with RRMS previously stable on natalizumab presents with subacute cognitive change and visual disturbances. MRI brain is obtained and reveals multiple subcortical white matter lesions involving the subcortical U-fibers, particularly in the parieto-occipital lobes. CSF is obtained and JC virus DNA is detected. What is the most appropriate next step in management?
    A. Start high-dose IV methylprednisolone
    B. Start treatment for HIV with antiretroviral therapy
    C. Begin treatment with pyrimethamine and sulfadiazine
    D. Discontinue natalizumab and begin plasmapheresis
    E. Start empiric coverage with ceftriaxone, vancomycin, and acyclovir

Correct answer: D

Explanation

This patient's presentation is consistent with progressive multifocal leukoencephalopathy (PML), an infection resulting from John Cunningham (JC) virus. While it typically affects patients with AIDS/HIV, the incidence in non-HIV patients is increasing. Natalizumab increases the risk of PML due to impaired immune surveillance in the CNS. The goal of apheresis treatment is to rapidly remove natalizumab and allow the body's own immune system to fight the JC virus infection. High-dose steroids (choice a) would be used if PML-IRIS (immune reconstitution inflammatory syndrome) were suspected. PML-IRIS usually presents in a delayed fashion (3 to 6 weeks) with new or worsening symptoms, which is not the case with this patient. There is no indication that this patient is HIV positive (choice b). Pyrimethamine and sulfadiazine is the treatment for toxoplasmosis (choice c).

Reference

Clifford DB, De Luca A, Simpson DM, Arendt G, Giovannoni G, Nath A. Natalizumab-associated progressive multifocal leukoencephalopathy in patients with multiple sclerosis: lessons from 28 cases. Lancet Neurol. 2010;9(4):438–46. https://doi.org/10.1016/S1474-4422(10)70028-4.

Linked questions: 37–38

37. A 32-year-old man with MS presents to your office for follow-up. He is being treated with ofatumumab. His neurological exam is stable and recent MRI shows no changes compared to prior. His major complaint is fatigue, described as easy fatigability, noting that he just "runs out of gas." He asks if there is any treatment for this. You recommend:
    A. Amantadine
    B. Modafinil
    C. Methylphenidate
    D. None of the above

Correct answer: D

Explanation

Fatigue is a major symptom of MS, considered an "invisible symptom" that can affect between 36.5–97% of patients with MS and in some patient surveys is considered the most disabling symptom of MS. MS fatigue can take various forms including asthenia, fatigability, and excessive sleepiness. Due to its major impact, various treatments have been tried over the years ranging from pharmaceutical interventions, behavioral modification, diet, and supplements. The literature is conflicting, but a randomized controlled trial conducted by Nourbakhsh et al. looked at some of the most commonly used pharmaceutical options. This study found that these agents were statistically and clinically no better than placebo, and a higher rate of adverse events were noted with the drugs.

Reference

Nourbakhsh B, Revirajan N, Morris B, Cordano C, Creasman J, Manguinao M, et al. Safety and efficacy of amantadine, modafinil, and methylphenidate for fatigue in multiple sclerosis: a randomised, placebo-controlled, crossover, double-blind trial. Lancet Neurol. 2021;20(1):38–48. https://doi.org/10.1016/S1474-4422(20)30354-9

Linked question

38. The patient from the prior question asks for some guidance, and you explain that some options with limited data for improvement of MS-related fatigue include the following:
    A. Exercise
    B. Mediterranean diet
    C. Cognitive behavioral therapy
    D. Ensuring adequate sleep hygiene
    E. Ruling out other medical and metabolic causes that may contribute
    F. All of the above

Correct answer: F

Explanation

MS fatigue can be difficult to treat. Physicians should always investigate additional factors that may contribute (impaired sleep or sleep disorders such as OSA, metabolic/medical abnormalities such as thyroid disease, vitamin B12 deficiency or anemia). Various non-pharmacological interventions have shown some statistical improvement in various fatigue measures including adoption of a Mediterranean diet, various forms of exercise, and cognitive behavioral therapy.

Reference

Diaz-Quiroz M, Chicue-Cuervo PC, Garcia-Moreno L, Gaviria-Carrillo M, Talero-Gutierrez C, Palacios-Espinosa X. Fatigue in multiple sclerosis: A scoping review of pharmacological and nonpharmacological interventions. Mult Scler J Exp Transl Clin. 2025;11(1):20552173241312527. https://doi.org/10.1177/20552173241312527.

Linked questions: 39–40

39. A 23-year-old woman with a history of MS calls the on-call answering service. You read in the chart that she was diagnosed after an episode of optic neuritis followed 3 months later by an episode of right arm weakness with MRI seen below. She was subsequently started on fingolimod which she has tolerated well, with clinical and radiologic stability. She calls, tearful, due to concern for a relapse, reporting recurrence of right upper extremity weakness.

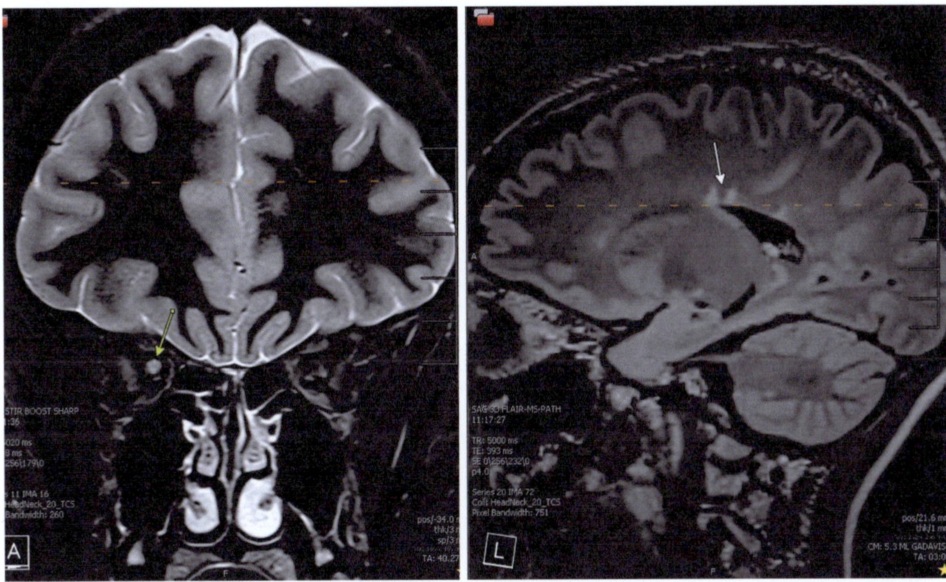

Left: Coronal STIR MRI orbits; Right: Sagittal FLAIR MRI brain. (Images courtesy of Dr. Vito Arena)

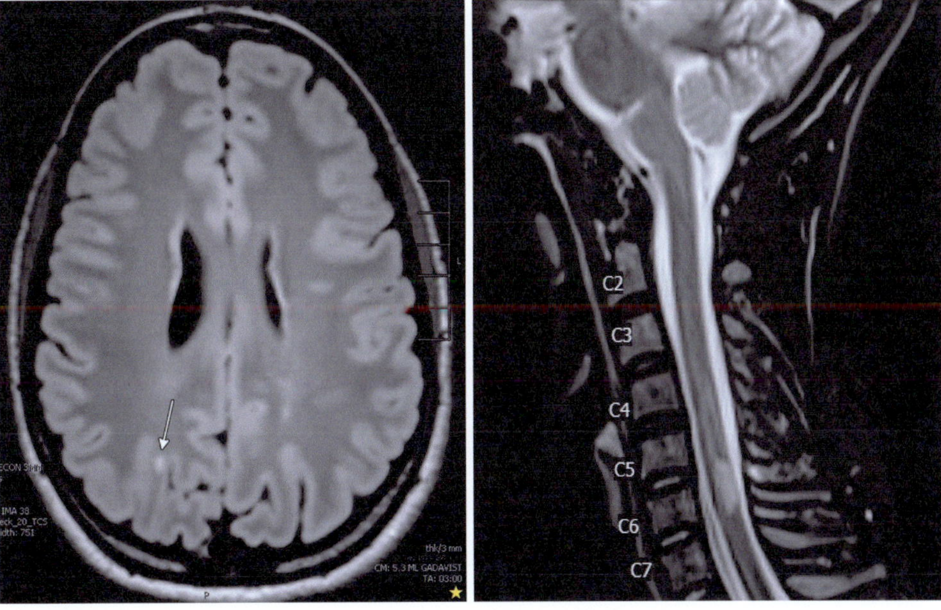

Left: Axial FLAIR MRI brain; Right: Sagittal STIR MRI spine. (Images courtesy of Dr. Vito Arena)

As the on-call physician, which is the best course of action?

   A. Send to the ER immediately for IV steroids
   B. Inquire about any stressors, infections, or environmental changes
   C. Recommend immediate change of her disease-modifying therapy
   D. Order an EMG/NCS

Correct answer: B

Linked question

40. She reports current symptoms of fever, chills, cough, rhinorrhea, and body aches. You direct her to an urgent care center where she tests positive for influenza A. What is the most likely clinical scenario?

   A. This is most likely a new clinical relapse
   B. This most likely represents transition to secondary progressive multiple sclerosis
   C. This is functional neurological disorder and patient should be referred for psychotherapy
   D. This is most likely a pseudorelapse. She should be counseled to monitor symptoms for resolution as she is treated for her flu with close follow-up in the clinic

Correct answer: D

Explanation (Questions 39 and 40)

Pseudorelapse in MS is a well-known phenomenon. Recrudescence of symptoms can be seen in the setting of various stressors, including social stress and anxiety, raised internal body temperature, infection, and fever. For this reason, it is prudent to consider these factors when a patient reports recurrent symptoms. Symptoms of pseudorelapse should be temporary and resolved with (or shortly thereafter) resolution of the stressors (e.g., resolution of illness/fever, cooling off after exercise).

Reference

Wang C, Ruiz A, Mao-Draayer Y. Assessment and Treatment Strategies for a Multiple Sclerosis Relapse. *J Immunol Clin Res*. 2018;5(1):1032.

Linked questions: 41–42

41. A 42-year-old woman with RRMS arrives for follow-up. She believes her walking speed is slowing down, confirmed on a timed 25-foot walk. Her examination reveals no other new or worsening deficits. She is interested in physical therapy, but also inquires if there are medications she can try. What is the mechanism of action of a first-line option?

   A. Sodium channel blockade
   B. Potassium channel blockade

   C. Modulation of GABA receptors
   D. Serotonin receptor antagonist
   E. Increased concentration of acetylcholine in the neuromuscular junction

Correct answer: B

Explanation

Dalfampridine (4-aminopyridine) is a potassium channel blocker that was approved in 2010 that has been shown to improve walking speed in some patients with MS. The largest trial ($n = 301$) of patients with any type of MS showed a 35% response rate (compared to 8% in the placebo group) as measured by improvement on timed 25-foot walk at 14 weeks (OR 4.75, 95% CI (2.08–10.86).

Reference

Goodman AD, Brown TR, Krupp LB, Schapiro RT, Schwid SR, Cohen R, et al. Sustained-release oral fampridine in multiple sclerosis: a randomised, double-blind, controlled trial. Lancet. 2009;373(9665):732–8. https://doi.org/10.1016/S0140-6736(09)60442-6

Linked question

42. What is an important side effect of dalfampridine that patients should be screened for and warned to watch for?

   A. Seizures
   B. Macular edema
   C. Facial flushing
   D. Diarrhea
   E. Irritability

Correct answer: A

Explanation

Dalfampridine is associated with a dose-dependent risk of seizures, including de novo in patients without a prior history. It is contraindicated in patients with a history of seizures. Other side effects include increased frequency of urinary tract infections, nausea, dizziness, headache, and insomnia.

Reference

Goodman AD, Brown TR, Krupp LB, Schapiro RT, Schwid SR, Cohen R, et al. Sustained-release oral fampridine in multiple sclerosis: a randomised, double-blind, controlled trial. Lancet. 2009;373(9665):732–8. https://doi.org/10.1016/S0140-6736(09)60442-6

43. A 59-year-old female patient with MS complains of sexual dysfunction, including decreased libido and anorgasmia. Her spasticity and depressive symptoms have improved compared to last visit. What is the best next step to address her concern?

A. Medication review
B. Referral to urogynecology
C. Referral to physical therapy for pelvic floor exercises
D. Referral for cognitive behavioral therapy
E. Prescribe bremelanotide

Correct answer: A

Explanation

Sexual dysfunction—including anorgasmia, erectile dysfunction, decreased libido, vaginal pain and dryness — is commonly reported in patients with multiple sclerosis. Etiologies to consider include autonomic dysfunction from spinal cord injury, cognitive or pelvic floor symptoms, and iatrogenic causes. Medications commonly prescribed for other MS symptoms have various sexual side effects, including selective serotonin reuptake inhibitors, antimuscarinics, baclofen, and tricyclic antidepressants, so medication review should be performed at every visit.

Reference

Zorzon M, Zivadinov R, Bosco A, Bragadin LM, Moretti R, Bonfigli L, et al. Sexual dysfunction in multiple sclerosis: a case-control study. I. Frequency and comparison of groups. Mult Scler. 1999;5(6):418–27. https://doi.org/10.1177/1352 45859900500i609.

44. A 42-year-old woman with MS reports daytime somnolence. She does not feel well-rested when waking up in the morning and has noted a mild holocephalic headache that improves throughout the day. She endorses frequent daytime naps and denies waking up often to urinate in the middle of the night. What is the appropriate next step?
    A. Provide reassurance
    B. Encourage regular aerobic exercise
    C. Order a polysomnography
    D. Prescribe a sleep aid
    E. Prescribe desmopressin

Correct answer: C

Explanation

Fatigue is a common symptom of MS, often experienced as exhaustion independent of physical activity that increases as the day progresses. Factors that can worsen or mimic MS-related fatigue include sleep disorders (obstructive sleep apnea, restless leg syndrome), depression, anemia, depression, and medication side effects. In this patient, the associated headache and nonrestorative sleep should prompt evaluation underlying obstructive sleep apnea with a polysomnography. Desmopressin may be indicated if poor sleep was secondary to nocturia. Regular aerobic exercise has

shown benefit in reducing MS-related fatigue. Once alternative etiologies have been ruled out or addressed, and conservative measures fail, a sleep aid may be considered.

References

Hensen HA, Krishnan AV, Eckert DJ. Sleep-Disordered Breathing in People with Multiple Sclerosis: Prevalence, Pathophysiological Mechanisms, and Disease Consequences. Front Neurol. 2017;8:740. https://doi.org/10.3389/fneur.2017.00740.

Veauthier C. Sleep disorders in multiple sclerosis. Review. Curr Neurol Neurosci Rep. 2015;15(5):21. https://doi.org/10.1007/s11910-015-0546-0.

Linked questions 45–47

You are evaluating three patients with MS in your outpatient clinic who complain of lower urinary tract symptoms. Infection has been ruled out and they have failed conservative management. Choose the appropriate first-line pharmacologic therapy.

45. A 56-year-old woman with secondary progressive MS (SPMS) has noted urinary urgency and multiple episodes of urinary incontinence. Post-void residual (PVR) is 50 mL.
    A. Terazosin
    B. Oxybutynin
    C. OnabotulinumtoxinA injections
    D. Desmopressin
    E. Nortriptyline

Correct answer: B

Explanation

Neurogenic bladder in MS can be divided into inability to store urine (e.g., from detrusor hyperactivity), difficulty emptying (e.g., from bladder hypoactivity, detrusor-sphincter dyssynergia), or a combination. Urinary urgency with normal PVR suggests difficulty storing urine, typically caused by demyelinating lesions in the frontal cortex. First-line treatment includes antimuscarinics (including oxybutynin). Second-line treatments include mirabegron (a β-3 adrenergic receptor agonist) and intradetrusor OnabotulinumtoxinA injections.

Reference

Tornic J, Panicker JN. The Management of Lower Urinary Tract Dysfunction in Multiple Sclerosis. Curr Neurol Neurosci Rep. 2018;18(8):54. https://doi.org/10.1007/s11910-018-0857-z.

46. A 65-year-old male with SPMS and benign prostatic hypertrophy notes a weak urinary stream, increased straining, and incomplete emptying. PVR is 310 mL.
    A. Terazosin
    B. Oxybutynin
    C. Botulinum toxin injections
    D. Desmopressin
    E. Nortriptyline
    Correct answer: A

Explanation

Incomplete emptying with an elevated PVR indicates impaired bladder emptying, for which intermittent self-catheterization is a cornerstone of management. In this patient with concurrent prostate-related voiding dysfunction, an α-1 blocker such as terazosin can be tried. Detrusor-sphincter dyssynergia (contraction of the detrusor muscle without urethral sphincter relaxation) is classically caused by spinal cord lesions above the sacral parasympathetic centers or in the pontine micturition center.

Reference

Tornic J, Panicker JN. The Management of Lower Urinary Tract Dysfunction in Multiple Sclerosis. Curr Neurol Neurosci Rep. 2018;18(8):54. https://doi.org/10.1007/s11910-018-0857-z.

47. A 42-year-old woman with RRMS complains of increased urinary frequency, particularly at night, which has significantly impacted her sleep.
    A. Terazosin
    B. Oxybutynin
    C. Botulinum toxin injections
    D. Desmopressin
    E. Nortriptyline
    Correct answer: D

Explanation

Desmopressin, a synthetic antidiuretic hormone analogue, is an effective management of nocturia in patients with MS. A meta-analysis showed reduced urinary frequency and increased uninterrupted sleep by an average of 2 hours.

Reference

Zahariou A, Karamouti M, Karagiannis G, Papaioannou P. Maximal bladder capacity is a positive predictor of response to desmopressin treatment in patients with MS and nocturia. Int Urol Nephrol. 2008;40(1):65–9. https://doi.org/10.1007/s11255-007-9232-8.

48. What class of medications is associated with CNS demyelination?
    A. Dopamine agonists
    B. Macrolide antibiotics
    C. Antiretroviral therapy
    D. Tumor necrosis factor-α (TNF-α) inhibitors
    E. Acetylcholinesterase inhibitors
    Correct answer: D

Explanation

Of the listed medication classes, only TNF-α inhibitors are associated with an increased risk of CNS demyelination.

Reference

Kunchok A, Aksamit AJ, Jr., Davis JM, 3rd, Kantarci OH, Keegan BM, Pittock SJ, et al. Association Between Tumor Necrosis Factor Inhibitor Exposure and Inflammatory Central Nervous System Events. JAMA Neurol. 2020;77(8):937–46. https://doi.org/10.1001/jamaneurol.2020.1162.

Linked questions: 49–52

49. A 44-year-old female without any significant past medical history presents with 2 days of progressively worsening weakness and numbness in her left arm. She has never had any similar symptoms and denies current headaches. On exam, she demonstrates 3+ reflexes in her upper extremities. Which of the following would be the best next step?
    A. MRI brain, cervical, and thoracic spine with and without contrast
    B. EMG and nerve conduction study
    C. CT head without contrast
    D. Lumbar puncture
    Correct answer: A

Explanation

MRI brain, cervical, and thoracic spine would be the most appropriate to evaluate for an upper motor neuron lesion.

Linked question

50. For the patient in the prior question, you obtain an MRI with the results shown below. Which of the following is the best next step in diagnostic workup? Axial MRI brain and sagittal MRI cervical spine. (Image source: Courtesy of Dr. Tyler Smith)

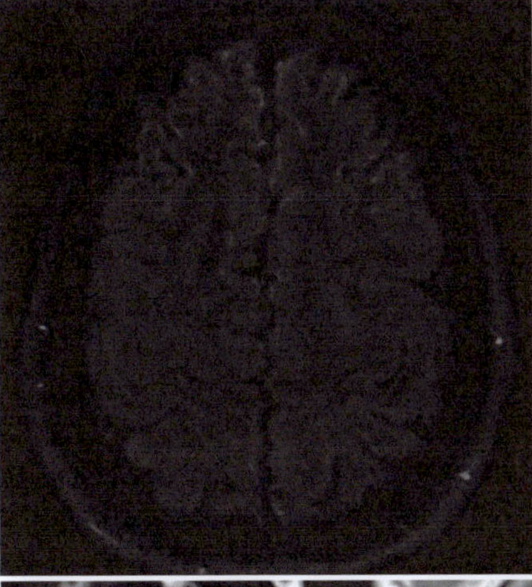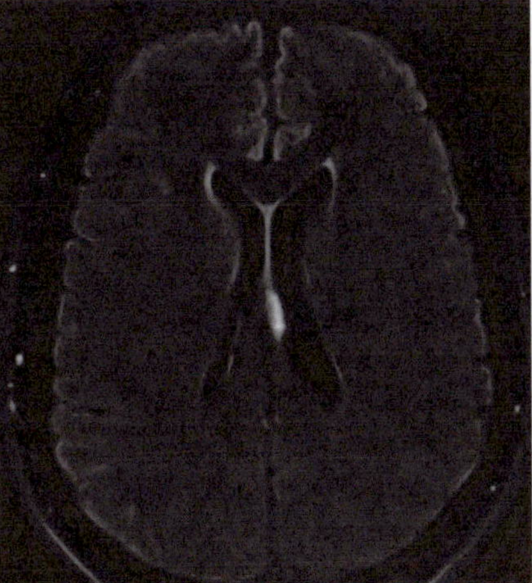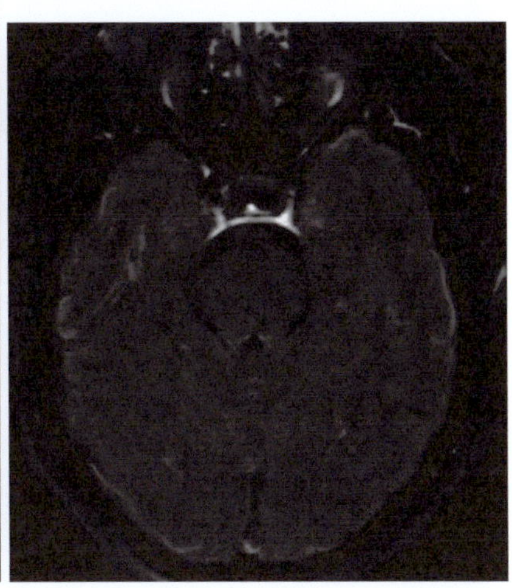

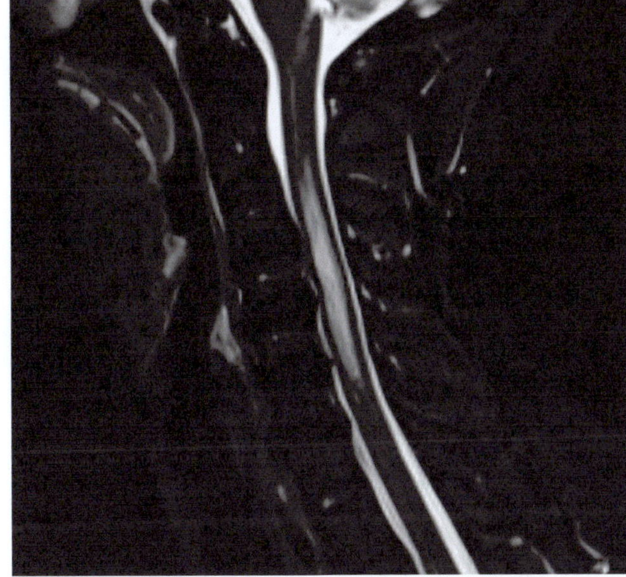

A. Serum aquaporin-4 IgG testing
B. Serum MOG antibody testing
C. Serum vitamin B12
D. Serum copper level
E. CSF testing for oligoclonal bands
F. Both (a) and (b)
G. Both (c) and (d)

Correct answer: F

with a longitudinally extensive transverse myelitis, so testing for both of these disease entities would be the best option.

References

Banwell B, Bennett JL, Marignier R, Kim HJ, Brilot F, Flanagan EP, et al. Diagnosis of myelin oligodendrocyte glycoprotein antibody-associated disease: International MOGAD Panel proposed criteria. Lancet Neurol. 2023;22(3):268–82. https://doi.org/10.1016/s1474-4422(22)00431-8.

Wingerchuk DM, Banwell B, Bennett JL, Cabre P, Carroll W, Chitnis T, et al. International consensus diagnostic criteria for neuromyelitis optica spectrum disorders. Neurology. 2015;85(2):177–89. https://doi.org/10.1212/wnl.0000000000001729.

Linked question

51. The patient from the prior question tests positive for aquaporin-4 IgG. Which of the following is the best next acute treatment?
    A. IV methylprednisolone
    B. IVIG
    C. Ocrelizumab
    D. Natalizumab

Correct answer: A

Explanation

This MRI demonstrates longitudinally extensive (spanning 3 or more vertebral segments) transverse myelitis centered in the cervical spine. While B12 and copper deficiencies are important to consider in the differential of noncompressive myelopathy, they are unlikely to present over the course of 2 days. While oligoclonal bands are commonly associated with multiple sclerosis, it is highly unusual to develop a longitudinally extensive transverse myelitis in MS. Meanwhile, both MOGAD and NMOSD can present with oligoclonal bands (although typically lower frequency than seen with MS). Both MOGAD and NMOSD can present acutely and

Explanation

IV methylprednisolone is the appropriate treatment for NMOSD relapse, typically at a dose of 1 g daily for 3 to 5 days. Depending on the severity, it would be reasonable to simultaneously administer plasma exchange (over time, it has become the authors' practice to use PLEX and IV methylprednisolone in most cases of NMOSD relapse). Ocrelizumab and natalizumab are DMTs used in the treatment of MS. Lastly, IVIG is used in the treatment of many neuroinflammatory disorders (including autoimmune encephalitis, ADEM, MOGAD), but is not considered first line for NMOSD.

Reference

Bonnan M, Valentino R, Debeugny S, Merle H, Fergé JL, Mehdaoui H, et al. Short delay to initiate plasma exchange is the strongest predictor of outcome in severe attacks of NMO spectrum disorders. J Neurol Neurosurg Psychiatry. 2018;89(4):346–51. https://doi.org/10.1136/jnnp-2017-316286.

Linked question

52. Which of the following would be the most appropriate long-term DMT for this individual (from prior question) with a new diagnosis of NMOSD?
    A. Natalizumab
    B. Teriflunomide
    C. Satralizumab
    D. Cladribine
    Correct answer: C

Explanation

The current FDA-approved therapies for NMOSD include satralizumab (IL-6 receptor blocker), ravulizumab (C5 inhibitor), eculizumab (C5 inhibitor), and inebilizumab (anti-CD19). The other therapies listed are used in the treatment of multiple sclerosis.

Reference

Kümpfel T, Giglhuber K, Aktas O, Ayzenberg I, Bellmann-Strobl J, Häußler V, et al. Update on the diagnosis and treatment of neuromyelitis optica spectrum disorders (NMOSD)—revised recommendations of the Neuromyelitis Optica Study Group (NEMOS). Part II: Attack therapy and long-term management. J Neurol. 2024;271(1):141–76. https://doi.org/10.1007/s00415-023-11910-z.

53. A 29-year-old female presents to the emergency room with intractable singultus for the past 2 weeks. She had undergone an extensive workup with her gastroenterologist that was unrevealing. You complete a brain MRI that shows a small focus of T2 hyperintensity with associated enhancement in the dorsal medulla. Her serum aquaporin-4 IgG testing is negative. Under the 2015 NMOSD diagnostic criteria, which of the following additional findings would be needed to confirm a diagnosis of NMOSD?
    A. Optic neuritis
    B. At least four oligoclonal bands unique to the CSF
    C. 90% of brain lesions demonstrating a central vein sign
    D. Positive MOG antibody in serum
    Correct answer: A

Explanation

The core clinical characteristics associated with NMOSD are optic neuritis, acute myelitis, area postrema syndrome, symptomatic narcolepsy or acute diencephalic clinical syndrome, and symptomatic cerebral syndrome with NMOSD-typical brain lesions. To receive a diagnosis of antibody-negative NMOSD, a patient must meet at least two core clinical characteristics. In this case, the patient likely has one lesion at the area postrema (dorsal medulla) leading to intractable hiccups, so an optic nerve lesion (involving more than half of the optic nerve or the optic chiasm) would satisfy this criterion.

Reference

Wingerchuk DM, Banwell B, Bennett JL, Cabre P, Carroll W, Chitnis T, et al. International consensus diagnostic criteria for neuromyelitis optica spectrum disorders. Neurology. 2015;85(2):177–89. https://doi.org/10.1212/WNL.0000000000001729.

54. Which of the following is true of NMOSD when compared to multiple sclerosis?
    A. NMOSD is less likely to have oligoclonal bands unique to the CSF
    B. NMOSD is more likely to manifest as progressive disease
    C. Both are demyelinating diseases
    D. Recovery from an exacerbation tends to better in NMOSD than MS
    Correct answer: A

Explanation

NMOSD is less likely to have oligoclonal bands unique to the CSF than multiple sclerosis. The possibility of progressive disease in NMOSD is the subject of debate and generally considered unlikely to occur. While multiple sclerosis is a demyelinating disease, NMOSD is an astrocytopathy. Relapses in NMOSD tend to be very severe and may require both plasma exchange and steroids for acute treatment.

Reference

Flanagan EP. Neuromyelitis Optica Spectrum Disorder and Other Non-Multiple Sclerosis Central Nervous System Inflammatory Diseases. Continuum (Minneap Minn). 2019;25(3):815–44. https://doi.org/10.1212/con.0000000000000742.

55. A 32-year-old female presents to the emergency room with left-sided blurry vision, painful eye movements, and photosensitivity. On exam she is found to have red desaturation and a relative afferent pupillary defect. Additionally, she has left arm weakness. Her MRI orbits are shown below. Which of the following is the most likely diagnosis?

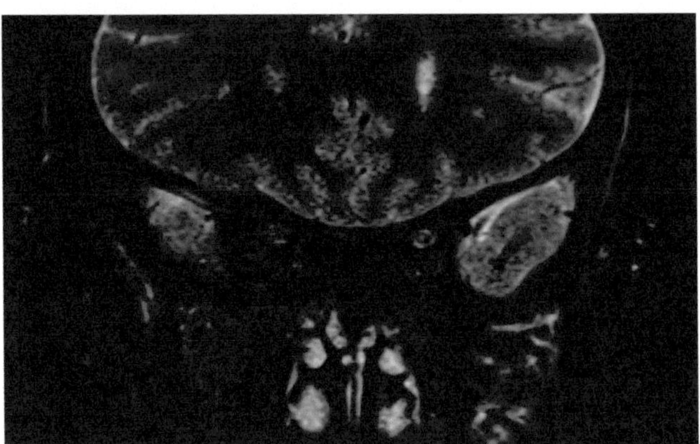

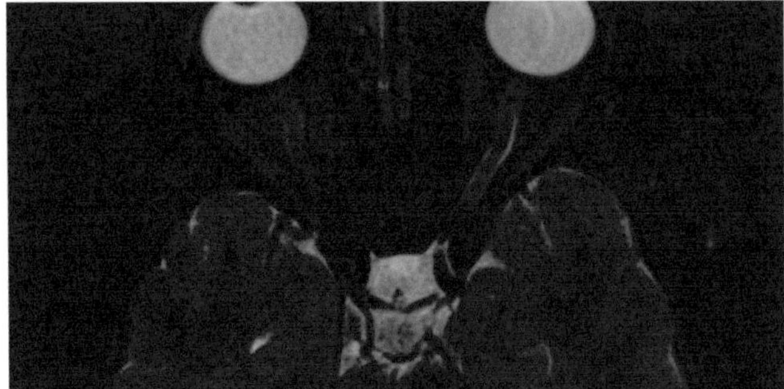

Coronal MRI brain and orbits. (Image source: Courtesy of Dr. Tyler Smith)

Axial MRI brain and orbits. (Image source: Courtesy of Dr. Tyler Smith)

A. Optic neuritis
B. Idiopathic intracranial hypertension
C. Optic nerve glioma
D. Giant cell arteritis

Correct answer: A

Explanation

These images show increased signal in the left optic nerve, compatible with optic neuritis given the clinical timeline provided. Giant cell arteritis would be highly unlikely in an individual that is 32 years of age. These images do not show a significant mass lesion as would be expected with an optic nerve glioma. Idiopathic intracranial hypertension would often have involvement of both optic nerves.

56. Which of the following is true of NMOSD, as compared to MS and MOGAD?
    A. NMOSD is more likely to have bilateral optic neuritis or optic chiasm involvement than MS.
    B. MS and NMOSD both have decreased rates of disease activity during pregnancy.
    C. NMOSD and MOGAD can both present as monophasic disease without risk of relapse.
    D. NMOSD has the lowest female–male ratio compared to MOGAD and MS.

Correct answer: A

Explanation

NMOSD is more likely to demonstrate bilateral optic neuritis and/or optic chiasm involvement compared to MS. While MS has a decreased likelihood of relapse during pregnancy, NMOSD tends to have an increased risk of relapse during pregnancy. While MOGAD can be monophasic (only one relapse), individuals with NMOSD are at risk of relapse indefinitely.

References

Flanagan EP. Neuromyelitis Optica Spectrum Disorder and Other Non-Multiple Sclerosis Central Nervous System Inflammatory Diseases. Continuum (Minneap Minn). 2019;25(3):815–44. https://doi.org/10.1212/con.0000000000000742.

Siriratnam P, Huda S, Butzkueven H, van der Walt A, Jokubaitis V, Monif M. Risks and outcomes of pregnancy in neuromyelitis optica spectrum disorder: A comprehensive review. Autoimmun Rev. 2024;23(2):103499. https://doi.org/10.1016/j.autrev.2023.103499

57. NMOSD is associated with aquaporin-4 IgG. On which of the following cells is aquaporin-4 most likely to be found?
    A. Astrocytes
    B. Interneurons
    C. Oligodendrocytes
    D. Purkinje cells

Correct answer: A

Explanation

Aquaporin-4 water channels are found on astrocytes, and NMOSD is considered an astrocytopathy.

Reference

Carnero Contentti E, Correale J. Neuromyelitis optica spectrum disorders: from pathophysiology to therapeutic strategies. J Neuroinflammation. 2021;18(1):208. https://doi.org/10.1186/s12974-021-02249-1.

Linked questions: 58–60

58. A 41-year-old woman with a history of migraines presents with new-onset blurred vision and painful eye movements. Symptoms started in the right eye, worsened over 2 days, and progressed to the left eye. She was seen by her ophthalmologist who was concerned for optic disc edema and referred her to the emergency department (ED). In the ED, MRI brain and orbits with contrast were completed showing bilateral optic nerve signal changes and contrast enhancement along with nerve sheath enhancement. MRI brain is otherwise unremarkable. Which of the following is your highest diagnostic suspicion?

A. MS
B. MOGAD
C. Neurosarcoidosis
D. Migraine
E. Idiopathic intracranial hypotension

Correct answer: B

Linked question

59. For the patient in the prior question, which of the following diagnostic tests do you expect to be the highest yield?
    A. MRI cervical and thoracic spine
    B. Lumbar puncture
    C. Serum MOG and aquaporin-4 antibodies
    D. Visual evoked potentials
    E. CT angiogram of head and neck

    Correct answer: C

Explanation (Questions 58 and 59)

Symptom description of subacute loss of vision with painful eye movements is classic for inflammatory optic neuritis. In this case, this history is concerning for bilateral optic neuritis. Rates of bilateral optic neuritis are highest in MOGAD, followed by NMOSD, and uncommonly occurs in MS. Other hints in the question stem point towards MOGAD-associated optic neuritis as well. Optic disc edema is most commonly seen in MOGAD-associated optic neuritis. Additionally, the report of nerve sheath enhancement suggests perineuritis, which is again more common in MOGAD than NMOSD or MS. Given this presence of bilateral optic neuritis and otherwise normal brain MRI, MS is unlikely. Though MOGAD is highest on the differential, aquaporin-4 antibody should also be checked given the difference in disease course and long-term management.

Reference

Sechi E, Cacciaguerra L, Chen JJ, et al. Myelin Oligodendrocyte Glycoprotein Antibody-Associated Disease (MOGAD): A Review of Clinical and MRI Features, Diagnosis, and Management. *Front Neurol.* 2022;13:885218. Published 2022 Jun 17. https://doi.org/10.3389/fneur.2022.885218

Linked question

60. You treat the patient with high-dose IV methylprednisolone with excellent visual recovery. She follows up with you in clinic. Hospital workup revealed lumbar puncture with normal cell count, protein, and glucose and negative oligoclonal bands. MRI C and T spine were negative for any lesions. Serum workup revealed a positive MOG antibody at a titer of 1:1000. You discuss next steps with the patient. Based on current evidence which of the following is true?
    A. MOGAD is always a relapsing condition and treatment should be started immediately
    B. Repeat MOG antibody as seroconversion to negative antibody status precludes further relapses
    C. Roughly half of MOG cases may be monophasic with the other experiencing disease relapses
    D. Do not start treatment as 80% of cases are monophasic
    E. None of the above are true

    Correct answer: C

Explanation

Approximately 40–50% of MOG cases are monophasic while 50–60% of cases experience relapses. While MOG seroconversion to negative may present a lower risk of relapse, this is not absolute or guaranteed to predict no further relapses. Furthermore, antibody testing can be influenced by acute treatments. There is no consensus guideline on when to start maintenance treatment for MOGAD at the time of publication. Since roughly half of cases may be monophasic, many physicians will monitor off treatment after a first attack and initiate long-term prophylactic therapy only after a second attack. However various clinical factors, such as attack type or incomplete recovery, are important to consider when deciding to initiate immunotherapy. Some emerging evidence on early treatment and subsequent disease course and clinical outcomes may argue for early treatment, but the intervention and duration of treatment is not well defined.

Reference

Sechi E, Cacciaguerra L, Chen JJ, Mariotto S, Fadda G, Dinoto A, et al. Myelin Oligodendrocyte Glycoprotein Antibody-Associated Disease (MOGAD): A Review of Clinical and MRI Features, Diagnosis, and Management. Front Neurol, 2022;13:885218. https://doi.org/10.3389/fneur.2022.885218.

61. Which of the following is *incorrect* regarding MOG antibody testing?
    A. MOG antibody testing is more sensitive in the serum compared to the CSF.
    B. The sensitivity and specify are roughly equivalent among various testing methodologies (i.e., cell-based assays and ELISA) and thus can be used interchangeably.
    C. Patients who are MOG antibody positive may seroconvert to negative on serial testing.
    D. Timing of antibody testing is important with regard to accuracy of testing.

    E. Immunotherapy such as steroids and PLEX may decrease the sensitivity of MOG antibody testing.

    F. Antibody titer is important with regard to the positive predictive value of the test.

Correct answer: B

Explanation

MOG antibody testing methodology is critical to the reliability of the results. The most reliable method is a live cell-based assay, which should be used whenever possible. Fixed cell-based assays, though not as reliable, are still substantially more sensitive and specific than ELISA which are of little value due to their poor performance. MOG antibody testing is more sensitive in the serum than the CSF, though a few studies have demonstrated that there may be a small proportion of patients that have been found to be positive in the CSF when serum testing is negative. Thus, CSF testing can be considered when there is high clinical suspicion and serum antibody testing is negative. Patients who initially test positive for MOG may seroconvert to negative after an initial attack. Some data suggest this may be associated with a lower risk of future relapse; however, it does not entirely eliminate risk of future relapses. When there is clinical suspicion, MOG antibody testing should be performed as close to the time of an attack as possible for most reliable results. Furthermore, testing prior to any immunotherapy is preferable as some treatments can impact the reliability of results. Delayed testing or testing after immunotherapy may fail to capture patients that are positive. In the case of initially negative testing, it is reasonable to test again at the time of future relapses. Lastly, antibody titer has been shown to be important in determining positive predictive value of a test with higher titers conveying greater PPV. A result is considered to be a "clear positive" with a titer of >/= 1:100. For this reason, pretest probability must be considered when ordering MOG antibody testing, as false positives with low titers can be seen in conditions such as MS.

References

Reindl M, Schanda K, Woodhall M, Tea F, Ramanathan S, Sagen J, et al. International multicenter examination of MOG antibody assays. Neurol Neuroimmunol Neuroinflamm. 2020;7(2). https://doi.org/10.1212/NXI.0000000000000674.

Sechi E, Buciuc M, Pittock SJ, et al. Positive Predictive Value of Myelin Oligodendrocyte Glycoprotein Autoantibody Testing. JAMA Neurol. 2021;78(6):741–746. https://doi.org/10.1001/jamaneurol.2021.0912

62. A 24-year-old man presents following a second episode of subacute vision loss with painful eye movements in his right eye in the last 2 years. MRI reveals findings consistent with acute right optic neuritis with radiological evidence of involvement of the left eye as well. It also reveals several small, scattered subcortical white matter lesions. Your workup reveals MOG antibody positivity at 1:1000 titer. You advise the patient that after treatment of this acute flare with IV steroids, you would recommend starting treatment to prevent further relapses. Which do you recommend?

    A. Fingolimod

    B. Monthly IVIG

    C. Natalizumab

    D. Dimethyl fumarate

    E. Eculizumab

Correct answer: B

Explanation

No definite treatment guidelines exist for MOGAD. Various immunotherapy agents have been used with variable benefit for relapse prevention. Pulse IVIG is a common and effective strategy for relapse prevention that is generally well-tolerated. Dosing varies but typically includes a loading dose of 2 g/kg spread over 2–5 days followed by a monthly maintenance dose (1 g/kg). Some retrospective data suggests relapse rate with IVIG was significantly lower compared to other treatments (rituximab, azathioprine, mycophenolate mofetil). Natalizumab and dimethyl fumarate are treatments for multiple sclerosis while eculizumab is an FDA-approved therapy for NMOSD.

Source

Chen JJ, Flanagan EP, Bhatti MT, Jitprapaikulsan J, Dubey D, Lopez Chiriboga ASS, et al. Steroid-sparing maintenance immunotherapy for MOG-IgG associated disorder. Neurology. 2020;95(2):e111-e20. https://doi.org/10.1212/WNL.0000000000009758.

63. Typical syndromes associated with adult-onset MOGAD include all of the following except:

    A. Optic neuritis

    B. Progressive myelopathy

    C. Myelitis

    D. Cerebral cortical encephalitis with seizures

    E. ADEM

    F. B and E

Correct answer: B

Explanation

The spectrum of presentations of MOGAD has evolved with time. The typical syndromes of MOGAD include:

- Optic neuritis: Often severe attacks, bilateral optic nerve commonly affected, typically affect anterior portion of the nerves and are longitudinally extensive. Can have associated perineuritis and moderate to severe nerve head edema and can be relapsing and steroid-dependent.

- Myelitis: Typically, single or multiple longitudinally extensive lesions but can be short segment with predilection for gray matter as well. Motor impairment can be severe but often recovers well. There is risk of residual sphincter and sexual dysfunction despite good motor recovery, and conus involvement is also suggestive of MOGAD.
- ADEM: this can be a presentation of MOGAD, but is more common in pediatric and adolescent patients.
- Cerebral monofocal or polyfocal deficits.
- Brainstem or cerebellar deficits: pons and large middle cerebellar peduncle lesions are typical.
- Cerebral cortical encephalitis often with seizures.

References

Banwell B, Bennett JL, Marignier R, Kim HJ, Brilot F, Flanagan EP, et al. Diagnosis of myelin oligodendrocyte glycoprotein antibody-associated disease: International MOGAD Panel proposed criteria. Lancet Neurol. 2023;22(3):268–82. https://doi.org/10.1016/S1474-4422(22)00431-8

Sechi E, Cacciaguerra L, Chen JJ, Mariotto S, Fadda G, Dinoto A, et al. Myelin Oligodendrocyte Glycoprotein Antibody-Associated Disease (MOGAD): A Review of Clinical and MRI Features, Diagnosis, and Management. Front Neurol. 2022;13:885218. https://doi.org/10.3389/fneur.2022.885218.

64. Which of the following is atypical of MOG-associated myelitis?
    A. Steroid-responsive
    B. Longitudinally extensive
    C. Often non-enhancing
    D. Tend to be central with predilection for gray matter
    E. Persistence on follow-up MRI

    Correct answer: E

Explanation

MOGAD-associated myelitis has several features which may help you distinguish it from other forms of myelitis.

Longitudinally extensive (≥ 3 vertebral segments) lesions are common. Patients can have multiple long lesions, though short segment myelitis can also be seen. MOGAD myelitis shows contrast enhancement 50% of the time. Lesions tend to affect the central cord with predilection for the gray matter, producing the radiologic findings of the "H-sign," though a quarter of cases may not affect the gray matter of the cord. Most cord lesions either completely resolve or reduce in size substantially following the initial relapse.

References

Banwell B, Bennett JL, Marignier R, Kim HJ, Brilot F, Flanagan EP, et al. Diagnosis of myelin oligodendrocyte glycoprotein antibody-associated disease: International MOGAD Panel proposed criteria. Lancet Neurol. 2023;22(3):268–82. https://doi.org/10.1016/S1474-4422(22)00431-8

Mariano R, Messina S, Kumar K, Kuker W, Leite MI, Palace J.Comparison of clinical outcomes of transverse myelitis among adults with myelin oligodendrocyte glycoprotein antibody vs aquaporin-4 antibody disease. JAMA Netw Open 2019; 2: e1912732.

Sechi E, Cacciaguerra L, Chen JJ, Mariotto S, Fadda G, Dinoto A, et al. Myelin Oligodendrocyte Glycoprotein Antibody-Associated Disease (MOGAD): A Review of Clinical and MRI Features, Diagnosis, and Management. Front Neurol. 2022;13:885218. https://doi.org/10.3389/fneur.2022.885218.

Sechi E, Krecke KN, Messina SA, et al. Comparison of MRI lesion evolution in different central nervous system demyelinating disorders. Neurology 2021; 97: e1097–109.

Linked questions: 65–66

65. A 7-year-old immunocompetent boy presents with 4 days of progressively worsening headache, somnolence, and right arm weakness. He recovered from an upper respiratory tract infection 2 weeks ago. His MRI is shown below. What is the most likely diagnosis?

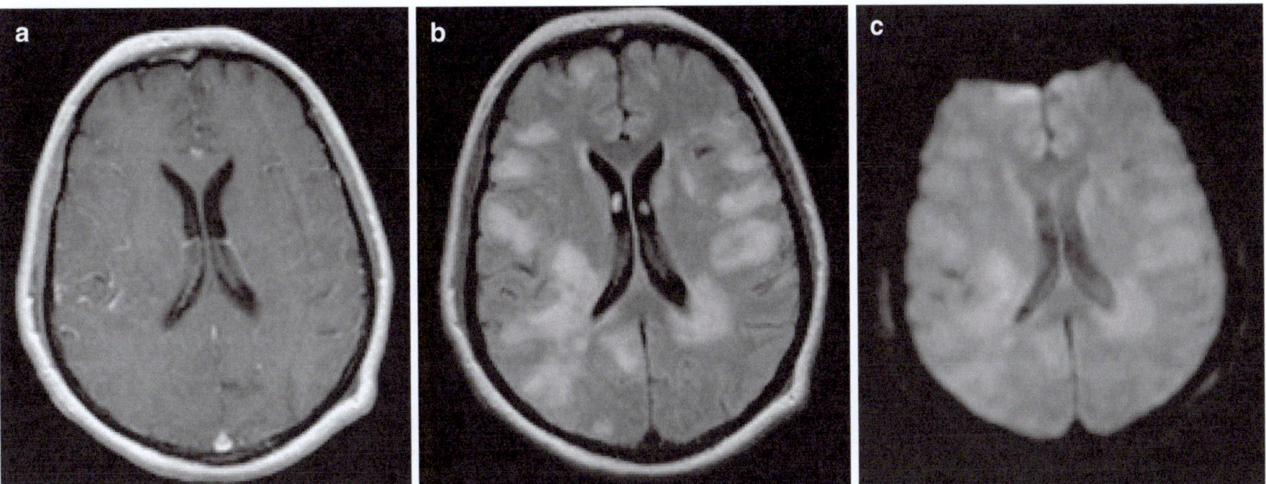

Axial MRI brain, (**a**) T1 Gd-enhanced, (**b**) T2-FLAIR, C) DWI. (Source: Huhn K, Lee DH, Linker RA, Kloska S, Huttner HB via SpringerPlus (2014). CC-BY 4.0 (https://creativecommons.org/licenses/by/4.0/). Image has not been modified from source. Please see full attribution with citation below in references section)

A. Progressive multifocal leukoencephalopathy (PML)
B. Toxoplasmosis
C. CNS lymphoma
D. Multiple sclerosis (MS)
E. Acute disseminated encephalomyelitis (ADEM)

Correct answer: E

Explanation

The most likely diagnosis is ADEM, which typically affects children and presents with encephalopathy and multifocal neurologic signs attributable to CNS lesions and is often preceded by a viral infection. As in this case, MRI may reveal bilateral, large, poorly-demarcated T2/fluid-attenuated inversion recovery (FLAIR) hyperintense lesions that can involve both white and gray matter. PML and toxoplasmosis would be unlikely in an immunocompetent host. Somnolence and headache are uncommon presenting features of MS. Although at times difficult to differentiate radiologically at time of first attack from MS, a diffuse bilateral lesion pattern favors ADEM.

References

Kamate M, Chetal V, Tonape V, Mahantshetti N, Hattiholi V. Central nervous system inflammatory demyelinating disorders of childhood. Ann Indian Acad Neurol. 2010;13(4):289–92. https://doi.org/10.4103/0972-2327.74204.

Ketelslegers IA, Neuteboom RF, Boon M, Catsman-Berrevoets CE, Hintzen RQ, Dutch Pediatric MSSG. A comparison of MRI criteria for diagnosing pediatric ADEM and MS. Neurology. 2010;74(18):1412–5. https://doi.org/10.1212/WNL.0b013e3181dc138b.

Huhn K, Lee DH, Linker RA, Kloska S, Huttner HB via SpringerPlus (2014). CC-BY 4.0 (https://creativecommons.org/licenses/by/4.0/). Image has not been modified from source.

Huhn K, Lee DH, Linker RA, Kloska S, Huttner HB. Pneumococcal-meningitis associated acute disseminated encephalomyelitis (ADEM)—case report of effective early immunotherapy. Springerplus. 2014;3:415. Published 2014 Aug 8. https://doi.org/10.1186/2193-1801-3-415

Linked question

66. He is started on 30 mg/kg daily of IV methylprednisolone. Five days later he shows no improvement. Which of the following may be the next best choice?
    A. Cyclophosphamide
    B. Bortezomib
    C. Intravenous immunoglobulin (IVIG)
    D. Natalizumab
    E. Rituximab

Correct answer: C

Explanation

First-line therapy for ADEM is high-dose intravenous glucocorticoids (e.g., methylprednisolone). If improvement is not seen within 5 days, therapy should be escalated to second-line therapy which includes intravenous immunoglobulin (IVIG) or plasma exchange (PLEX). IVIG is often preferred due to availability, relative safety, and ease of administration with PLEX reserved for use in more fulminant courses. Cyclophosphamide can be considered in refractory cases. The other options listed are second- and third-line immunotherapies used in other disorders, such as autoimmune encephalitis.

Linked questions: 67–68

67. A 13-year-old boy presents with subacute onset of right hemiplegia and ADEM or MS is suspected. Which of the following findings, if present on MRI brain would make ADEM *less* likely?
    A. Hypointense lesions on T1 sequence
    B. Deep gray matter involvement
    C. Poorly demarcated lesions
    D. Enhancement with gadolinium
    E. Bilateral cerebral hemisphere involvement
    Correct answer: A

Explanation

Brain MRI findings that are more suggestive of MS over ADEM during a first clinical demyelinating event are hypointense lesions on T1 imaging, absence of bilateral diffuse lesions, absence of gray matter involvement, and multiple periventricular lesions.

Reference

Krupp LB, Tardieu M, Amato MP, Banwell B, Chitnis T, Dale RC, et al. International Pediatric Multiple Sclerosis Study Group criteria for pediatric multiple sclerosis and immune-mediated central nervous system demyelinating disorders: revisions to the 2007 definitions. Mult Scler. 2013;19(10):1261–7. https://doi.org/10.1177/1352458513484547.

Linked question

68. The patient from the prior question is ultimately diagnosed with ADEM. Which of the following antibodies is most likely to be positive in a patient presenting with ADEM?
    A. Aquaporin-4 IgG
    B. N methyl-D-aspartate receptor IgG
    C. Gamma-Aminobutyric Acid Receptor, Type A IgG
    D. MOG IgG
    E. Glutamic Acid Decarboxylase 65 IgG
    Correct answer: D

Explanation

Up to 50% of pediatric patients presenting with ADEM have MOG antibodies. Antibodies against aquaporin-4 are found in neuromyelitis optica spectrum disorders, which most often present with optic neuritis and transverse myelitis. The other choices are antibodies seen in various forms of autoimmune encephalitis, which is unlikely in this patient presenting with isolated weakness.

Reference

Bruijstens AL, Lechner C, Flet-Berliac L, Deiva K, Neuteboom RF, Hemingway C, et al. E.U. paediatric MOG consortium consensus: Part one—Classification of clinical phenotypes of paediatric myelin oligodendrocyte glycoprotein antibody-associated disorders. Eur J Paediatr Neurol. 2020;29:2–13. https://doi.org/10.1016/j.ejpn.2020.10.006

69. What clinical features may be helpful in supporting a diagnosis of MS over MOGAD?
    A. Presence of fever
    B. Prodromal viral infection
    C. Impaired consciousness
    D. Development of asymptomatic lesions
    Correct answer: D

Explanation

Both MS and MOGAD should be considered in the differential diagnoses when a patient presents with symptoms and signs attributable to CNS demyelination. It is quite rare for patients with NMOSD and MOGAD to develop asymptomatic lesions, compared to patients with MS.

Reference

Camera V, Holm-Mercer L, Ali AAH, Messina S, Horvat T, Kuker W, et al. Frequency of New Silent MRI Lesions in Myelin Oligodendrocyte Glycoprotein Antibody Disease and Aquaporin-4 Antibody Neuromyelitis Optica Spectrum Disorder. JAMA Netw Open. 2021;4(12):e2137833. https://doi.org/10.1001/jamanetworkopen.2021.37833.

70. A 57-year-old male presents to the clinic with 6 months of gradually progressive weakness and numbness in her legs. On examination you note symmetric hyperreflexia. His prior neurologist administered a 5-day course of IV steroids, but this made his symptoms worse. MRI brain is unremarkable. Which of the following findings would you suspect on workup?
    A. 6 Oligoclonal bands unique to CSF
    B. Flow voids on spine MRI
    C. Nerve root enhancement
    D. Spinal cord atrophy
    Correct answer: B

Explanation

Flow voids on spinal MRI can be associated with a spinal dural AV fistula (sDAVF). SDAVFs tend to affect males, present later in life, and worsen with steroids and exertion. SDAVF may also demonstrate a "missing piece sign" on spine MRI, which is an abrupt, discrete region of nonenhancement within a long segment of intense spinal cord enhancement.

Reference

Zalewski NL, Rabinstein AA, Brinjikji W, Kaufmann TJ, Nasr D, Ruff MW, et al. Unique Gadolinium Enhancement Pattern in Spinal Dural Arteriovenous Fistulas. JAMA Neurol. 2018;75(12):1542–5. https://doi.org/10.1001/jamaneurol.2018.2605.

Linked questions: 71–72

71. A 23-year-old male presents to your clinic for a second opinion. He reports that neck flexion causes an electric shock to spread down his back to his lumbar spine. What is the best next step and expected finding?
    A. MRI cervical spine; T2 hyperintense cord lesion.
    B. MRI brain; dilated ventricles.
    C. MRI lumbar spine; nerve root enhancement.
    D. CT head and neck; vertebral artery dissection.
    Correct answer: A

Explanation

The description of a sudden electric shock-like sensation beginning in the neck and extending down the spine, sometimes radiating to the arms and legs, is typical for a cervical cord lesion. The other findings listed would not be expected to produce this sensory phenomenon.

Linked question

72. Which of the following is the correct term for this clinical finding in the prior question?
    A. Uhthoff's phenomenon
    B. Lhermitte's sign
    C. Positive Spurling's test
    D. Hoffman's sign
    Correct answer: B

Explanation

This is known as Lhermitte's sign, and it is often provoked by neck flexion. Uhotff's phenomenon is seen in patients with MS, described as a temporary worsening in previous neurologic symptoms with an increase in body temperature (e.g., ambient, infection). Hoffman's sign is a reflexive flexion and abduction of the thumb when the nail of the middle finger is flicked downward. Although not always pathologic, it can indicate corticospinal tract dysfunction, particularly in the cervical spinal cord. Spurling's test is a provocative maneuver to assess cervical radiculopathy in which the examiner extends, laterally flexes, then applies axial pressure to the patient's head.

73. Which of the following statements is *incorrect*?
    A. Spinal cord MS lesions tend to be short and peripheral in location.
    B. NMOSD cord lesions tend to be longer than two vertebral bodies in length.
    C. An enhancing spinal cord lesion always indicates an active autoimmune etiology.
    D. Spinal cord lesions in MOGAD can affect the conus medullaris.
    Correct answer: C

Explanation

An enhancing cord lesion does not necessarily indicate an autoimmune cause. One example is the "pancake sign" seen in spondylotic myelopathy, which is flat, transverse enhancement seen on axial and sagittal sequences immediately below the point of maximal stenosis. Enhancement can also be seen in sDAVF, described as a "missing piece sign," which is an abrupt, discrete region of nonenhancement within a long segment of intense spinal cord enhancement.

References

Jidal M, Horache K, Messaoud O, Fikri M, Kettani NE, Jiddane M, et al. The "pancake-like" enhancement in cervical spondylotic myelopathy. Radiol Case Rep. 2024;19(8):3503–7. https://doi.org/10.1016/j.radcr.2024.05.013.

Zalewski NL, Rabinstein AA, Brinjikji W, Kaufmann TJ, Nasr D, Ruff MW, et al. Unique Gadolinium Enhancement Pattern in Spinal Dural Arteriovenous Fistulas. JAMA Neurol. 2018;75(12):1542–5. https://doi.org/10.1001/jamaneurol.2018.2605.

Linked questions: 74–77

74. A 57-year-old black man with a history of hypertension presents to your office with 6 months of progressive gait dysfunction. Your exam reveals intact cranial nerves and upper extremity sensorimotor function but bilateral lower extremity weakness, evidence of dorsal column dysfunction, lower extremity spasticity, and Babinski reflex. Differential diagnosis includes all of the following except.
    A. Primary progressive MS
    B. Spinal dural AV-fistula
    C. Spinal cord infarct
    D. Vitamin B12 deficiency associated myelopathy
    E. Neurosarcoidosis
    Correct answer: C

Explanation

The patient is presenting with a clinical picture of a chronic progressive myelopathy as evidenced by the time course of symptoms and exam with upper motor neuron findings localizable to the spinal cord. A spinal cord infarct would not be in the differential diagnosis as it classically presents with hyperacute onset of symptoms. The other options listed are causes of subacute or chronic myelopathies.

Reference

Zalewski NL, Rabinstein AA, Krecke KN, Brown RD, Jr., Wijdicks EFM, Weinshenker BG, et al. Characteristics of Spontaneous Spinal Cord Infarction and Proposed Diagnostic Criteria. JAMA Neurol. 2019;76(1):56–63. https://doi.org/10.1001/jamaneurol.2018.2734

Linked question

75. You obtain an MRI of the spine showing the following:

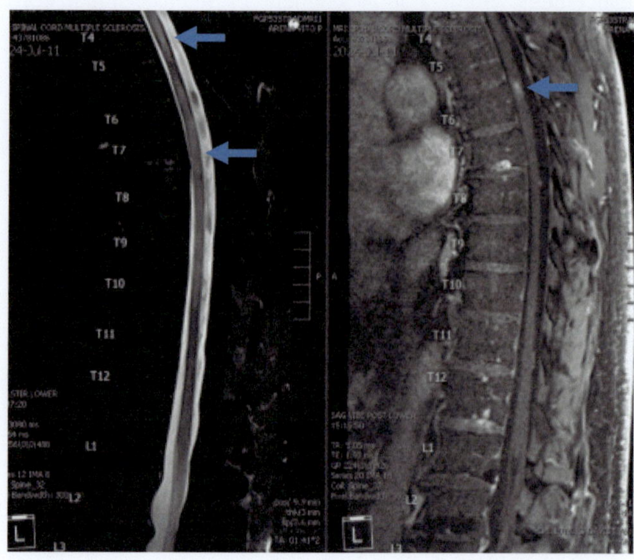

Left Sagittal STIR MRI of lower thoracic spine; Right: Sagittal post-contrast MRI of lower thoracic spine. (Images courtesy of Dr. Vito Arena)

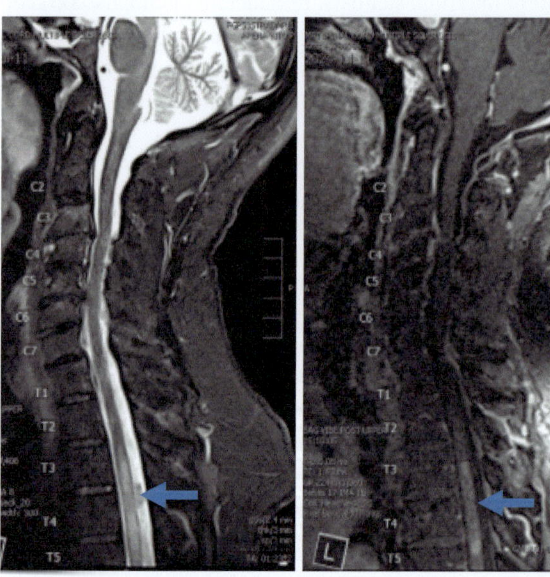

Left: Sagittal STIR MRI of cervical and upper thoracic spine; Right: Sagittal post-contrast MRI of cervical and upper thoracic spine. (Images courtesy of Dr. Vito Arena)

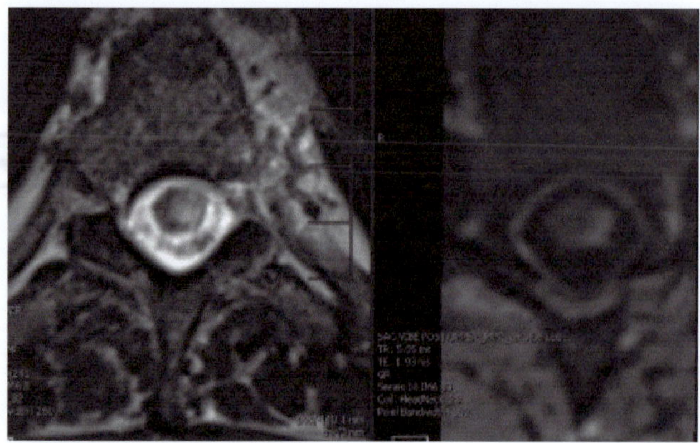

Left: Axial T2 MRI spine; Right: Axial post-contrast MRI spine. (Images courtesy of Dr. Vito Arena)

Additional studies include normal MRI brain and normal/negative serum ANA, Sjogren's antibodies, anti-dsDNA antibodies, HTLV antibodies, Lyme antibodies, vitamin B12, copper, MOG antibody, and aquaporin-4 antibody. Lumbar puncture reveals 25 white blood cells per mm³, protein of 50 mg/dL, elevated IgG synthesis rate with matching oligoclonal bands in the CSF and serum, and elevated CD4:8 ratio on flow cytometry of 6.5:1. What next test might be most helpful?

A. Serum MPO and ANCA for evidence of vasculitis
B. CT chest to assess for hilar lymphadenopathy
C. Spinal angiography to assess for spinal dural AVF
D. OCT to evaluate for thinning of the optic nerves
E. NCS/EMG to assess for peripheral neuropathy

Correct answer: B

Explanation

The patient is presenting with a progressive myelopathy with MRI imaging showing a longitudinally extensive transverse myelitis. Typical causes of such have been ruled out with serum testing. LP shows an inflammatory profile. Vasculitis would be an atypical cause for such a presentation. The presentation and LP make a vascular process less likely. OCT would not help refine the diagnosis further. CT chest demonstrating hilar lymphadenopathy might suggest a systemic process such as sarcoidosis and potentially a site to biopsy.

References

Bradshaw MJ, Pawate S, Koth LL, Cho TA, Gelfand JM. Neurosarcoidosis: Pathophysiology, Diagnosis, and Treatment. Neurol Neuroimmunol Neuroinflamm.

2021;8(6). https://doi.org/10.1212/nxi.0000000000001084

Stern BJ, Royal W, 3rd, Gelfand JM, Clifford DB, Tavee J, Pawate S, et al. Definition and Consensus Diagnostic Criteria for Neurosarcoidosis: From the Neurosarcoidosis Consortium Consensus Group. JAMA Neurol. 2018;75(12):1546–53. https://doi.org/10.1001/jamaneurol.2018.2295

Linked question

76. A biopsy of the hilar lymph nodes is performed on the patient in the prior question, as shown below. This biopsy identifies a(n):
    A. Non-necrotizing granuloma
    B. Eosinophilic palisading granulomas
    C. Neutrophil invasion of medium-sized arteries
    D. Storiform fibrosis
    Correct answer: A

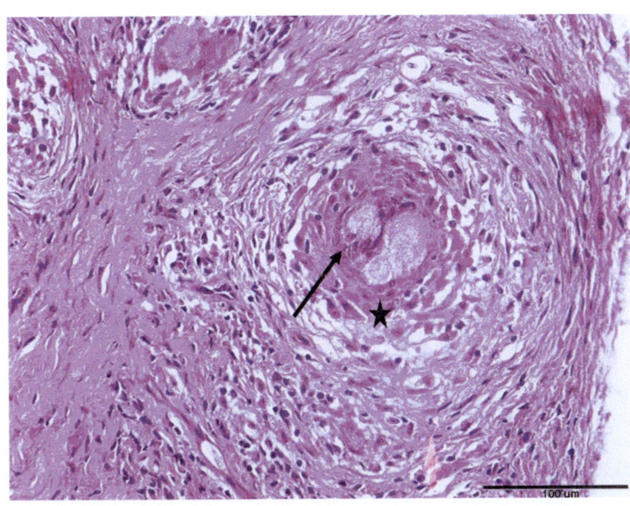

(Source: Henrichs, M-P., Streitburger, A., Surke, C., Dierkes, C., Hardes, J. CC-BY 2.0 (https://creativecommons.org/licenses/by/2.0/), via BMC Research Notes. Image has not been modified from source. Please see full attribution with citation below in references section for this question.)

Explanation

The hallmark histopathologic findings of sarcoidosis are the non-necrotizing (non-caseating) granuloma without evidence of infectious organisms. The core of the granuloma is composed of macrophages, giant cells, epithelioid cells, and CD4+ T cells while the crust is formed of predominantly CD8+ T lymphocytes and B cells. Activated T cells accumulate at sites of inflammation and produce various cytokines and chemokines, including TNF, which is a major driver of the formation and maturation of the granuloma. Eosinophilic

palisading granulomas can be found in eosinophilic granulomatosis with polyangiitis. Neutrophil invasion of medium-sized arteries can be seen in vasculitis. Storiform fibrosis is a key feature of IgG-4 disease.

References

Bradshaw MJ, Pawate S, Koth LL, Cho TA, Gelfand JM. Neurosarcoidosis: Pathophysiology, Diagnosis, and Treatment. Neurol Neuroimmunol Neuroinflamm. 2021;8(6). https://doi.org/10.1212/nxi.0000000000001084.

Henrichs MP, Streitbürger A, Gosheger G, Surke C, Dierkes C, Hardes J. Scar sarcoidosis on a finger mimicking a rapidly growing soft tissue tumour: a case report. BMC Res Notes. 2012;5:545. https://doi.org/10.1186/1756-0500-5-545.

Stern BJ, Royal W, 3rd, Gelfand JM, Clifford DB, Tavee J, Pawate S, et al. Definition and Consensus Diagnostic Criteria for Neurosarcoidosis: From the Neurosarcoidosis Consortium Consensus Group. JAMA Neurol. 2018;75(12):1546–53. https://doi.org/10.1001/jamaneurol.2018.2295.

Linked question

77. For the patient in the prior question, you make a diagnosis of
    A. Possible neurosarcoidosis
    B. Probable neurosarcoidosis
    C. Definite neurosarcoidosis
    D. Tuberculosis
    Correct answer: B

Explanation

The patient is presenting with a typical syndrome of neurosarcoidosis, supporting features in the form of typical MRI, supportive lumbar puncture results, and negative testing for alternative diagnosis. He has extraneural biopsy-proven sarcoidosis in the hilar lymph nodes, but no biopsy of a central nervous system site has been completed. By the 2018 diagnostic criteria, this is probable neurosarcoidosis. A diagnosis of definite neurosarcoidosis can be made when the above conditions are met and there is biopsy of the neurological site of involvement demonstrating sarcoidosis (i.e., non-necrotizing granulomas).

Reference

Stern BJ, Royal W, 3rd, Gelfand JM, Clifford DB, Tavee J, Pawate S, et al. Definition and Consensus Diagnostic Criteria for Neurosarcoidosis: From the Neurosarcoidosis Consortium Consensus Group. JAMA Neurol. 2018;75(12):1546–53. https://doi.org/10.1001/jamaneurol.2018.2295.

78. Typical MRI features of neurosarcoid-associated transverse myelitis include all the following except:
    A. Longitudinally extensive
    B. Central canal and posterior subpial enhancement leading to an appearance known as the "trident sign"
    C. Persistent enhancement for >3 months
    D. Cervical region is most commonly affected
    Correct answer: D

Explanation

Myelopathy is one of the classic syndromes of neurosarcoidosis, with the thoracic region most commonly affected followed by the cervical region. Patients often present with lower extremity sensory and motor symptoms that progress over months. The most common imaging presentation is a longitudinally extensive transverse myelitis. Other manifestations include short tumefactive myelitis and spinal meningitis or meningoradiculitis. MRI features include intramedullary T2 hyperintensity with various enhancement patterns. Dorsal subpial enhancement extending circumferentially, along with central canal enhancement extending to the dorsal cord, create what is known as the "trident sign" best visualized on axial sequences. Enhancement that persists for >3 months can be a clue towards neurosarcoidosis. Steroids remain the mainstay of treatment of neurosarcoidosis, but additional steroid-sparing agents are often used. Given the severity of neurosarcoid-associated myelopathy, early initiation of anti-TNF agents, such as infliximab, is often used.

References

Bradshaw MJ, Pawate S, Koth LL, Cho TA, Gelfand JM. Neurosarcoidosis: Pathophysiology, Diagnosis, and Treatment. Neurol Neuroimmunol Neuroinflamm. 2021;8(6). https://doi.org/10.1212/nxi.0000000000001084.

Murphy OC, Salazar-Camelo A, Jimenez JA, Barreras P, Reyes MI, Garcia MA, et al. Clinical and MRI phenotypes of sarcoidosis-associated myelopathy. Neurol Neuroimmunol Neuroinflamm. 2020;7(4). https://doi.org/10.1212/nxi.0000000000000722.

79. Sites of nervous system involvement in neurosarcoidosis include:
    A. Cranial nerves
    B. Brain parenchyma
    C. Meninges
    D. Spinal cord
    E. Peripheral nerves
    F. A, C, and D
    G. A, B, C, and D
    H. All of the above
    Correct answer: H

Explanation

Sarcoidosis is sometimes referred to as "the great mimicker" or the "great imitator" due to its many and varied clinical manifestations. This is often thought to be true for neurosarcoidosis as well due its multifarious neurological manifestations. However, there are typical presentations that coincide with the anatomical site of involvement. It behooves the good neurologist to be aware of the possible sites of involvement and the typical manifestations therein. Typical manifestations include:

- Cranial neuropathy: Mononeuropathy or multiple cranial neuropathy (i.e., polyneuritis cranialis)
- Parenchymal involvement: Seizures, encephalopathy, mass lesions with focal deficits, and endocrine dysfunction from hypothalamic or pituitary involvement. Rarely can cause vasculitis and stroke
- Meninges: Subacute leptomeningitis or pachymeningitis, meningeal mass lesions mimicking meningioma
- Spinal cord: Longitudinally extensive lesion with a progressive myelopathy, short segment tumefactive myelitis
- Peripheral nerves: Large fiber neuropathy

References

Bradshaw MJ, Pawate S, Koth LL, Cho TA, Gelfand JM. Neurosarcoidosis: Pathophysiology, Diagnosis, and Treatment. Neurol Neuroimmunol Neuroinflamm. 2021;8(6). https://doi.org/10.1212/nxi.0000000000001084.

Stern BJ, Royal W, 3rd, Gelfand JM, Clifford DB, Tavee J, Pawate S, et al. Definition and Consensus Diagnostic Criteria for Neurosarcoidosis: From the Neurosarcoidosis Consortium Consensus Group. JAMA Neurol. 2018;75(12):1546–53. https://doi.org/10.1001/jamaneurol.2018.2295.

80. A 31-year-old woman with MS presents to clinic for routine follow-up. Her disease has been stable on ocrelizumab for the last 4 years with stable MRI. She is interested in pursuing pregnancy. Which of the following about MS and pregnancy is *incorrect*?
    A. Rates of relapse are relatively lower during pregnancy
    B. Rates of relapse are elevated in the first 3–6 months postpartum

C. Breastfeeding is protective against postpartum relapse risk

D. The risk of MS in an offspring is 7–8% with one affected parent

Correct answer: D

Explanation

As many patients with MS are women of childbearing age, aspects of fertility, pregnancy planning, and pre- and post-partum counseling are critical. Historically, women with MS were counseled against pregnancy, but more recent data has led to a paradigm shift. Women with MS should follow standard obstetric advice. A common concern is risk of MS to offspring of a parent with MS. This has been estimated at 2–3% with one affected parent and higher with two affected parents. Several studies have demonstrated a relative decrease in relapse risk during pregnancy with an increased relapse risk in the first 3–6 months postpartum, with rates subsequently returning to prepartum rates. Relapse risk may be influenced by DMT, and therefore one must consider efficacy, recommended washout period prior to conception, and medication dynamics (e.g., risk of rebound disease with discontinuation of certain DMTs). Exclusive breastfeeding has a protective effect on postpartum relapse risk. Therefore, postpartum DMT choice is also important, and one must consider exposure to offspring via breastmilk of various DMTs.

References

Confavreux C, Hutchinson M, Hours MM, Cortinovis-Tourniaire P, Moreau T. Rate of pregnancy-related relapse in multiple sclerosis. Pregnancy in Multiple Sclerosis Group. N Engl J Med. 1998;339(5):285–91. https://doi.org/10.1056/NEJM199807303390501.

Houtchens MK, Edwards NC, Phillips AL. Relapses and disease-modifying drug treatment in pregnancy and live birth in US women with MS. Neurology. 2018;91(17):e1570–e1578. https://doi.org/10.1212/WNL.0000000000006382.

Langer-Gould A, Smith JB, Albers KB, et al. Pregnancy-related relapses and breastfeeding in a contemporary multiple sclerosis cohort. Neurology. 2020;94(18):e1939–e1949. https://doi.org/10.1212/WNL.0000000000009374.

Yeh WZ, Widyastuti PA, Van der Walt A, et al. Natalizumab, Fingolimod and Dimethyl Fumarate Use and Pregnancy-Related Relapse and Disability in Women With Multiple Sclerosis. Neurology. 2021;96(24):e2989 e3002. Published 2021 Jun 15. https://doi.org/10.1212/WNL.0000000000012084

81. A 28-year-old woman presents with a 4-day history of blurred vision and pain with eye movement in her right eye. Visual acuity is 20/200 in the affected eye, and a relative afferent pupillary defect is present. Fundoscopic exam is normal. MRI of the brain and orbits shows high T2 signal and contrast enhancement of the right optic nerve and one non-enhancing periventricular white matter lesion. Based on the findings of the Optic Neuritis Treatment Trial, which of the following is the most appropriate initial management?

A. Oral prednisone 1mg/kg for 14 days

B. High-dose intravenous methylprednisolone followed by an oral prednisone taper

C. Plasmapheresis

D. Intravenous immunoglobulin (IVIG)

E. Initiate a high efficacy disease-modifying therapy for MS

Correct answer: B

Explanation

The Optic Neuritis Treatment Trial (ONTT, 1992) was a large, randomized controlled trial that compared different treatments for acute optic neuritis - 1) high-dose IV methylprednisolone (1 g/day for 3 days) followed by an oral prednisone taper (1 mg/kg/day for 11 days), 2) oral prednisone (1 mg/kg/day) for 14 days, and 3) placebo. Treatment with IV steroids hastened visual recovery compared to placebo, but there was no statistical difference in final visual acuity at 6 months and 10 years. Furthermore, oral prednisone at this dose was no better than placebo and was associated with a higher risk of recurrent optic neuritis. As such, demyelinating optic neuritis is typically treated with 3 to 5 days of high-dose IV methylprednisolone.

Reference

Beck RW, Cleary PA, Anderson MM, Jr., Keltner JL, Shults WT, Kaufman DI, et al. A randomized, controlled trial of corticosteroids in the treatment of acute optic neuritis. The Optic Neuritis Study Group. N Engl J Med. 1992;326(9):581-8. https://doi.org/10.1056/NEJM199202273260901.

Linked questions: 82–83

82. A 41-year-old right-handed man with RRMS presents with subacute onset left arm numbness and weakness. An outpatient MRI confirms a new T2 hyperintense lesion in the cervical spinal cord with associated enhancement. He is hesitant to be admitted for a course of IV steroids because of childcare concerns and asks about an alternative, if possible. Which of the following is correct?

A. Oral corticosteroids are less effective than intravenous corticosteroids for MS relapse and should not be used
B. Oral corticosteroids are equally effective as intravenous methylprednisolone for MS relapses and can be considered in appropriate patients
C. Plasma exchange is a first-line therapy for all acute MS relapses, thus warranting inpatient admission
D. Oral corticosteroids are only effective in optic nerve or cerebral lesions, not spinal cord lesions

Correct answer: B

Explanation

The COPOUSEP Trial (2015) was a pivotal study in the treatment of MS relapses. It was a randomized, controlled, double-blind, non-inferiority trial that compared high-dose oral methylprednisolone to high-dose IV methylprednisolone (both 1000 mg/day) for acute relapses. It demonstrated that oral administration was not inferior to intravenous administration at improving disability scores at 28 days. This data supports the use of oral steroids in appropriate patients. Plasma exchange (choice c) is typically used in steroid-refractory or severe MS relapses.

Reference

Le Page E, Veillard D, Laplaud DA, Hamonic S, Wardi R, Lebrun C, et al. Oral versus intravenous high-dose methylprednisolone for treatment of relapses in patients with multiple sclerosis (COPOUSEP): a randomised, controlled, double-blind, non-inferiority trial. Lancet. 2015;386(9997):974-81. https://doi.org/10.1016/S0140-6736(15)61137-0.

Linked question

83. You prescribe the patient in the prior question a 5-day course of high-dose oral steroids. Which side effect should you counsel him is *more* commonly seen with oral steroids when compared to intravenous steroids?
    A. Anxiety
    B. Palpitations
    C. Metallic taste
    D. Nausea
    E. Insomnia

Correct answer: E

Explanation

All of these adverse effects – anxiety, palpitations, metallic taste, nausea, and insomnia – were reported by participants in both the intravenous and oral methylprednisolone group of the COPOUSEP trial. However, there was only a statistically significant difference in the incidence of insomnia at day 28. Insomnia was reported by 77 of 100 patients (77%) in the oral prednisolone group and 63 of 99 patients (64%) in the intravenous group ($p = 0.0390$).

Reference

Le Page E, Veillard D, Laplaud DA, Hamonic S, Wardi R, Lebrun C, et al. Oral versus intravenous high-dose methylprednisolone for treatment of relapses in patients with multiple sclerosis (COPOUSEP): a randomised, controlled, double-blind, non-inferiority trial. Lancet. 2015;386(9997):974-81. https://doi.org/10.1016/S0140-6736(15)61137-0.

84. What is the estimated lifetime prevalence of depression in patients with MS?
    A. 1%
    B. 10%
    C. 25%
    D. 50%
    E. 75%

Correct answer: D

Explanation

There is a high rate of depression in patients with multiple sclerosis when compared to the general population. Across multiple studies, annual prevalence is estimated at 20% and lifetime prevalence is estimated at 50%. Multiple factors associated with MS likely contribute to this, including pain, fatigue, anxiety, and cognitive impairment.

Reference

Siegert RJ, Abernethy DA. Depression in multiple sclerosis: a review. J Neurol Neurosurg Psychiatry. 2005;76(4):469-75. https://doi.org/10.1136/jnnp.2004.054635.

Eddie Louie and Scott Weisenberg

1. A 6-year-old boy from an under-vaccinated community presents with sudden onset asymmetric weakness in his right leg, accompanied by fever and myalgia in late winter. Examination reveals decreased muscle tone, absent deep tendon reflexes, and no sensory deficits. CSF analysis shows mild pleocytosis with elevated protein and normal glucose. Which of the following is the most likely causative agent?
   A. Enterovirus D68
   B. Poliovirus
   C. Guillain-Barré syndrome
   D. West Nile virus
   E. Herpes simplex virus (HSV)
   Correct answer: B

Explanation

The history and examination strongly support the diagnosis of poliovirus. Poliovirus is an enterovirus transmitted via the fecal-oral or respiratory route, affecting anterior horn cells, leading to acute flaccid paralysis without sensory loss. Diagnosis is via stool/throat PCR, and prevention is through inactivated poliovirus vaccination. Enterovirus D 68 can cause acute flaccid paralysis especially in children and is usually associated with respiratory symptoms and occurs in the late summer to the fall. West Nile virus is a flavivirus and can also present with an acute flaccid paralysis but is associated with mosquito bites and not likely to occur in winter. Guillain-Barre can cause acute flaccid paralysis but usually affects both the motor and sensory nerves. Herpes simplex virus resides mainly in sensory nerves and rarely associated with acute flaccid paralysis.

Reference

Wolbert JG, Rajnik M, Swinkels HM, Higginbotham K. Poliomyelitis. StatPearls. Treasure Island (FL): StatPearls Publishing Copyright © 2025, StatPearls Publishing LLC.; 2025.

2. A 60-year-old man with leukemia on chemotherapy presents with fevers, headache, confusion, neutropenia, and focal left-sided weakness. MRI brain shows multiple ring-enhancing lesions. Biopsy with GMS stain as below. What is the most likely diagnosis?

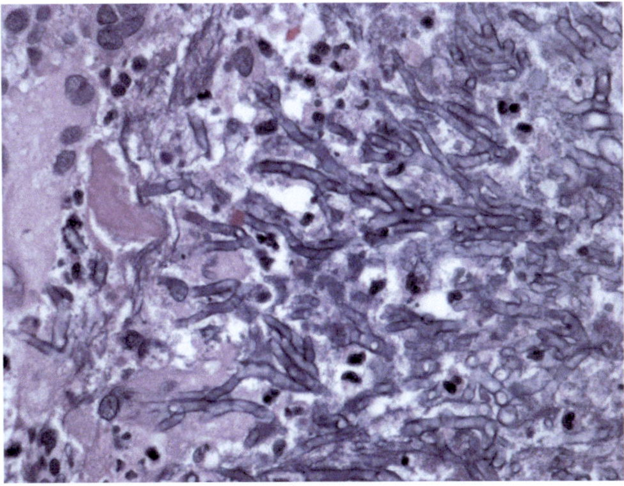

Biopsy, GMS staining. (Source: Bonagiri, P. R., Raman, A., Hassan, S., Ramsey, A. CC-BY 4.0 (https://creativecommons.org/licenses/by/4 0/) via *Cureus*. Image has not been modified from source. Please see full attribution with citation below in references section for this question.)

E. Louie (✉) · S. Weisenberg
Department of Medicine, NYU Grossman School of Medicine,
New York, NY, USA
e-mail: eddie.louie@nyulangone.org; scott.weisenberg@
nyulangone.org

A. Cryptococcal meningoencephalitis
B. Tuberculous meningitis
C. Toxoplasmosis
D. Cerebral aspergillosis
E. Bacterial brain abscess

Correct answer: D

Explanation

Cerebral aspergillosis occurs in immunocompromised patients and presents with ring-enhancing brain lesions. Histopathology shows acute-angle branching septate hyphae which is pathognomonic for *Aspergillus*. Voriconazole is the treatment of choice. Isavuconazole is a newer antifungal that is being studied and appears to be effective. Cryptococcus does not usually present with ring-enhancing lesions even in immunocompromised patients, and the pathology shows round to oval encapsulated yeasts with narrow-based budding. CNS toxoplasmosis can present with multiple enhancing lesions but is most commonly seen in patients with AIDS, and the biopsy does not show acute-angle branching hyphae. Tuberculous meningitis does not usually present with multiple ring-enhancing lesions. CT scan in patients with tuberculous meningitis may be abnormal but when present show basal meningeal enhancement and enhancing lesions (tuberculomas). A bacterial brain abscess is possible but the biopsy revealed fungal elements.

References

Bonagiri PR, Raman A, Hassan S, Ramsey A. CNS Aspergillosis: A Downside of Corticosteroid Use. Cureus. 2024;16(6):e62018. https://doi.org/10.7759/cureus.62018.

Dahan A, CNS aspergillosis. Case study, Radiopaedia.org (Accessed on 15 Apr 2025) https://doi.org/10.53347/rID-74204

Schwartz S, Kontoyiannis DP, Harrison T, Ruhnke M. Advances in the diagnosis and treatment of fungal infections of the CNS. Lancet Neurol. 2018;17(4):362–72. https://doi.org/10.1016/s1474-4422(18)30030-9.

Serris A, Rautemaa-Richardson R, Laranjinha JD, Candoni A, Garcia-Vidal C, Alastruey-Izquierdo A, et al. European Study of Cerebral Aspergillosis treated with Isavuconazole (ESCAI): A study by the ESCMID Fungal Infection Study Group. Clin Infect Dis. 2024;79(4):936–43. https://doi.org/10.1093/cid/ciae371.

Linked questions: 3–4

3. A 26-year-old woman with recently diagnosed ulcerative colitis and started on prednisone presents with a week of fever, headache, neck stiffness, and confusion. She frequently consumes deli meats. CSF analysis shows elevated white blood cell count with a neutrophilic predominance, high protein, and low glucose. MRI reveals brainstem involvement. What would the gram stain likely show?
   A. Gram positive diplococci
   B. Gram negative diplococci
   C. Gram negative rods
   D. Gram positive rods

Correct answer: D

Linked question

4. For the patient from the previous question, which of the following is the most likely causative organism?
   A. Streptococcus pneumoniae
   B. Listeria monocytogenes
   C. Neisseria meningitidis
   D. Cryptococcus neoformans
   E. Mycobacterium tuberculosis

Correct answer: B

Questions 3 and 4 Explanation

Listeria monocytogenes is a gram-positive rod that can cause meningoencephalitis in neonates, pregnant women, the elderly, and immunocompromised individuals. It is transmitted via contaminated food (e.g., unpasteurized dairy, deli meats). Unlike other bacterial meningitides such as *Streptococcus pneumoni*ae and *Neisseria meningitidis*, *Listeria* has a predilection for the brainstem (rhomboencephalitis), leading to cranial nerve deficits and ataxia. Treatment is ampicillin plus/minus gentamicin. On gram stain, *Streptococcus pneumoniae* appears as gram-positive lancet-shaped diplococci while *Neisseria meningitides* appears as gram-negative diplococci. CSF in *Cryptococcus neoformans* and *Mycobacterium tuberculosis* usually has a lymphocytic predominance.

Treatment: Ampicillin + gentamicin (for synergy in severe cases).

References

Brouwer MC, van de Beek D, Heckenberg SG, Spanjaard L, de Gans J. Community-acquired Listeria monocytogenes meningitis in adults. Clin Infect Dis. 2006;43(10):1233–8. https://doi.org/10.1086/508462.

Calder JA. Listeria meningitis in adults. Lancet. 1997;350(9074):307–8. https://doi.org/10.1016/s0140-6736(05)63384-3.

Rogalla D, Bomar PA. Listeria Monocytogenes. StatPearls. Treasure Island (FL): StatPearls Publishing Copyright © 2025, StatPearls Publishing LLC.; 2025.

Linked questions: 5–6

5. *A 45-year-old man with poorly* controlled diabetes presents with headache, facial pain, and left eye proptosis. Examination reveals ophthalmoplegia, decreased vision, and a necrotic eschar over the nasal mucosa. Blood results reveal glucose 450, bicarbonate 12, pH 7.1, and urine was positive for ketones. MRI reveals cavernous sinus involvement. Biopsy nasal mucosa reveals broad, non-septate hyphae with right angle branching. What is the most likely pathogen?
   A. Candida albicans
   B. Aspergillus fumigatus
   C. Mucormycosis
   D. Staphylococcus aureus
   Correct answer: C

Linked question

6. For the patient in the prior question, what is the most appropriate treatment?
   A. Voriconazole
   B. Amphotericin B and surgical debridement
   C. Fluconazole
   D. Caspofungin
   E. Acyclovir
   Correct answer: B

Questions 5 and 6 Explanation
Mucormycosis (caused by *Rhizopus* and *Mucor*) is life-threatening and presents with rhinocerebral spread, necrotic eschars, and cavernous sinus invasion. Mucormycosis is usually seen in patients with poorly controlled diabetes with ketoacidosis, immunocompromised patients, and patients with hemochromatosis. Histopathology showing broad non-septate hyphae with right angle branching is pathognomonic for mucormycosis. Liposomal amphotericin B and surgical debridement are required. Antifungal treatment alone is not adequate. Fluconazole is not active against mucormycosis. Acyclovir is an antiviral. *Aspergillus* and *Staphylococcus aureus* can present with invasive sinus infections and lead to cavernous sinus thrombosis, but the history, examination, and findings on pathology are most consistent with mucormycosis.

References
Sharma A, Goel A. Mucormycosis: risk factors, diagnosis, treatments, and challenges during COVID-19 pandemic. Folia Microbiol (Praha). 2022;67(3):363–87. https://doi.org/10.1007/s12223-021-00934-5.

Sigera LSM, Denning DW. A Systematic Review of the Therapeutic Outcome of Mucormycosis. Open Forum Infect Dis. 2024;11(1):ofad704. https://doi.org/10.1093/ofid/ofad704.

7. A 55-year-old previously healthy man presents with progressive cognitive decline, personality changes, and dysarthria over the past year. He has a history of untreated syphilis 15 years ago. Neurological examination reveals hyperreflexia, pupils that accommodated but did not constrict to light, and a broad-based gait. MRI shows atrophy, and CSF analysis is pending. What is the most likely diagnosis?

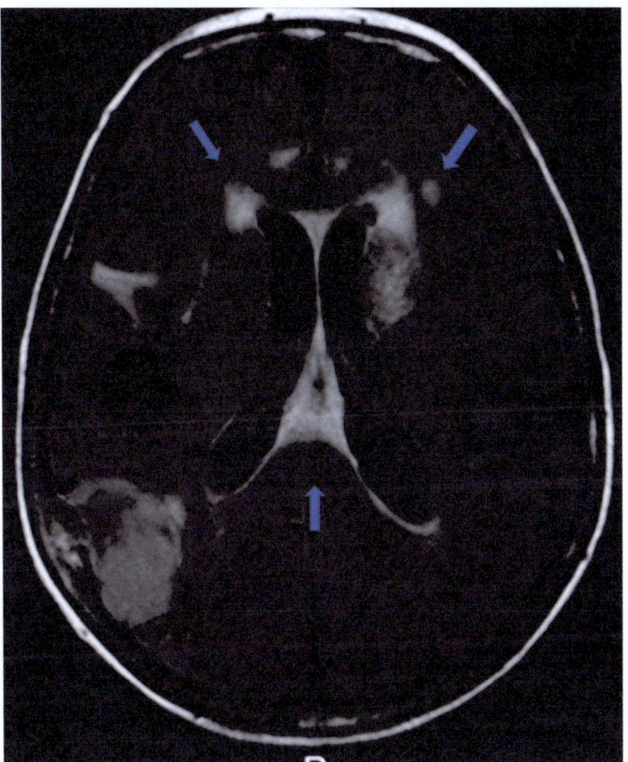

Axial MRI brain (for purpose of this question, please disregard incidental R parietal meningioma). (Source: Jancar, N., Simões, M., Gonçalves, F., Duro, J., Aguiar, P. CC-BY 4.0 (https://creativecommons.org/licenses/by/4.0/) via *Cureus*. Image has not been modified from source. Please see full attribution with citation below in references section for this question.)

   A. Tabes dorsalis
   B. Neurosyphilis (General paresis)
   C. Progressive multifocal leukoencephalopathy (PML)
   D. Alzheimer's disease
   E. HIV-associated dementia
   Correct answer: B

Explanation

Given his history of untreated syphilis and presentation, the most likely diagnosis is neurosyphilis. Neurosyphilis occurs when *Treponema pallidum* invades the central nervous system. If syphilis is left untreated, it can manifest in different forms many years later. One is general paresis (dementia paralytica) where patients present with neuropsychiatric symptoms such as dementia, personality changes, Argyll Robertson pupils (pupils that accommodate but did not constrict to light), dysarthria, hyperreflexia, and seizures. It is associated with cortical atrophy, nonspecific t2 hyperintensities, infarcts on MRI, and a positive CSF VDRL test. Tabes dorsalis is another late manifestation of syphilis characterized by sensory ataxia, lancinating pains, and loss of proprioception due to dorsal column degeneration. This patient's symptoms and findings are more consistent with general paresis. The recommended treatment is high-dose IV penicillin G for 10–14 days. Progressive multifocal leukoencephalopathy (PML) and HIV-associated dementia is seen in immunocompromised patients. PML is due to JC virus and is characterized by progressive damage of white matter of the brain. Alzheimer's dementia can lead to a similar presentation, but Argyll Robertson pupils is mainly seen with neurosyphilis.

References

Hamill MM, Ghanem KG, Tuddenham S. State-of-the-Art Review: Neurosyphilis. Clin Infect Dis. 2024;78(5):e57–e68. https://doi.org/10.1093/cid/ciad437.

Jancar N, Simões M, Gonçalves F, Duro J, Aguiar P. Neurosyphilis: The Great Imitator. Cureus. 2022;14(12):e32747. https://doi.org/10.7759/cureus.32747.

U.S. Centers for Disease Control and Prevention - Neurosyphilis, Ocular Syphilis, & Otosyphilis. https://www.cdc.gov/syphilis/hcp/neurosyphilis-ocular-syphilis-otosyphilis/index.html#cdc_generic_section_4-evaluation-and-treatment (2024). Accessed July 20 2025.

8. A 16-year-old boy presents with progressive cognitive decline, myoclonic jerks, and behavioral changes over the past several months. His parents elected not to have their son receive any vaccines. They report that he had a measles infection at the age of 4. EEG reveals periodic high-voltage discharges repetitive polyspike and sharp and slow wave complexes. MRI shows periventricular white matter hyperintensities. CSF analysis demonstrates elevated measles IgG antibodies. What is the most likely diagnosis?
A. Creutzfeldt-Jakob disease (CJD)
B. Subacute sclerosing panencephalitis (SSPE)
C. Autoimmune encephalitis
D. Progressive multifocal leukoencephalopathy (PML)
E. Acute disseminated encephalomyelitis (ADEM)

Correct answer: B

Explanation

SSPE is a rare but fatal progressive neurodegenerative disease caused by persistent measles virus infection. It typically occurs years after an initial measles infection, especially in those who were infected at a young age and did not receive vaccination. It is characterized by cognitive decline, myoclonus, seizures, and progressive neurological deterioration. Creutzfeldt-Jakob disease is a prion disease and usually rapidly progressive. Autoimmune encephalitis can have a similar presentation, but the elevated measles IgG antibodies in the CSF and EEG findings confirm the diagnosis of SSPE. ADEM is an acute, inflammatory, and demyelinating disease that can follow a vaccination or viral illness which he did not have. Progressive multifocal leukoencephalopathy (PML) is due to JC virus and seen in immunocompromised patients and is characterized by progressive damage of white matter of the brain

References

Adams and Victor's Principles of Neurology (11th Edition). Discusses the neurological complications of measles, including SSPE. ISBN: 978-0071794794

Campbell H, Lopez Bernal J, Bukasa A, Andrews N, Baker E, Maunder P, et al. A Re-emergence of Subacute Sclerosing Panencephalitis in the United Kingdom. Pediatr Infect Dis J. 2023;42(1):82–4. https://doi.org/10.1097/inf.0000000000003744.

Mandell, Douglas, and Bennett's Principles and Practice of Infectious Diseases (ninth Edition). Comprehensive review of measles virus and SSPE pathogenesis. ISBN: 978-0323482554

Mubbashir Z, Tharwani ZH, Kambar T, Munawar S, Raphael O, Siddiqui I, et al. Subacute Sclerosing Panencephalitis: Impact on Public Health, Current Insights, and Future Perspectives. Brain Behav. 2025;15(2):e70292. https://doi.org/10.1002/brb3.70292.

U.S. Centers for Disease Control and Prevention - Clinical Overview of Measles. https://www.cdc.gov/measles/hcp/clinical-overview/index.html (2025). Accessed July 20 2025.

9. A 67-year-old man presents in late summer with fever, confusion, and lower extremity flaccid paralysis. No respiratory or gastrointestinal symptoms. He recently camped in rural New York State and had multiple mosquito bites. No travel outside of the United States. CSF shows mild lymphocytic pleocytosis, elevated protein, and normal glucose. MRI is unremarkable. What is the most likely diagnosis?
   A. Herpes simplex virus encephalitis
   B. Guillain-Barré syndrome
   C. West Nile virus neuroinvasive disease
   D. Acute flaccid myelitis due to enterovirus D68
   E. Tick-borne encephalitis

Correct answer: C

Explanation

West Nile virus (a flavivirus) causes neuroinvasive disease with encephalitis, asymmetric flaccid paralysis, and areflexia. CSF IgM confirms diagnosis. Supportive care is the mainstay of treatment. Herpes simplex virus encephalitis usually presents acutely with fevers and altered mental status and seizures and does not usually cause lower extremity flaccid paralysis. Guillain-Barre syndrome does not typically present with fevers and confusion. Enterovirus D68 can cause acute flaccid paralysis especially in children and is usually associated with respiratory symptoms and usually occurs in late summer and early fall. Tick-borne encephalitis is also due to flavivirus and transmitted by ticks but not found in the United States. It is endemic in parts of Europe and Asia.

References

Habarugira G, Suen WW, Hobson-Peters J, Hall RA, Bielefeldt-Ohmann H. West Nile Virus: An Update on Pathobiology, Epidemiology, Diagnostics, Control and "One Health" Implications. Pathogens. 2020;9(7). https://doi.org/10.3390/pathogens9070589.

Sejvar James J. West Nile Virus Infection. Microbiology Spectrum. 2016;4(3):10.1128/microbiolspec. ei10–0021–2016. https://doi.org/10.1128/microbiolspec.ei10-0021-2016.

10. A 55-year-old man from the Ohio River Valley with Crohn's disease on adalimunab presents with chronic headache, fever, and weight loss. He reports night sweats and progressive confusion over the past 2 months. MRI brain shows basal meningeal enhancement, and CSF analysis reveals lymphocytic pleocytosis, elevated protein, and low glucose. Fungal culture is pending. Which of the following is the most likely diagnosis?
    A. Cryptococcal meningitis
    B. Tuberculous meningitis
    C. Histoplasma capsulatum meningitis
    D. Coccidioidal meningitis
    E. Bacterial meningitis

Correct answer: C

Explanation

Histoplasmosis is caused by *Histoplasma capsulatum*, a dimorphic fungus endemic to the Ohio and Mississippi River Valleys. It primarily affects immunocompromised individuals and can lead to chronic meningitis, characterized by basilar meningitis, hydrocephalus, and cranial neuropathies. Diagnosis is confirmed with a positive CSF histoplasma antigen, fungal culture, or PCR. Cryptococcus, mycobacteria tuberculosis, and coccidioidomycosis can all present in a similar way. The only clue that would make histoplasmosis more likely is that the patient was from the Ohio River Valley. A bacterial meningitis would present with a neutrophilic pleocytosis in the CSF.

Treatment: Liposomal amphotericin B followed by prolonged itraconazole therapy.

References

Ramírez JA, Reyes-Montes MDR, Rodríguez-Arellanes G, Pérez-Torres A, Taylor ML. Central Nervous System Histoplasmosis: An Updated Insight. Pathogens. 2023;12(5). https://doi.org/10.3390/pathogens12050681.

Wheat J, Myint T, Guo Y, Kemmer P, Hage C, Terry C, et al. Central nervous system histoplasmosis: Multicenter retrospective study on clinical features, diagnostic approach and outcome of treatment. Medicine (Baltimore). 2018;97(13):e0245. https://doi.org/10.1097/md.0000000000010245.

11. A 42-year-old man with a history of untreated HIV presents with progressive confusion, memory loss, and difficulty walking over the past 2 months. His CD4 count is 45 cells/μL. MRI of the brain is shown below. Which of the following is the most likely diagnosis?

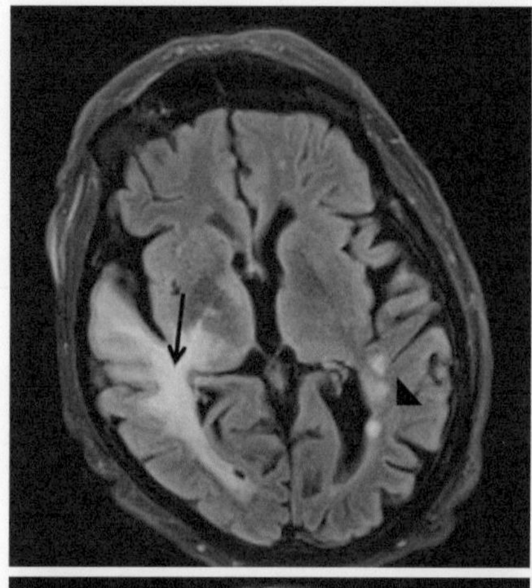
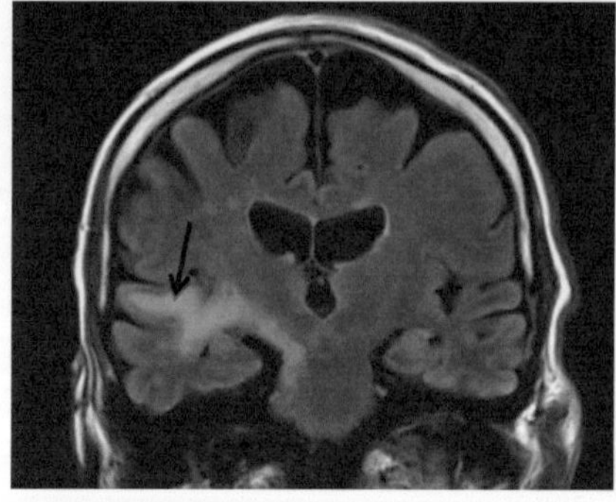
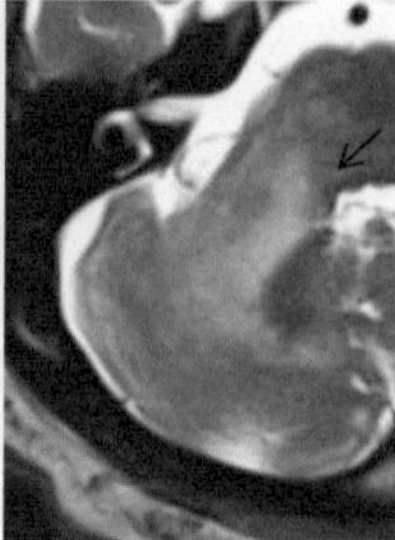

Axial (top left), coronal (bottom left), and axial (bottom right) MRI brain sections. (Source: Kmezic, I, Weinberg, J., Hauzenberger, D., Hashim, F., Kollia, E., Klimkowska, M., Nennesmo, I., Paucar, M. CC-BY 4.0 (https://creativecommons.org/licenses/by/4.0/) via *Cerebellum & Ataxias*. Image has been cropped from source. Please see full attribution with citation below in references section for this question.)

A. Progressive multifocal leukoencephalopathy (PML)
B. Cryptococcal meningitis
C. Primary CNS lymphoma
D. HIV-associated neurocognitive disorder (HAND)
E. Toxoplasmic encephalitis

Correct answer: A

Explanation

PML is caused by reactivation of the JC virus in immunocompromised individuals, particularly those with AIDS (CD4 <200). It presents with insidious cognitive decline, motor deficits, and ataxia. MRI findings of PML include asymmetric, non-enhancing white matter lesions without mass effect. CSF PCR for JC virus can confirm the diagnosis. HAND would be the next most likely diagnosis. HAND encompasses a spectrum of neurocognitive impairments associated with HIV, ranging from asymptomatic neurocognitive impairment to HIV-associated dementia. It is common in patients with CD4 <200. MRI findings include mild cortical atrophy and white matter changes. Choices B, C, and E can all be seen in HIV patients with low CD4 counts, but the MRI findings here are not usually seen with these choices.

References

Gaillard F, Progressive Multifocal Leukoencephalopathy (PML). Case Study, Radiopaedia.org https://doi.org/10.53347/rID-22071

Kmezic I, Weinberg J, Hauzenberger D, Hashim F, Kollia E, Klimkowska M, et al. An unusual cause of fatal rapid-onset ataxia plus syndrome. Cerebellum Ataxias. 2017;4:5. https://doi.org/10.1186/s40673-017-0063-9.

Nshimiyimana JF, Onsongo S. Progressive Multifocal Leukoencephalopathy confined to the posterior fossa as the presenting manifestation of HIV in a paediatric patient. IDCases. 2024;37:e02064. https://doi.org/10.1016/j.idcr.2024.e02064.

Patel K, Dutta A, Roger M. An Atypical Presentation of Progressive Multifocal Leukoencephalopathy With Newly Diagnosed HIV Infection. Annals of Internal Medicine: Clinical Cases. 2023;2. https://doi.org/10.7326/aimcc.2022.0809.

12. A 36-year-old woman with advanced HIV (CD4 count 30 cells/μL) presents with new-onset seizures and confusion. MRI is shown below. Serology is positive for *Toxoplasma gondii* IgG. What is the next best step in management?

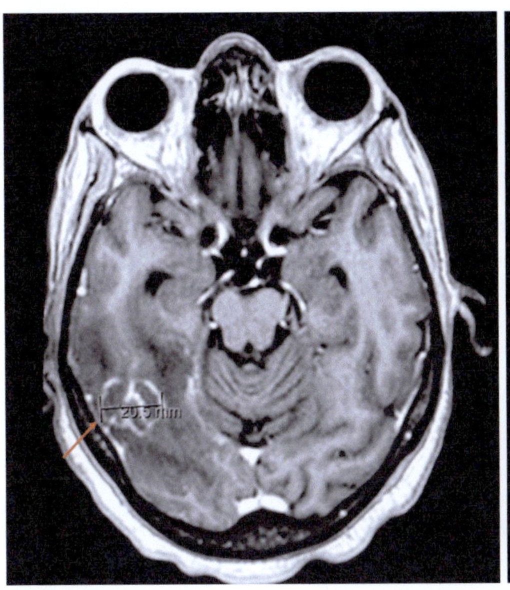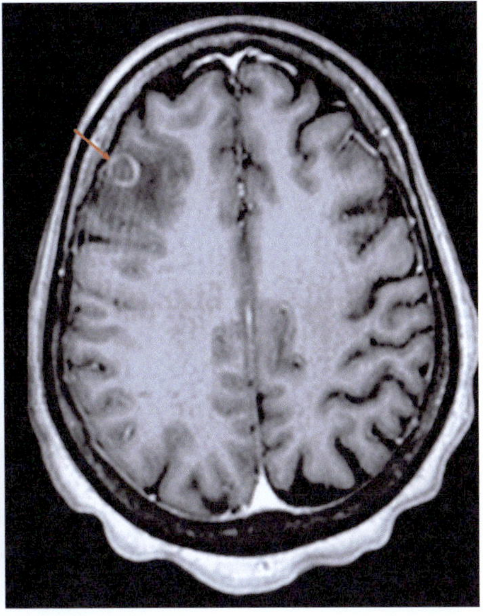

(**a, b**) axial MRI brain. (Source: Alves, D., Sobrosa, P., Passos, R. M., Silva, F., Ferreira, A., da Silva, R. C., Silva, D. CC-BY 4.0 (https://creativecommons.org/licenses/by/4.0/) via *Cureus*. Image has not been modified from source. Please see full attribution with citation below in references section for this question.)

A. Start pyrimethamine, sulfadiazine, and leucovorin
B. Perform a brain biopsy
C. Initiate IV amphotericin B
D. Start antiretroviral therapy immediately
E. Administer IV dexamethasone and observe

Correct answer: A

Explanation

Toxoplasmosis encephalitis is a common CNS opportunistic infection in AIDS patients with CD4 <100. It presents with focal neurological deficits and seizures. MRI findings include multiple ring-enhancing lesions, sometimes nodular enhancing lesions, typically in the basal ganglia. Given MRI findings and positive serology for toxoplasmosis, empiric treatment with pyrimethamine, sulfadiazine, and leucovorin should be initiated. If there is no improvement in 10–14 days, a brain biopsy should be considered to evaluate for lymphoma and other etiologies. Starting antiretroviral therapy immediately should also be done, but treating for toxoplasmosis is the better answer. Treating with amphotericin or starting dexamethasone alone is not appropriate given his findings which strongly suggest toxoplasmosis encephalitis.

References

Alves D, Sobrosa P, Morais Passos R, Silva F, Ferreira A, Corga da Silva R, et al. Cerebral Toxoplasmosis Mimicking a Brain Neoplasm in an Inaugural HIV-Positive Patient: The Importance of Early Decision-Making and Background Assessment in the Emergency Department. Cureus. 2025;17(1):e76936. https://doi.org/10.7759/cureus.76936.

Luft BJ, Chua A. Central Nervous System Toxoplasmosis in HIV Pathogenesis, Diagnosis, and Therapy. Curr Infect Dis Rep. 2000;2(4):358–62. https://doi.org/10.1007/s11908-000-0016-x.

13. A 40-year-old man with HIV presents with progressive cognitive decline, forgetfulness, and difficulty concentrating over several months. His CD4 count is 150 cells/µL. MRI shows mild cerebral atrophy without focal lesions. CSF studies are unremarkable. Syphilis IgG antibody is negative. What is the most likely diagnosis?

    A. HIV-associated neurocognitive disorder (HAND)
    B. Primary CNS lymphoma
    C. Progressive multifocal leukoencephalopathy (PML)
    D. Neurosyphilis
    E. Cryptococcal meningitis

    Correct answer: A

Explanation

HIV-associated neurocognitive disorder (HAND) encompasses a spectrum of neurocognitive impairments associated with HIV, ranging from mild neurocognitive impairment to HIV-associated dementia. It is common in patients with CD4 <200, even with ART. MRI findings include mild cortical atrophy and white matter changes. Diagnosis is clinical, and management includes optimizing ART. Primary CNS lymphoma usually presents with supratentorial, single, or multiple contrast-enhancing lesions on imaging. PML presents with non-enhancing white matter changes with no mass effect on imaging. Neurosyphilis is less likely given negative syphilis IgG antibody and normal CSF studies. Cryptococcal meningitis usually presents with abnormal CSF studies.

Reference

A Healthcare Provider's Guide to HIV-Associated Neurocognitive Disorder (HAND): Diagnosis, pharmacologic management and other considerations. UCSF Weill Institute for Neurosciences. Accessed July 20 2025.

14. A 55-year-old previously healthy woman presents with rapidly progressive dementia, myoclonus, and ataxia over the past 3 months. EEG shows periodic sharp wave complexes and MRI (see image below). CSF was sent for biomarkers. Syphilis IgG antibody is negative. What is the most likely diagnosis?

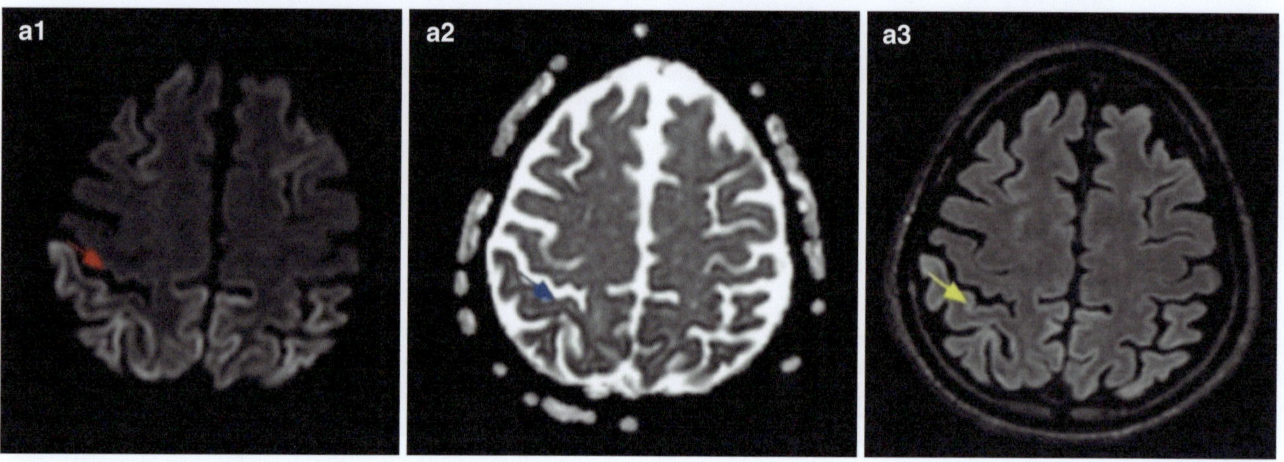

Axial MRI brain—diffusion weighted (A1), apparent diffusion coefficient (A2), and T2 FLAIR (A3) sequences. (Source: Rai, B, Nandish, S. Randall, M., Rajgopal, A. CC-BY 4.0 (https://creativecommons.org/licenses/by/4.0/) via *Cureus*. Image has been cropped from source. Please see full attribution with citation below in references section for this question.)

A. Creutzfeldt-Jakob disease (CJD)
B. HSV encephalitis
C. Progressive multifocal leukoencephalopathy (PML)
D. Neurosyphilis
E. Autoimmune encephalitis

Correct answer: A

Explanation

Creutzfeldt-Jakob disease (CJD) is a prion disease characterized by rapidly progressive dementia, myoclonus, and ataxia. It is diagnosed based on clinical features, EEG (periodic sharp wave complexes), MRI (cortical ribboning and basal ganglia hyperintensities), CSF biomarkers such as 14-3-3 protein, and a positive CSF real-time quaking-induced conversion (RT-QuIC). There is no effective treatment, and the disease is universally fatal within months. HSV encephalitis most commonly presents acute onset of fevers, altered mental status, and seizures. Imaging in patients with PML show non-enhancing white matter changes with no mass effect. Neurosyphilis can present with dementia but over a longer period of time and is less likely in this case given negative syphilis IgG antibody. Given MRI and EEG findings, autoimmune encephalitis is less likely.

References

Desai P, Sporadic Creutzfeldt Jakob Disease. Case Study, Radiopaedia.org (Accessed on 17 Apr 2025) https://doi.org/10.53347/rID-10043

Noor H, Baqai MH, Naveed H, Naveed T, Rehman SS, Aslam MS, et al. Creutzfeldt-Jakob disease: A comprehensive review of current understanding and research. J Neurol Sci. 2024;467:123293. https://doi.org/10.1016/j.jns.2024.123293.

Rai B, Nandish S, Randall M, Rajgopal A. Insights Into Creutzfeldt-Jakob Disease With a Case Series From a District General Hospital and a Literature Review. Cureus. 2025;17. https://doi.org/10.7759/cureus.92026.

Zerr I, Kallenberg K, Summers DM, Romero C, Taratuto A, Heinemann U, et al. Updated clinical diagnostic criteria for sporadic Creutzfeldt-Jakob disease. Brain. 2009;132(Pt 10):2659–68. https://doi.org/10.1093/brain/awp191.

15. A 5-year-old child in West Texas presents with fever, cough, conjunctivitis, and a maculopapular rash that started on the face and spread downward. The child was never given any vaccines as his parents were concerned that vaccines would lead to autism. A few days later, he develops altered mental status and seizures. CSF analysis shows normal glucose, mildly elevated protein, and a lymphocytic pleocytosis. MRI reveals hyperintensities in the subcortical white matter. What is the most likely diagnosis?

A. Acute disseminated encephalomyelitis (ADEM)
B. Measles encephalitis
C. Subacute sclerosing panencephalitis (SSPE)
D. Herpes simplex encephalitis
E. Bacterial meningitis

Correct answer: B

Explanation

Measles encephalitis is an acute CNS complication of measles virus infection that typically occurs within days of the rash. It presents with fever, headache, altered mental status, and seizures. CSF findings show a lymphocytic pleocytosis, elevated protein, and normal glucose. MRI may show diffuse or focal hyperintensities in the subcortical white matter. Treatment is supportive, as there is no specific antiviral therapy. Prevention through measles vaccination (MMR vaccine) is essential. ADEM is a postinfectious autoimmune response that can occur after measles but not seen during the acute infection. SSPE develops many years after the acute infection with measles. Herpes simplex encephalitis does not present with cough, conjunctivitis, and a maculopapular rash. The presentation and CSF findings are not suggestive of a bacterial meningitis (neutrophilic pleocytosis, low glucose).

References

Fisher DL, Defres S, Solomon T. Measles-induced encephalitis. Qjm. 2015;108(3):177–82. https://doi.org/10.1093/qjmed/hcu113.

Patterson MC. Neurological Complications of Measles (Rubeola). Curr Neurol Neurosci Rep. 2020;20(2):2. https://doi.org/10.1007/s11910-020-1023-y.

16. A 45-year-old man presents with a 2-week history of headache, fever, and progressive right-sided weakness. He has a history of chronic sinusitis. MRI is shown below. What is the most appropriate next step in management?

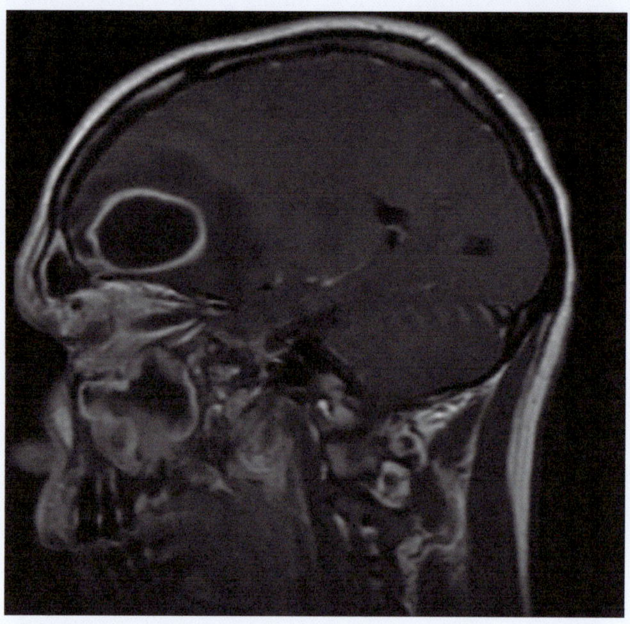

Sagittal MRI brain. (Source: Traficante, D., Riss, A., Hochman, S. CC-BY 4.0 (https://creativecommons.org/licenses/by/4.0/) via *International Journal of Emergency Medicine.* Image has not been modified from source. Please see full attribution with citation below in references section for this question.)

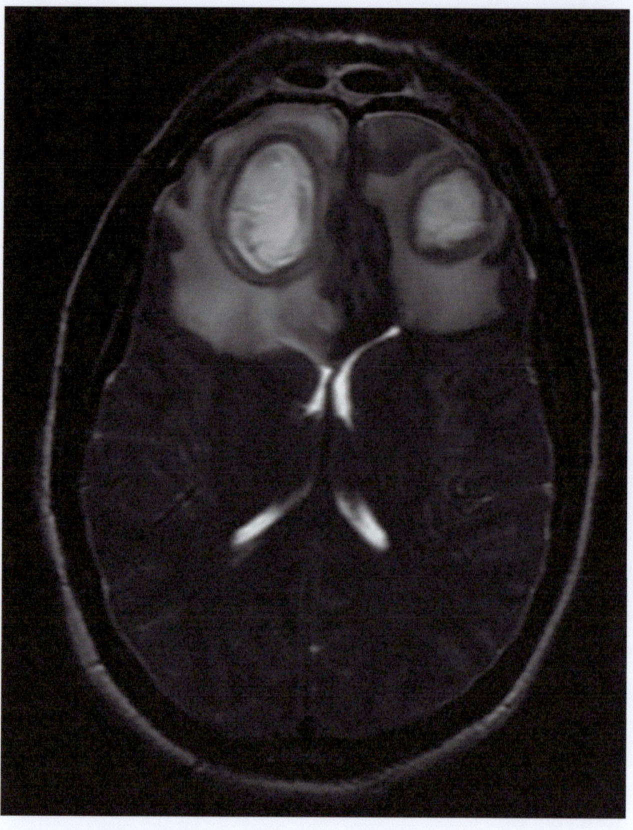

Axial MRI brain. (Source: Traficante, D., Riss, A., Hochman, S. CC-BY 4.0 (https://creativecommons.org/licenses/by/4.0/) via International Journal of Emergency Medicine. Image has not been modified from source. Please see full attribution with citation below in references section for this question.)

A. Lumbar puncture
B. Empiric IV antibiotics and surgical drainage
C. High-dose corticosteroids alone
D. Oral antibiotics and close monitoring
E. Anticoagulation therapy

Correct answer: B

Explanation

The patient's symptoms, imaging findings, and history of chronic sinusitis suggest a brain abscess. Lumbar puncture is often contraindicated due to the risk of herniation in cases of significant mass effect. Corticosteroids alone are not sufficient without addressing the underlying infection. Oral antibiotics and monitoring are inadequate for a lesion of this size. Most bacterial brain abscesses require intravenous antibiotics. Anticoagulation therapy is not indicated in brain abscess management.

References

Brouwer MC, Tunkel AR, McKhann GM, 2nd, van de Beek D. Brain abscess. N Engl J Med. 2014;371(5):447–56. https://doi.org/10.1056/NEJMra1301635.

Gaillard F, Le L, Silverstone L, et al. Cerebral abscess. Reference article, Radiopaedia.org https://doi.org/10.53347/rID-6677.

Traficante D, Riss A, Hochman S. Bifrontal brain abscesses secondary to orbital cellulitis and sinusitis extension. Int J Emerg Med. 2016;9(1):23. https://doi.org/10.1186/s12245-016-0117-4.

17. A 30-year-old woman presents with a 5-day history of progressively worsening headache, periorbital swelling, and fever. She reports a recent history of a painful pimple on her nose and sinusitis. Examination reveals proptosis, chemosis, cranial nerve VI palsy, as well as impaired sensation in the distribution of the ipsilateral maxillary branch of the trigeminal nerve. What is the most appropriate initial management?

    A. Empiric IV antibiotics and possible anticoagulation
    B. Lumbar puncture for CSF analysis
    C. Surgical thrombectomy
    D. High-dose corticosteroids alone
    E. Observation and symptomatic treatment

Correct answer: A

Explanation

Cavernous sinus thrombosis (CST) is a life-threatening condition usually resulting from facial or sinus infections. The presence of periorbital swelling, proptosis, cranial nerve palsy, and a known facial infection strongly suggests CST. Broad-spectrum IV antibiotics should be started immediately to cover *Staphylococcus aureus* and *Streptococcus* spp. Gram negative organisms like *Klebsiella* and anaerobes may also cause CST and should be covered with the appropriate antibiotic regimen. Anticoagulation is often recommended to prevent further thrombus propagation though evidence is limited. Lumbar puncture is usually not needed unless meningitis is suspected. Surgical thrombectomy is usually not done due to technical difficulty and lack of evidence of benefit. High-dose corticosteroids alone and observation are not appropriate as the infection needs to be treated with antibiotics.

References

Ali S. Cavernous Sinus Thrombosis: Efficiently Recognizing and Treating a Life-Threatening Condition. Cureus. 2021;13(8):e17339. https://doi.org/10.7759/cureus.17339.

D'Souza D, Jones J, Saber M, et al. Cavernous sinus thrombosis. Reference article, Radiopaedia.org https://doi.org/10.53347/rID-1065

18. A 55-year-old man with a history of diabetes and recent spine surgery presents with severe back pain, fever, and progressive lower extremity weakness over the past 3 days. On examination, he has tenderness over the thoracolumbar region of his spine and difficulty walking. MRI T2 with contrast reveals a rim-enhancing epidural collection compressing the spinal canal. What is the most appropriate next step in management?

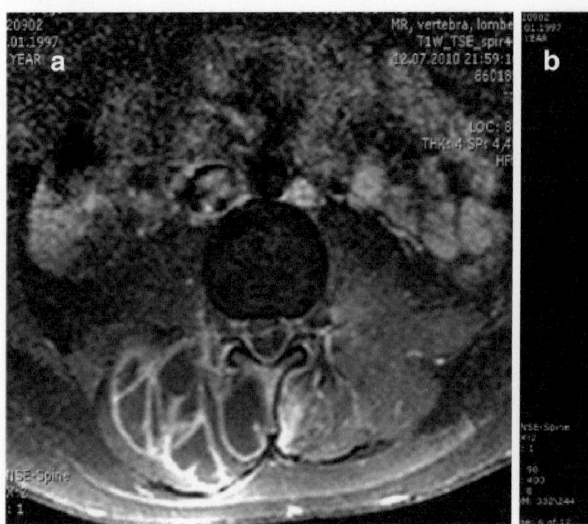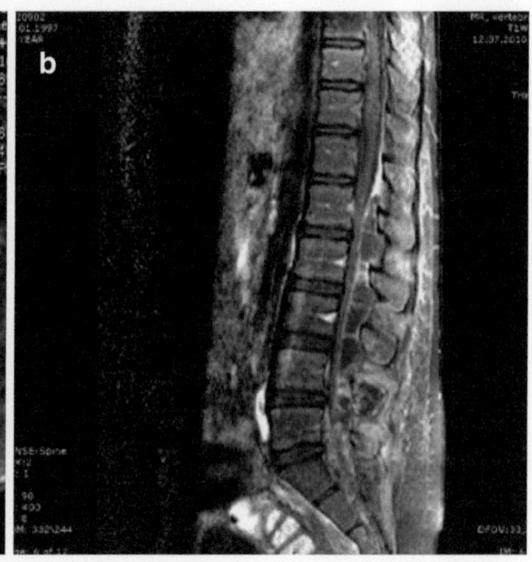

Axial (**a**) and sagittal (**b**) spine MRI. (Source: Aycan, A., Aktas, O. Y., Guzey, F. K., Tufan, A., Isler, C., Aycan N., Gulsen, I., Arslan, H. CC-BY 4.0 (https://creativecommons.org/licenses/by/4.0/) via *Case* *Reports in Infectious Disease*. Image has not been modified from source. Please see full attribution with citation below in references section for this question.)

A. Empiric IV antibiotics and urgent surgical decompression
B. Oral antibiotics and close outpatient follow-up
C. High-dose corticosteroids only
D. Observation and pain management
E. Lumbar puncture for CSF analysis

Correct answer: A

Explanation

Spinal epidural abscess (SEA) is a medical and surgical emergency that can lead to irreversible neurological damage if not promptly treated. The classic triad of back pain, fever, and neurological deficits suggests SEA. MRI is the diagnostic gold standard. Empiric antibiotics should cover *Staphylococcus aureus*, including MRSA, and gram-negative organisms. Surgical decompression is indicated in cases with neurological deficits to prevent permanent disability. Oral antibiotics and outpatient follow-up are inappropriate due to the risk of rapid deterioration. Corticosteroids alone and observation and pain management are not sufficient as the infection must be treated to prevent sepsis and progressive neurological symptoms. Lumbar puncture is not necessary and could increase the risk of worsening cord compression and lead to seeding of the CSF and meningitis.

References

Aycan A, Aktas OY, Guzey FK, Tufan A, Isler C, Aycan N, et al. Rapidly Progressive Spontaneous Spinal Epidural Abscess. Case Rep Infect Dis. 2016;2016:7958291. https://doi.org/10.1155/2016/7958291.

Darouiche RO. Spinal epidural abscess. N Engl J Med. 2006;355(19):2012–20. https://doi.org/10.1056/NEJMra055111.

Tetsuka S, Suzuki T, Ogawa T, Hashimoto R, Kato H. Spinal Epidural Abscess: A Review Highlighting Early Diagnosis and Management. Jma j. 2020;3(1):29–40. https://doi.org/10.31662/jmaj.2019-0038.

19. A 42-year-old man from China presents with a 3-week history of headache, low-grade fever, night sweats, and weight loss. He also reports new-onset confusion and difficulty walking. MRI with contrast is shown below. CSF analysis reveals elevated protein, low glucose, and lymphocytic pleocytosis. What is the most appropriate treatment?

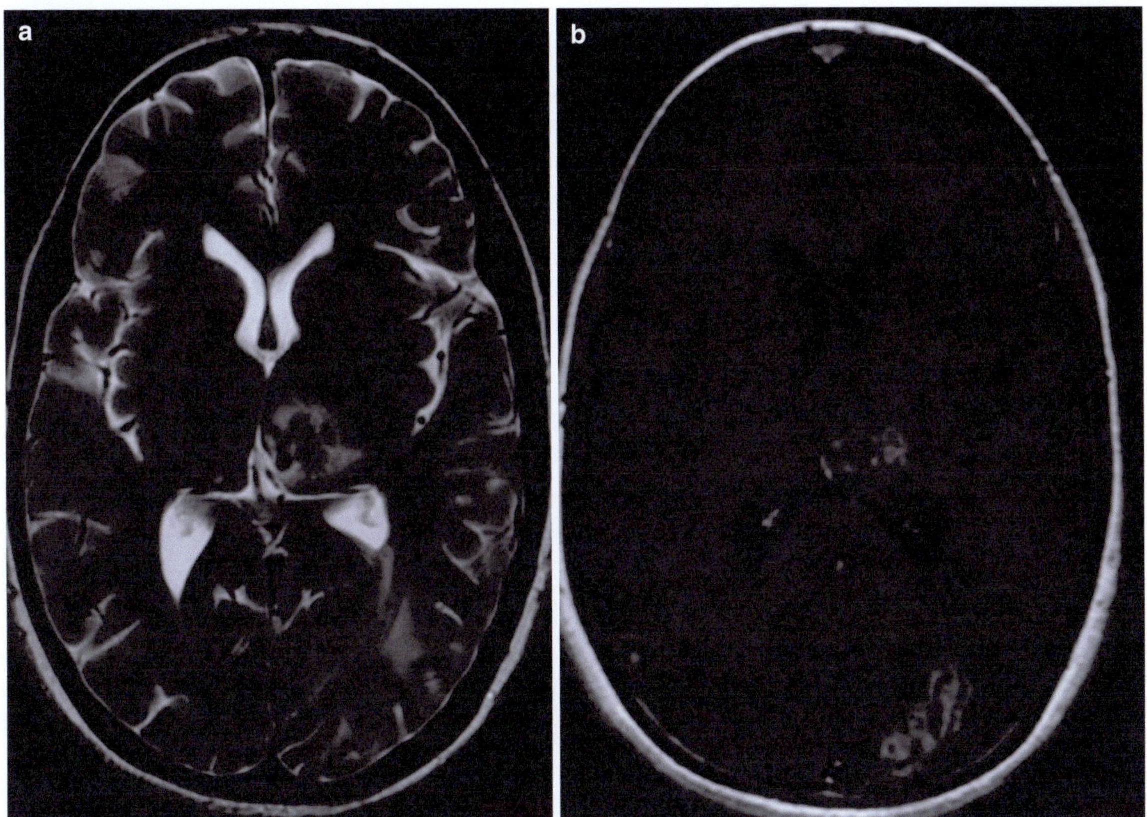

Axial MRI brain. (Source: Patel, T., Meena, V. K., Khandekar, A., K., Rachani, K., Meena, P., Shukla, D. CC-BY 4.0 (https://creativecommons.org/licenses/by/4.0/) via *Cureus*. Image has been cropped from source. Please see full attribution with citation below in references section for this question.)

A. IV ceftriaxone and vancomycin
B. IV acyclovir
C. Rifampin, isoniazid, pyrazinamide, and ethambutol with corticosteroids
D. High-dose corticosteroids alone
E. IV amphotericin B

Correct answer: C

Explanation

Tuberculous meningitis presents with subacute symptoms, basal meningeal enhancement, hydrocephalus, and CSF findings of elevated protein, low glucose, and lymphocytic pleocytosis. The first-line treatment includes a 4-drug antituberculous regimen along with corticosteroids to reduce inflammation. The 3-week history goes against a bacterial meningitis and herpes encephalitis so A and B are not correct. High-dose corticosteroids alone do not address the probable infection which is likely given MRI and CSF findings. A fungal meningitis is possible but less likely given his presentation.

References

Dian S, Hermawan R, van Laarhoven A, Immaculata S, Achmad TH, Ruslami R, et al. Brain MRI findings in relation to clinical characteristics and outcome of tuberculous meningitis. PLoS One. 2020;15(11):e0241974. https://doi.org/10.1371/journal.pone.0241974.

Patel T, Meena VK, Khandekar AK, Rachani K, Meena P, Shukla D. Diverse Manifestations of Central Nervous System Tuberculosis: Magnetic Resonance Imaging (MRI) Presentations and Laboratory Investigations in a Cohort Study. Cureus. 2025;17(6):e87077. https://doi.org/10.7759/cureus.87077.

Wilkinson RJ, Rohlwink U, Misra UK, van Crevel R, Mai NTH, Dooley KE, et al. Tuberculous meningitis. Nat Rev. Neurol. 2017;13(10):581–98. https://doi.org/10.1038/nrneurol.2017.120.

20. 65-year-old man presents with fever, cough, neck stiffness, heart murmur, and altered mental status. Chest x-ray reveals consolidation in the left lower lobe. CSF analysis shows elevated WBCs (predominantly neutrophils), low glucose, and elevated protein and negative herpes simplex PCR. What is the most likely causative organism?

A. *Streptococcus pneumoniae*
B. Herpes simplex virus
C. *Cryptococcus neoformans*
D. *Mycobacterium tuberculosis*

Correct answer: A

Explanation

Streptococcus pneumoniae is the most common cause of bacterial meningitis in adults. Patients with streptococcal pneumoniae meningitis may also present with pneumonia and endocarditis (Austrian's triad). Herpes simplex encephalitis does not present with pneumonia, and negative herpes simplex PCR makes it less likely. The CSF in cryptococcus and tuberculous meningitis usually shows a lymphocytic predominance.

References

Austrian R. Pneumococcal endocarditis, meningitis, and rupture of the aortic valve. AMA Arch Intern Med. 1957;99(4):539–44.

Hasbun R. Progress and Challenges in Bacterial Meningitis: A Review. Jama. 2022;328(21):2147–54. https://doi.org/10.1001/jama.2022.20521.

21. A 29-year-old man presents with progressive weakness in his legs over the past 3 days. He recently recovered from a diarrheal illness 1 week ago. On exam, he has symmetric lower extremity weakness, areflexia, and diminished vibration sense in his feet. His vital capacity is within normal limits. Lumbar puncture shows elevated protein with normal cell count.

Which of the following is the most appropriate next step in treatment?
A. Administer high-dose corticosteroids
B. Begin intravenous immunoglobulin (IVIG) therapy
C. Observe and monitor for respiratory compromise
D. Start broad-spectrum antibiotics
E. Perform plasmapheresis and IVIG concurrently

Correct answer: B

Explanation

This patient has Guillain-Barré Syndrome (GBS), likely triggered by *Campylobacter jejuni* (post-infectious). Classic signs include ascending symmetric weakness, areflexia, and albuminocytologic dissociation in CSF (elevated protein, normal WBC). Treatment is with IVIG or plasmapheresis but not both simultaneously. Corticosteroids are not recommended and may even be harmful. Observation in this patient without treatment for his GBS may increase risk for respiratory compromise GBS is an autoimmune condition and there is no need for antibiotics.

Reference

Bellanti R, Rinaldi S. Guillain-Barré syndrome: a comprehensive review. Eur J Neurol. 2024;31(8):e16365. https://doi.org/10.1111/ene.16365.

22. A 45-year-old man from Massachusetts presents with a 5-day history of facial droop on the right side, headache, neck stiffness, and fatigue. He denies rash. He recently returned from a hiking trip in rural Massachusetts 3 weeks ago. On exam, he has right-sided lower motor neuron facial weakness, normal limb strength, and mild photophobia. MRI is unremarkable. Lumbar puncture shows lymphocytic pleocytosis with mildly elevated protein and normal glucose. Serum Lyme ELISA is positive; western blot is pending. Which of the following is the most appropriate next step in management?

A. Oral doxycycline for 14–28 day
B. High-dose IV corticosteroids
C. IV ceftriaxone for 14–28 days
D. Repeat Lyme serology in 2 weeks
E. Empiric acyclovir and await test results

Correct answer: C

Explanation

This patient shows signs of early disseminated Lyme disease with neurologic involvement, including facial nerve palsy and aseptic meningitis and abnormal CSF. These findings support neuroborreliosis. The recommended treatment for neuroborreliosis is IV ceftriaxone or in less severe cases oral doxycycline. Steroids are not indicated in treating neuroborreliosis. Repeat Lyme serology can be done but would not change his management. History does not suggest a herpes infection so E is incorrect.

References

Halperin JJ. Nervous system Lyme disease. Infect Dis Clin North Am. 2015;29(2):241–53. https://doi.org/10.1016/j.idc.2015.02.002.

U.S. Centers for Disease Control and Prevention - Clinical Care and Treatment of Neurologic Lyme Disease. https://www.cdc.gov/lyme/hcp/clinical-care/neurologic-lyme-disease.html (2025). Accessed July 202025.

23. A 42-year-old woman is brought to the emergency department after being found confused at home. Her family reports that she had a headache, low-grade fever, and nausea for 2 days. This morning, she became disoriented and began speaking incoherently. On exam, she is febrile (38.9 °C), disoriented to time and place, and intermittently agitated. She is unable to follow complex commands. No nuchal rigidity is noted.

    MRI brain is shown below.

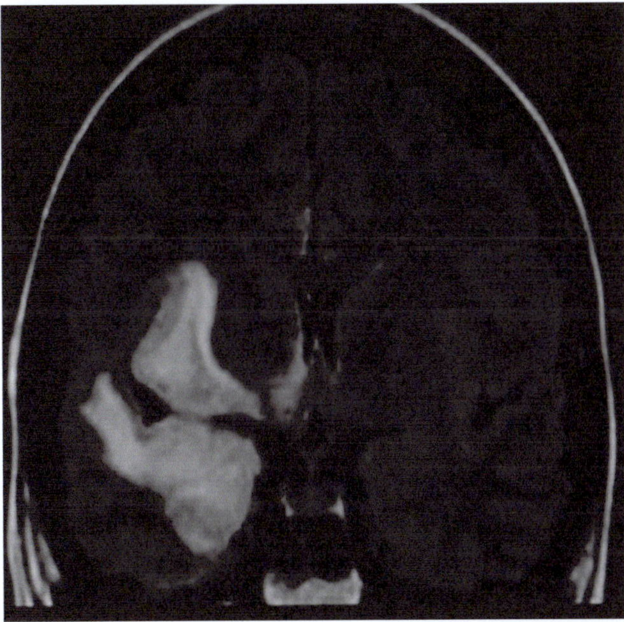

Coronal MRI brain. (Source: Defres, S., Keller, S. S., Das, K., Vidyasagar, R., Parkes, L. M., Burnside, G., Griffiths, M., Kopelman, M., Roberts, N., Solomon, T., ENCEPH UK study group. CC-BY 4.0 (https://creativecommons.org/licenses/by/4.0/) via *PLoS One*. Image has been cropped from source. Please see full attribution with citation below in references section for this question.)

Lumbar puncture reveals:

- WBC: 120/mm^3 (90% lymphocytes)
- Protein: 95 mg/dL
- Glucose: 60 mg/dL (serum glucose: 100 mg/dL)

Which of the following is the most appropriate next step in management?

   A. Begin IV ceftriaxone, vancomycin, and dexamethasone

   B. Wait for CSF HSV PCR results before starting treatment

   C. Administer IV acyclovir immediately

   D. Order EEG and defer treatment until results return

   E. Start high-dose corticosteroids for suspected autoimmune encephalitis

Correct answer: C

Explanation

Patient has classic signs of herpes simplex virus (HSV) encephalitis which is the most common cause of sporadic fatal encephalitis in the United States. She presents with acute onset of confusion, aphasia, fever, MRI with temporal lobe involvement, and CSF with lymphocytic pleocytosis and elevated protein. A bacterial meningitis is not likely given her MRI and CSF findings, so she does not need antibiotics. Delaying treatment pending definitive diagnosis significantly increases morbidity and mortality. Autoimmune encephalitis is possible, but findings are more consistent with HSV encephalitis and HSV should be ruled out prior to starting steroids.

References

Dawes L, HSV Encephalitis. Case Study, Radiopaedia.org. https://doi.org/10.53347/rID-3444

Defres S, Keller SS, Das K, Vidyasagar R, Parkes LM, Burnside G, et al. A Feasibility Study of Quantifying Longitudinal Brain Changes in Herpes Simplex Virus (HSV) Encephalitis Using Magnetic Resonance Imaging (MRI) and Stereology. PLoS One. 2017;12(1):e0170215. https://doi.org/10.1371/journal.pone.0170215.

Matthews E, Beckham JD, Piquet AL, Tyler KL, Chauhan L, Pastula DM. Herpesvirus-Associated Encephalitis: an Update. Curr Trop Med Rep. 2022;9(3):92–100. https://doi.org/10.1007/s40475-022-00255-8.

Tyler KL. Acute Viral Encephalitis. N Engl J Med. 2018;379(6):557–66. https://doi.org/10.1056/NEJMra1708714.

Whitley RJ. Herpes simplex encephalitis: adolescents and adults. Antiviral Res. 2006;71(2–3):141–8. https://doi.org/10.1016/j.antiviral.2006.04.002.

24. A 25-year-old man is brought to the emergency department by ambulance after a neighbor found him confused in the hallway of his apartment building. He is febrile (38.9 °C), mildly disoriented, and intermittently agitated. He answers "no" when asked about sexual activity, drug use, dietary exposures, or contact with animals, but provides no elaboration. He says "yes" when asked about having fevers and, with limited questioning, reports these have lasted a few days.

Neurologic exam shows increased muscular tone, hyperreflexia, bilateral extensor plantar responses, and fasciculations. Cranial nerves are intact. Skin exam is unremarkable. There is no nuchal rigidity or focal weakness.

His wallet contains only an expired driver's license indicating organ donor status. He is otherwise unidentified. His sister, contacted through emergency contacts, reports he recently returned from a 1-month trip across Southeast Asia where he visited common tourist sites in large cities, where he stayed in hotels and ate mostly in restaurants, though he may have tried street food once or twice. He had been documenting his travels via social media. He did not go to rural areas. She received a text from him upon arrival back in the United States 1 week ago. He was preparing to begin law school in 2 weeks and was searching for an apartment in Washington, D.C. She describes him as generally risk-averse and thinks it is unlikely that he had new sexual contacts.

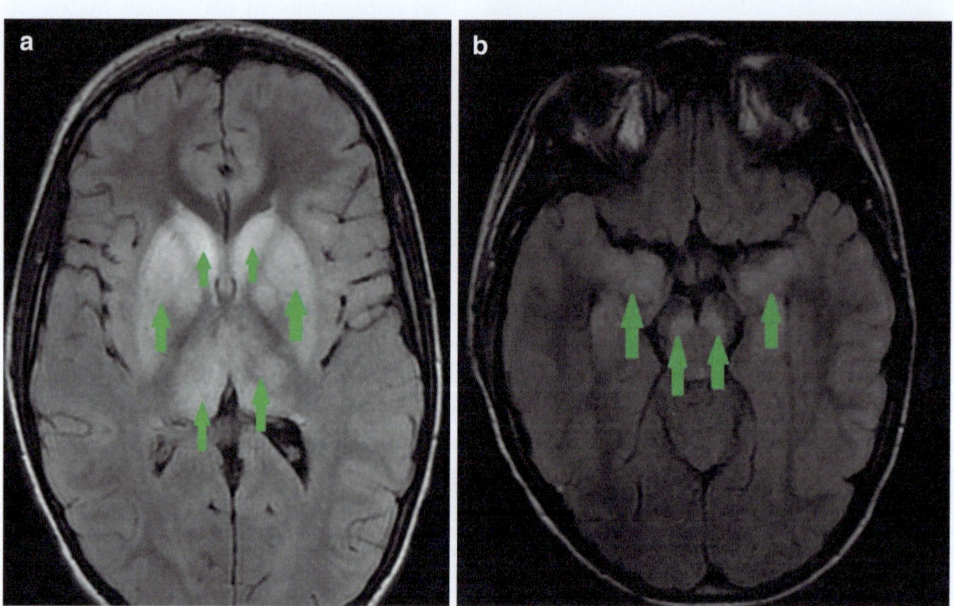

Axial MRI brain (**a**, **b**). (Source: Chahbi, Z., Adnor, S., Bigi, S., Salek, M., Wakrim, S. CC-BY 4.0 (https://creativecommons.org/licenses/by/4.0/) via *Radiology Case Reports*. Image has not been modified from source. Please see full attribution with citation below in references section for this question.)

CSF Analysis:

- Opening pressure: 180 mm H$_2$O
- WBC: 18/μL (80% lymphocytes)
- Protein: 60 mg/dL
- Glucose: 58 mg/dL (serum glucose: 100 mg/dL)
- Gram stain and cultures: Negative
- Toxicology screen: Negative
- HIV and syphilis serologies: Pending

Which of the following is the most likely diagnosis?
  A. Rabies
  B. Japanese encephalitis
  C. Dengue fever
  D. Tuberculosis meningitis
  E. Acute drug intoxication or withdrawal
  F. HIV-associated encephalopathy

Correct answer: A

Explanation

A. *Rabies—Correct.*

This is the most likely diagnosis. Rabies should be considered in any encephalopathic returning traveler from a rabies-endemic region (which includes most of Asia, particularly Southeast Asia), even when a history of animal bite is not available. The majority of human rabies cases globally result from dog bites, and even minor or unnoticed exposures (e.g., scratches or contact with infected saliva) may transmit the virus. The patient's disorientation, agitation, abnormal reflexes, and MRI findings (often including increased T2 signal in basal ganglia, brainstem, thalami) are classic for encephalitic rabies. CSF often shows mild lymphocytic pleocytosis, as in this case. The recent travel is the key epidemiologic clue.

B. *Japanese encephalitis—Incorrect.*

This mosquito-borne flavivirus is most common in rural and agricultural areas of Southeast Asia. The patient primarily stayed in urban settings. Although Japanese encephalitis can present similarly with fever and altered mental status, the hippocampal and brainstem MRI findings are not typical (thalamic lesions are more characteristic), and most urban travelers are not exposed to the high-risk environments required for transmission.

C. *Dengue fever—Incorrect.*

Dengue is common in Southeast Asia and often presents with fever, myalgias, and rash, but encephalopathy is rare and typically only occurs in severe cases involving hemorrhage or vascular leak syndrome. This patient has no rash, hypotension, or thrombocytopenia, and his MRI findings and neurologic exam do not support this diagnosis.

D. *Acute drug intoxication or withdrawal—Incorrect.*

While drug intoxication or withdrawal can cause confusion and agitation, this patient's exam shows objective upper motor neuron signs (hyperreflexia, extensor plantar responses, fasciculations), imaging abnormalities, and CSF pleocytosis, none of which are typical for toxic-metabolic encephalopathy. His tox screen is negative, and there is no supporting collateral history of substance use.

E. *HIV-associated encephalopathy—Incorrect.*

HIV can lead to neurological complications, especially in advanced disease. However, these conditions are typically subacute or chronic and are associated with marked immunosuppression. There is no history of immunodeficiency, and this presentation lacks features of acute retroviral syndrome or HIV-associated neurocognitive disorders.

References

Chahbi Z, Adnor S, Bigi S, Salek M, Wakrim S. MRI findings in human rabies: A case report on the importance of neuroimaging when biological tests are inconclusive. Radiology Case Reports. 2025;20(7):3281–6. https://doi.org/10.1016/j.radcr.2025.03.056.

Hemachudha T, Ugolini G, Wacharapluesadee S, Sungkarat W, Shuangshoti S, Laothamatas J. Human rabies: neuropathogenesis, diagnosis, and management. Lancet Neurol. 2013;12(5):498–513. https://doi.org/10.1016/s1474-4422(13)70038-3.

Linked questions: 25–26

25. A 36-year-old woman presents with severe frontal headache, neck stiffness, photophobia, nausea, and two episodes of vomiting that began 3 days after returning from a 2-week vacation in Thailand. She spent most of her time relaxing on the beach, drank alcohol moderately, and had no new sexual partners. During the trip, she was in good health overall, except for 2 days of self-limited diarrhea. She also recalls having had numerous mosquito bites. Her dietary history includes consumption of raw seafood, snails, shellfish, salads, and potentially untreated water. She denies rash or confusion. She has no chronic medical conditions and takes no medications.

On Examination:

- *General*: Alert and oriented, appears uncomfortable due to headache
- *Vital signs*: T 37.9 °C, HR 88 bpm, BP 118/72 mm Hg, RR 14, SpO$_2$ 99% on room air
- *Neck*: Stiffness present; Brudzinski and Kernig signs equivocal
- *Neurologic*: Cranial nerves intact, no focal deficits, no papilledema
- *Skin*: No rash or eschar
- *Abdomen*: Soft, non-tender, no organomegaly

Laboratory and Imaging Findings:
Serum

- CBC: WBC 10,200/mm^3 with 12% eosinophils (absolute eosinophil count: 1224/mm^3)
- ESR: 28 mm/hr
- CRP: 6.1 mg/L
- HIV, RPR, and malaria antigen tests: Negative
- Stool O&P and Strongyloides IgG: Negative

CSF Analysis (Lumbar Puncture):

- Opening pressure: Not recorded
- WBC: 500 cells/mm^3 with 50% eosinophils (~250 eos/mm^3)
- Glucose: 65 mg/dL
- Protein: 70 mg/dL
- Gram stain, culture, HSV PCR, enterovirus PCR: All negative

Neuroimaging:

- Non-contrast CT head: Normal
- MRI brain: Normal

What is the most likely diagnosis?
    A. Neurocysticercosis
    B. Guillain-Barré Syndrome
    C. Viral meningitis
    D. Bacterial meningitis
    E. Eosinophilic meningitis due to *Angiostrongylus cantonensis*

Correct answer: E

Explanation

A. *Neurocysticercosis*:
Would likely present with seizures or focal deficits. Imaging is typically abnormal, with calcifications or cysts. CSF eosinophilia is not this prominent.

B. *Guillain-Barré Syndrome*:
Presents with ascending weakness and areflexia. CSF shows albuminocytologic dissociation (elevated protein, low WBC count). The CSF findings here are incompatible.

C. *Viral Meningitis*:
Typically lymphocytic pleocytosis, not eosinophilia. Also, less likely with high eosinophil count in both CSF and peripheral blood.

D. *Bacterial Meningitis*:
Neutrophilic pleocytosis, high protein, and low glucose are expected. This case features eosinophils, normal glucose, and only mild protein elevation.

E. *Eosinophilic Meningitis due to Angiostrongylus cantonensis (Correct)*:
This is a common parasitic cause of eosinophilic meningitis in Thailand. Infection occurs via ingestion of raw snails or contaminated produce. Her exposure history, marked CSF eosinophilia, and typical symptom onset support this diagnosis. The mosquito bites and diarrhea are incidental unless coinfection is suspected, which is not supported here.

Linked question

26. For the patient in the prior question, what is the most appropriate initial management for this patient?

    A. High-dose intravenous ceftriaxone
    B. Oral albendazole alone
    C. Supportive care with analgesics and corticosteroids
    D. Intravenous acyclovir
    E. Empiric amphotericin B

Correct answer: C

Explanation

Mainstay treatment for eosinophilic meningitis due to *Angiostrongylus cantonensis* is supportive: corticosteroids (e.g., prednisone or dexamethasone) for inflammation, and analgesics for pain relief. Albendazole may be considered in prolonged or severe cases but is controversial during the acute phase. Antibacterial, antiviral, and antifungal treatments are not appropriate here.

References

Prociv P, Turner M. Neuroangiostrongyliasis: The "Subarachnoid Phase" and Its Implications for Anthelminthic Therapy. Am J Trop Med Hyg. 2018;98(2):353–9. https://doi.org/10.4269/ajtmh.17-0206.

Slom TJ, Cortese MM, Gerber SI, Jones RC, Holtz TH, Lopez AS, et al. An outbreak of eosinophilic meningitis caused by Angiostrongylus cantonensis in travelers returning from the Caribbean. N Engl J Med. 2002;346(9):668–75. https://doi.org/10.1056/NEJMoa012462.

Tsai HC, Liu YC, Kunin CM, Lai PH, Lee SS, Chen YS, et al. Eosinophilic meningitis caused by Angiostrongylus cantonensis associated with eating raw snails: correlation of brain magnetic resonance imaging scans with clinical findings. Am J Trop Med Hyg. 2003;68(3):281–5.

Linked questions: 27–28

27. A 39-year-old woman originally from Mexico, who immigrated to San Diego 3 years ago, presents to the emergency department following a generalized tonic-clonic seizure. She denies fever, headache, or any focal neurological symptoms. Her past medical history is unremarkable. She is HIV-negative on recent testing and married and works as a cook in a local restaurant. A non-contrast CT of the head shows a single, well-circumscribed calcified lesion in the left parietal lobe. MRI confirms the calcified nature of the lesion without evidence of surrounding edema or additional abnormalities. She is diagnosed with neurocysticercosis based on clinical history and imaging findings. What is the most appropriate next step in the management of this patient?

    A. Albendazole and dexamethasone
    B. Observation only
    C. Albendazole alone
    D. Surgical resection
    E. Dexamethasone and praziquantel
    Correct answer: B

Explanation

The correct approach for managing a patient with a single calcified neurocysticercosis lesion is observation without antiparasitic or anti-inflammatory therapy. Calcified lesions represent dead parasites and are not associated with active infection. Treating such lesions with antiparasitic agents has not been shown to improve outcomes and may provoke inflammation, increasing seizure risk. The clinical focus should instead be on seizure control using antiepileptic medications as needed, without initiating albendazole or corticosteroids.

Incorrect answers:

- A. The combination of albendazole and dexamethasone is appropriate only in cases where there are viable (non-calcified) cysts, particularly multiple lesions, or lesions with edema. This patient has a single, inactive lesion without inflammation.

C. Albendazole monotherapy is similarly inappropriate, as antiparasitic drugs are not beneficial for calcified lesions.

Option D, surgical resection, is reserved for large lesions causing mass effect, hydrocephalus, or refractory seizures, none of which apply here.

Option E, dexamethasone with praziquantel, is also used for viable cysts and carries no benefit in the context of a calcified, non-inflammatory lesion.

Linked question

28. For the patient in the prior question, what is the most appropriate next step to reduce the risk of *Taenia solium* transmission to others, given her occupation as a restaurant cook?

    A. Test close family members for seizures
    B. Refer to neurosurgery
    C. Check her stool for *Taenia solium* eggs
    D. Test for HIV again
    E. Repeat MRI in 1 week
    Correct answer: C

Explanation

Although neurocysticercosis occurs when a person ingests *T. solium* eggs, it is important to assess whether this patient is also a carrier of the adult intestinal tapeworm, which sheds eggs capable of infecting others. Since she works as a cook, there is a significant public health concern. If she harbors an adult tapeworm, she could potentially infect coworkers or customers. Therefore, stool testing for *T. solium* eggs is essential. None of the other options address the public health risk posed by possible tapeworm carriage.

***Taenia solium* Summary (Questions 27–28):**
This case highlights the management of a patient with calcified neurocysticercosis, a condition that commonly results from prior *Taenia solium* infection and presents with seizures. In the absence of active or viable lesions, antiparasitic therapy is not indicated. Calcified lesions signify a resolved infection, and the focus of treatment is on seizure control with antiepileptic drugs. There is no role for albendazole, praziquantel, corticosteroids, or surgical intervention in the absence of inflammation, mass effect, or hydrocephalus. Importantly, because the patient works as a cook, it is critical to evaluate for adult tapeworm carriage through stool testing, as she may be a source of infection to others if she is excret-

ing *T. solium* eggs. This follow-up step addresses the public health aspect of neurocysticercosis and the broader implications of food-handler-related transmission risk.

Questions 27–28 Reference

White AC, Jr., Coyle CM, Rajshekhar V, Singh G, Hauser WA, Mohanty A, et al. Diagnosis and Treatment of Neurocysticercosis: 2017 Clinical Practice Guidelines by the Infectious Diseases Society of America (IDSA) and the American Society of Tropical Medicine and Hygiene (ASTMH). Clin Infect Dis. 2018;66(8):e49–e75. https://doi.org/10.1093/cid/cix1084.

29. An 18-year-old male presents to the emergency department with acute mental status changes and fever over the past 2 days. He had been on vacation with his grandparents in Florida for the past 2 weeks, where he engaged in hunting, fishing, hiking, and swimming in a freshwater lake near their home. He went hunting with friends but did not hit or touch any animals or animal skins. He also reports numerous bug bites to his grandmother, though he is unsure of the insect type. He has no long-term medical conditions and has been otherwise healthy. His family reports severe headaches, nausea, confusion, and increasing irritability. On examination, he is febrile (102 °F / 38.9 °C) and exhibits signs of meningeal irritation.

Lumbar puncture:

- WBC: >5000 cells/mm^3
- RBC: >10,000 cells/mm^3
- Protein: 200 mg/dL
- Glucose: 30 mg/dL (serum glucose 100 mg/dL)
- ICP: 29 cm H$_2$O
- Gram stain: Negative
- Meningitis panel: Negative

What is the most likely diagnosis?
A. Viral meningitis
B. Bacterial meningitis
C. Herpes simplex virus encephalitis
D. Primary amoebic meningoencephalitis (*Naegleria fowleri*)
E. Anthrax

Correct answer: D

Explanation

A. Viral meningitis: Less likely with such elevated WBC, RBC, and low glucose.

B. Bacterial meningitis: Negative Gram stain and high RBCs make this less likely.
C. HSV encephalitis: Often affects the temporal lobes and confirmed via PCR; CSF profile not typical.
D. Primary amoebic meningoencephalitis (PAM): Classic after swimming in warm freshwater, with high CSF WBCs, RBCs, low glucose, and negative standard tests.
E. Anthrax: No direct animal exposure or cutaneous/pulmonary signs; not supported by exposure history.

Summary of Key Points for Primary Amoebic Meningoencephalitis

Primary amoebic meningoencephalitis (PAM) is caused by *Naegleria fowleri*, a thermophilic amoeba found in warm freshwater. It typically affects healthy young individuals following exposure to lakes, ponds, or hot springs. The clinical course is rapidly progressive, presenting with fever, headache, nausea, and neurological decline. CSF shows a neutrophilic pleocytosis, high RBC count, low glucose, and elevated protein—often mimicking bacterial meningitis but with negative Gram stain. Wet prep microscopy of CSF is a key early diagnostic tool. Despite intensive care and experimental treatments (e.g., amphotericin plus miltefosine plus other medications), the mortality rate remains extremely high.

Reference

CDC: Naegleria fowleri Infections. https://www.cdc.gov/naegleria/about/index.html (2025). Accessed 2 Jun 2025.

30. A 37-year-old woman from western Massachusetts presents in early June with progressive confusion and word-finding difficulty that began 4 days ago. A week prior, she experienced low-grade fever and generalized body aches for 2–3 days that resolved without treatment. This was followed by headaches and gradual worsening confusion. Her family also notes a fine tremor and mild unsteadiness of gait.

She is otherwise healthy and was recently treated for Lyme disease with doxycycline. She is a vegetarian, hikes daily with her dogs, and frequently visits local farms.

Neurologic exam: Mild disorientation, fine postural tremor in both hands, slightly wide-based gait.

MRI brain: Normal

CSF: Lymphocytic plcocytosis, mildly elevated protein, normal glucose

CBC: WBC 6.8 × 10^9/L, hemoglobin 13.2 g/dL, platelets 245 × 10^9/L

Which of the following is the most likely cause of her symptoms?

A. Epstein-Barr virus (EBV)
B. Babesiosis
C. Meningococcal meningitis
D. Powassan virus
E. West Nile virus
Correct answer: D

Explanation

Powassan virus is a tick-borne flavivirus endemic to the northeastern United States, including Massachusetts. It is transmitted by *Ixodes scapularis* ticks—the same vector as Lyme disease. Cases peak in late spring to early summer and often begin with a nonspecific febrile prodrome, followed days later by neurologic symptoms, including confusion, tremor, and encephalopathy.

This patient's seasonal and geographic exposure, recent tick-borne illness, prodrome followed by neurologic progression, and normal MRI with CSF findings consistent with viral encephalitis support the diagnosis. Her normal blood counts (particularly WBC and platelets) make alternative diagnoses like Babesia or bacterial meningitis less likely.

Rising incidence: The number of Powassan virus cases has increased in recent years, with more than 40 confirmed cases reported in 2022—the highest number to date (as of publication).

Incorrect answers:

A. Epstein-Barr Virus (EBV):

   Typically causes infectious mononucleosis with sore throat, lymphadenopathy, and fatigue. Rarely causes isolated encephalitis in immunocompetent adults.

B. Babesiosis:

   A tick-borne protozoan infection that typically causes hemolytic anemia, thrombocytopenia, and fever. Neuroinvasive disease is not typical. This patient's normal hemoglobin and platelets make Babesia unlikely.

C. Meningococcal Meningitis:

   Presents acutely with high fever, neck stiffness, and rapid deterioration. CSF usually shows neutrophilic pleocytosis, low glucose, and elevated protein. The patient's afebrile status, subacute progression, and CSF profile are inconsistent with bacterial meningitis.

E. West Nile Virus:

   Neuroinvasive disease typically affects older adults and occurs in late summer to early fall. The timing (early June) and demographic make this less likely.

References

CDC: Data and Maps for Powassan. https://www.cdc.gov/powassan/data-maps/index.html (2024). Accessed 2 Jun 2025 2025.

Hermance ME, Thangamani S. Powassan Virus: An Emerging Arbovirus of Public Health Concern in North America. Vector Borne Zoonotic Dis. 2017;17(7):453–62. https://doi.org/10.1089/vbz.2017.2110.

Linked questions: 31–32

31. A 29-year-old medical student travels to Malawi for a 4-week global health elective. During his stay, he treats patients with malaria, tuberculosis, HIV, and a variety of other diseases and eats local food from both the hospital cafeteria and neighborhood restaurants. He takes atovaquone-proguanil for malaria prophylaxis. On weekends, he swims in a local freshwater lake with friends. He is generally healthy and is engaged to his long-term female partner. He denies any bites or direct animal exposures, though at the end of the rotation he went on a 3-day safari in Kenya.

   Four weeks after returning to the United States, he develops fevers, cough, urticaria, and malaise. Two weeks later, he presents with new-onset bladder dysfunction and progressive lower extremity weakness. MRI of the spine shows longitudinally extensive transverse myelitis involving the thoracic cord.

Which of the following is the most likely diagnosis?
   A. Acute HIV seroconversion
   B. Tuberculous meningomyelitis
   C. West Nile virus infection
   D. Schistosomal myeloradiculopathy
   E. Guillain-Barré syndrome
Correct answer: D

Explanation

This patient's freshwater exposure in an endemic region (Uganda) is classic for *Schistosoma mansoni* or *S. haematobium*. These parasites can lead to spinal cord granulomatous inflammation, often presenting weeks after exposure with cauda equina syndrome or transverse myelitis, as seen here. MRI shows longitudinally extensive lesions and conus medullaris enhancement.

• Neurologic complications occur due to egg deposition and inflammatory response in the spinal cord.

- Though he took malaria prophylaxis, this does not prevent schistosomiasis, which is acquired via skin penetration from infested freshwater.

Incorrect answers:

A. Acute HIV seroconversion: May cause fever, rash, and aseptic meningitis, but rarely causes transverse myelitis or bladder dysfunction this early.
B. Tuberculous meningomyelitis: Can cause chronic spinal involvement, but usually evolves more indolently. He had no respiratory symptoms, and TB spine involvement more often causes vertebral destruction and epidural abscess.
C. West Nile virus: May cause flaccid paralysis, but usually not a transverse myelitis pattern or bladder involvement. It also typically follows mosquito exposure rather than freshwater.
E. Guillain-Barré syndrome: This affects peripheral nerves and typically causes ascending weakness and areflexia, without spinal cord lesions on MRI.

Linked question

32. Which of the following activities presents the highest risk for acquiring *Schistosoma* infection that can later cause neurologic disease?
    A. Drinking unpasteurized milk
    B. Eating undercooked freshwater fish
    C. Walking barefoot in contaminated soil
    D. Swimming or wading in freshwater lakes or rivers in endemic regions
    E. Close contact with infected individuals
    Correct answer: D

Explanation

Swimming or wading in freshwater is the primary mode of exposure for *Schistosoma* species. Cercariae –free-swimming larvae released by infected freshwater snails—penetrate intact human skin, typically during activities like swimming, bathing, or wading in infested water.

Incorrect answers:

A. Drinking unpasteurized milk—Unpasteurized milk can transmit a variety of pathogens including *Brucella* species, but not *Schistosoma* species.
B. Eating undercooked fish—This is a risk for other parasites (e.g., *Opisthorchis*, *Clonorchis*), but not schistosomiasis.
C. Walking barefoot in soil—Associated with hookworm, *Strongyloides*, and larva migrans, but not schistosomiasis.
E. Person-to-person contact—Schistosomiasis is not spread via direct contact; humans acquire it from environmental exposure to water containing cercariae.

Questions 31–32 References

Ferrari TC, Moreira PR. Neuroschistosomiasis: clinical symptoms and pathogenesis. Lancet Neurol. 2011;10(9):853–64. https://doi.org/10.1016/s1474-4422(11)70170-3.
Pittella JE. Neuroschistosomiasis. Brain Pathol. 1997;7(1):649–62. https://doi.org/10.1111/j.1750-3639.1997.tb01080.x.

Linked questions: 33–34

33. A 28-year-old woman from Ecuador, who has lived in Texas for 4 years, presents to the emergency department after her first generalized seizure. She has no fever, no focal neurologic deficits, and no systemic symptoms. She is HIV-negative, denies drug or alcohol use, and has no significant medical history.

    CT head reveals several parenchymal cystic lesions, each showing the characteristic "hole-with-dot" sign (scolex), surrounded by mild perilesional edema. There is no evidence of subarachnoid or ventricular involvement. There are also no signs of hydrocephalus or increased intracranial pressure.

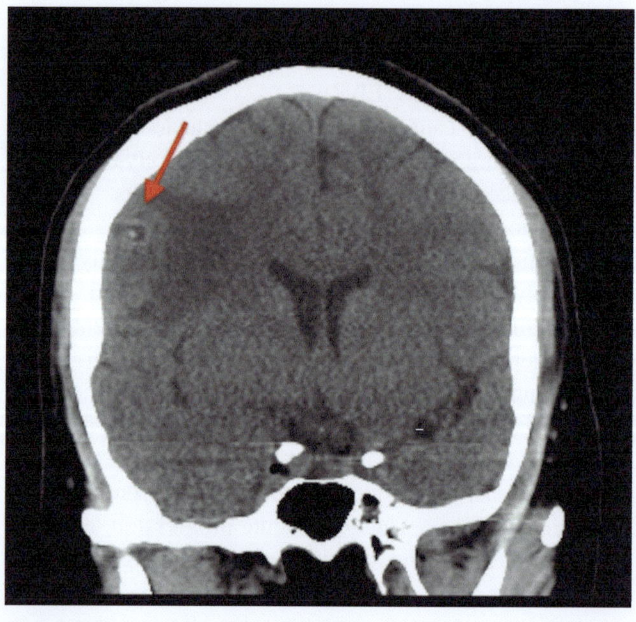

Coronal CT head. (Source: Gonzalez, S., Medina-Perez, R., Herrera, D., Rullan, J. M. A., Lopez, J. L. CC-BY 4.0 (https://creativecommons.org/licenses/by/4.0/) via *Cureus*. Image has not been modified from source. Please see full attribution with citation below in references section for this question.)

What is the most appropriate initial management for this patient?

A. Albendazole and corticosteroids only
B. Praziquantel monotherapy
C. Albendazole plus praziquantel with corticosteroids and antiepileptic therapy
D. Corticosteroids alone
E. Observation only

Correct answer: C

Explanation

This patient presents with viable parenchymal neurocysticercosis, as evidenced by the MRI showing active cysts with scolex and surrounding edema. According to the 2017 IDSA/ASTMH guidelines, patients with ≥2 viable cysts benefit most from combination antiparasitic therapy with albendazole plus praziquantel, which has superior efficacy compared to monotherapy. Corticosteroids (e.g., dexamethasone or prednisone) are prescribed concurrently to limit inflammation and reduce the risk of worsening cerebral edema during cysticidal therapy. Antiepileptic drugs are indicated due to seizure presentation.

There is no evidence of calcified cysts, and the absence of subarachnoid or intraventricular disease allows for safe initiation of antiparasitic therapy.

Incorrect answers:

A. Albendazole and corticosteroids only:
Monotherapy is less effective for multiple viable cysts and is not preferred when more than two lesions are present.

B. Praziquantel monotherapy:
Praziquantel is less effective than albendazole, and monotherapy is inferior to combination therapy. It also interacts unfavorably with steroids.

D. Corticosteroids alone:
This may reduce inflammation, but does not treat the underlying parasitic infection, and fails to address the seizure risk.

E. Observation only:
This is not appropriate for a symptomatic patient with confirmed viable cysts, which require active treatment.

Linked question

34. Which of the following are contraindications to initiating antiparasitic therapy in neurocysticercosis?
    A. Hydrocephalus due to intraventricular cysts
    B. Marked cerebral edema and signs of elevated intracranial pressure
    C. A and B
    D. None of the above

    Correct answer: C

Explanation

Antiparasitic therapy can trigger robust inflammation during cyst death, which may worsen intracranial pressure. In cases with intraventricular cysts, hydrocephalus, or significant cerebral edema, therapy is delayed until intracranial pressure is stabilized—typically using steroids, CSF diversion (e.g., shunt), or neurosurgery.

References (questions 33–34)

Gonzalez S, Medina-Perez R, Herrera D, Acosta Rullan JM, Lopez JL. The Role of Serial Imaging in Neurocysticercosis for Disease Resolution. Cureus. 2021;13(7):e16790. https://doi.org/10.7759/cureus.16790.

White AC, Jr., Coyle CM, Rajshekhar V, Singh G, Hauser WA, Mohanty A, et al. Diagnosis and Treatment of Neurocysticercosis: 2017 Clinical Practice Guidelines by the Infectious Diseases Society of America (IDSA) and the American Society of Tropical Medicine and Hygiene (ASTMH). Clin Infect Dis. 2018;66(8):e49–e75. https://doi.org/10.1093/cid/cix1084.

Linked questions: 35–36

35. A 42-year-old woman from Miami presents with a 2-week history of worsening headaches, now accompanied by nausea and two episodes of vomiting. She reports a several-week history of non-productive cough and intermittent fevers though these resolved a month ago. She received two courses of antibiotics during that time without immediate improvement.

    She is was previously healthy and had traveled to Phoenix and the Grand Canyon in Arizona, staying in a hotel in Phoenix and a lodge at the Grand Canyon. She engaged in short hikes in the Grand Canyon and Flagstaff areas. Her medical history includes type 2 diabetes.

    On examination, she is febrile (38.5 °C) and appears lethargic. Neurological examination reveals mild neck stiffness, disorientation to time and place, and no focal motor deficits.

Investigations:

- Chest X-ray: Right lower lobe infiltrate
- Peripheral WBC count: 13,000 cells/μL (with 6% eosinophils)
- CSF analysis:
  - Opening pressure: 230 mm H_2O
  - WBC count: 800 cells/μL (lymphocytic predominance, with 4% eosinophils)
  - Protein: 145 mg/dL
  - Glucose: 42 mg/dL (serum glucose 90 mg/dL)
  - Gram stain: Negative
  - Fungal culture: Pending

Which of the following is the most likely diagnosis?

A. Sin Nombre virus infection
B. Plague meningitis
C. Coccidioidomycosis meningitis
D. Meningococcal meningitis
E. Histoplasmosis meningitis

Correct answer: C

Explanation

The patient's recent travel to an endemic area (Arizona), initial respiratory symptoms, chest infiltrate, peripheral and CSF eosinophilia, and CSF findings (lymphocytic pleocytosis, elevated protein, mild hypoglycorrhachia) are characteristic of coccidioidomycosis meningitis. Coccidioides immitis is endemic to the southwestern United States, and meningitis is a severe extrapulmonary manifestation.

Incorrect answers:

A. Sin Nombre virus infection: This hantavirus primarily causes hantavirus pulmonary syndrome, characterized by fever, myalgia, and acute respiratory distress, not meningitis. CSF findings are typically unremarkable in such cases.
B. Plague meningitis: Plague meningitis is rare and usually presents with acute onset of high fever, nuchal rigidity, and altered mental status. It is associated with exposure to rodents or fleas, which is not indicated in this case. Additionally, CSF findings often show neutrophilic pleocytosis rather than lymphocytic.
D. Meningococcal meningitis: Typically presents acutely with high fever, neck stiffness, and altered mental status. CSF analysis usually reveals neutrophilic pleocytosis, very low glucose, and elevated protein. Peripheral eosinophilia is not characteristic.
E. Histoplasmosis meningitis: More common in immunocompromised individuals and endemic to the Ohio and Mississippi River valleys. CSF findings may be similar, but peripheral eosinophilia is uncommon, and there is no reported travel history to endemic areas.

Linked question

36. What is the most appropriate treatment for this patient in the prior question?
    A. Observation without antifungal therapy
    B. Oral fluconazole 400–1200 mg daily
    C. Intravenous amphotericin B alone
    D. Intrathecal amphotericin B alone
    E. Short course of corticosteroids

    Correct answer: B

Explanation

According to the Infectious Diseases Society of America (IDSA) guidelines, the treatment of choice for coccidioidomycosis meningitis is oral fluconazole at doses ranging from 400 to 1200 mg daily, often continued for life to prevent relapse. Intrathecal amphotericin B is no longer first line, and IV amphotericin CSF penetration is inadequate. Itraconazole is an alternative but requires monitoring for absorption and has more drug interactions. Corticosteroids are not standard treatment and may worsen fungal infections. Observation is appropriate for mild pulmonary coccidioidomycosis but not for CNS involvement, which requires prompt antifungal therapy.

Summary for Questions 35–36

This case illustrates coccidioidomycosis meningitis in a patient with recent travel to an endemic area. Key features include a preceding respiratory illness, peripheral and CSF eosinophilia, and characteristic CSF findings. Diagnosis is confirmed with complement fixation titers.

Reference

Galgiani JN, Ampel NM, Blair JE, Catanzaro A, Geertsma F, Hoover SE, et al. 2016 Infectious Diseases Society of America (IDSA) Clinical Practice Guideline for the Treatment of Coccidioidomycosis. Clin Infect Dis. 2016;63(6):e112–46. https://doi.org/10.1093/cid/ciw360.

Linked questions: 37–38

37. A 63-year-old male presents to the emergency department with a 3-week history of progressively worsening headaches and intermittent fever. He also reports a 2-month history of unintentional weight loss, persistent diarrhea, and night sweats. On examination, he appears chronically ill, with temporal wasting and oral thrush. He has mild cervical and axillary lymphadenopathy, but his lungs are clear to auscultation and he is afebrile at the time of examination. Initial laboratory studies reveal a CD4 count of 42 cells/mm^3 and a positive HIV antigen/antibody combination test. Brain imaging is unremarkable. A lumbar puncture is about to be performed. What is the most likely cause of his symptoms?
    A. Cryptococcal meningitis
    B. Primary CNS lymphoma
    C. Tuberculosis meningitis
    D. Bacterial meningitis
    E. Viral meningitis

    Correct answer: A

Explanation

This patient presents with signs of advanced, untreated HIV infection, including wasting, oral candidiasis, and systemic symptoms like weight loss and diarrhea. His subacute presentation with headaches and fever, coupled with a very low CD4 count, strongly suggests cryptococcal meningitis, the most common cause of chronic meningitis in patients with AIDS. This case highlights the importance of considering opportunistic infections in patients presenting with systemic illness and neurological symptoms, particularly in those without a prior HIV diagnosis.

Cryptococcus neoformans is an encapsulated yeast that causes subacute to chronic meningitis, most often in patients with advanced HIV/AIDS. Common symptoms include fever, headache, malaise, and altered mental status. Risk factors include a CD4 count <100 cells/mm³, weight loss, chronic diarrhea, oral thrush, and lymphadenopathy—features all present in this patient. India ink staining or cryptococcal antigen testing of the CSF can confirm the diagnosis. Prompt initiation of antifungal therapy is critical.

Incorrect answers:

B. Primary CNS lymphoma—Less likely. While CNS lymphoma may occur in patients with AIDS, it usually presents with focal neurological deficits and mass lesions on imaging, which are absent here. Also, lymphoma does not typically cause meningitis-like symptoms or fever.

C. Tuberculosis meningitis—Possible but less likely. TB meningitis can present similarly but often evolves more insidiously and may show basal meningeal enhancement or hydrocephalus on imaging. Positive CSF acid-fast bacilli stains or PCR would be needed for diagnosis.

D. Bacterial meningitis—Typically presents acutely with marked neck stiffness, photophobia, and altered mental status. In HIV patients, it is less common than cryptococcal meningitis, particularly in those with very low CD4 counts.

E. Viral meningitis—Usually presents more mildly and is less common as a severe complication in patients with advanced AIDS. It is a diagnosis of exclusion when more serious causes like cryptococcus have been ruled out.

Linked question

38. A 25-year-old man presents with a 3-week history of progressively worsening headaches, photophobia, nausea, and recent confusion. He was diagnosed with HIV 2 weeks ago but has not yet started antiretroviral therapy. He has no known history of opportunistic infections.

On exam, he is febrile (38.1 °C), somnolent but arousable, and oriented only to his name. He has mild neck stiffness but no focal neurological deficits. Funduscopic exam reveals no papilledema.

Laboratory studies:

- WBC count: 3200/μL
- CD4 count: 10 cells/μL
- HIV viral load: 540,000 copies/mL
- Serum cryptococcal antigen: Positive

CSF analysis (after LP):

- Opening pressure: 330 mm H₂O
- WBC count: 75 cells/μL (lymphocyte predominant)
- Protein: 115 mg/dL
- Glucose: 35 mg/dL (serum glucose 95 mg/dL)
- India ink stain: Positive for encapsulated yeast
- Cryptococcal antigen (CSF): Positive

What is the most appropriate treatment for this patient in the prior question?

A. Oral fluconazole 800 mg daily
B. IV amphotericin B plus oral flucytosine
C. Start ART immediately
D. Acetazolamide and supportive care
E. Repeat lumbar punctures only, without antifungal therapy until pressure is lower

Correct answer: B

Explanation

This patient has HIV-associated cryptococcal meningitis, confirmed by serum and CSF cryptococcal antigen and India ink positivity. The appropriate initial treatment is induction therapy with:

- IV liposomal amphotericin B (3–4 mg/kg daily)
- Oral flucytosine (25 mg/kg four times daily)

This regimen is given for at least 2 weeks, followed by consolidation with high-dose fluconazole. This combination has been shown to reduce fungal burden and mortality, especially in patients with very low CD4 counts.

Incorrect Answers:

A. Oral fluconazole 800 mg daily—Fluconazole is used for consolidation and maintenance, not for induction in severe cryptococcal meningitis. Monotherapy at this stage is associated with poorer outcomes.

C. Start ART immediately—Initiating antiretroviral therapy during acute cryptococcal meningitis increases the risk of immune reconstitution inflammatory syndrome (IRIS) and mortality. ART should be delayed for 4–6 weeks after antifungal therapy begins.

D. Acetazolamide and supportive care—Acetazolamide is not indicated for cryptococcal meningitis and may worsen dehydration and acidosis. Intracranial pressure should be managed by serial lumbar punctures, not acetazolamide.

E. Repeat lumbar punctures only, without antifungal therapy—While therapeutic LPs are crucial for managing elevated intracranial pressure, they do not replace antifungal treatment. Both are essential components of care.

Summary for Questions 37–38

- *Diagnosis*: HIV-associated cryptococcal meningitis
- *CSF clues*: Elevated opening pressure, lymphocytic pleocytosis, low glucose, positive India ink
- *Treatment*: IV amphotericin B + oral flucytosine
- *Delay ART*: Begin after 4–6 weeks to avoid IRIS
- *ICP Management*: Serial lumbar punctures targeting pressure <20 cm H_2O or 50% reduction from baseline

References for Questions 37–38

Bicanic T, Harrison TS. Cryptococcal meningitis. Br Med Bull. 2004;72:99–118. https://doi.org/10.1093/bmb/ldh043.

Panel on Guidelines for the Prevention and Treatment of Opportunistic Infections in Adults and Adolescents With HIV. Guidelines for the Prevention and Treatment of Opportunistic Infections in Adults and Adolescents With HIV. National Institutes of Health, HIV Medicine Association, and Infectious Diseases Society of America. https://clinicalinfo.hiv.gov/en/guidelines/adult-and-adolescent-opportunistic-infection. Accessed July 20 2025.

Perfect JR, Dismukes WE, Dromer F, Goldman DL, Graybill JR, Hamill RJ, et al. Clinical practice guidelines for the management of cryptococcal disease: 2010 update by the Infectious Diseases Society of America. Clin Infect Dis. 2010;50(3):291–322. https://doi.org/10.1086/649858.

Linked questions: 39–40

39. A 55-year-old female originally from rural Vietnam, residing in Oregon for the past 20 years, presents to the emergency department with fever, headache, and progressive confusion. On arrival, she is febrile (38.7 °C) and disoriented and has neck stiffness. Her mental status declines rapidly, and she is intubated for airway protection.

    Her daughter states that she was previously healthy and had not traveled outside the United States since immigrating. She had recently been treated at an urgent care center for poison ivy, where she was prescribed both topical and oral prednisone. The household includes two pet cats, but no recent known infections. She has no history of HIV, cancer, or other known immunocompromising conditions.

CSF Analysis:

- Opening pressure: 290 mm H_2O
- WBC count: 3200 cells/mm^3
  - Differential: 80% neutrophils, 0% eosinophils
- Glucose: 25 mg/dL
- Protein: 190 mg/dL
- Gram stain: Gram-negative rods
- CSF culture and blood cultures: Pending
- CT head (non-contrast): Unremarkable

What is the most likely diagnosis?
A. Bacillary angiomatosis
B. Leptospirosis
C. Neurocysticercosis
D. *Strongyloides* hyperinfection precipitated by steroid use
E. Tuberculous meningitis
Correct answer: D

Explanations
Strongyloides stercoralis can persist for decades via autoinfection. Immunosuppression—particularly with corticosteroids—can trigger hyperinfection, leading to larval dissemination and translocation of gut flora, especially Gram-negative bacteria (e.g., *E. coli*), into the bloodstream and CNS. The CSF profile is consistent with bacterial meningitis, and lack of eosinophilia is expected in severe disseminated cases.

Incorrect answers:
A. Bacillary angiomatosis
Typically caused by *Bartonella henselae* or *B. quintana*, this condition primarily presents with cutaneous lesions in immunocompromised hosts (often HIV-positive). CNS involvement is rare. Gram-negative rods in CSF are not characteristic.
B. Leptospirosis
Can affect the CNS but usually includes hepatic and renal dysfunction. CSF findings are not typically dominated by neutrophils, and Gram-negative rods are not part of the expected Gram stain.
C. Neurocysticercosis
Presents with seizures or signs of chronic intracranial pressure, not acute meningitis. Imaging often shows cysts or calcifications. CSF may show eosinophils but not Gram-negative rods. No recent travel or seizures were reported.

E. Tuberculous meningitis

Typically causes a subacute illness with lymphocytic CSF, elevated protein, and low glucose. Gram-negative rods are not expected, and progression is usually more gradual.

Important Clinical Note

The absence of eosinophilia does not rule out parasitic infection. In *Strongyloides* hyperinfection, eosinophilia is often absent due to overwhelming immunosuppression and systemic bacterial superinfection.

Linked question

40. Given that *Strongyloides stercoralis* is endemic in Southeast Asia but the patient in the prior question has lived in Oregon for 20 years, where and when was she most likely infected?
    A. During recent gardening activities in Oregon
    B. From a household contact with pinworm
    C. During her childhood or early adult life in rural Vietnam
    D. From uncooked fish consumed recently in Oregon
    E. From contaminated hospital water during recent emergency room visit

    Correct answer: C.

Explanation

Strongyloides stercoralis can persist for decades due to its *autoinfective lifecycle*, even without reexposure. Infection during childhood or early adulthood in an endemic area (e.g., Vietnam) is the most likely source. *Hyperinfection syndrome may emerge years later*, especially after immunosuppressive events like steroid use.

Reference

Keiser PB, Nutman TB. Strongyloides stercoralis in the Immunocompromised Population. Clin Microbiol Rev. 2004;17(1):208–17. https://doi.org/10.1128/cmr.17.1.208-217.2004.

Linked questions: 41–42

41. A 19-year-old previously healthy male presents with progressive confusion and difficulty walking after returning from a 2-week hiking trip through the Czech Republic, Switzerland, and Hungary. He stayed in mountain lodges and hostels, consumed local food but no unpasteurized dairy, and had one new sexual contact during the trip (with condom use). His travel companions remain asymptomatic.

He initially experienced fever, malaise, and body aches for 3–4 days, followed by a brief period of improvement.

Several days later, he developed recurrent fever, headache, photophobia, mild confusion, and an unsteady gait. On neurologic examination, he shows slowed processing and mild ataxia, but no focal motor or cranial nerve deficits. A brain MRI is normal.

CSF analysis reveals:

- Opening pressure: Normal
- White blood cell count: 100/mm^3 with 80% lymphocytes
- Protein: Mildly elevated
- Glucose: Normal

What is the most likely diagnosis?
A. Tick-borne encephalitis
B. Neurosyphilis
C. Viral meningitis
D. Multiple sclerosis
E. Delirium due to substance use

Correct answer: A

Explanation

Tick-borne encephalitis (TBE) is a viral infection caused by a flavivirus transmitted primarily through *Ixodes* tick bites. It is endemic in Central and Eastern Europe, including the countries the patient visited. The infection classically follows a biphasic course. The first phase includes nonspecific symptoms such as fever, fatigue, and myalgia. This is followed by an asymptomatic interval and then a second phase of central nervous system involvement, presenting with meningitis, encephalitis, or ataxia.

This patient's biphasic clinical course, recent travel to endemic regions, and neurologic symptoms are highly suggestive of TBE. The cerebrospinal fluid profile—lymphocytic pleocytosis with mildly elevated protein and normal glucose—is typical of viral meningoencephalitis, particularly in the setting of TBE. Early in the disease, neuroimaging may be normal. The incubation period is typically 4–28 days, with most patients becoming symptomatic 7–14 days after exposure.

Incorrect answers:
B. Neurosyphilis presents in a subacute manner and often involves cranial nerve deficits, tabes dorsalis, or cognitive impairment. There is no history of untreated syphilis or supportive CSF findings in this case.
C. Viral meningitis could present similarly in CSF profile, but does not usually follow a biphasic pattern or lead to progressive encephalitic symptoms. TBE has a distinct epidemiologic and clinical profile.
D. Multiple sclerosis (MS) typically involves focal neurologic deficits such as optic neuritis or sensory loss. It rarely presents with encephalitis. Fevers and systemic

symptoms would be a red flag in the diagnostic workup of MS and suggest an alternative diagnosis; CSF WBC count tends to be lower in MS.

E. Delirium due to substance use is not supported by this patient's history or lab findings. The CSF profile is inconsistent with a toxic or metabolic cause of confusion.

Linked question

42. What is the most effective strategy to prevent tick-borne encephalitis in travelers to endemic regions?
    A. Daily doxycycline during travel
    B. Tick-borne encephalitis vaccination prior to travel
    C. Insect repellents containing DEET only
    D. Avoidance of all uncooked meats and dairy
    E. Yellow fever vaccination

Correct answer: B

Explanation

Vaccination is the most effective preventive measure for travelers visiting TBE-endemic regions, especially those engaging in outdoor activities. While DEET and protective clothing help reduce tick exposure, vaccination offers more reliable protection. Unpasteurized dairy is a rare transmission route, and yellow fever vaccination is unrelated.

Summary for Questions 41–42

Tick-borne encephalitis should be considered in travelers who develop neurologic symptoms—including headache, confusion, photophobia, or ataxia—after returning from endemic regions in Central or Eastern Europe. The virus is typically transmitted by *Ixodes* ticks, with an incubation period of 4–28 days. The illness follows a characteristic biphasic course, beginning with nonspecific febrile symptoms, followed by a neurologic phase. Cerebrospinal fluid often shows lymphocytic pleocytosis, elevated protein, and normal glucose. Imaging may be normal early on. Diagnosis is confirmed by TBEV-specific IgM and IgG antibodies in serum or CSF. Vaccination is the most effective preventive strategy, particularly for outdoor travelers.

Reference

Kunze U. Report of the 20th annual meeting of the International Scientific Working Group on Tick-Borne Encephalitis (ISW-TBE): ISW-TBE: 20 years of commitment and still challenges ahead. Ticks Tick Borne Dis. 2019;10(1):13–7. https://doi.org/10.1016/j.ttbdis.2018.08.004.

43. A 72-year-old man presents to the emergency department in South Africa in March with fever, aphasia, and confusion. He arrived directly from the United States the previous evening for a 2-week safari. His symptoms began mid-flight, starting with fever and headache, progressing to mild confusion and expressive aphasia shortly after landing.

His medical history includes well-controlled hypertension. He received the yellow fever vaccine 8 days ago in preparation for this trip based on his travel agent's strong recommendation. His wife reports he had a minor bite from a neighbor's 8-year-old Golden Retriever (fully vaccinated) 2 weeks ago in Oregon. The dog is reportedly healthy and behaving normally. The patient has not traveled outside the United States in recent years, including no recent trips to rabies- or malaria-endemic regions. He and his wife live in Connecticut.

On Examination:

- Temperature: 38.7 °C
- Neurologic exam: Disoriented to time, +expressive aphasia, no neck stiffness, cranial nerves intact, slowed but spontaneous movement in all extremities
- No photophobia, rash, or meningeal signs

Key Laboratory and CSF Findings:

- CBC:
    – WBC 5000/μL with normal differential
    – Platelets: 110,000/μL
- ALT/AST: Mildly elevated
- CT head: Normal
- CSF opening pressure: 17 cm H_2O
- CSF WBC: 30/mm^3 (80% lymphocytes)
- CSF protein: 75 mg/dL
- CSF glucose: 60 mg/dL (serum glucose: 100 mg/dL)
- CSF Gram stain: Negative

Which of the following is the most likely diagnosis?
A. Yellow fever vaccine-associated neurotropic disease (YEL-AND)
B. Malaria
C. West Nile virus infection
D. Rabies
E. Japanese encephalitis

Correct answer: A

Explanation

This elderly patient presents with fever, aphasia, and altered mental status, with CSF lymphocytic pleocytosis and mild hepatic enzyme elevation—within the 8-day window following yellow fever vaccination. This patient's presentation is classic for yellow fever vaccine-associated neurotropic disease (YEL-AND), a rare but serious complication occurring typically 4–30 days after vaccination, especially in adults over age 60. Symptoms include encephalitis, meningitis, Guillain-Barré-like syndromes, or focal neurologic deficits. CSF usually shows lymphocytic pleocytosis with elevated protein and normal glucose. This case highlights the importance of understanding regional vaccine requirements, as yellow fever vaccination was not indicated for travel to South Africa (South Africa does not have endemic yellow fever). Despite its risks in some populations, the vaccine remains highly safe and effective when appropriately used.

While the yellow fever vaccine is highly effective and safe for most people, certain groups—including those over age 60, infants under 6 months, and individuals with thymic disorders—have an increased risk for vaccine-associated neurotropic (YEL-AND) or viscerotropic disease (YEL-AVD).

Incorrect answers:

B. Malaria:

Symptoms began on arrival in South Africa, making new infection impossible, and there is no recent travel to endemic areas. The patient has not left the United States for decades, so relapse from *P. vivax* or *P. ovale* is also extremely unlikely.

C. West Nile virus infection:

March is low season for mosquito-borne transmission in the Eastern United States, and West Nile is not endemic in South Africa. Incubation is usually 2–14 days postexposure, which does not fit.

D. Rabies:

While he was bitten by a dog, the dog was vaccinated, the bite was minor, and the dog is alive and well 2 weeks later.

E. Japanese encephalitis:

There is no history of travel to Asia, where the virus is endemic. This condition is not found in South Africa and has an incubation of 5–15 days.

References

Lindsey NP, Rabe IB, Miller ER, Fischer M, Staples JE. Adverse event reports following yellow fever vaccination, 2007-13. J Travel Med. 2016;23(5). https://doi.org/10.1093/jtm/taw045.

U.S. Centers for Disease Control and Prevention - Yellow Fever Vaccine Information for Healthcare Providers. https://www.cdc.gov/yellow-fever/hcp/vaccine/index.html (2025). Accessed July 20 2025.

44. A 55-year-old man presents to the emergency department with intermittent fever, pleuritic chest pain, and progressive confusion that began approximately 2 weeks ago. His wife reports that he has been increasingly somnolent and unable to focus over the past few days.

He lives in Manhattan, works in finance, and is married with three children. The family recently returned from a 3-week safari through South Africa, Malawi, and Tanzania, where they visited game reserves and rural areas.

On presentation, he is febrile (38.9 °C), disoriented to time and place, and tachycardic. He has no focal motor deficits, but his neurologic exam reveals impaired attention, somnolence, and an ataxic gait. A full skin examination was deferred until he could be moved from the emergency department hallway but his family says he has a large scab like lesion on his left upper leg.

Laboratory Findings:

- *WBC count: 11,400/μL*
- *Hemoglobin: 10.2 g/dL*
- *Platelet count: 86,000/μL*
- *Peripheral smear: No organisms seen inside red blood cells. There are wavy extracellular organisms with a nucleus and kinetoplasts.*
- *Malaria rapid antigen test: Negative*
- *CSF*:
  - *Elevated protein*
  - *Lymphocytic pleocytosis*
  - *Gram stain negative*

What is the most likely diagnosis?
A. HIV/AIDS
B. Acute respiratory infection (e.g., pneumonia)
C. Malaria
D. Bacterial endocarditis
E. East African trypanosomiasis
F. Neurosarcoidosis

Correct answer: E

Explanation

East African trypanosomiasis (*T. brucei rhodesiense*), also known as acute African sleeping sickness, is transmitted by tsetse flies and occurs in East and South Africa. This form is more fulminant than West African trypanosomiasis (*T. brucei gambiense*). Hallmarks include:

- Acute febrile illness with rapid CNS progression (e.g., confusion, ataxia, somnolence)
- Thrombocytopenia, anemia, and lymphocytic CSF pleocytosis with trypanosomes
- Potential cardiopulmonary symptoms due to systemic involvement
- History of travel to endemic regions such as Tanzania, Malawi, and South Africa

His acute illness, worsening encephalopathy, and the recent safari exposure in endemic regions should raise suspicion for East African trypanosomiasis.

Incorrect answers:

A. HIV/AIDS:

HIV can cause chronic neurocognitive disorders, but acute confusion, CSF trypanosomes, and hematologic findings (thrombocytopenia) are inconsistent with either acute retroviral syndrome or untreated HIV in isolation.

B. Acute Respiratory Infection (e.g., Pneumonia):

Does not account for neurological deterioration, CSF findings, or parasitic infection. No cough or pulmonary infiltrates are noted.

C. Malaria:

Falciparum malaria may cause encephalopathy, but the malaria rapid test is negative, and trypanosomes, not plasmodia, were observed. Additionally, the clinical course is more progressive than typical cerebral malaria.

D. Bacterial Endocarditis:

Could potentially explain fever and confusion due to embolic stroke, but there is no murmur, no known risk factors (e.g., IV drug use), and parasitemia, and CSF findings are incompatible with this diagnosis.

F. Neurosarcoidosis:

While it can cause meningitis-like symptoms, this condition typically affects younger adults, progresses more insidiously, and would not explain trypanosomes in CSF or the travel-related exposure.

Reference

Kennedy PG. Clinical features, diagnosis, and treatment of human African trypanosomiasis (sleeping sickness). Lancet Neurol. 2013;12(2):186–94. https://doi.org/10.1016/s1474-4422(12)70296-x.

45. A 65-year-old woman presents to the emergency department with altered mental status. She recently retired from her job as a social worker in Washington, D.C., and returned 2 days ago from a month-long backpacking trip through South Asia, including rural areas of northern India, Bangladesh, southern India, and Sri Lanka. Her medical history includes coronary artery disease and hyperlipidemia.

One week before presentation, she developed high-grade fever, myalgias, and headache. Over the past 2 days, she has become increasingly confused and lethargic.

On exam, she is febrile (39.3 °C) and disoriented (GCS 13) and shows no focal neurological deficits. A faint maculopapular rash is noted on the trunk, and a black eschar is visible in the left axilla. No nuchal rigidity is present.

Laboratory Findings:

- WBC: 6800/mm^3 (normal differential)
- Hemoglobin: 11.0 g/dL
- Platelets: 78,000/μL
- AST: 162 U/L, ALT: 104 U/L
- Creatinine: 1.3 mg/dL

Lumbar Puncture:

- Opening pressure: Normal
- CSF WBC: 25/mm^3 (lymphocytic predominance)
- Protein: 85 mg/dL
- Glucose: 58 mg/dL (serum glucose 90 mg/dL)

Which of the following diagnoses is most likely given her presentation?

A. Scrub typhus (*Orientia tsutsugamushi*)
B. Dengue fever
C. Malaria
D. Japanese encephalitis
E. Typhoid fever

Correct answer: A

Explanation

This patient presents with a classic syndrome of scrub typhus. Scrub typhus is a mite-borne rickettsial infection caused by *Orientia tsutsugamushi*. It is transmitted by chigger mite larvae (*Leptotrombidium* species) and endemic to rural areas within the "tsutsugamushi triangle" of South and Southeast Asia. Clinical clues include fever, rash, eschar, transaminitis, thrombocytopenia, and lymphocytic pleocytosis in the CSF. Neurologic manifestations may include confusion, encephalitis, or meningoencephalitis, particularly in older adults. Diagnosis is suggested by travel history and clinical features and confirmed by PCR or IgM serology. Because early treatment improves outcomes, empiric therapy with doxycycline should be initiated when scrub typhus is suspected, even before confirmatory testing.

Although other diagnoses are plausible, scrub typhus is the most likely in this case given the combination of eschar, rash, thrombocytopenia, CNS findings, and travel history. Diagnostic confirmation can be made via PCR or IgM serology, but treatment should be initiated empirically if suspected.

Incorrect answers:

B. Dengue fever:

Can cause fever, rash, and thrombocytopenia, but encephalopathy is rare, and eschar is not typical.

C. Malaria:

May cause altered mental status in cerebral malaria, but is usually more acute in onset, and eschar and rash are not seen. Diagnosis requires blood smear or antigen testing.

D. Japanese encephalitis:

Can cause fever and confusion but is transmitted by mosquitoes, and rarely associated with rash, eschar, or transaminitis. It often presents with seizures or focal neurologic signs.

E. Typhoid fever:

Neuropsychiatric symptoms like "typhoid encephalopathy" may occur, but the presence of eschar, rash, and the CSF profile make scrub typhus more likely.

Reference

Wang Q, Ma T, Ding F, Lim A, Takaya S, Saraswati K, et al. Global and regional seroprevalence, incidence, mortality of, and risk factors for scrub typhus: A systematic review and meta-analysis. Int J Infect Dis. 2024;146:107151. https://doi.org/10.1016/j.ijid.2024.107151.

Brain and Spinal Trauma and Spinal Diseases

Jessica Lin

1. A 34-year-old man was brought into the emergency room after being hit by a car in a high-velocity accident while riding a motorcycle. On exam, he is hypotensive and with flaccid paralysis in all four extremities. Which of the following signs or symptoms would NOT be consistent with neurogenic shock?
   A. Bradycardia
   B. Tachycardia
   C. Hypotension
   D. Flushed skin
   E. MRI showing edema and hemorrhage in the cervical spine

   Correct answer: B

Explanation

Neurogenic shock, a type of distributive shock, is due to loss of sympathetic outflow from injury to the spinal cord above T6. The sympathetic dysfunction and unopposed vagal activity causes hypotension, bradycardia, and vasodilation. Pooling of venous blood due to vasodilation can lead to flushed skin and warm extremities. Imaging of the spine can show different mechanisms of injury to the cervical or upper thoracic spine, including compressive extramedullary or intramedullary lesions.

Reference

Massaro AF. Approach to the patient with shock. In: Loscalzo J, Fauci A, Kasper D, Hauser S, Longo D, Jameson J, editors. Harrison's Principles of Internal Medicine. 21st ed. McGraw-Hill Education; 2022.

2. A 28-year-old man is brought to the emergency department after an accidental fall off the rooftop. His blood pressure is 75/43 mm Hg, and the heart rate is 45 bpm. Extremities are warm. On exam he is awake and alert, but there is complete paralysis of the lower extremities, and there is sensory loss below the T4 level. CT of the spine shows a T4 burst vertebral fracture with spinal fragments in the spinal canal compressing the thoracic cord. Which of the following is the most appropriate initial step in management?
   A. Administer intravenous high-dose methylprednisolone
   B. Immediate surgical decompression
   C. Start norepinephrine infusion
   D. Intubation to prevent impending respiratory failure
   E. Obtain MRI spine to evaluate for epidural hematoma

   Correct answer: C

Explanation

This patient has neurogenic shock, with hypotension and bradycardia. His extremities are warm due to vasodilation and pooling of venous blood. It is important to stabilize his hemodynamics first and foremost. Surgical decompression is necessary and should ideally occur within 24 h, but should occur after hemodynamic stabilization. Administration of high-dose glucocorticoids after acute spinal cord injury is not recommended by multiple medical societies, including the Congress of Neurological Surgeons and the American College of Surgeons, due to lack of high-level evidence and well-documented risk.

Unless there was direct trauma to the lungs, thoracic spinal cord injury should not lead to respiratory failure, and so intubation for that purpose is not indicated. MRI of the spine should ultimately be obtained, but is not the most important first step in management.

J. Lin (✉)
Department of Neurology, NYU Langone Health,
New York, NY, USA
e-mail: jessica.lin@nyulangone.org

T. E. Smith, V. Arena (eds.), *Essential Neurology Board Review Q & A*, https://doi.org/10.1007/978-3-032-17213-6_8

References

American College of Surgeons Committee on Trauma. Best practices guidelines: spine injury. American College of Surgeons. 2022. https://www.facs.org/media/k45gikqv/spine_injury_guidelines.pdf. Accessed 25 May 2025

Fehlings MG, Tetreault LA, Hachem L, Evaniew N, Ganau M, McKenna SL, et al. An update of a clinical practice guideline for the management of patients with acute spinal cord injury: recommendations on the role and timing of decompressive surgery. Global Spine J. 2024;14(3_suppl):174S–186S. https://doi.org/10.1177/21925682231181883

Hurlbert RJ, Hadley MN, Walters BC, Aarabi B, Dhall SS, Gelb DE, et al. Pharmacological therapy for acute spinal cord injury. Neurosurgery. 2013;72 Suppl 2:93–105. https://doi.org/10.1227/NEU.0b013e31827765c6

Massaro AF. Approach to the patient with shock. In: Loscalzo J, Fauci A, Kasper D, Hauser S, Longo D, Jameson J, editors. Harrison's Principles of Internal Medicine. 21st ed. McGraw-Hill Education; 2022.

3. A 24-year-old man presents to the emergency room after falling down a flight of stairs. He is awake and responsive, but has flaccid paralysis and sensory loss of all four extremities. On exam he also has absent deep tendon reflexes in the extremities, and a bladder scan revealed 800 cc of urine in the bladder. MRI of the cervical spine shows some edema in the high central cervical cord. Which of the following is an INCORRECT statement?
   A. The bulbocavernosus reflex is likely lost
   B. He might have priapism
   C. He might develop respiratory failure
   D. He has spinal shock
   E. The loss of reflexes will likely be permanent

Correct answer: E

Explanation

This patient has spinal shock, which is a loss of reflexes, motor, and sensory function below the level of spinal cord injury that is usually temporary. The loss of function happens almost immediately and tends to return over the next few weeks. Spinal shock should be differentiated from neurogenic shock, which is a type of distributive shock due to loss of sympathetic outflow. In spinal shock, there can be atonic paralysis of bowel and bladder and loss of the bulbocavernosus reflex, and priapism can be seen in male patients. Due to the high cervical injury, this patient is at risk of respiratory compromise from diaphragm dysfunction.

Reference

Ropper AH, Samuels MA, Klein JP, Prasad S. Diseases of the spinal cord. In: Ropper AH, Samuels MA, Klein JP, Prasad S, editors. Adams and Victor's Principles of Neurology. 12th ed. McGraw-Hill Education; 2023.

Linked questions: 4–6

4. A 25-year-old woman fell from a 4-story high balcony. Upon arrival to the emergency room, she was found to be in severe hemodynamic and respiratory distress. Neurologic exam was notable for dilated and sluggishly reactive pupils, unresponsiveness to tactile or noxious stimuli, and lack of motor movement. After intubation and stabilization of hemodynamics, imaging of the brain and cervical spine was obtained. Brain CT showed multifocal hemorrhages in the epidural, subdural, and parenchymal spaces, with diffuse edema and downward herniation. Cervical spine CT showed near-complete transection at the C2 level. Which of the following is INCORRECT?
   A. Consider placement of an external ventricular drain
   B. Consider placement of a parenchymal intracranial pressure monitor
   C. Consider decompressive craniectomy
   D. Aim for mean arterial pressure of 65 mmHg or lower, due to intracranial hemorrhage
   E. Consider administration of hypertonic saline

Correct answer: D

Explanation

Per the Brain Trauma Foundation guidelines, patients with severe traumatic brain injury and a Glasgow Coma Scale of less than 9 should be considered for intracranial pressure (ICP) monitoring. There are different options available for intracranial pressure monitoring, including an external ventricular drain, which can be both diagnostic and therapeutic, or an intraparenchymal device, sometimes called an ICP bolt.

Given the findings of downward herniation on imaging with a correlating clinical exam, hyperosmolar therapy such as hypertonic saline or mannitol should be given, and early decompressive craniectomy should also be considered.

Cerebral perfusion pressure (CPP) is the difference between the mean arterial pressure (MAP) and ICP. As ICP becomes elevated, CPP decreases, predisposing the brain to hypoperfusion. To avoid this, hypotension should be avoided, and the target CPP should be between 60 and 70 mmHg. Occasionally, pressors are used to maintain this target CPP.

In addition to consideration of CPP, maintenance of spinal cord perfusion is also important in patients with acute spinal cord injury. In isolated acute spinal cord injury, consider maintaining the MAP between 85 and 90 mmHg. However, since there is concomitant severe brain injury and intracranial hemorrhage in this patient, this high MAP goal should probably be avoided in this particular case.

References

American College of Surgeons Committee on Trauma. Best practices guidelines: spine injury. American College of Surgeons. 2022. https://www.facs.org/media/k45gikqv/spine_injury_guidelines.pdf. Accessed 14 May 2025

Carney N, Totten AM, O'Reilly C, Ullman JS, Hawryluk GW, Bell MJ, et al. Guidelines for the management of severe traumatic brain injury, fourth edition. Neurosurgery. 2017; 80(1):6–15. https://doi.org/10.1227/NEU.0000000000001432

Ryken TC, Hurlbert RJ, Hadley MN, Aarabi B, Dhall SS, Gelb DE, et al. The acute cardiopulmonary management of patients with cervical spinal cord injuries. Neurosurgery. 2013;72 Suppl 2:84–92. https://doi.org/10.1227/NEU.0b013e318276ee16

Linked question

5. For the patient in the prior question, an external ventricular drain was placed. Intracranial pressure was noted to be 33 mmHg. Which of the following should NOT be instituted as part of her management?
   A. Frequent holding of sedatives for neurologic exam
   B. Hypertonic saline
   C. Anesthetic drip
   D. Paralysis
   E. Strict temperature control
   Correct answer: A

Explanation

This patient has elevated intracranial pressures (ICPs) that should be treated. ICPs greater than 22 mmHg are associated with increased mortality. Nonsurgical options include hyperosmolar therapy such as hypertonic saline or mannitol, sedation and analgesia, paralysis, and temperature control (in particular, avoidance of fever, which can increase ICP). Increased drainage of cerebrospinal fluid from the external ventricular device can be considered. Frequently holding sedatives in this patient who is likely in pain and discomfort from her injuries and intubation will cause further elevations of her ICPs, which should be avoided.

References

Carney N, Totten AM, O'Reilly C, Ullman JS, Hawryluk GW, Bell MJ, et al. Guidelines for the management of severe traumatic brain injury, fourth edition. Neurosurgery. 2017; 80(1):6–15. https://doi.org/10.1227/NEU.0000000000001432

Cook AM, Morgan Jones G, Hawryluk GWJ, Mailloux P, McLaughlin D, Papangelou A, et al. Guidelines for the acute treatment of cerebral edema in neurocritical care patients. Neurocrit Care. 2020;32(3):647–66. https://doi.org/10.1007/s12028-020-00959-7

Tripathy S, Ahmad SR. Raised intracranial pressure syndrome: a stepwise approach. Indian J Crit Care Med. 2019;23(Suppl 2):S129–S135. https://doi.org/10.5005/jp-journals-10071-23190

Linked question

6. Over the next 72 h, the patient in the prior question progresses to lose cranial nerve function on bedside testing despite escalating medical management for high intracranial pressures. Her pupils are dilated and nonreactive to light. The corneal, oculovestibular, cough, and gag reflexes are absent. There is no mental status or motor response to noxious stimuli. She has developed severe acute respiratory distress syndrome and on 100% oxygen on the ventilator, with oxygen saturations around 90%. Decompressive hemicraniectomy was not pursued given the likely poor functional outcome with the extent of brain and high cervical cord injuries. What is the most appropriate next step in management?
   A. Declare brain death
   B. Perform an apnea test
   C. Obtain radionuclide cerebral scintigraphy
   D. Test the oculocephalic reflex
   E. Obtain consent from family to perform a brain death evaluation
   Correct answer: C

Explanation

Given the clinical exam, there is high suspicion that this patient has progressed to brain death. However, there is not enough information or testing yet to declare brain death. It is generally not required to obtain consent from family to perform a brain death evaluation, although discussing the intention to perform brain death evaluation with the family is recommended. Oculocephalic reflex testing should not be performed in this patient with cervical spine instability. The oculovestibular reflex tests the same cranial nerves, and if absent bilaterally, is sufficient in this case. While an apnea test is a part of the usual brain death evaluation, due to the patient's high oxygen requirements, she would not be able to tolerate an apnea test and it should not be performed. In addition, given the high cervical cord injury, it would not be clear whether apnea in this case is due to brain death or due to the cord injury.

Ancillary testing such as with radionuclide cerebral scintigraphy is required to confirm brain death in this case. Other available forms of ancillary testing include transcranial Doppler ultrasonography and conventional 4-vessel catheter angiography. Currently, EEG, CT angiography, and MR angiography are not acceptable forms of ancillary testing.

There are other situations where ancillary testing might be needed. These include facial or ear trauma that precludes a complete bedside cranial nerve evaluation, severe metabolic derangements that cannot be corrected, or limb movements that may or may not be spinally mediated.

Reference

Greer DM, Kirschen MP, Lewis A, Gronseth GS, Rae-Grant A, Ashwal S, et al. Pediatric and adult brain death/death by neurologic criteria consensus guideline. Neurology. 2023;101(24):1112–32. https://doi.org/10.1212/WNL.0000000000207740

7. A 45-year-old man was hit by a car while crossing the street. He was brought to the emergency room by emergency medical services. His Glasgow Coma Scale (GCS) was 7. On exam, he has intermittent bilateral decorticate motor posturing. His systolic blood pressure hovers around 85 mmHg. Initial head CT obtained is unremarkable. Which of the following is NOT a reason for placement of an intracranial pressure monitor in this patient?
   A. Age greater than 40
   B. GCS less than 9
   C. Bilateral motor posturing
   D. Systolic blood pressure less than 90 mmHg
   E. Unremarkable head CT
   Correct answer: E

Explanation

As per the Brain Trauma Foundation guidelines, in general, patients with a GCS less than 9 with an abnormal head CT should be considered for intracranial pressure (ICP) monitoring. If the head CT is unremarkable, ICP monitoring should still be considered in patients with a GCS less than 9 if they have at least two of the following characteristics: age greater than 40 years, unilateral or bilateral motor posturing, or systolic blood pressure less than 90 mmHg. Patients with low systemic blood pressures are at higher risk of brain tissue ischemia in the setting of traumatic brain injury and loss of cerebral autoregulation, and it is important to monitor their ICPs to maintain adequate cerebral perfusion pressures. Cerebral perfusion pressure is the difference between the mean arterial pressure and intracranial pressure.

Reference

Carney N, Totten AM, O'Reilly C, Ullman JS, Hawryluk GW, Bell MJ, et al. Guidelines for the management of severe traumatic brain injury, fourth edition. Neurosurgery. 2017; 80(1):6–15. https://doi.org/10.1227/NEU.0000000000001432

8. A 65-year-old man was found down and unresponsive at home by his daughter, who called emergency medical services. He was found pulseless, with telemetry showing pulseless electrical activity, and cardiopulmonary resuscitation was initiated. Return of spontaneous circulation was obtained after 45 min. Patient remained nonresponsive over the next 2 days, and neurologic exam was notable for an enucleated right eye, dilated and nonreactive left pupil, absent corneal reflexes, absent oculovestibular reflexes, absent cough and gag reflexes, and no movement to noxious stimuli. He has developed hypothermia with a temperature of 34 °C. He has increased diuresis and has a sodium level of 172 mEq/L. Head CT shows the following:

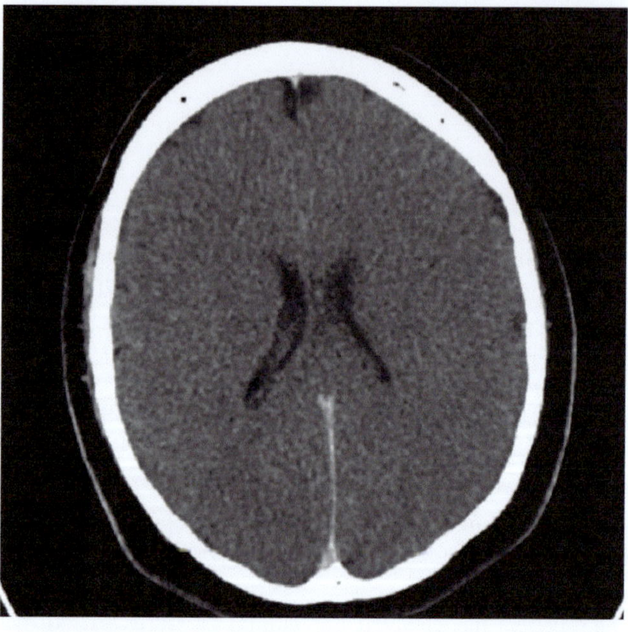

Axial CT head. (Source: Meillier, A., Heller, C. CC-BY 3.0 (https://creativecommons.org/licenses/by/3.0/) via *Case Reports in Medicine*. Image has not been modified. Please see full attribution with citation below in references section for this question.)

What is NOT an appropriate next step in management?

   A. Warm the patient to a body temperature of ≥36 °C
   B. Check levels of sedative drugs/medications
   C. Initiate prognostic discussions with family members
   D. Perform an apnea test
   E. Give free water
   Correct answer: D

Explanation

The patient's bedside clinical exam is concerning for brain death. However, a few issues should be addressed first prior to performing an apnea test to evaluate for brain death. Per the American Academy of Neurology guidelines, core body temperature should be maintained at or above 36 °C before pursuing brain death evaluation. If a patient's body temperature has been below 35.5 °C, the clinician should wait at least 24 h after rewarming before brain death evaluation. The severe hypernatremia likely developed due to central diabetes insipidus and lack of antidiuretic hormone and should also be corrected with free water or hypotonic saline prior to brain death evaluation. If the patient has been on sedative medications, checking available drug levels is appropriate to ensure that there is no pharmacologic reason for a depressed mental status. Given the poor neurologic exam and extensive anoxic injury seen on head imaging, initiating prognostic discussions with family members is appropriate.

References

Greer DM, Kirschen MP, Lewis A, Gronseth GS, Rae-Grant A, Ashwal S, et al. Pediatric and adult brain death/death by neurologic criteria consensus guideline. Neurology. 2023;101(24):1112–32. https://doi.org/10.1212/WNL.0000000000207740

Meillier A, Heller C. Acute cyanide poisoning: hydroxocobalamin and sodium thiosulfate treatments with two outcomes following one exposure event. Case Rep Med. 2015;2015:217951. https://doi.org/10.1155/2015/217951

Linked question

9. All medications that could suppress central nervous system functioning have been stopped, and drug levels that could be obtained were within therapeutic or subtherapeutic range. The patient has been rewarmed and is now normothermic, and the sodium level has been corrected to 149 mEq/L with free water. Due to concern for brain death, an apnea test was performed. There was no spontaneous breathing effort noted, and the partial pressure of carbon dioxide ($PaCO_2$) increased from 35 to 64 mm Hg on the arterial blood gas. What is an appropriate next step in this patient?
   A. Transcranial Doppler ultrasonography
   B. Computed tomography angiography
   C. Electroencephalogram (EEG)
   D. Auditory evoked potentials (AEPs)
   E. Somatosensory evoked potentials (SEPs)
   F. Declare brain death
   Correct answer: A

Explanation

The patient's apnea test is consistent with apnea given that (1) no respiratory effort was noted, (2) the $PaCO_2$ increased by at least 20 mmHg above the pre-apnea test baseline, and (3) the $PaCO_2$ level post-apnea test is at least 60 mmHg. Given that the patient has an enucleated eye, the absence of bilateral pupillary reflexes cannot be confirmed, and ancillary testing is needed prior to declaring brain death. Out of the listed tests, transcranial Doppler ultrasonography is the only currently acceptable ancillary test. Other available ancillary tests not listed here include 4-vessel catheter angiography and radionuclide cerebral scintigraphy. Electroencephalogram only assesses function of the cerebral hemispheres and not the brainstem. Auditory evoked potentials and somatosensory evoked potentials only evaluate certain parts of the brainstem and cortex.

Reference

Greer DM, Kirschen MP, Lewis A, Gronseth GS, Rae-Grant A, Ashwal S, et al. Pediatric and adult brain death/death by neurologic criteria consensus guideline. Neurology. 2023;101(24):1112–32. https://doi.org/10.1212/WNL.0000000000207740

10. A 3-month-old infant was brought into the emergency room with severe respiratory distress leading to cardiac arrest. Neurologic exam remained poor after 24 h of admission, and bedside testing is concerning for brain death. Head imaging obtained showed catastrophic anoxic injury involving the cerebral hemispheres and brainstem. Which of the following statements is accurate?
    A. 1 brain death evaluation is sufficient to declare brain death
    B. 1 apnea test is sufficient to declare brain death
    C. Apnea testing is not required in brain death declaration of pediatric patients
    D. Sucking or rooting reflex must be absent to be consistent with brain death
    E. The parameters for blood pressure requirements prior to brain death evaluation are the same for adult and pediatric patients
    Correct answer: D

Explanation

There are a few differences in brain death evaluation between adult and pediatric patients, as put forth by the American Academy of Neurology. In infants younger than 6 months, it must be determined that there is no primitive sucking or rooting reflex. The sucking reflex becomes a voluntary response at around the age of 4 months, while the rooting reflex disappears between the ages of 3 and 6 months. In pediatric patients, clinicians should maintain systolic blood pressure (SBP) and mean arterial pressure (MAP) ≥ fifth percentile for age, while in adults, SBP should be ≥100 mmHg and MAP ≥75 mmHg. In pediatric patients, two separate brain death evaluations, including the apnea test, by two different clinicians should be performed.

Reference

Greer DM, Kirschen MP, Lewis A, Gronseth GS, Rae-Grant A, Ashwal S, et al. Pediatric and adult brain death/death by neurologic criteria consensus guideline. Neurology. 2023;101(24):1112–32. https://doi.org/10.1212/WNL.0000000000207740

11. A 19-year-old man was brought in after being found unresponsive on a park bench. There are signs of trauma on his face and scalp. Head CT was unremarkable. Brain MRI obtained showed the following. What is the mechanism of injury?

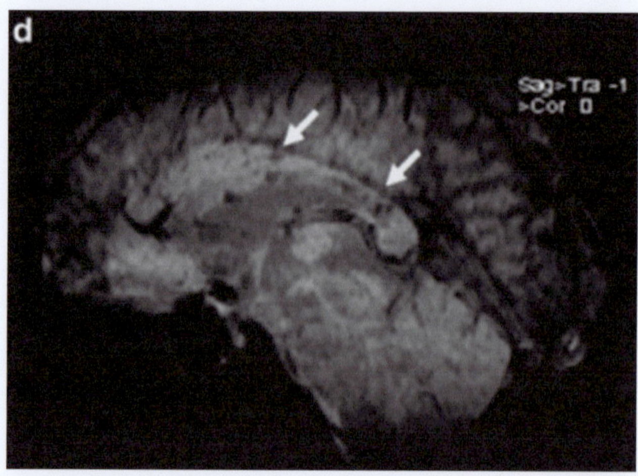

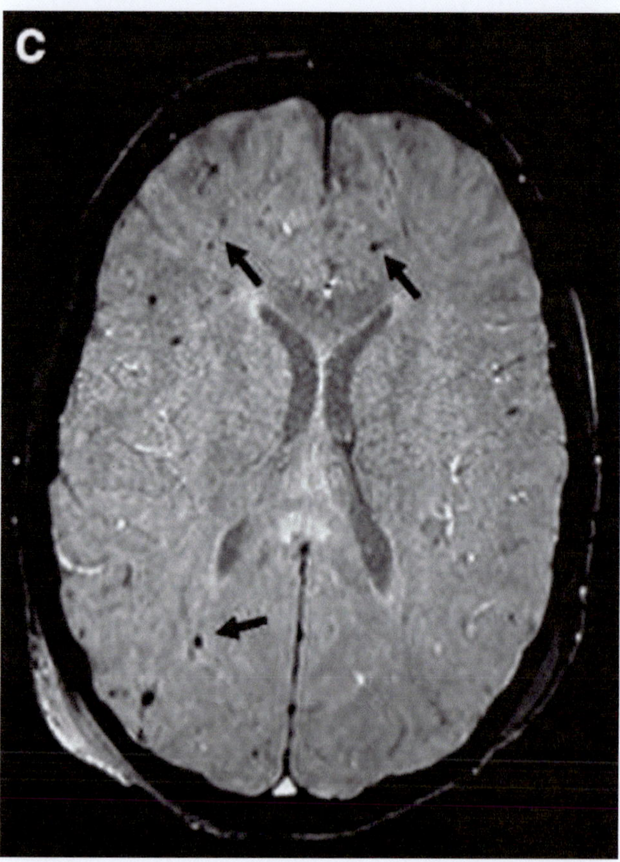

Axial and sagittal MRI brain. (Source: Gasparotti, R., Pinelli, L., Liserre, R. CC-BY 2.0 (https://creativecommons.org/licenses/by/2.0/) via *Insights Imaging*. Images have been cropped from original. Please see full attribution with citation below in references section for this question.)

   A. Shearing force on axons
   B. Ischemia from cardioembolism
   C. Vessel inflammation
   D. Amyloid deposition
   E. Air embolism

Correct answer: A

Explanation

These are susceptibility-weighted images (SWI) on MRI showing multiple microhemorrhages in the white matter, at the gray-white matter junction, and in the corpus callosum. This is compatible with diffuse axonal injury, which is due to shearing forces on axons caused by rapid deceleration or acceleration of the brain. This most often occurs at the gray-white matter junction, brainstem, and corpus callosum. These lesions might not be detectable on head CT. 3 Tesla MRI might reveal even more lesions not appreciated on 1.5 Tesla MRI.

Acute ischemia would be best detected on diffusion-weighted imaging and would not appear dark on SWI unless there was hemorrhagic conversion. Vessel inflammation can be best detected on vessel wall imaging. The sequelae of vessel inflammation can be seen as hyperintense T2/FLAIR white matter lesions, and occasionally, hemorrhagic lesions may be seen on SWI. However, the presentation of facial and scalp trauma here makes traumatic axonal injury more likely. Amyloid deposition cannot be directly detected on MRI. Cerebral amyloid angiopathy also presents as multiple microhemorrhages, typically in a lobar distribution in the cortical and subcortical regions, but the age and presentation of the patient would make this an unlikely diagnosis. While air emboli appear dark on SWI, corresponding hypodense lesions would have appeared on head CT.

References

Adams JH, Doyle D, Ford I, Gennarelli TA, Graham DI, McLellan DR. Diffuse axonal injury in head injury: definition, diagnosis and grading. Histopathology. 1989;15(1):49–59. https://doi.org/10.1111/j.1365-2559.1989.tb03040.x

Gasparotti R, Pinelli L, Liserre R. New MR sequences in daily practice: susceptibility weighted imaging. A pictorial essay. Insights Imaging. 2011;2(3):335–347. https://doi.org/10.1007/s13244-011-0086-3

Humble SS, Wilson LD, Wang L, Long DA, Smith MA, Siktberg JC, et al. Prognosis of diffuse axonal injury with traumatic brain injury. J Trauma Acute Care Surg. 2018;85(1):155–59. https://doi.org/10.1097/TA.0000000000001852

Luccichenti G, Giugni E, Péran P, Cherubini A, Barba C, Bivona U, et al. 3 Tesla is twice as sensitive as 1.5 Tesla magnetic resonance imaging in the assessment of diffuse axonal injury in traumatic brain injury patients. Funct Neurol. 2010;25(2):109–14.

12. A 42-year-old man presents to the emergency room 1 week after falling down the stairs due to worsening headache and new left leg weakness. Head CT obtained is shown below. What is the likely etiology of his new left leg weakness?

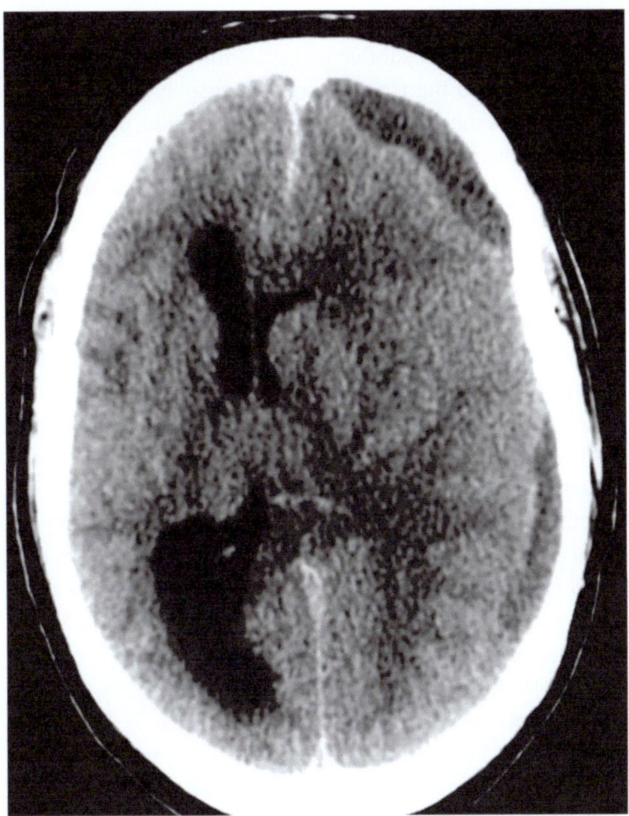

Axial CT head. (Source: Persson, M. E., Thelin, E. P., Bellander, B. CC-BY 3.0 (https://creativecommons.org/licenses/by/3.0/) via *Frontiers in Neurology*. Image is not modified from original. Please see full attribution with citation below in references section for this question.)

A. Uncal herniation
B. Embolic stroke of the right anterior cerebral artery
C. Subfalcine herniation
D. Central herniation
E. Tonsillar herniation

Correct answer: C

Explanation

This CT scan shows subfalcine herniation of the left cerebral hemisphere into the right cerebral hemisphere. This occurs when there is increased mass effect on one side, causing herniation of the ipsilateral cingulate gyrus under the falx. This can sometimes lead to compression of the contralateral anterior cerebral artery, in this case, the right anterior cerebral artery, causing ischemia and subsequent left leg weakness. This should prompt immediate neurosurgical consult for surgical decompression. While this can result in a stroke, the mechanism is not embolic in nature (and thus B is incorrect).

Uncal herniation occurs when the uncus of the medial temporal lobe herniates through the tentorium cerebelli, which separates the cerebral hemispheres from the posterior fossa. Central herniation is a central downward herniation through the tentorium. Lastly, tonsillar herniation occurs when cerebellar tonsils herniate through the foramen magnum, which can occur with either supratentorial or infratentorial lesions.

References

Persson ME, Thelin EP, Bellander BM. Case report: extreme levels of serum S-100B in a patient with chronic subdural hematoma. Front Neurol. 2012;3:170. https://doi.org/10.3389/fneur.2012.00170

Posner JB, Saper CB, Schiff ND, Claassen J. Structural causes of stupor and coma. In: Posner JB, Saper CB, Schiff ND, Claassen J, editors. Plum and Posner's diagnosis and treatment of stupor and coma. fifth ed. New York: Oxford University Press; 2019. p. 94–124.

13. A 28-year-old woman presents after a fall with head strike from horseback riding. On exam she is obtunded, with a dilated and nonreactive right pupil and flaccid weakness on the right. Her heart rate is in the 50s, blood pressure is 182/95 mm Hg, and she has an abnormal respiratory pattern. Which of the following is an INCORRECT statement?
    A. Consider empiric hyperosmolar therapy prior to head CT
    B. She has increased intracranial pressure
    C. Initial management includes elevating the head of bed to 30 degrees
    D. Prolonged hyperventilation can lead to cerebral ischemia
    E. The dilated right pupil and right-sided weakness cannot be from the same lesion

Correct answer: E

Explanation

The dilated right pupil and right-sided weakness can possibly be from a right-sided uncal herniation with Kernohan's phenomenon. Usually, uncal herniation results in an ipsilateral dilated and nonreactive pupil from compression of the ipsilateral oculomotor nerve and contralateral hemiparesis from compression of the ipsilateral cerebral peduncle and corticospinal tract. However, occasionally the midbrain is pushed across midline, and the contralateral cerebral peduncle is compressed by the tentorial notch, resulting in ipsilateral weakness.

The patient's presentation is consistent with increased intracranial pressure, supported by the exam and Cushing's triad: hypertension, bradycardia, and irregular respirations. It is reasonable to administer empiric hyperosmolar therapy even prior to confirmation with a head CT scan due to imminent fatality. Initial management also includes elevating the head of bed to 30 degrees and consideration of induced hyperventilation after intubation to vasoconstrict the cerebral blood vessels and decrease blood flow, therefore decreasing intracranial pressure. Since cerebral blood flow is decreased with hyperventilation, prolonged hyperventilation can potentially lead to cerebral ischemia. Hyperventilation should be temporary, often used as a holding measure until more definitive management such as surgical decompression can be implemented.

References

Posner JB, Saper CB, Schiff ND, Claassen J. Structural causes of stupor and coma. In: Posner JB, Saper CB, Schiff ND, Claassen J, editors. Plum and Posner's diagnosis and treatment of stupor and coma. fifth ed. New York: Oxford University Press; 2019. p. 94–124.

Ropper AH, Samuels MA, Klein JP, Prasad S. Disorders of the autonomic nervous system, respiration, and swallowing. In: Ropper AH, Samuels MA, Klein JP, Prasad S, editors. Adams and Victor's Principles of Neurology. 12th ed. McGraw-Hill Education; 2023.

14. Which of the following is NOT evaluated on the Glasgow Coma Scale?
    A. Eye-opening
    B. Respiratory pattern
    C. Motor response to noxious stimulation
    D. Motor response to verbal command
    E. Verbal response

Correct answer: B

Explanation

The Glasgow Coma Scale (GCS) was first defined in 1974 in The Lancet as an attempt to provide a standardized description of different states of impaired consciousness. The GCS consists of three different components: best eye-opening response, best verbal response, and best motor response. Possible scores range from 3 to 15, with a lower score indicating a worse clinical presentation. Respiratory pattern is not evaluated in the GCS, but is evaluated on the Full Outline of UnResponsiveness (FOUR) score. The FOUR score provides a more detailed description of patients with impaired consciousness and ranges from scores of 0 to 16, with a lower score indicating higher clinical severity. Like the GCS, it includes assessment of eye and motor response, but it also includes assessment of brainstem reflexes and respiratory pattern.

References

Teasdale G, Jennett B. Assessment of coma and impaired consciousness: a practical scale. Lancet. 1974;2(7872):81–4. https://doi.org/10.1016/s0140-6736(74)91639-0

Teasdale G, Maas A, Lecky F, Manley G, Stocchetti N, Murray G. The Glasgow Coma Scale at 40 years: standing the test of time. Lancet Neurol. 2014;13(8):844–54. https://doi.org/10.1016/S1474-4422(14)70120-6

Wijdicks EF, Bamlet WR, Maramattom BV, Manno EM, McClelland RL. Validation of a new coma scale: the FOUR score. Ann Neurol. 2005;58(4):585–93. https://doi.org/10.1002/ana.20611

15. A 75-year-old man with hypertension, poorly-controlled diabetes mellitus, atrial fibrillation on anticoagulation, and prior ischemic strokes presents with a right-sided headache and left arm and leg weakness after tripping and falling with head strike on the sidewalk. Head CT obtained shows a 1.5 cm right-sided subdural hematoma with 1 cm of midline shift. He was given prothrombin complex concentrate for anticoagulation reversal and undergoes a craniotomy and hematoma evacuation with improvement of his symptoms. 3 weeks later, he represents with new headache, as well as redevelopment of left arm and leg weakness. Head CT shows an isodense right-sided subdural hematoma with 0.5 cm midline shift. He has not yet restarted anticoagulation. A burr hole was performed and a subdural drain placed, with resolution of his symptoms. What is the most appropriate next step in management to consider?
    A. Craniotomy and hematoma evacuation
    B. Restart anticoagulation immediately
    C. Middle meningeal artery embolization
    D. Start dexamethasone
    E. Re-dose prothrombin complex concentrate
    Correct answer: C

Explanation

The patient has presented with a symptomatic subacute subdural hematoma that is a recurrence of a prior subdural hematoma. An appropriate next step is to consider a right middle meningeal artery (MMA) embolization, based on recent randomized controlled studies showing a decrease in hematoma recurrence or progression when middle meningeal artery embolization is performed in conjunction with surgical and nonsurgical standard of care in patients with subacute to chronic subdural hematomas. Recurrence of subdural hematomas is thought to be partly due to fragile neovasculature in the subdural space that is supplied by the middle meningeal artery.

Since this patient responded well to burr hole evacuation, craniotomy and hematoma evacuation is not necessary and would not be appropriate. Redosing prothrombin complex concentrate would also not be appropriate as patient has not been on anticoagulation. While restarting anticoagulation can be considered down the line, it should not be restarted immediately. There are some studies showing possible benefit of dexamethasone in decreasing subdural hematoma recurrence rate, but data is conflicting, and given this patient's uncontrolled diabetes mellitus, it would not be the best next step in management.

References

Davies JM, Knopman J, Mokin M, Hassan AE, Harbaugh RE, Khalessi A, et al. Adjunctive middle meningeal artery embolization for subdural hematoma. N Engl J Med. 2024;391(20):1890–1900. https://doi.org/10.1056/NEJMoa2313472

Fiorella D, Monteith SJ, Hanel R, Atchie B, Boo S, McTaggart RA, et al. Embolization of the middle meningeal artery for chronic subdural hematoma. N Engl J Med. 2025;392(9):855–64. https://doi.org/10.1056/NEJMoa2409845

Hutchinson PJ, Edlmann E, Bulters D, Zolnourian A, Holton P, Suttner N, et al. Trial of dexamethasone for chronic subdural hematoma. N Engl J Med. 2020;383(27):2616–27. https://doi.org/10.1056/NEJMoa2020473

Liu J, Ni W, Zuo Q, Yang H, Peng Y, Lin Z, et al. Middle meningeal artery embolization for nonacute subdural hematoma. N Engl J Med. 2024;391(20):1901–12. https://doi.org/10.1056/NEJMoa2401201

Miah IP, Holl DC, Blaauw J, Lingsma HF, den Hertog HM, Jacobs B, et al. Dexamethasone versus surgery for chronic subdural hematoma. N Engl J Med. 2023;388(24):2230–40. https://doi.org/10.1056/NEJMoa2216767

16. A 30-year-old man with no significant medical history is brought into the emergency room by his partner after a physical assault with blunt trauma to the head. On exam, he is disoriented and slightly lethargic, but otherwise appears to have a normal cranial nerve and motor exam. Head CT obtained is shown below. A CT angiogram is obtained which does not show any aneurysm or vascular injury. He is admitted to the neurologic intensive care unit for close monitoring. On the third day of admission, he develops new right-sided weakness and aphasia. A stat head CT is obtained, which is similar compared to prior. A CT angiogram is subsequently obtained. What is the most likely finding on the CT angiogram?

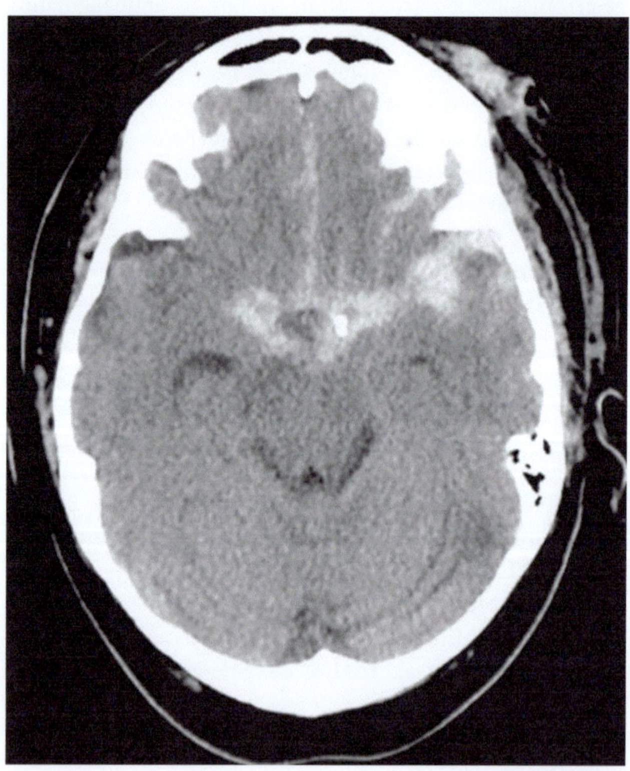

Axial CT head. (Lasry, O., Marcoux, J. CC-BY 4.0 (https://creativecommons.org/licenses/by/4.0/) via *SpringerPlus*. Image has not been modified from original. Please see full attribution with citation below in references section for this question.)

A. Middle cerebral artery vessel occlusion
B. Middle cerebral artery dissection
C. Middle cerebral artery aneurysm
D. A normal CT angiogram—the patient is having a seizure
E. Middle cerebral artery vasospasm

Correct answer: E

Explanation

The patient is most likely having vasospasm of the middle cerebral artery due to the thick subarachnoid hemorrhage (SAH). While cerebral vasospasm after traumatic SAH is less studied and recognized than in aneurysmal SAH, it is not an uncommon occurrence and seems to occur earlier than in aneurysmal SAH. Whereas vasospasm after aneurysmal SAH occurs mainly in day 3–14 after the hemorrhage, it seems to occur earlier in traumatic SAH with the highest risk peaking before day 7. It is less likely that the patient has a large vessel occlusion of the middle cerebral artery given that he is otherwise young and healthy, and initial CT angiogram did not show any evidence of large vessel injury or disease. While the patient is at risk of having seizures after a traumatic SAH, the clinical presentation is more suspicious for a vascular etiology.

References

Al-Mufti F, Amuluru K, Changa A, Lander M, Patel N, Wajswol E, et al. Traumatic brain injury and intracranial hemorrhage-induced cerebral vasospasm: a systematic review. Neurosurg Focus. 2017;43(5):E14. https://doi.org/10.3171/2017.8.FOCUS17431

Izzy S, Muehlschlegel S. Cerebral vasospasm after aneurysmal subarachnoid hemorrhage and traumatic brain injury. Curr Treat Options Neurol. 2014;16(1):278. https://doi.org/10.1007/s11940-013-0278-x

Lasry O, Marcoux J. The use of intravenous milrinone to treat cerebral vasospasm following traumatic subarachnoid hemorrhage. Springerplus. 2014 Oct 27;3:633. https://doi.org/10.1186/2193-1801-3-633

17. A 42-year-old woman with a strict vegan diet presents with worsening gait and balance issues. She describes that these issues are especially prominent in the dark. On exam she is noted to have a stomping gait. Which of the following statements is INCORRECT?

A. A patient with pernicious anemia might have similar symptoms
B. Imaging will likely reveal abnormalities in the cerebellum

C. Romberg testing is likely abnormal
D. Syphilis testing should be performed
E. This condition might be associated with lateral corticospinal tract dysfunction

Correct answer: B

Explanation

A gait and coordination disorder that is more prominent in the dark, along with a stomping gait, suggests a sensory ataxia. The issues are more prominent in the dark because of removal of visual input, such as with Romberg testing (which will likely be abnormal in this case). Other expected exam findings would be loss of vibratory and proprioceptive sensation, decreased reflexes, and possibly motor weakness. In this patient with a strict vegan diet, the symptoms are likely due to vitamin B12 deficiency, causing dorsal column dysfunction. Pernicious anemia is another possible cause of vitamin B12 deficiency. The patient should also be asked about nitrous oxide use, which can lead to a functional B12 deficiency. Neurosyphilis and tabes dorsalis should be on the differential as well. Occasionally, the lateral corticospinal tracts are also involved, resulting in subacute combined degeneration. The cerebellum is not typically affected in vitamin B12 deficiency.

Reference

Ropper AH, Samuels MA, Klein JP, Prasad S. Diseases of the nervous system caused by nutritional deficiency. In: Ropper AH, Samuels MA, Klein JP, Prasad S, editors. Adams and Victor's Principles of Neurology. 12th ed. McGraw-Hill Education; 2023.

18. A 64-year-old man presents with progressive difficulties using his hands. He describes feeling weak and often dropping things and has difficulty with opening bottles and jars and also with fine finger movements such as buttoning his clothes. He also complains of frequent tripping and feeling unsteady on his feet. On exam, he has decreased vibratory and proprioceptive sensation, spasticity, and mild weakness in the arms and legs. Deep tendon reflexes are increased. He has a positive Romberg test, a stomping gait, and difficulty with tandem gait. Which of the following is the most UNLIKELY diagnosis?
    A. Vitamin B12 deficiency
    B. Tropical spastic paraparesis
    C. Zinc toxicity

D. Copper deficiency
E. West Nile myelitis

Correct answer: E

Explanation

Based on the exam, spinal motor and sensory tracts, in particular, the corticospinal tracts and dorsal columns, are both affected in this patient. Conditions with a predilection for the lateral corticospinal tracts and dorsal columns include both metabolic and infectious causes and include vitamin B12 deficiency, copper deficiency, and tropical spastic paraparesis from human T-cell lymphotropic virus type 1 (HTLV-1) infection of the spinal cord. Zinc toxicity can affect copper absorption, leading to copper deficiency. This can be seen in excess zinc supplementation, or with excess use of certain denture creams that contain zinc.

On the other hand, West Nile virus has a predilection for the anterior horn cells and causes an acute flaccid paralysis. Of note, West Nile virus can also cause a meningoencephalitis. West Nile infection typically occurs in the summer and early fall. Enteroviruses, including coxsackievirus, enterovirus D68, and poliovirus, also have a predilection for the anterior horn cells.

References

Ropper AH, Samuels MA, Klein JP, Prasad S. Diseases of the nervous system caused by nutritional deficiency. In: Ropper AH, Samuels MA, Klein JP, Prasad S, editors. Adams and Victor's Principles of Neurology. 12th ed. McGraw-Hill Education; 2023.

Ropper AH, Samuels MA, Klein JP, Prasad S. Diseases of the spinal cord. In: Ropper AH, Samuels MA, Klein JP, Prasad S, editors. Adams and Victor's Principles of Neurology. 12th ed. McGraw-Hill Education; 2023.

Ropper AH, Samuels MA, Klein JP, Prasad S. Viral infections of the nervous system, chronic meningitis and prion disease. In: Ropper AH, Samuels MA, Klein JP, Prasad S, editors. Adams and Victor's Principles of Neurology. 12th ed. McGraw-Hill Education; 2023.

19. A 45-year-old man from China presents with 3 months of progressive mid-back pain, low-grade fevers, night sweats, and new onset of bilateral leg weakness and numbness. On exam, there is increased tone and slight weakness in bilateral lower extremities and increased patellar and ankle deep tendon reflexes. There is a sensory level at T9. MRI obtained of the thoracic spine is shown below. Which of the following is an INCORRECT statement?

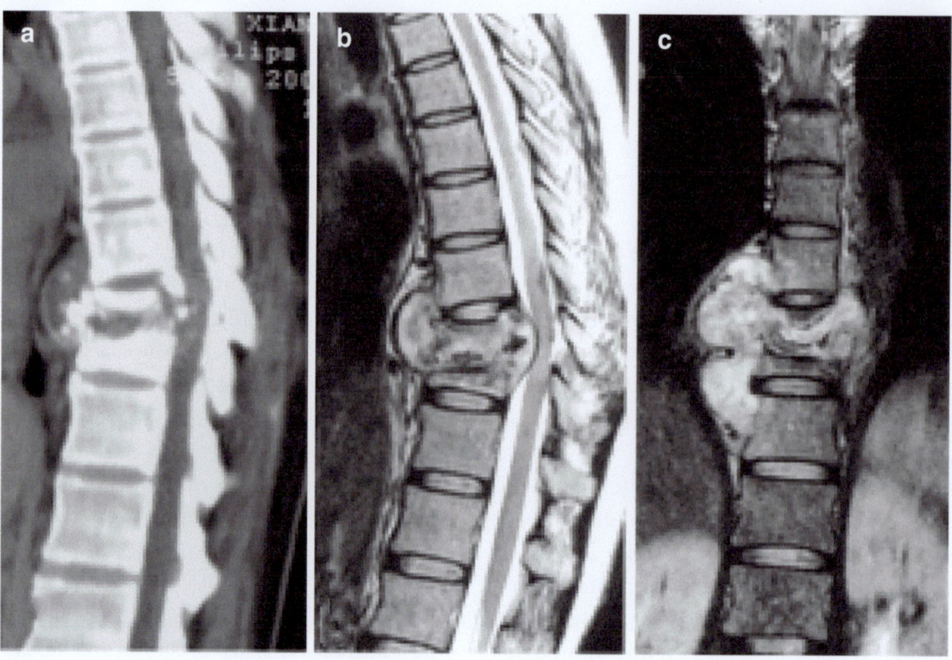

Sagittal CT spine (**a**), sagittal (**b**), and coronal (**c**) MRI spine. (Source: Zeng, H., Zhang, P., Xiongjie, S., Luo, C., Xu, Z., Zhang, Y., Liu, Z., Wang, X. CC-BY 4.0 (https://creativecommons.org/licenses/by/4.0/) via *BMC Musculoskeletal Disorders*. Image has been cropped from original. Please see full attribution with citation below in references section for this question.)

A. Angular kyphosis is often seen in this condition due to collapse of vertebral bodies or intervertebral discs
B. The thoracic or lumbar spine are most often affected in this condition
C. Initiation of broad-spectrum antibiotics like vancomycin and piperacillin/tazobactam is the most appropriate next step in management
D. The initial site of disease was likely in the lungs
E. Initiation of rifampin, isoniazid, pyrazinamide, and ethambutol is an appropriate next step in management

Correct answer: C

Explanation

This patient has spinal tuberculosis, or Pott's disease, which is characterized by abscess formation and vertebral body osteomyelitis with spread to the intervertebral discs. The thoracic and upper lumbar segments are most commonly affected. Collapse of the intervertebral discs or vertebral bodies can lead to angular kyphosis, also known as a gibbus deformity. Myelopathy can occur due to compression by an abscess or due to deformities of the vertebral structures themselves. Pott's disease typically occurs after primary infection of the lungs. Initiation of antituberculous therapy is the most appropriate next step in management.

References

Raviglione MC, Gori A. Tuberculosis. In: Loscalzo J, Fauci A, Kasper D, Hauser S, Longo D, Jameson J, editors. Harrison's Principles of Internal Medicine. 21st ed. McGraw-Hill Education; 2022.

Ropper AH, Samuels MA, Klein JP, Prasad S. Bacterial, fungal, spirochetal, and parasitic infections of the nervous system. In: Ropper AH, Samuels MA, Klein JP, Prasad S, editors. Adams and Victor's Principles of Neurology. 12th ed. McGraw-Hill Education; 2023.

Zeng H, Zhang P, Shen X, Luo C, Xu Z, Zhang Y, et al. One-stage posterior-only approach in surgical treatment of single-segment thoracic spinal tuberculosis with neurological deficits in adults: a retrospective study of 34 cases. BMC Musculoskelet Disord. 2015;16:186. https://doi.org/10.1186/s12891-015-0640-0

20. A 55-year-old man presents with worsening low back pain, trouble with walking, and difficulty with urination. On exam, he has weakness and patchy sensory loss in the distal lower extremities that is relatively symmetric. There is decreased sensation in the perianal region and a decreased rectal tone. The patellar reflexes are absent, but the Achilles reflexes are increased. Which of the following is the most likely diagnosis?

A. Conus medullaris syndrome
B. Cauda equina syndrome
C. L5 radiculopathy
D. Lumbosacral plexopathy
E. Acute inflammatory demyelinating polyradiculoneuropathy

Correct answer: A

Explanation

This patient has symmetric exam findings in the bilateral lower extremities with upper and lower motor neuron signs. Because of the bilateral symptoms and increased Achilles reflexes, this is not consistent with a radiculopathy. While bilateral lumbosacral plexopathies might be possible, the increased Achilles reflexes are not consistent with a plexopathy. The increased Achilles reflexes are also not consistent with an acute inflammatory demyelinating polyradiculoneuropathy.

In both cauda equina and conus medullaris syndromes, there might be urinary or stool retention or overflow incontinence, decreased rectal tone, sexual dysfunction, or saddle anesthesia. However, a pure cauda equina lesion affecting only the nerve roots should result in decreased or absent deep tendon reflexes, thus making a conus medullaris syndrome the most appropriate answer here. Depending on the location and extent of a lesion in the conus medullaris, reflexes in the lower extremities may be normal, increased, decreased, or absent. In addition, findings in cauda equina syndrome are often more asymmetrical than in conus medullaris syndrome.

References

Mandigo CE, Kaiser MG, Angevine PD. Traumatic spinal cord injury. In: Louis ED, Mayer SA, Noble JM, editors. Merritt's neurology. 14th ed. Wolters Kluwer; 2022.

Ropper AH, Samuels MA, Klein JP, Prasad S. Diseases of the spinal cord. In: Ropper AH, Samuels MA, Klein JP, Prasad S, editors. Adams and Victor's Principles of Neurology. 12th ed. McGraw-Hill Education; 2023.

21. A 75-year-old man with hypertension, hyperlipidemia, and coronary artery disease develops acute onset back pain and lower extremity weakness immediately after abdominal aortic surgery. On exam there is severe, symmetric, bilateral weakness and absent deep tendon reflexes in the lower extremities. Which of the following is a CORRECT statement?
    A. The artery of Adamkiewicz most often arises from the right aorta
    B. MRI of the spinal cord is often normal in the hyperacute phase
    C. This condition most often occurs in the cervical cord

D. The vertebral bodies are not affected in this condition
E. The dorsal and ventral spinal cord are likely equally affected

Correct answer: B

Explanation

This patient has suffered a spinal cord infarction in the setting of abdominal aortic surgery. This could be due to intraoperative occlusion, atheroembolism, or aortic dissection. Spinal cord infarct is relatively rare and occurs most often in the thoracolumbar region. This is because the cervical cord has a more robust vascular supply to the anterior and posterior spinal arteries, originating in branches of the subclavian arteries, including the vertebral arteries, thyrocervical trunk, and costocervical trunk. On the other hand, there is one major radiculomedullary artery, the artery of Adamkiewicz, supplying the thoracolumbar cord. This artery typically arises from the left side of the aorta between T9 and L2. The radiculomedullary arteries branch from segmental arteries, which come off the aorta.

Additionally, spinal cord infarcts more often occur in the ventral two-thirds of the spinal cord, the territory supplied by the singular anterior spinal artery. The dorsal one-third of the cord is supplied by two posterior spinal arteries, one on each side. Given the severe lower extremity weakness in this patient, he likely has an anterior spinal cord infarct. Additional exam findings would include loss of pain and temperature due to involvement of the spinothalamic tracts.

MRI is often normal in the hyperacute phase, and imaging findings may not show up until a few days later. Typical findings include restriction on diffusion-weighted imaging and a hyperintense signal on T2 and STIR. There might also be enlargement of the cord from edema. Occasionally, the only radiographic findings early after onset might be T2 hyperintense signals in the vertebral bodies adjacent to the segment of cord infarct, consistent with vertebral body infarction. The vertebral bodies also derive vascular supply from the segmental and radicular arteries.

References

Costamagna G, Meneri M, Abati E, Brusa R, Velardo D, Gagliardi D, et al. Hyperacute extensive spinal cord infarction and negative spine magnetic resonance imaging: a case report and review of the literature. Medicine (Baltimore). 2020;99(43):e22900. https://doi.org/10.1097/MD.0000000000022900

Faig J, Busse O, Salbeck R. Vertebral body infarction as a confirmatory sign of spinal cord ischemic stroke: report of three cases and review of the literature. Stroke. 1998;29(1):239–43. https://doi.org/10.1161/01.str.29.1.239

Lazorthes G, Gouaze A, Zadeh JO, Santini JJ, Lazorthes Y, Burdin P. Arterial vascularization of the spinal cord. Recent studies of the anastomotic substitution pathways. J Neurosurg. 1971;35(3):253–62. https://doi.org/10.3171/jns.1971.35.3.0253

Ropper AH, Samuels MA, Klein JP, Prasad S. Diseases of the spinal cord. In: Ropper AH, Samuels MA, Klein JP, Prasad S, editors. Adams and Victor's Principles of Neurology. 12th ed. McGraw-Hill Education; 2023.

Vargas MI, Gariani J, Sztajzel R, Barnaure-Nachbar I, Delattre BM, Lovblad KO, et al. Spinal cord ischemia: practical imaging tips, pearls, and pitfalls. AJNR Am J Neuroradiol. 2015;36(5):825–30. https://doi.org/10.3174/ajnr.A4118

Yuh WT, Marsh EE 3rd, Wang AK, Russell JW, Chiang F, Koci TM, et al. MR imaging of spinal cord and vertebral body infarction. AJNR Am J Neuroradiol. 1992;13(1):145–54.

22. Which of the following is an INCORRECT statement about the vascular supply of the spinal cord?
    A. The cervical cord vascular supply originates from the subclavian arteries
    B. The largest anterior radiculomedullary artery is the artery of Adamkiewicz
    C. The vertebral arteries feed only the anterior spinal artery, but not the posterior spinal arteries
    D. The anterior spinal artery supplies the ventral two-thirds of the spinal cord
    E. The vertebral arteries feed both the anterior spinal artery and posterior spinal arteries

Correct answer: C

Explanation

The cervical cord has a robust vascular supply from branches of the subclavian arteries, including the vertebral arteries, thyrocervical trunk, and costocervical trunk. The vertebral arteries feed into both the anterior spinal artery and posterior spinal arteries in the cervical region. The posterior spinal arteries can come off directly from the vertebral arteries, or from the posterior inferior cerebellar arteries. The singular anterior spinal artery supplies the ventral two-thirds of the spinal cord, while two posterior spinal arteries supply the dorsal one-third of the cord. The lower two-thirds of the spinal cord, or the thoracolumbar region, is mainly supplied by a large singular anterior radiculomedullary artery known as the artery of Adamkiewicz. This artery typically arises from the left side of the aorta between T9 and L2.

References

Lazorthes G, Gouaze A, Zadeh JO, Santini JJ, Lazorthes Y, Burdin P. Arterial vascularization of the spinal cord. Recent studies of the anastomotic substitution pathways. J Neurosurg. 1971;35(3):253–62. https://doi.org/10.3171/jns.1971.35.3.0253

Miyasaka K, Asano T, Ushikoshi S, Hida K, Koyanagi I. Vascular anatomy of the spinal cord and classification of spinal arteriovenous malformations. Interv Neuroradiol. 2000;6 Suppl 1(Suppl 1):195–8. https://doi.org/10.1177/159101990000060S131

Ropper AH, Samuels MA, Klein JP, Prasad S. Diseases of the spinal cord. In: Ropper AH, Samuels MA, Klein JP, Prasad S, editors. Adams and Victor's Principles of Neurology. 12th ed. McGraw-Hill Education; 2023.

23. A 22-year-old healthy man presents with sudden onset low back pain followed by rapidly progressive bilateral lower extremity weakness and numbness 1 h after a surfing lesson. He is also unable to urinate. On exam, he has flaccid paraplegia of the lower extremities, a sensory level at T10, and absent lower extremity deep tendon reflexes. An MRI of the thoracic spine shows a longitudinal T2 hyperintense lesion in the thoracic spinal cord. Which of the following is the most likely underlying mechanism of his condition?
    A. Traumatic spinal cord contusion
    B. Syrinx formation
    C. Demyelination
    D. Hyperextension-induced spinal cord ischemia
    E. Venous infarction from spinal arteriovenous malformation rupture

Correct answer: D

Explanation

Surfer's myelopathy is a rare, nontraumatic spinal cord injury typically seen in novice surfers shortly after surfing. It is thought to result from ischemia of the spinal cord, usually in the thoracic region, due to prolonged hyperextension of the back while lying prone on the surfboard. This position may lead to compromised blood flow through the anterior spinal artery or its feeders. Patients typically present with acute back pain, rapidly followed by bilateral weakness and sensory loss in the lower extremities. MRI of the spine will show a longitudinally extensive T2 hyperintensity. Restricted diffusion can also be seen if diffusion-weighted images are obtained.

References

Choi J, Seok HY, Kim Y, Kim BJ. Surfer's myelopathy mimicking infectious myelitis. J Clin Neurol. 2017;13(2):207–8. https://doi.org/10.3988/jcn.2017.13.2.207

Freedman BA, Malone DG, Rasmussen PA, Cage JM, Benzel EC. Surfer's myelopathy: a rare form of spinal cord infarction in novice surfers: a systematic review. Neurosurgery. 2016;78(5):602–11. https://doi.org/10.1227/NEU.0000000000001089

Ropper AH, Samuels MA, Klein JP, Prasad S. Diseases of the spinal cord. In: Ropper AH, Samuels MA, Klein JP, Prasad S, editors. Adams and Victor's Principles of Neurology. 12th ed. McGraw-Hill Education; 2023.

24. A 58-year-old man presents with a 6-month history of progressive difficulty walking, numbness in the legs, and urinary urgency. He also reports dull, achy back pain. On exam, there is spasticity and weakness of the lower extremities and a mid-thoracic sensory level. MRI of the thoracic spine obtained is shown below. What is the most appropriate next step in management?

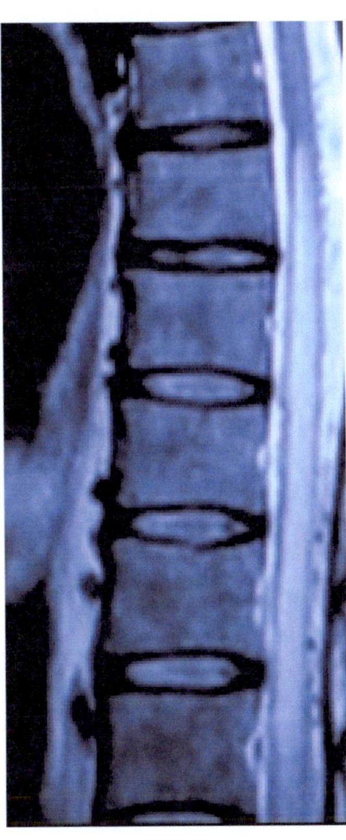

Sagittal MRI spine. (Source: Chen, S., Ma, Y., Liang, P., Wang, X., Peng, C., Bian, L., Liu, J., Zhang, H., Ling, F. CC-BY 4.0 (https://creativecommons.org/licenses/by/4.0/) via *Medicine*. Image has been cropped from original. Please see full attribution with citation below in references section for this question.)

A. Administer high-dose intravenous corticosteroids
B. Start broad-spectrum antibiotics
C. Referral to neuro-oncology
D. Perform a lumbar puncture and send cerebrospinal fluid for analysis
E. Obtain spinal angiography

Correct answer: E

Explanation

This is a sagittal T2-weighted image of the thoracic spine showing a longitudinal hyperintense T2 signal abnormality in the central cord, as well as multiple intradural flow voids. The imaging is suspicious for cord edema and expansion due to venous congestion from a spinal vascular malformation, such as an arteriovenous malformation or dural arteriovenous fistula. The most appropriate next step in management would be to obtain spinal angiography for confirmation and potential embolization treatment. Surgical resection might be necessary if endovascular treatment fails.

Spinal vascular malformations present most commonly in middle-aged and elderly men and present with a progressive myelopathy with gait disturbance and lower extremity paresthesias and weakness. Spinal dural arteriovenous fistulas are more common than intramedullary arteriovenous malformations and are usually acquired, whereas the arteriovenous malformations are likely congenital.

While transverse myelitis can have a similar appearance of a longitudinal T2 hyperintensity on MRI, the clinical history of this patient makes this an unlikely diagnosis.

References

Apostolova M, Nasser S, Kodsi S. A rare case of spinal dural arteriovenous fistula. Neurol Int. 2012;4(3):e19. https://doi.org/10.4081/ni.2012.e19

Chen S, Ma Y, Liang P, Wang X, Peng C, Bian L, et al. Hyperbaric oxygen therapy for postoperative spinal dural arterio-venous fistula patients: an observational cohort study. Medicine (Baltimore). 2016;95(37):e4555. https://doi.org/10.1097/MD.0000000000004555

Ropper AH, Samuels MA, Klein JP, Prasad S. Diseases of the spinal cord. In: Ropper AH, Samuels MA, Klein JP, Prasad S, editors. Adams and Victor's Principles of Neurology. 12th ed. McGraw-Hill Education; 2023.

25. A 34-year-old scuba diver presents to the emergency department 2 h after completion of a deep dive. He reports mid-back pain and numbness and weakness in both legs. On exam, he has severe weakness in the lower extremities and diminished pinprick sensation below the umbilicus. MRI of the spine is unremarkable. Which of the following is the most appropriate next step in management?

A. High-dose intravenous corticosteroids
B. Emergent spinal cord angiography
C. Hyperbaric oxygen therapy
D. Intravenous immunoglobulin therapy
E. Supportive care and close observation

Correct answer: C

Explanation

Decompression illness occurs after rapid ascent, such as during scuba diving or high-altitude aviation. This is due to formation of inert gas bubbles, especially nitrogen, that were previously dissolved within tissues that can cause vessel occlusion, typically of small veins. When this occurs in spinal vessels, it can cause a severe ischemic myelopathy.

MRI of the spine is often normal, but can show a T2 hyperintense lesion or diffusion restriction. Risk factors include longer or deeper submersions, breath-holding, warm temperatures during the dive, or cold temperatures after the dive. Emergent management focuses on hyperbaric oxygen therapy, which allows gas dissolution from tissues, and increases oxygen delivery to ischemic organs.

References

Gempp E, Blatteau JE. Risk factors and treatment outcome in scuba divers with spinal cord decompression sickness. J Crit Care. 2010;25(2):236–42. https://doi.org/10.1016/j.jcrc.2009.05.011

Leach MR, Zammit C. Decompression illness. In: Louis ED, Mayer SA, Noble JM, editors. Merritt's neurology. 14th ed. Wolters Kluwer; 2022.

Vann RD, Butler FK, Mitchell SJ, Moon RE. Decompression illness. Lancet. 2011;377(9760):153–64. https://doi.org/10.1016/S0140-6736(10)61085-9

26. A 5-month-old baby boy is brought to the emergency department with lethargy, vomiting, and seizures. His parents report that he was "fussy" earlier in the day. The history provided by the parents is inconsistent. He is afebrile. Exam is notable for a bulging anterior fontanelle, decreased level of consciousness, and bruising in the shape of a handprint along the thorax and back. There is no external evidence of head injury. Cranial ultrasound is concerning for intracerebral hemorrhage. Which of the following statements is the LEAST correct?

    A. There is likely an epidural hematoma with skull fracture
    B. Neurosurgery should be consulted
    C. Child Protective Services should be contacted
    D. Retinal hemorrhages might be present on fundoscopic exam
    E. Neurological outcome is likely poor

Correct answer: A

Explanation

This patient's history and presentation is suspicious for shaken baby syndrome from child abuse. The inconsistent history provided by the parents is concerning. There is likely intracerebral hemorrhage and swelling from accelerating and decelerating shearing forces intracranially, resulting in a bulging anterior fontanelle, decreased consciousness, and seizures. The bruising along the thorax and back is likely from being held tightly. Retinal hemorrhages might be found on fundoscopic exam and may be due to rotational forces. Neurologic prognosis is usually poor in these patients. Neurosurgery should be consulted immediately for possible surgical intervention. It is the physician's duty to report any suspected child abuse or neglect to Child Protective Services, known as mandated reporting. An epidural hematoma with a skull fracture would only be present if there was direct head trauma, which is often not the case in shaken baby syndrome, and is therefore the least correct answer here.

Reference

Piña-Garza JE, James KC. Altered states of consciousness. In: Piña-Garza JE, James KC, editors. Fenichel's clinical pediatric neurology: a signs and symptoms approach. ninth ed. Elsevier, Inc.;2025. p. 61–94

27. A 54-year-old man was brought to clinic by his wife for 4–5 years of progressive cognitive decline and behavioral changes. His wife reports worsening impulsivity, mood swings, and episodes of aggressive behavior. He also has short-term memory loss and poor attention. He is a retired professional football player with many incidents of head trauma over his career. On exam, he has impaired recall, mild executive dysfunction, and impaired attention. MRI of the brain shows an enlarged cavum septum pellucidum, but otherwise appears unremarkable. Which of the following neuropathological findings is most characteristic of his suspected condition?

    A. Amyloid-beta plaques in the hippocampus
    B. Lewy bodies in the substantia nigra
    C. TDP-43 inclusions in the motor cortex
    D. Perivascular accumulation of phosphorylated tau at the depths of cortical sulci
    E. Pick bodies in the frontal cortex

Correct answer: D

Explanation

This patient likely has chronic traumatic encephalopathy from repeated concussive and sub-concussive head injuries during his football career. Patients can present initially with mainly cognitive issues or behavioral and mood changes. There is often a history of chronic headache as well. Most patients have progressive decline, such as in other neurodegenerative conditions. MRI is often normal early on, but can show cortical atrophy in the frontal and medial temporal lobes, enlarged third and lateral ventricles, enlarged cavum septum pellucidum, and mammillary body atrophy. The pathognomonic pathological finding in chronic traumatic encephalopathy is the accumulation of phosphorylated tau in neurons and glial cells around small vessels at the depths of cortical sulci.

Amyloid-beta plaques in the hippocampus are most characteristic of Alzheimer's disease. Lewy bodies in the substantia nigra are consistent with Parkinson's disease or dementia with Lewy bodies. TDP-43 inclusions can be seen in amyotrophic lateral sclerosis or a subset of frontotemporal lobar degeneration. Pick bodies are found in the tau subtype of frontotemporal lobar degeneration.

References

Alosco ML, Culhane J, Mez J. Neuroimaging biomarkers of chronic traumatic encephalopathy: targets for the academic memory disorders clinic. Neurotherapeutics. 2021;18(2):772–91. https://doi.org/10.1007/s13311-021-01028-3

McKee AC, Stein TD, Huber BR, Crary JF, Bieniek K, Dickson D, et al. Chronic traumatic encephalopathy (CTE): criteria for neuropathological diagnosis and relationship to repetitive head impacts. Acta Neuropathol. 2023;145(4):371 94. https://doi.org/10.1007/s00401-023-02540-w

Sparks P, Lawrence T, Hinze S. Neuroimaging in the diagnosis of chronic traumatic encephalopathy: a systematic review. Clin J Sport Med. 2020;30 Suppl 1:S1-S10. https://doi.org/10.1097/JSM.0000000000000541

Stern RA, Daneshvar DH, Baugh CM, Seichepine DR, Montenigro PH, Riley DO, et al. Clinical presentation of chronic traumatic encephalopathy. Neurology. 2013;81(13):1122–9. https://doi.org/10.1212/WNL.0b013e3182a55f7f

Linked questions: 28–29

28. A 32-year-old man presents with a 5-year history of progressive gait difficulties, leg stiffness, and urinary difficulty. He also reports darkening patches on the skin. His medical history is significant for multiple hospital admissions throughout his childhood and teenage years for hypotension and hypoglycemia in the setting of respiratory illnesses. There are multiple family members, especially biologically male relatives, with gait impairment and neuropathy. On exam, he has spastic paraparesis, increased deep tendon reflexes in the lower

extremities, and impaired vibratory sensation in the feet. There is also skin hyperpigmentation. MRI of the thoracic spine is shown below. Which of the following is the most likely diagnosis?

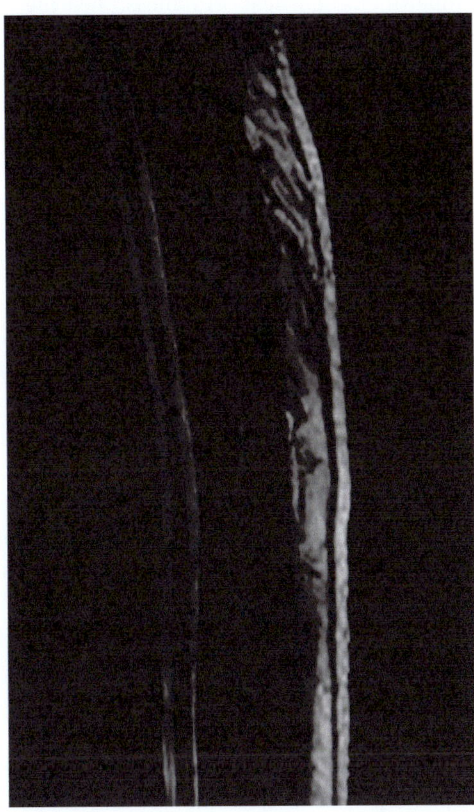

Sagittal MRI spine. (Source: Li, J., Wang, H., He, Z., Wang, X., Tang, J., Huang, D. CC-BY 4.0 (https://creativecommons.org/licenses/by/4.0/) via *BMC Neurology*. Image cropped from original. Please see full attribution with citation below in references section for this question.)

A. Hereditary spastic paraparesis
B. Adrenomyeloneuropathy
C. Primary lateral sclerosis
D. Subacute combined degeneration
E. Tropical spastic paraparesis

Correct answer: B

Explanation

This patient has developed gait difficulties and urinary dysfunction in young adulthood, along with a family history of abnormal gait and neuropathy. He also has a history concerning for adrenal insufficiency, resulting in episodes of hypoglycemia and hypotension, particularly in the setting of an acute infection. Additionally, he has skin hyperpigmentation. His MRI shows atrophy of the thoracic cord. This presentation is highly suspicious for adrenomyeloneuropathy, which is typically an X-linked inherited condition that presents in the third to fifth decades of life. There is a related condition, adrenoleukodystrophy, which presents during childhood, with cognitive impairment, cortical blindness, hearing loss, and seizures.

The other conditions listed here can also present with progressive spasticity, lower extremity weakness, and hyperreflexia, but would not be accompanied by signs of adrenal insufficiency. Sensory loss would not be expected in primary lateral sclerosis, as it is a condition that affects the motor neurons only. Human T-cell lymphotropic virus type 1 (HTLV-1), which can cause tropical spastic paraparesis, has a predilection for white matter of the thoracic spinal cord. It is endemic to different regions including Central and South America, the Caribbean, southern Japan, and Africa. Hereditary spastic paraparesis is a heterogeneous group of disorders and is mainly inherited in an autosomal dominant fashion, but can also have autosomal recessive or X-linked inheritance. It can present in childhood or adulthood. The spectrum of presentation is varied, with an uncomplicated form consisting of spastic paraparesis, urinary dysfunction, and dorsal column dysfunction. Complex forms of hereditary spastic paraparesis may present with seizures, cognitive decline, and extrapyramidal symptoms.

References

Gessain A, Ramassamy JL, Afonso PV, Cassar O. Geographic distribution, clinical epidemiology and genetic diversity of the human oncogenic retrovirus HTLV-1 in Africa, the world's largest endemic area. Front Immunol. 2023;14:1043600. https://doi.org/10.3389/fimmu.2023.1043600

Li J, Wang H, He Z, Wang X, Tang J, Huang D. Clinical, neuroimaging, biochemical, and genetic features in six Chinese patients with adrenomyeloneuropathy. BMC Neurol. 2019;19(1):227. https://doi.org/10.1186/s12883-019-1449-5

Piña-Garza JE, James KC. Paraplegia and quadriplegia. In: Piña-Garza JE, James KC, editors. Fenichel's clinical pediatric neurology: a signs and symptoms approach. 9th ed. Elsevier, Inc.;2025. p. 539–69

Ropper AH, Samuels MA, Klein JP, Prasad S. Inherited metabolic diseases of the nervous system. In: Ropper AH, Samuels MA, Klein JP, Prasad S, editors. Adams and Victor's Principles of Neurology. 12th ed. McGraw-Hill Education; 2023.

Ropper AH, Samuels MA, Klein JP, Prasad S. Diseases of the spinal cord. In: Ropper AH, Samuels MA, Klein JP, Prasad S, editors. Adams and Victor's Principles of Neurology. 12th ed. McGraw-Hill Education; 2023.

Verdonck K, González E, Van Dooren S, Vandamme AM, Vanham G, Gotuzzo E. Human T-lymphotropic virus 1: recent knowledge about an ancient infection. Lancet Infect Dis. 2007;7(4):266–81. https://doi.org/10.1016/S1473-3099(07)70081-6

Linked question

29. Additional work-up for the patient in the prior question is pursued. Which of the following is an INCORRECT statement?
    A. Levels of very long chain fatty acids are elevated
    B. Genetic mutation will be found on the ABCD1 gene
    C. There is a deficiency in arylsulfatase A
    D. Levels of cortisol and adrenocorticotropic hormone will be consistent with adrenal insufficiency
    E. Electrodiagnostic studies will show polyneuropathy

Correct answer: C

Explanation

Adrenomyeloneuropathy and its related condition, adrenoleukodystrophy, are due to impaired peroxisomal oxidation of very long chain fatty acids, leading to their accumulation in the brain and adrenal glands. Serum levels of very long chain fatty acids will be elevated when checked. The mutation occurs in the gene that codes the peroxisomal membrane transporter ABCD1. Given this patient's history with episodes of hypoglycemia, hypotension, and skin hyperpigmentation, levels of cortisol and adrenocorticotropic hormone should be checked, which would likely be consistent with adrenal insufficiency. Electrodiagnostic studies performed will likely show evidence of sensorimotor polyneuropathy, particularly in the lower extremities.

Arylsulfatase A deficiency is found in metachromatic leukodystrophy.

References

Chaudhry V, Moser HW, Cornblath DR. Nerve conduction studies in adrenomyeloneuropathy. J Neurol Neurosurg Psychiatry. 1996;61(2):181–5. https://doi.org/10.1136/jnnp.61.2.181

Ropper AH, Samuels MA, Klein JP, Prasad S. Inherited metabolic diseases of the nervous system. In: Ropper AH, Samuels MA, Klein JP, Prasad S, editors. Adams and Victor's Principles of Neurology. 12th ed. McGraw-Hill Education; 2023.

van Geel BM, Koelman JH, Barth PG, Ongerboer de Visser BW. Peripheral nerve abnormalities in adrenomyeloneuropathy: a clinical and electrodiagnostic study. Neurology. 1996;46(1):112–8. https://doi.org/10.1212/wnl.46.1.112

30. A 45-year-old woman without any significant medical history presents with progressively worsening headaches for 2 weeks. Her headaches noticeably improve upon lying down and worsen after standing up. She denies any recent head trauma or infectious symptoms. On neurologic exam, she is awake, alert, and without any focal findings. A brain MRI obtained shows bilateral subdural hematomas, each about 5 millimeters in width, without any midline shift. There is also diffuse, smooth pachymeningeal enhancement and low-lying cerebellar tonsils. Which of the following is the most appropriate next step in management?
    A. Bilateral craniotomy for subdural evacuation
    B. Bilateral burr holes and placement of subdural drains
    C. Angiography of the brain
    D. Angiography of the spine
    E. MRI of the spine

Correct answer: E

Explanation

An orthostatic headache is highly suspicious for intracranial hypotension. The MRI findings of symmetric bilateral subdural hematomas without any history of trauma, diffusely smooth pachymeningeal enhancement, and low-lying cerebellar tonsils are consistent with intracranial hypotension. Other possible findings on MRI include venous engorgement and pituitary enlargement. The most common cause of spontaneous intracranial hypotension is a cerebrospinal fluid (CSF) leak from a spinal dural tear, typically from a disc herniation or spinal osteophytes. This is known as a type 1 CSF leak. A type 2 CSF leak is due to a meningeal diverticulum. A type 3 CSF leak is due to a CSF-venous fistula, causing CSF to leak into the venous system. The most appropriate next step here is to image the spine to look for an epidural CSF collection that would be consistent with a type 1 CSF leak. This can be done with an MRI, or a CT myelogram, of the spine. In type 2 and 3 CSF leaks, specialized dynamic myelograms can be performed to detect the location of the diverticulum or CSF-venous fistula. Once a CSF leak has been confirmed, initial management consists of conservative measures, such as bed rest and increased intake of fluids and caffeine, as well as an epidural blood patch. More severe cases may require surgical repair of the dura, and CSF-venous fistulas can be treated endovascularly or surgically.

Surgical evacuation of the subdural hematomas is not indicated here given the small size and the lack of attributable symptoms, and recurrence of the subdural hematomas is likely without first treating the cause of the intracranial hypotension.

References

Dobrocky T, Nicholson P, Häni L, Mordasini P, Krings T, Brinjikji W, et al. Spontaneous intracranial hypotension: searching for the CSF leak. Lancet Neurol. 2022;21(4):369–80. https://doi.org/10.1016/S1474-4422(21)00423-3

Schievink WI. Spontaneous intracranial hypotension. N Engl J Med. 2021;385(23):2173–78. https://doi.org/10.1056/NEJMra2101561

Neuro-ophthalmology

Scott Grossman

Linked questions: 1–2

1. A 60-year-old woman presents for clinical complaint of imbalance, dizziness, and a sense of oscillation in her visual world which worsens in extremes of horizontal gaze (oscillopsia). On examination, she has downbeat nystagmus which is worse when looking to the sides. Saccades are normal in speed and her fundus exam is normal. Structural MRI is unrevealing. Genetic testing should be sent in this case to rule out what condition?
   A. SCA2
   B. SCA3
   C. SCA7
   D. SCA8
   E. SCA27b
   Correct answer: E

Explanation
SCA27B results from a GAA repeat expansion in the FGF14 gene and was first identified in 2023. This appears to be an important cause of late-onset spinocerebellar ataxias that were previously characterized as idiopathic. Median age of onset has been 55 years, and the clinical phenotype has been predominantly downbeat nystagmus with some patients having a phenotype that overlaps with cerebellar ataxia, neuropathy, and vestibular areflexia syndrome (CANVAS).

Reference
Pellerin D, Danzi MC, Wilke C, Renaud M, Fazal S, Dicaire MJ, et al. Deep Intronic FGF14 GAA Repeat Expansion in Late-Onset Cerebellar Ataxia. N Engl J Med. 2023; 388(2):128–41. https://doi.org/10.1056/NEJMoa2207406.

Linked question

2. For this same 60-year-old patient, the best medication to aide in symptomatic treatment has what mechanism of action?
   A. Potassium channel blockade
   B. Sodium channel blockade
   C. Reduced uptake of acetylcholine from the neuromuscular junction
   D. Anti-NMDA receptor antagonist
   E. Anti-GABA activity
   Correct answer: A

Explanation
Dalfampridine (4-aminopyridine) is a potassium channel blocker that has been shown to reduce clinical effect of downbeat nystagmus and improve the velocity of the slow phase of the nystagmus. This medication has also been approved for use to improve walking speed in MS.

Reference
Wilke C, Pellerin D, Mengel D, Traschütz A, Danzi MC, Dicaire MJ, et al. GAA-FGF14 ataxia (SCA27B): phenotypic profile, natural history progression and 4-aminopyridine treatment response. Brain. 2023;146(10): 4144–57. https://doi.org/10.1093/brain/awad157.

Linked questions: 3–4

3. A 32-year-old man with a history of multiple sclerosis (MS) with recurrent episodes of optic neuritis presents with worsening visual acuity. His MRI shows no actively

S. Grossman (✉)
Departments of Neurology and Ophthalmology, New York University Grossman School of Medicine, New York, NY, USA
e-mail: scott.grossman@nyulangone.org

demyelinating lesions, but his visual acuity is 20/100 on the right eye and 20/80 on the left. His exam is notable for constant slow phase ellipsoid eye movements with predominant horizontal directionality. What is his most likely nystagmus pattern?

A. Acquired pendular nystagmus
B. Gaze-evoked nystagmus
C. Opsoclonus
D. Ocular flutter
E. Rebound nystagmus

Correct answer: A

Explanation

Acquired pendular nystagmus (APN) is most frequently present in patients with MS with up to 4% of MS patients showing APN. APN can manifest with either binocular or monocular involvement. The pathophysiology is unclear but may reflect brain stem disease and correlate with optic nerve function, most likely reflecting abnormal brain stem feedback circuits for eye position.

Reference

Tilikete C, Jasse L, Pelisson D, Vukusic S, Durand-Dubief F, Urquizar C, et al. Acquired pendular nystagmus in multiple sclerosis and oculopalatal tremor. Neurology. 2011;76(19):1650–7. https://doi.org/10.1212/WNL.0b013e318219fa9c

Linked question

4. Of the following choices, which medication is most likely to improve the visual acuity of the patient in the prior question?
A. Levetiracetam
B. Valproic acid
C. Gabapentin
D. Zonisamide
E. Dalfampridine

Correct answer: C

Explanation

Gabapentin (along with memantine) is the medication of choice to improve visual acuity and oscillopsia from acquired pendular nystagmus (APN). Dalfampridine is indicated for downbeat nystagmus, whereas other medications listed have more limited utility in the treatment of nystagmus.

Reference

Averbuch-Heller L, Tusa RJ, Fuhry L, Rottach KG, Ganser GL, Heide W, et al. A double-blind controlled study of gabapentin and baclofen as treatment for acquired nystagmus. Ann Neurol. 1997;41(6):818–25. https://doi.org/10.1002/ana.410410620

Linked questions: 5–6

5. A 45-year-old man has a 4-year history of headaches and the following visual field.

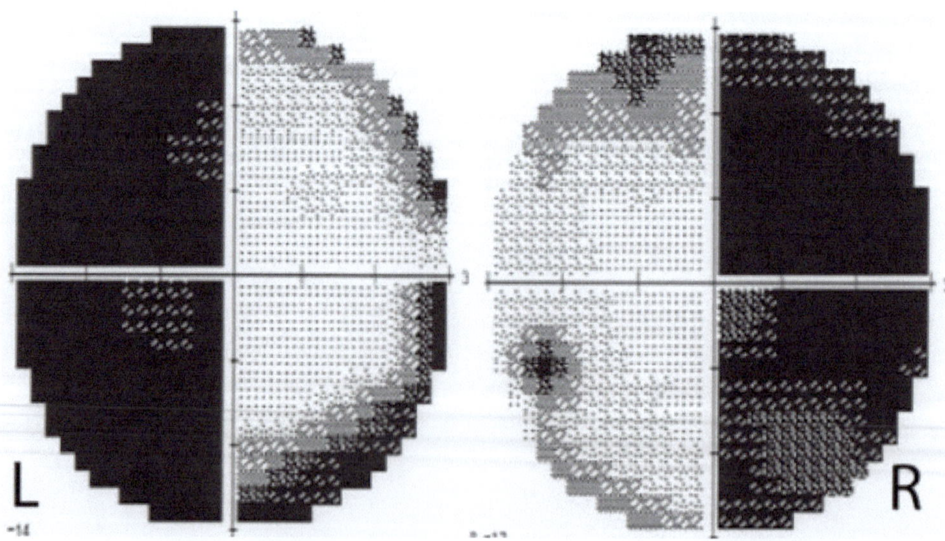

Visual fields. (Image source: Dhandapani, S., Negm, H. M., Cohen, S., Anand, V. K., Schwartz, T. H. CC-BY 3.0 (https://creativecommons.org/licenses/by/3.0/) via *Cureus*. Image has not been modified from source. Please see full attribution with citation below in references section for this question.)

He is brought to the emergency department by his husband with a thunderclap headache and new complaint of double vision. Ocular motility exam is notable for deficits in adduction, elevation, and depression of the left eye, and the eyelid is droopy. What medication class is essential to initiate in this setting?

A. Growth hormone
B. Corticosteroids
C. Antihypertensives
D. Anti-seizure medication
E. Analgesics

Correct answer: B

Explanation

Pituitary apoplexy is a life-threating emergency in which the blood supply of the pituitary adenoma is outstripped by growth of the tumor. Infarct of the tumor can lead to hemorrhage and can be associated with thunderclap headache and ophthalmoplegia as well as change in mental status. Adrenal crisis in this setting is an emergency, and corticosteroids should be initiated early.

References

Almutairi MM, Thamer GM, Alharthi KF, Ali HJ, Ahmed AE. Pituitary Apoplexy: A Rare but Critical Emergency in Neuroendocrinology. Cureus. 2025;17(1):e77970. https://doi.org/10.7759/cureus.77970

Dhandapani S, Negm IIM, Cohen S, Anand VK, Schwartz TH. Endonasal Endoscopic Transsphenoidal Resection of Tuberculum Sella Meningioma with Anterior Cerebral Artery Encasement. Cureus. 2015;7(8):e311. https://doi.org/10.7759/cureus.311

Linked question

6. In the same patient from the prior question, what structure accounts for his ocular motility defects?
   A. Nuclear third nerve palsy
   B. Fascicular third nerve palsy
   C. Third nerve palsy in the cavernous sinus
   D. Sixth nerve palsy in the cavernous sinus
   E. Superior divisional third nerve palsy

   Correct answer: C

Explanation

Apoplexy can result in ophthalmoplegia in several ways, but one common scenario is rupture of sellar tissue into the cavernous sinus; specifically, this can result in local injury to the third cranial nerve as it courses superiorly within the cavernous sinus. The sixth cranial nerve is free floating in the center of the cavernous sinus, making it more vulnerable in instances of gradual increased pressure such as cavernous sinus lymphoma.

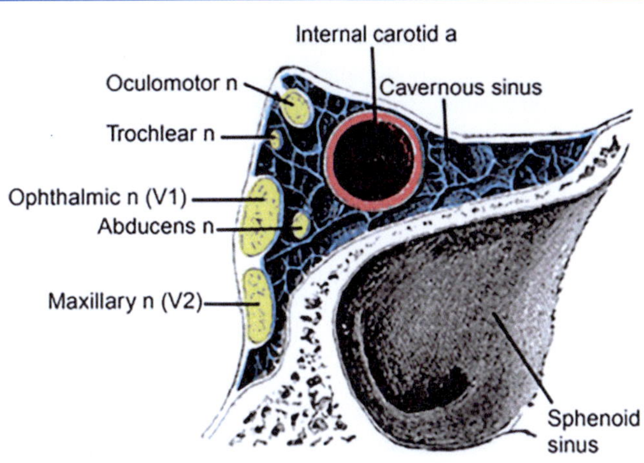

Cavernous sinus anatomy. Reprinted from: Encyclopedia of the Eye, Second edition, Baker, M. J., Lee, M. S., Orbital Vascular Anatomy, 510–521, 2025, with permission from Elsevier. Originally adapted from Gray's Anatomy, 20th edition, copyright expired

Reference

Capatina C, Inder W, Karavitaki N, Wass JA. Management of endocrine disease: pituitary tumour apoplexy. Eur J Endocrinol. 2015 May;172(5):R179–90. https://doi.org/10.1530/EJE-14-0794. Epub 2014 Dec 1. PMID: 25452466.

Encyclopedia of the Eye, Second edition, Baker, M. J., Lee, M. S., Orbital Vascular Anatomy, 510–521, 2025, with permission from Elsevier. Originally adapted from Gray's Anatomy, 20th edition, copyright expired.

7. A 26-year-old man with no medical history gets into a high-speed car crash, and you are called to evaluate him in the hospital for headache and progressive right eye chemosis, proptosis, and double vision which is present only when both eyes are open. His exam is notable for proptotic appearance of the right eye and complete ophthalmoplegia of the right eye. What is his most likely diagnosis?
   A. Cavernous sinus thrombosis
   B. Subdural hemorrhage
   C. Traumatic cranial neuropathy from shearing effect
   D. Subarachnoid hemorrhage
   E. Carotid-cavernous fistula

   Correct answer: E

Explanation

High-flow carotid-cavernous fistulae (CCF) result from a direct connection between the cavernous segment of the carotid artery and the cavernous sinus. Typically, they are traumatic in origin and tend to present with progressive proptosis, chemosis, and ophthalmoplegia. Complete ophthalmoplegia results in manual injury to the CN III, CN IV, and CN V in the cavernous sinus. Low-flow CCFs refer to dural fistulae leading to indirect communication between the carotid and the cavernous sinus and are less classically associated with trauma.

Reference

de Keizer R. Carotid-cavernous and orbital arteriovenous fistulas: ocular features, diagnostic and hemodynamic considerations in relation to visual impairment and morbidity. Orbit. 2003;22(2):121–42. https://doi.org/10.1076/orbi.22.2.121.14315

8. A 12-year-old boy presents to the emergency room with bilateral blurry vision and headaches, as well as an event concerning for first generalized tonic-clonic convulsion of life. He undergoes lumbar puncture which shows low-grade pleocytosis and elevated opening pressure to 30-cm H2O. His MRI shows bilateral optic perineuritis that extends along the majority of the optic nerve. What is the most likely diagnosis?
   A. Multiple sclerosis (MS)
   B. Pediatric idiopathic intracranial hypertension (IIH)
   C. Myelin oligodendrocyte glycoprotein antibody-associated disease (MOGAD)
   D. Neuromyelitis optica spectrum disorder (NMOSD)
   E. Optic pathway glioma
   Correct answer: C

Explanation

MOGAD is an increasingly appreciated cause of bilateral optic neuritis in children. Typical imaging features include longitudinal bilateral optic perineuritis. Seizures can be a presenting feature given cortical involvement of intraparenchymal lesions. Increased intracranial pressure at time of initial presentation has also been described. Approximately 50% of MOGAD clinical courses will be monophasic, and 50% of MOGAD-associated optic neuritis will be bilateral, though much is still being discovered about this novel entity.

Reference

Jurynczyk M, Messina S, Woodhall MR, Raza N, Everett R, Roca-Fernandez A, et al. Clinical presentation and prognosis in MOG-antibody disease: a UK study. Brain. 2017;140(12):3128–38. https://doi.org/10.1093/brain/awx276

9. In optic neuritis, which of the following disorders is most likely to present with optic disc edema that may be appreciable by fundoscopy or optical coherence tomography (OCT)?
   A. MOGAD
   B. NMOSD
   C. Multiple sclerosis
   D. Idiopathic optic neuritis
   Correct answer: A

Explanation

Several clues about the clinical presentation and examination in optic neuritis favor one etiology over others. In MOGAD-associated optic neuritis, pain often precedes vision loss and may be reported as headache in children. The visual nadir is lower, and optic disc edema is found in up to 86% of MOGAD optic neuritis attacks. Disc edema in MOGAD may also be severe enough to cause associated hemorrhages in the peripapillary region.

Reference

Chen JJ, Flanagan EP, Jitprapaikulsan J, López-Chiriboga ASS, Fryer JP, Leavitt JA, et al. Myelin Oligodendrocyte Glycoprotein Antibody-Positive Optic Neuritis: Clinical Characteristics, Radiologic Clues, and Outcome. Am J Ophthalmol. 2018;195:8–15. https://doi.org/10.1016/j.ajo.2018.07.020

10. A 24-year-old man is stabbed with an ice pick in his temple while on the subway platform. His MRI of the orbit reveals complete transection of the optic nerve on the right eye, but his globe and anterior segment remain intact. What is the most likely appearance of his pupillary exam in ambient lighting conditions?
    A. Large pupil on the right eye, small pupil on the left eye
    B. Bilateral large pupil
    C. Bilateral small pupil
    D. Bilateral midrange pupil consistent with physiologic pupil size
    E. Large pupil on the left eye and small pupil on the right eye
    Correct answer: D

Explanation

Complete transection of the optic nerve should lead to a number of abnormalities on the pupillary exam, but in ambient lighting conditions at rest, the pupil size should remain symmetric and physiologic. Pupillary constriction is mediated via the parasympathetic nerve fibers of the third cranial nerve, while pupillary dilation is mediated via the sympathetic pathway that originates in the hypothalamus and consists of three neurons. Neither should be affected in pure transection of the optic nerve.

Reference

Digre KB. Principles and techniques of examination of the pupils, accommodation and lacrimation. In: Walsh and Hoyt Clinical Neuro-ophthalmology, 6th ed, Miller NR, Newman NJ, Biousse V, Kerrison JB (Eds), Williams & Wilkins, Baltimore 2005. p.715.

Linked questions: 11–12

11. A 22-year-old woman develops right-sided neck pain after a yoga class. She looks in the mirror the following morning, feels her pupils are asymmetric, and then comes into the office to be evaluated. She is found to have anisocoria greater in the dark with the smaller pupil on the right, as well as 1–2 mm of ptosis on the right eye. She is otherwise neurologically non-focal. Where is her lesion?
    A. Vertebral artery on the right
    B. Vertebral artery on the left
    C. Internal carotid artery on the right
    D. Internal carotid artery on the left
    E. Posterior communicating artery on the right
    Correct answer: C

Explanation

This is a Horner's syndrome with pupillary asymmetry (anisocoria) that is greater in the dark due to a failure of the miotic pupil to relax, due to injury of the sympathetic chain as it courses along the internal carotid on the right. This is a stretch injury. Posterior communicating artery aneurysm would lead to a third nerve palsy; vertebral artery injury or lesion may lead to Wallenberg syndrome which can include a Horner syndrome but would also involve other findings on physical exam.

Reference

Kardon, R. Anatomy and physiology of the autonomic nervous system. In: Walsh and Hoyt Clinical Neuro-ophthalmology, 6th ed, Miller, NR, Newman, NJ, Biousse, V, Kerrison, JB (Eds), Williams & Wilkins, Baltimore 2005. p.649.

Linked question

12. At this time, what would be the most appropriate initial test as part of the workup for the patient in the prior question?
    A. Cocaine drop testing
    B. Apraclonidine drop testing
    C. MR angiogram of the neck
    D. Non-contrast head CT
    E. Dilute pilocarpine drop testing
    Correct answer: C

Explanation

This patient needs urgent angiographic imaging to evaluate for carotid artery dissection. Apraclonidine drop testing may be helpful but may not be as useful in the acute setting before denervation supersensitivity develops. Cocaine testing is rarely done clinically in the modern era. Non-contrast head CT would not be as high yield here as angiographic imaging to rule out a life-threatening emergency.

Reference

Morales J, Brown SM, Abdul-Rahim AS, Crosson CE. Ocular effects of apraclonidine in Horner syndrome. Arch Ophthalmol. 2000;118(7):951–4.

13. A 40-year-old woman is evaluated in clinic for incidentally discovered anisocoria. Her right pupil is 5 mm in the dark and 2 mm in the light with a brisk reaction to light and to near convergence. Her left pupil is 4 mm and fixed to light, though it goes to 2.5 mm to accommodation at near. When evaluated under a slit lamp examination, she is found to have sectoral paralysis of the pupillary sphincter. What is the location of the lesion causing her injury?
    A. Third cranial nerve
    B. Sympathetic chain in the lung apex
    C. Dorsal midbrain
    D. Optic nerve
    E. Parasympathetic ciliary ganglion
    Correct answer: E

Explanation

Adie's tonic pupil is a pupil with parasympathetic denervation that constricts poorly to light but is more reactive to accommodation at near and classically stays tonically constricted before redilating slowly when exposed to dark lighting environment (the "tonic" in tonic pupil). Reviewing old photographs can be helpful in the diagnostic process.

Reference

Thompson HS. Adie's syndrome: some new observations. Trans Am Ophthalmol Soc. 1977;75:587–626.

14. A 52-year-old woman develops galactorrhea. She has had headaches for several years that are different than her baseline migraine and undergoes brain MRI with and without gadolinium that shows a sellar mass compressing the optic chiasm. Of these, what is her most likely visual field pattern?
    A. Bi-superonasal quadrantanopsia
    B. Bi-superotemporal quadrantanopsia
    C. Bi inferonasal quadrantanopsia
    D. Bi-inferotemporal quadrantanopsia
    E. Bilateral enlarged blind spot
    Correct answer: B

Explanation

In the setting of sellar mass and galactorrhea, the most likely diagnosis is pituitary adenoma. The anatomy of the optic chiasm and pituitary/stalk is such that the pituitary sits below the chiasm. Therefore, the most likely early visual field defect before bitemporal hemianopsia seen in advanced cases is more likely to be bi-superotemporal defects because the inferior aspect of the chiasm is compressed and elevated early.

Reference

Molitch ME. Nonfunctioning pituitary tumors and pituitary incidentalomas. Endocrinol Metab Clin North Am. 2008;37(1):151–71, xi. https://doi.org/10.1016/j.ecl.2007.10.011

15. A 67-year-old diabetic man develops double vision that is vertical and binocular. He is diagnosed with an ischemic cranial neuropathy of his right fourth cranial nerve. In which context will his double vision be improved?
    A. Left head tilt
    B. Left gaze
    C. Down gaze
    D. Right head tilt
    E. Chin-up head position
    Correct answer: A

Explanation

The fourth cranial nerve mainly incyclotorts and depresses the eye and has some abducting action. Development of acute ocular motor nerve palsy from ischemia in the setting of diabetes is common and can involve the third, fourth, or sixth cranial nerves. The action of the fourth would lead this patient's double vision to be worse in attempted left gaze, down gaze, and right head tilt. He may develop a left head tilt to compensate for his relatively excyclotorted right eye, therefore bringing his fully functioning left eye into an incyclotorted position to meet the excyclotorted right eye. He may also develop a chin tuck position to resolve vertical double by maintaining relative upgaze.

Reference

Kline LB, Demer JL, Vaphiades MS, Tavakoli M. Disorders of the Fourth Cranial Nerve. J Neuroophthalmol. 2021;41(2):176–93. https://doi.org/10.1097/wno.0000000000001261

16. On MRI of the brain, a 28-year-old woman with new headache is found to have a sphenoid wing meningioma with compression of the area where the right optic nerve and optic chiasm meet. What is her most likely pattern of visual field loss on formal testing?
    A. Left eye central scotoma and right eye superior temporal defect
    B. Right eye central scotoma and left eye superior temporal defect

C. Bitemporal depressions
D. Binasal depressions
E. Bilateral central scotoma
Correct answer: B

Explanation

"Junctional scotoma" is a visual field pattern that results from a focal lesion to the area where the optic nerve meets the chiasm and is frequently referable to sellar lesions including pituitary adenomas, as well as craniopharyngiomas and sphenoid wing meningiomas. At the point of compression, the ipsilateral optic nerve is compressed leading to a central scotoma in that eye, while the contralateral crossing inferior nasal retinal fibers are also affected, accounting for the contralateral superotemporal depression. Formal visual field testing is typically required to diagnose a junctional scotoma.

Reference

Foroozan R. Chiasmal syndromes. Curr Opin Ophthalmol. 2003;14(6):325–31. https://doi.org/10.1097/00055735-200312000-00002

Linked questions: 17–20

17. A 24-year-old woman has put on 50 pounds over the past year and over the past several months have developed a sense of blurry vision as well as pulsatile tinnitus. She also has horizontal binocular diplopia that is worse at distance and headaches that are worse in the morning and have woken her from sleep, as well as transient daily episodes of greying out of her vision that are brought on by the Valsalva maneuver. Which of these clinical complaints are most ominous for her long-term visual outcome?
    A. Pulsatile tinnitus
    B. Double vision
    C. Headaches
    D. Transient visual obscurations (greying out of vision)
    E. Blurry vision
    Correct answer: D

Explanation

In idiopathic intracranial hypertension (IIH), the CSF pressure is elevated with normal constituents and without other alternative identifiable cause. There is some heterogeneity in the clinical presentation of IIH but the IIH Study Group defined several features that predict treatment failure, including male sex, high-grade papilledema, and decreased visual acuity at baseline. Transient greying out of vision (transient visual obscurations) are one symptom that portends poor visual outcome.

Reference

Wall M, Falardeau J, Fletcher WA, Granadier RJ, Lam BL, Longmuir RA, et al. Risk factors for poor visual outcome in patients with idiopathic intracranial hypertension. Neurology. 2015;85(9):799–805. https://doi.org/10.1212/wnl.0000000000001896

Linked question

18. In this same patient from the prior question, lumbar puncture is performed and demonstrates opening pressure of 32-cm H2O, though her visual field is full and she is deemed not at risk for rapid loss of vision over the next 4 weeks ("fulminant IIH.") What is the most important approach to treatment for long-term remission of the disease?
    A. Early treatment with acetazolamide
    B. Stenting of the transverse sinuses
    C. Optic nerve sheath fenestration
    D. Weight loss of goal 10–15% of body weight at time of diagnosis
    E. CSF shunting procedure
    Correct answer: D

Explanation

In the absence of "fulminant IIH," defined as likely incipient vision loss within the following 4 weeks, the most appropriate approach for patients with newly diagnosed IIH is weight loss with an ultimate goal of 10–15% of body weight from time of diagnosis. The IIH randomized controlled weight trial (IIH:WT) established that weight loss with bariatric surgery significantly reduced intracranial pressure compared with a conventional weight management program. In general, the greater the weight loss, the more the team found a reduction in intracranial pressure. The amount of weight loss needed for remission is not entirely known, though one study noted 5–15% body weight gain in the year preceding diagnosis of IIH and up to 15% of body weight loss required to put IIH into remission.

Reference

Mollan SP, Mitchell JL, Yiangou A, Ottridge RS, Alimajstorovic Z, Cartwright DM, et al. Association of Amount of Weight Lost After Bariatric Surgery With Intracranial Pressure in Women With Idiopathic Intracranial Hypertension. Neurology. 2022;99(11):e1090–e9. https://doi.org/10.1212/wnl.0000000000200839

Linked question

19. In this same patient from the prior question, which of the following medications would *not* be concerning as part of the patient's history for iatrogenic increase in intracranial pressure?

A. Isotretinoin
B. Doxycycline
C. Levonorgestrel implant
D. Minocycline
E. Furosemide
Correct answer: E

Explanation

Each of these medications has been found to have an association with iatrogenic increase in intracranial pressure other than furosemide. Furosemide, a diuretic, has anecdotal support as a third-line agent in the management of IIH and can serve as an adjunctive treatment to first-line agents like acetazolamide.

Reference

Mollan SP, Davies B, Silver NC, Shaw S, Mallucci CL, Wakerley BR, et al. Idiopathic intracranial hypertension: consensus guidelines on management. J Neurol Neurosurg Psychiatry. 2018;89(10):1088–100. https://doi.org/10.1136/jnnp-2017-317440

Linked question

20. If this prior patient were instead 8 years old and presented with similar symptoms, which of the following statements would apply?
    A. The pressure required to make a diagnosis of pediatric IIH is lower than in adults.
    B. The pressure required to make a diagnosis of pediatric IIH is higher than in adults.
    C. The pressure required to make a diagnosis of pediatric IIH is the same as in adults.
    D. There is no such diagnosis as pediatric IIH.
    Correct answer: B

Explanation

Pediatric IIH is a rare entity, but diagnostic criteria have recently been promulgated that include a CSF opening pressure of greater than or equal to 28 centimeters of water. This is higher than the reference range for adults which is 25 centimeters of water. A 2-year single-center retrospective study from 2010 established for the first time that on a reference population basis of otherwise healthy children the 90th percentile of CSF opening pressure was found to be 28 centimeters of water.

Citation

Avery RA, Shah SS, Licht DJ, Seiden JA, Huh JW, Boswinkel J, et al. Reference range for cerebrospinal fluid opening pressure in children. N Engl J Med. 2010;363(9):891–3. https://doi.org/10.1056/NEJMc1004957

Friedman DI, Liu GT, Digre KB. Revised diagnostic criteria for the pseudotumor cerebri syndrome in adults and children. Neurology. 2013;81(13):1159–65. https://doi.org/10.1212/WNL.0b013e3182a55f17

21. A 68-year-old woman with a history of lupus develops double vision. Her eyes are found to be proptotic, and she is ultimately diagnosed with Graves' disease. On MRI of the orbits, what part of the orbital anatomy is most likely to show abnormalities?
    A. Muscle belly
    B. Muscle tendon
    C. Annulus of Zinn
    D. Sclera
    Correct answer: A

Explanation

Enlargement of extraocular muscle bodies and expansion of fatty connective tissues are radiographically evident in patients with Graves' ophthalmopathy. Graves' disease is common with annual incidence of approximately 1 in 1000. Expanded orbital tissues push the globe forward causing ocular misalignment and binocular diplopia. Extraocular muscle cells are intact in early active disease, and muscle bodies are primarily expanded in thyroid eye disease (TED) due to the accumulation of hydrophilic glycosaminoglycans and edema.

Reference

Garrity JA, Bahn RS. Pathogenesis of graves ophthalmopathy: implications for prediction, prevention, and treatment. Am J Ophthalmol. 2006;142(1):147–53. https://doi.org/10.1016/j.ajo.2006.02.047

22. Which extraocular muscle is *least* likely to show hypertrophy in thyroid eye disease (TED)?
    A. Inferior rectus
    B. Medial rectus
    C. Superior rectus
    D. Lateral rectus
    Correct answer: D

Explanation

Extraocular muscles in thyroid eye disease (TED) are involved in a predictable manner and can lend support to diagnosis in the setting of imaging abnormalities of the orbit. One study reviewed 54 patients (108 orbits) and found that motility restriction was greatest in the direction of the inferior and medial rectus. The lateral rectus is typically least involved in the progression of TED; therefore, the most likely answer is D.

Reference

Dagi LR, Zoumalan CI, Konrad H, Trokel SL, Kazim M. Correlation between extraocular muscle size and motility restriction in thyroid eye disease. Ophthalmic Plast Reconstr Surg. 2011;27(2):102–10. https://doi.org/10.1097/IOP.0b013e3181e9a063

Linked questions: 23–24

23. A 25-year-old woman presents to the emergency department with 2 days of blurry vision, supraorbital pain, and pain with eye movements of the left eye. She is found to have an afferent pupillary defect and red desaturation on color testing. She is diagnosed with idiopathic optic neuritis and is given a course of IV methylprednisolone. What is the way that this intervention is most likely to affect her vision?
    A. She will have improved structural integrity of the optic nerve in the long run on structural measures using OCT of the retinal nerve fiber layer.
    B. She will have improved acuity in the long run.
    C. She will have the same visual recovery but will get there faster.
    D. Her vision will be worse in the short term but equal in the long term.
    E. It will improve her pain but will not affect her vision.
    Correct answer: C

Explanation

The Optic Neuritis Treatment Trial (ONTT) enrolled 457 patients between July 1988 and June 1991 and randomized patients to either intravenous methylprednisolone followed by oral prednisone, oral prednisone alone, and oral placebo. Visual field and contrast sensitivity were the primary measures of outcome, while visual acuity and color vision were secondary measures. Ultimately, this trial demonstrated that IV methylprednisolone hastened visual recovery relative to placebo but did not ultimately affect visual outcome.

Reference

Beck RW, Cleary PA, Anderson MM, Jr., Keltner JL, Shults WT, Kaufman DI, et al. A randomized, controlled trial of corticosteroids in the treatment of acute optic neuritis. The Optic Neuritis Study Group. N Engl J Med. 1992;326(9):581–8. https://doi.org/10.1056/nejm199202273260901

Linked question

24. If this same patient in the prior question is given oral steroids, what is the most likely adverse visual outcome compared to her getting intravenous steroids?
    A. Worse color saturation at 1 year compared to placebo
    B. Worse visual acuity at 1 year compared to placebo
    C. Increased risk of recurrent episodes of optic neuritis

D. Upper gastrointestinal bleed
E. Greater rate of development of multiple sclerosis
Correct answer: C

Explanation
In the ONTT, an important and newly reported adverse outcome for the group that received oral steroids was increased rate of recurrent episode of optic neuritis. This was true relative to both the placebo group and the intravenous methylprednisolone group. For this reason, oral steroids are not recommended as treatment for acute optic neuritis. There was no significant difference in the ultimate rate of development of multiple sclerosis or worsened visual outcome.

Reference
Beck RW, Cleary PA, Anderson MM, Jr., Keltner JL, Shults WT, Kaufman DI, et al. A randomized, controlled trial of corticosteroids in the treatment of acute optic neuritis. The Optic Neuritis Study Group. N Engl J Med. 1992;326(9):581–8.   https://doi.org/10.1056/nejm199202273260901

Linked questions: 25–27

25. A 19-year-old man develops severe bilateral sequential vision loss, first in his right eye and then in his left, which is painless and has only improved minimally after a course of intravenous methylprednisolone to the range of 20/400 in each eye. What is his most likely diagnosis?
    A. Optic neuritis
    B. Leber's hereditary optic neuropathy (LHON)
    C. Compressive optic neuropathy from glioblastoma multiforme
    D. Metabolic optic neuropathy from B12 deficiency
    E. MOGAD
    Correct answer: B

Explanation
Leber's hereditary optic neuropathy (LHON) is typically associated with a mitochondrial DNA (mtDNA) point mutation and is inherited maternally. LHON classically manifests clinically with bilateral sequential subacute optic neuropathy with severe acuity losses, most frequently in young men. It is the first human disease to be defined by a point mutation in mtDNA and leads to loss of retinal ganglion cells

Linked question

26. In this same patient from the prior question, if genetic testing is sent, what mutation is *least* likely present?
    A. 3460G>A in gene MT-ND1
    B. 11778G>A in the gene MT-ND4

C. 14484T>C in the gene MT-ND6
D. 14221A>G in the gene MT-ND5
Correct answer: D

Explanation
Three genetic variants account for around 90% of individuals with LHON, 3460G>A, 11778G>A, and 14484T>C. These are missense mutations that lead to defects in the electron transport chain. The specific pathogenesis of LHON remains incompletely understood. Favorable outcomes are associated with the 11778 mutation.

Reference
Brown MD, Sun F, Wallace DC. Clustering of Caucasian Leber hereditary optic neuropathy patients containing the 11778 or 14484 mutations on an mtDNA lineage. Am J Hum Genet. 1997;60(2):381–7.

Linked question

27. Recent clinical trials for LHON have demonstrated support for which of the following agents early in the disease course?
    A. Idebenone
    B. Magnesium
    C. Cyanocobalamin
    D. Riboflavin
    E. Folate
    Correct answer: A

Explanation
Three recent clinical studies, RHODOS, RHODOS-OFU, and LEROS, have suggested that idebenone should be started early in patients with LHON. Treatment benefit from a novel intraocular injectable agent, lenadogene nolparvovec, leads to a visual course that significantly differs from the published natural history of LHON and leads to improvement relative to the use of idebenone.

Reference
Chen BS, Newman NJ. Clinical trials in Leber hereditary optic neuropathy: outcomes and opportunities. Curr Opin Neurol.   2025;38(1):79–86.   https://doi.org/10.1097/wco.0000000000001343

Linked questions: 28–29

28. A 62-year-old man develops acute onset of vision loss on awakening, consisting of an inferior altitudinal defect of the left eye with blurry vision centrally that is painless. His fundoscopic exam reveals grade II disc edema of the left eye with associated hemorrhages, his right eye

vision is normal, but he has a reduced cup-to-disc ratio in that eye. What is his most likely diagnosis?
A. Optic neuritis
B. Central retinal artery occlusion (CRAO)
C. Central retinal vein occlusion (CRVO)
D. LHON
E. Non-arteritic ischemic optic neuropathy (NAION)
Correct answer: E

Explanation

Non-arteritic ischemic optic neuropathy (NAION) classically presents in late middle age with painless inferior altitudinal field loss and other markers of optic neuropathy. Important risk factors for NAION include a so-called disc at risk in the fellow eye of a decreased cup-to-disc ratio (<0.3), as well as metabolic risk factors and obstructive sleep apnea. CRAO and CRVO may also present with acute vision loss, but the exam would be different than in this case, whereas optic neuritis is typically painful and may not involve optic disc edema, and LHON is typically in younger individuals and involves bilateral sequential vision loss.

Reference

Patel JN, Miller NR. Non-arteritic anterior ischaemic optic neuropathy causes sudden-onset painless loss of vision. Lancet. 2024;404(10447):67. https://doi.org/10.1016/s0140-6736(24)01358-8

Linked question

29. What is the most important modifiable risk factor in the prior case?
A. Atrial fibrillation screening
B. Carotid stenosis screening
C. Intracranial hypertension screening
D. Cerebral vasculitis screening
E. Obstructive sleep apnea screening
Correct answer: E

Explanation

In NAION, the most important modifiable risk factors include elimination of exacerbating medications such as PDE-5 inhibitors as well as smoking cessation. However, obstructive sleep apnea (OSA) has been shown to have a strong association with NAION in several population studies, and referral for sleep study is indicated to screen for OSA in all individuals presenting with signs and symptoms consistent with NAION.

Reference

Miller NR. Current concepts in the diagnosis, pathogenesis, and management of non-arteritic anterior ischemic optic

neuropathy. J Neuroophthalmol. 2011;31(2):e1–3. https://doi.org/10.1097/WNO.0b013e31821f955c

Linked questions: 30–31

30. An 85-year-old woman presents with transient episodes of visual greying out in her left eye. On review of systems, she also notes pain in both temporal regions of her head, fatigue in her proximal arms, and recent episodes of night sweats. When she eats steak for dinner, she also notes jaw fatigue and must take breaks. What is the most important action to take immediately for visual protection in this patient?
A. Temporal artery biopsy
B. Treatment with infusion of tocilizumab
C. Start high-dose oral prednisone
D. Send inflammatory markers (ESR, CRP)
E. Lumbar puncture for opening pressure
Correct answer: C

Explanation

In giant cell arteritis (GCA), transient episodes of visual blacking or greying out portend imminent vision loss and must be treated as a neuro-ophthalmic emergency. In GCA, the temporal arteries become inflamed and narrowed, leading to transient and then permanent ischemic damage to the optic nerves which is irreversible once it occurs (arteritic ischemic optic neuropathy). There is a significant association with polymyalgia rheumatica (PMR), and this patient has several canonical symptoms including jaw claudication and temporal tenderness.

Reference

Liu GT. Visual loss: optic neuropathies. In: Neuro-Ophthalmology: Diagnosis and Management, Liu GT, Volpe NJ, Galetta SL (Eds), WB Saunders, Philadelphia 2001.

Linked question

31. The most appropriate evidence-based long-term maintenance therapy for this patient in the prior question is:
A. Tocilizumab
B. Rituximab
C. Monthly IVIg
D. Daily oral 60 mg of prednisone in perpetuity
E. Ocrelizumab
Correct answer: A

Explanation

The most evidence-based long-term maintenance therapy for biopsy-proven GCA is tocilizumab, an anti-IL-6 agent, based on a large clinical trial published in 2017. Long-term steroids may be effective, but the side effect profile is often intolerable for many older adults with GCA. The other agents would not be considered first line. Sustained remission in the 2017 trial at week 52 occurred in 56% of the patients treated with tocilizumab weekly and in 53% of those treated with tocilizumab every other week. Only 14–18% of those in the placebo groups achieved sustained remission.

Reference

Stone JH, Tuckwell K, Dimonaco S, Klearman M, Aringer M, Blockmans D, et al. Trial of Tocilizumab in Giant-Cell Arteritis. N Engl J Med. 2017;377(4):317–28. https://doi.org/10.1056/NEJMoa1613849

32. A 53-year-old woman develops episodes of 30–60 min of imbalance, at times accompanied by headache or muffled hearing. She has always been a carsick person. She notices episodes more during times when the barometric pressure is dropping. She also notes attacks of hearing loss. Her workup is notable for normal brain MRI with and without gadolinium as well as low-frequency sensorineural hearing loss of the left ear on audiogram. Which of the following features are least suggestive of vestibular migraine as etiology of her symptoms?
    A. Carsickness
    B. 60-minute-long episodes of imbalance
    C. Low-frequency SNHL of the left ear
    D. Episodes triggered by barometric pressure drop
    E. Normal brain MRI
    Correct answer: C

Explanation

Meniere's disease is defined by diagnostic criteria that include episodes of minute- to hour-long periods of imbalance as well as low-frequency SNHL on audiogram and fluctuating aural symptoms. The low-frequency SNHL loss is definitional for Meniere's disease and would not be expected in a diagnosis of vestibular migraine. Vestibular migraine and Meniere's disease may have a normal brain MRI. Vestibular migraine is more likely associated with carsickness and triggered by barometric pressure drop.

Reference

Lopez-Escamez JA, Carey J, Chung WH, Goebel JA, Magnusson M, Mandalà M, et al. Diagnostic criteria for Menière's disease. J Vestib Res. 2015;25(1):1–7. https://doi.org/10.3233/ves-150549

33. An 82-year-old woman develops episodes of second- to minute-long violent room-spinning. They started when she woke up and turned over in bed. When she sits completely still, she is relatively asymptomatic but head movement, including going from sitting to standing or standing to lying, triggers a violent episode. On examination, she has upbeat torsional nystagmus to the right shoulder when she lies down quickly on an exam table with her right ear down. What is the most likely localization of her pathology?
    A. Left posterior semicircular canal
    B. Right posterior semicircular canal
    C. Left horizontal canal
    D. Right horizontal canal
    E. Left anterior canal
    Correct answer: B

Explanation

Benign paroxysmal positional vertigo (BPPV) is characterized by the presence of otoconia into the sensory component of the vestibular apparatus, the semicircular canals. Because of the relative position of the canals to the cupula, the posterior canal is typically most frequently involved, and patients will complain of disturbing violent room-spinning sensation typically triggered by change in head position. The Dix-Hallpike maneuver can be used to accurately diagnose posterior canal BPPV, and examiners should position the patient's head 45 degrees toward either direction, lie them back quickly with each ear down, and observe the eyes for crescendo of upbeat torsional nystagmus toward the ear in the down position. This is diagnostic for posterior canal BPPV on that same side as the down-facing ear.

Reference

Dix MR, Hallpike CS. The pathology, symptomatology and diagnosis of certain common disorders of the vestibular system. Ann Otol Rhinol Laryngol. 1952;61(4):987–1016. https://doi.org/10.1177/000348945206100403

Linked questions: 34–35

34. A 40-year-old man presents to the emergency department (ED) with complaint of continuous sense of room-spinning and in the ED is diagnosed with the "acute vestibular syndrome." Which of the following features are most consistent with a peripheral pattern of the acute vestibular syndrome, implying a relatively benign prognosis if left untreated?
    A. Unidirectional nystagmus that diminishes toward the left and increases to the right
    B. Upbeat nystagmus
    C. Direction-changing nystagmus in the horizontal plane
    D. Vertical correction of eye position during cross-cover testing
    E. Normal head impulse testing
    Correct answer: A

Explanation

Alexander's law holds that in acute vestibular loss, spontaneous nystagmus shows the fast phase toward the healthy ear and that nystagmus is greatest when gaze is directed toward the fast phase and diminishes away from the fast phase. This would be consistent with a peripheral pattern of vestibular loss such as vestibular neuritis. By contrast, upbeat nystagmus and direction-changing nystagmus are typically central in origin. Abnormal head impulse testing also suggests a peripheral etiology of the acute vestibular syndrome, while normal head impulse testing can suggest central etiology. A skew deviation (option D) would also suggest brain stem or central origin.

Reference

Kattah JC, Talkad AV, Wang DZ, Hsieh YH, Newman-Toker DE. HINTS to diagnose stroke in the acute vestibular syndrome: three-step bedside oculomotor examination more sensitive than early MRI diffusion-weighted imaging. Stroke. 2009;40(11):3504–10. https://doi.org/10.1161/strokeaha.109.551234

Linked question

35. For the patient in the prior question, MRI shows enhancement of the eighth cranial nerve and no parenchymal abnormality. What is the most likely diagnosis?
    A. BPPV
    B. Vestibular neuritis
    C. Meniere's disease
    D. Brain stem stroke
    E. Labyrinthine infarct
    Correct answer: B

Explanation

Vestibular neuritis is characterized by inflammation, typically thought to be of viral origin, of the eighth cranial nerve. It is the second-most frequent cause of peripheral vestibular vertigo after BPPV. Evidence derived from clinical trials has given conflicting evidence, but many clinicians opt to give glucocorticoids and antiviral by oral dosing. In the long-term, vestibular physical therapy remains a linchpin of treatment given vestibular neuropathy that can result from vestibular neuritis.

Reference

Strupp M, Zingler VC, Arbusow V, Niklas D, Maag KP, Dieterich M, et al. Methylprednisolone, valacyclovir, or the combination for vestibular neuritis. N Engl J Med. 2004;351(4):354–61. https://doi.org/10.1056/NEJMoa033280

36. Which of the following patients is defined as having a skew deviation?
    A. An 18-year-old boy with breakdown of congenital fourth nerve palsy
    B. A 42-year-old woman with superior divisional third nerve palsy from meningioma
    C. A 37-year-old with posterior communicating artery aneurysm and compressive pupil-involving third nerve palsy
    D. A 75-year-old man with vertical double vision and punctate medullary infarct
    E. A 42-year-old with vertical double vision and positive acetylcholine receptor antibody testing and single-fiber repetitive stimulation EMG
    Correct answer: D

Explanation

A skew deviation is defined as vertical misalignment of the eyes related to derangement in the parenchyma of the posterior fossa that are supranuclear. By definition, a third or fourth nerve palsy resulting in vertical ocular misalignment is not a skew deviation. Diplopia alone would also not be considered a skew deviation.

Reference

Jauregui-Renaud K, Faldon M, Clarke A, Bronstein AM, Gresty MA. Skew deviation of the eyes in normal human subjects induced by semicircular canal stimulation. Neurosci Lett. 1996;205(2):135–7. https://doi.org/10.1016/0304-3940(96)12372-7

Amanda Zhao, Thomas Flagiello, and Jiyeon Son

1. A 45-year-old woman presents to her outpatient primary care doctor for gait instability and bilateral leg numbness. On exam, she is noted to have a wide-based and spastic gait, distal, length-dependent sensory loss, and impaired vibration and proprioception in the bilateral toes. MRI of her spine is displayed below. Medical history is notable for Roux-en-Y gastric surgery 1 year ago. Vitamin B12 and methylmalonic acid levels are normal. Based on the provided history, what is the most likely cause of this patient's symptoms?

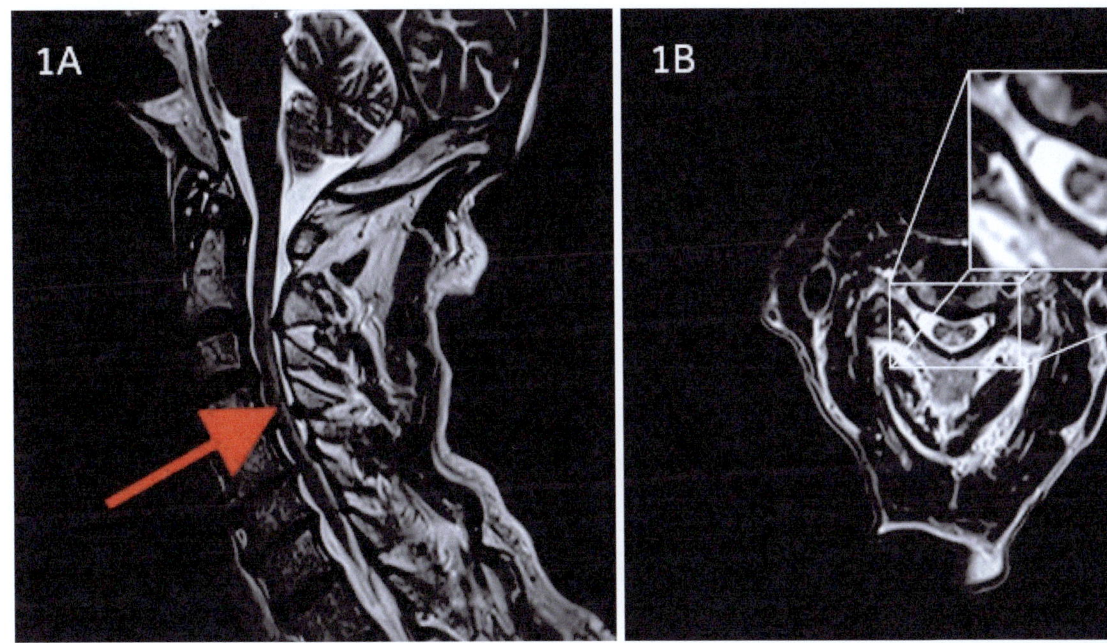

Sagittal STIR and axial T2 MRI images of the cervical spine. (Source: Marotta DA, Mason MC, Abraham BM, Kesserwani H. via Cureus. CC BY 4.0 (https://creativecommons.org/licenses/by/4.0/). Image has not been modified from source. Please see full attribution with citation below in references section for this question.)

A. Zhao · T. Flagiello · J. Son (✉)
Department of Neurology, NYU Langone Health,
New York, NY, USA
e-mail: amanda.zhao@nyulangone.org;
thomas.flagiello@nyulangone.org; jiyeon.son@nyulangone.org

© The Author(s), under exclusive license to Springer Nature Switzerland AG 2026
T. E. Smith, V. Arena (eds.), *Essential Neurology Board Review Q & A*, https://doi.org/10.1007/978-3-032-17213-6_10

A. Vitamin E deficiency
B. Copper deficiency
C. Zinc deficiency
D. ATP7B gene mutation
E. Vitamin B12 deficiency

Correct answer: B

Explanation

This patient presents with symptoms and signs consistent with subacute combined degeneration, which can result from both vitamin B12 deficiency and copper deficiency. They may present with similar imaging findings, and both deficiencies should be tested for in a patient with concurrent myelopathic and peripheral neuropathic signs as they are often clinically indistinguishable. In this case, the patient's B12 and methylmalonic acid levels are normal, making vitamin B12 (A) deficiency unlikely. Etiologies for copper deficiency myelopathy include malabsorption (either due to gastric surgery or due to congenital malabsorption syndromes) or zinc overload, for which this patient does not endorse any history (C). MRI may show long segment T2 hyperintensities in the cervical or thoracic dorsal columns as in this patient or less commonly lateral corticospinal tract abnormalities but may also be normal in half of all patients. A mutation of the ATP7B gene on chromosome 13 is associated with Wilson's disease, a condition of ceruloplasmin deficiency resulting in excessive copper accumulation in the liver and brain. The most common neurologic manifestations of Wilson's disease are tremor, dystonia, and ataxia (D). Vitamin E deficiency is typically associated with symptoms similar to spinocerebellar ataxia (A).

References

Marotta DA, Mason MC, Abraham BM, Kesserwani H. Myeloneuropathy in the Setting of Hypocupremia: An Overview of Copper-Related Pathophysiology. Cureus. 2021;13(7):e16254. Published 2021 Jul 8. https://doi.org/10.7759/cureus.16254

Roessler FC, Wolff S. Rapid healing of a patient with dramatic subacute combined degeneration of spinal cord: a case report. BMC Res Notes. 2017;10(1):18. https://doi.org/10.1186/s13104-016-2344-4

Saji AM, Lui F, De Jesus O. Spinal Cord Subacute Combined Degeneration. StatPearls. Treasure Island (FL) 2025.

Linked questions: 2–3

2. A patient is brought in by his wife for altered mental status. He was noted to have a cough 1 week before presentation and several days afterward complained of difficulty concentrating at work and progressive daytime sleepiness. On exam, the patient is somnolent but able to hold his hands out briefly with notable asterixis and cogwheel rigidity. His abdomen is distended with multiple spider angiomas and enlarged abdominal veins, and he has gynecomastia. Serum ammonia level is normal. The patient's MRI is shown below. Which of the following should *not* be a part of this patient's treatment plan?

A. Liver transplant
B. Disaccharide lactulose
C. Infectious evaluation
D. Emergent transjugular intrahepatic portosystemic shunt procedure
E. Rifaximin

Correct answer: D

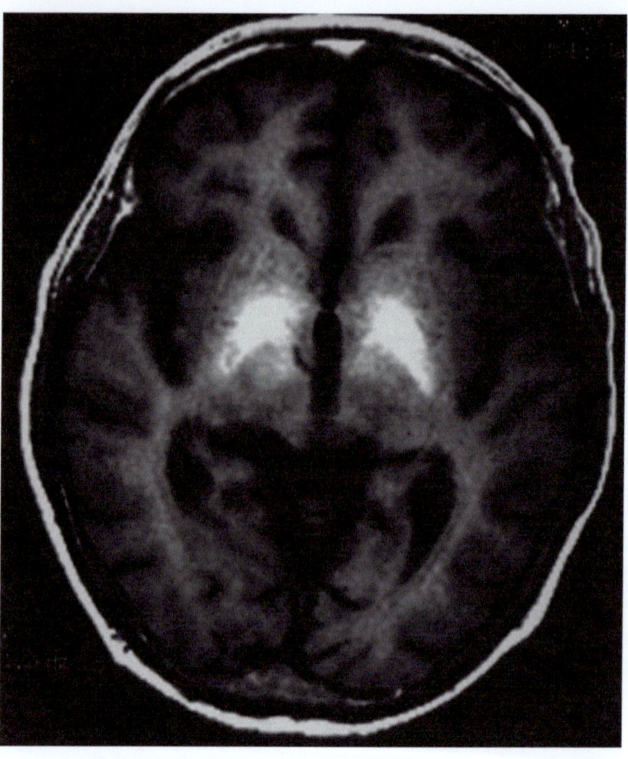

Axial FLAIR brain MRI. (Source: Yamamoto T, Abe K, Anjiki H, Ishii T, Kuyama Y. via Journal of Clinical Medicine Research. CC BY 2.0 (https://creativecommons.org/licenses/by/2.0/). Image has not been modified from original. Please see full attribution with citation below in references section for this question.)

Explanation

This patient is presenting with classic features of hepatic encephalopathy, which can be seen in any patient with liver cirrhosis. It typically presents as changes in wakefulness and attention, as well as cognition (simple calculations), but left untreated it can progress to somnolence or obtundation. Asterixis is not specific to hepatic encephalopathy and can also be seen in many other systemic disorders. Ammonia is often elevated but can also be normal and does not typically correlate with disease severity. MRI may show bilateral hyperintensities in the basal ganglia, in particular the globus pallidi, and EEG may show triphasic waves. Management should involve treatment of any precipitating factors (GI bleed; hyponatremia; hypoglycemia; benzodiazepine or alcohol use; infection such as pneumonia, UTI, or bacterial peritonitis; or hepatic/portal vein thrombosis) (C). It should also include reducing ammonia absorption from the colon using disaccharide lactulose (B) with antibiotics such as neomycin or rifaximin (E). Liver transplantation is curative (A). Transjugular intrahepatic portosystemic shunt (TIPS) procedures can precipitate hepatic encephalopathy due to increased shunting of ammonia into the systemic circulation and should be avoided (D).

References

Diesing TS. Neurologic Manifestations of Gastrointestinal and Nutritional Disorders. Continuum (Minneap Minn). 2023;29(3):708–33. https://doi.org/10.1212/CON.0000000000001235

Yamamoto T, Abe K, Anjiki H, Ishii T, Kuyama Y. Metronidazole-induced neurotoxicity developed in liver cirrhosis. J Clin Med Res. 2012;4(4):295–8. https://doi.org/10.4021/jocmr893w

Linked question

3. Which of the following imaging findings would you *not* expect in the prior patient?
   A. Diffusion restriction in the cortical ribbon
   B. FLAIR hyperintensity of globus pallidus
   C. Cerebral edema on CT head without contrast
   D. T2/FLAIR hyperintensity of bilateral mamillary bodies
   E. T2/FLAIR hyperintensity of bilateral thalami
   Correct answer: D

Explanation

In cases of hepatic encephalopathy, MRI may show bilateral, symmetric hyperintensities in the basal ganglia (particularly the globus pallidus), diffusion restriction in the cortex (particularly in the insula) (A), and bilateral thalamic hyperintensity. Mamillary body hyperintensity is classically associated with thiamine deficiency (D). CT imaging may show cerebral edema in severe cases (C), but MRI is superior.

4. A 43-year-old woman with medical history of hypertension, diabetes mellitus, and hyperlipidemia presents for acute onset involuntary right arm and right leg movements starting this morning. On exam, she is noted to have constant movement of her right arm and leg, with intermittent, higher amplitude flinging movements of her arm. Strength exam to confrontation and sensory exam are otherwise normal. MRI is shown below. What is the most likely treatment for this patient's condition?

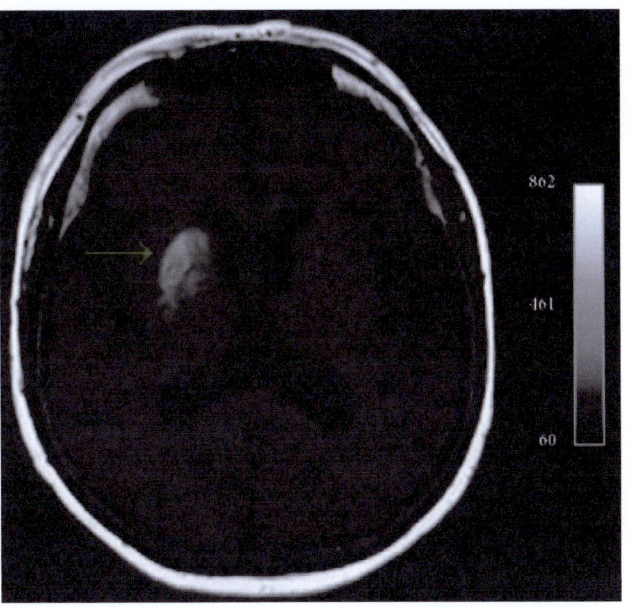

Axial T1 brain MRI. (Source: Suárez-Vega VM, Sánchez Almaraz C, Bernardo AI, Rodríguez-Díaz R, Díez Barrio A, Martín Gil L. via Case Reports in Radiology. CC BY 4.0 (https://creativecommons.org/licenses/by/4.0/). Image has not been modified from original. Please see full attribution with citation below in references section for this question.)

A. Aspirin load
B. Glycemic control
C. Trihexyphenidyl and IV Benadryl
D. IV tenecteplase
E. Chelation therapy
Correct answer: B

Explanation

Acute onset hemichorea with or without hemiballismus can be caused by poor glucose control, typically seen with blood glucose greater than 400 mg/dL and HgbA1c greater than 13% at presentation. While typically unilateral, it may be bilateral in 10% of patients. MRI is most notable for unilateral putamenal and caudate hyperintensity on T1- and sometimes T2-weighted images (as seen in the figure). Symptoms typically improve in days to weeks with glycemic control (B). While acute basal ganglia infarct could result in acute onset hemichorea on the contralateral side, it would typically present as diffusion restriction and not as T1 hyperintensity (A, D). Acute dystonic reactions are another example of an acute onset hyperkinetic movement disorder, but the patient does not have any relevant medication history, and this condition would also not be associated with the imaging findings provided (C). Wilson's disease can be associated with hemichorea but would not occur on this acute timescale (E).

References

Reda H. Neurologic Complications of Endocrine Disorders. Continuum (Minneap Minn). 2023;29(3):887–902. https://doi.org/10.1212/CON.0000000000001262

Suárez-Vega VM, Sánchez Almaraz C, Bernardo AI, Rodríguez-Díaz R, Díez Barrio A, Martín Gil L. CT and MR Unilateral Brain Features Secondary to Nonketotic Hyperglycemia Presenting as Hemichorea-Hemiballism. Case Rep Radiol. 2016;2016:5727138. https://doi.org/10.1155/2016/5727138

5. A 38-year-old man with history of substance use is brought in by EMS after being found confused in the street. Collateral from family reveals that for the last two months they've noted personality changes (no longer interacting with friends or family, not leaving his apartment), abnormal hand and arm tremors, and unsteadiness on his feet with multiple falls. On exam, the patient follows one-step commands but initiates no actions on his own, and is mute. His tone is spastic. Brain MRI reveals widespread and symmetric T2/FLAIR hyperintensities involving the posterior limbs of the internal capsules extending inferiorly to the pons as well as the cerebellar white matter and middle cerebellar peduncles. What toxic ingestion is most likely the cause of this patient's symptoms?
   A. Ketamine
   B. Kratom
   C. Delta-8 THC
   D. Bath salts
   E. Inhaled heroin vapor
   Correct answer: E

Explanation

Opioid use can result in detrimental CNS effects through hypoxic-ischemic injury from respiratory depression as well as a toxic spongiform leukoencephalopathy. This is typically associated with repeated exposure to black tar heroin fumes, which is produced through a method of consumption called "chasing the dragon," where tar is placed on aluminum foil and heated from below. This heroin-induced leukoencephalopathy often begins with cerebellar signs and motor restlessness and can progress to pyramidal signs, spasms, hypotonic paresis, or potentially death. Diffuse bilateral white matter FLAIR hyperintensities are typically seen on MRI, particularly in the posterior limb of the internal capsules, cerebellum, splenium of the corpus callosum, and midbrain white matter tracts. Kratom is a class of drugs that is made from the leaves of a tropical tree, which is typically consumed orally either in tea or in pills. It is a hallucinogen and also has mild opioid agonist properties (B). Ketamine is an N-methyl-d-aspartate (NMDA) receptor antagonist that can cause mild euphoria in lower doses and agitation and psychomotor retardation in higher doses (A). It may also precipitate new hallucinosis, delusions, or catatonia. Delta-8 THC is a psychoactive cannabinoid compound that is a less potent isomer of delta-9 THC (the primary component found in the marijuana plant). It can cause acute encephalopathy in high doses and has been associated with cerebrovascular complications in addition to being a risk factor for reversible cerebral vasoconstriction syndrome (RCVS) (C). Bath salts are a synthetic cathinone, which is a compound found naturally and which can produce a euphoric effect. Severe intoxication with bath salts may cause agitation (sometimes associated with violence), hallucinosis, and paranoia.

Reference

Howard, Jonathan, and Anuradha Singh. Neurology Image-Based Clinical Review. Springer Publishing Company, 28 Aug. 2016.

6. A 42-year-old male presents with headache and vision change. His physical exam reveals enlargement of his hands, feet, and facial features. His laboratory studies show pan hypopituitarism and an elevated serum insulin-like growth factor 1 (IGF-1). MRI of the pituitary reveals a pituitary adenoma. Which of these is least likely to be related to the patient's condition?
   A. Bitemporal hemianopsia
   B. Obstructive sleep apnea
   C. Median neuropathy
   D. Generalized sensory neuropathy
   E. Muscle pseudohypertrophy
   F. Cognitive impairment
   Correct answer: D

Explanation

This patient has clinical signs of excess growth hormone, which most commonly is due to growth hormone-secreting pituitary macroadenomas. These macroadenomas can cause headache and visual field deficits (A). Obstructive sleep apnea may result from tonsillar and adenoidal hypertrophy (B), which are both examples of visceromegaly associated with excess growth hormone. Median and ulnar mononeuropathies are also reported in 20–40% of patients, which is conjectured to be due to peripheral nerve edema and nerve entrapment (C). Generalized sensory and motor peripheral neuropathies (D) have also been seen in patients with excess growth hormone. Cognitive impairment, in particular impairments in learning, attention, and executive function, is also seen with acromegaly (E). Muscle pseudohypertrophy is not typically associated with acromegaly but may be seen with hypothyroidism (D).

7. A 53-year-old man with end-stage renal disease presents for urgent dialysis in the setting of chronic noncompliance. Prior to dialysis, labs are notable for BUN 150 mmol/L, glucose of 158 mg/dL, and sodium of 130 mg/dL. During dialysis, he acutely becomes somnolent, prompting activation of a stroke code. Labs are initially notable for BUN 51 mmol/L, glucose 128 mg/dL, and sodium 135 mmol/dL. Head CT is notable only for microvascular disease and diffuse cerebral edema. Continuous EEG monitoring is initiated and shows generalized delta slowing. The patient remains altered for the remainder of the day but returns to baseline the following morning. What is the most likely cause of the patient's acute mental status change?
   A. Cerebral ischemia due to intradialytic hypotension
   B. Blood-brain barrier disruption due to rapid correction of plasma urea
   C. Plasma hypertonicity due to rapid sodium correction
   D. Glucose loss to dialysate
   E. Inadequate clearance of uremic toxins

Correct answer: B

Explanation

Dialysis disequilibrium syndrome often occurs in patients being initiated on dialysis but can also occur at other points during treatment. Symptoms include acute encephalopathy, elevated intracranial pressure, and seizures. The mechanism is thought to be due to rapid shifts in osmotic gradients, with the sudden drop in blood urea nitrogen causing movement of water into the brain resulting in cerebral edema. This syndrome more commonly occurs with intermittent dialysis due to more rapid shifts. Cerebral ischemia, in particular watershed infarcts, may result from large volume shifts in dialysis sessions and global reduction in cerebral blood flow (A); however, the patient's hours of encephalopathy followed by return to baseline the following morning would be less typical for an infarct. Osmotic demyelination syndrome may also present as acute onset encephalopathy. This results from overly aggressive correction of hyponatremia, causing rapid water shifts out of cells and subsequent cellular injury (C). It typically presents with evidence of pontine damage on imaging (typically on MRI) rather than diffuse cerebral edema. Glucose-free or low-glucose dialysate solutions may be associated with intradialytic hypoglycemia (D); the patient's blood glucose is normal. Hypocalcemia during dialysis may result from the use of low-calcium dialysate and the use of citrate anticoagulation during dialysis (which can chelate calcium); however, hypocalcemia more commonly presents with neuromuscular symptoms such as paresthesias, cramps, and spasms. Uremic encephalopathy is an unlikely cause of the patient's symptoms given improvement in BUN (E).

Reference

Ghoshal S. Renal and Electrolyte Disorders and the Nervous System. Continuum (Minneap Minn). 2023;29(3):797–825. https://doi.org/10.1212/CON.0000000000001286

8. A 57-year-old man with history of polysubstance use disorder presents with acute encephalopathy and gait issues. On exam, he is noted to have bidirectional horizontal nystagmus with significant anterograde amnesia and confabulation. He is given IV thiamine with improvement in encephalopathy and gait dysfunction but continues to have significant memory impairment. Which of the following processes could explain these ongoing symptoms?
   A. Hemorrhagic necrosis of bilateral thalami and mammillary bodies
   B. Cortical laminar necrosis
   C. Demyelination of the corpus callosum
   D. Accumulation of copper in basal ganglia
   E. NAD+ depletion in the pons and midbrain

Correct answer: A

Explanation

Laminar necrosis in the hippocampus and neocortex can be seen with hypoglycemia, but presentation with extraocular movement and gait abnormalities would be less typical, and symptoms would not be expected to improve with thiamine (B). Chronic alcohol use is sometimes associated with Marchiafava-Bignami disease, a progressive neurologic disease that typically presents as nonspecific motor and cognitive disturbances or hemispheric disconnection syndrome; it is also associated with seizures (C). Pathology typically reveals demyelination and necrosis of the corpus callosum. Basal ganglia copper accumulation occurs with Wilson's disease, which can cause extraocular movement abnormalities (e.g., hypometric saccades, vertical saccade impairment, and impaired vertical gaze), gait disturbance (due to basal ganglia involvement), and cognitive impairment (frontal syndrome, subcortical dementia) (D); however, symptoms would not be expected to improve symptoms, and the patient's prominent memory symptoms are less typical. NAD+ depletion of the pons and midbrain is associated with pellagra or severe niacin (vitamin B3) deficiency (E). Pellagra classically presents with cutaneous, gastrointestinal, and neuropsychiatric symptoms. Frontotemporal atrophy and ventricular enlargement are most commonly seen on brain imaging.

Reference

de Oliveira AM, Paulino MV, Vieira AP, McKinney AM, da Rocha AJ, Dos Santos GT, Leite CD, Godoy LF, Lucato

LT. Imaging patterns of toxic and metabolic brain disorders. Radiographics. 2019 Oct;39(6):1672–95.

9. A 65-year-old woman presents with a 3-month history of difficulty with fine motor tasks, progressive gait instability, and distal paresthesias. On exam, she has a broad-based gait, significantly impaired vibration and joint position sense in her feet and hands, and patchy sensory loss. When testing pronator drift, you notice involuntary finger movements as if she is playing the piano, and on Romberg testing, she immediately falls when closing her eyes. Motor strength is completely preserved. Although she denies any prescription medications, on further questioning, she states she has been taking a vitamin supplement that she read online will "improve brain health" and "boost energy." MRI of her brain and total spine are unremarkable, and she is pending a nerve conduction study. What is the most likely etiology of her presentation?
   A. Vitamin E toxicity
   B. Vitamin A toxicity
   C. Vitamin B6 toxicity
   D. Vitamin B1 toxicity
   E. Copper deficiency due to zinc excess
   Correct answer: C

Explanation

This constellation of signs (involuntary finger movements consistent with pseudoathetosis, positive Romberg testing, reduced vibratory and position sense, intact motor function) and symptoms (gait instability, loss of dexterity, paresthesias) is consistent with a sensory ganglionopathy. This is a pure sensory neuropathy involving the dorsal root ganglion. Of the options listed, only vitamin B6 excess is linked to the development of a sensory ganglionopathy. Nerve conduction studies reveal reduced amplitude of sensory nerve action potentials (SNAPs), oftentimes asymmetric, with normal conduction velocities. Motor nerve conduction studies are classically normal. Other important causes of sensory ganglionopathy to remember are paraneoplastic (anti-Hu, anti-amphiphysin), autoimmune (Sjogren's syndrome), toxic (platinum-based chemotherapy), and infectious (HIV).

Reference

Amato AA, Ropper AH. Sensory Ganglionopathy. N Engl J Med. 2020;383(17):1657–62. https://doi.org/10.1056/NEJMra2023935

10. A 19-year-old man is brought to the emergency department from a music festival after he had a witnessed generalized tonic-clonic seizure. His friends are not being forthright about any substances consumed but note that he's been drinking a lot of water to stay hydrated. On exam, he is somnolent and disoriented but does not have an appreciable focal deficit. Workup is notable for serum sodium of 113 mmol/L (normal serum sodium range 135–45 mmol/L), plasma osmolality of 255 mOsm/kg (normal plasma osmolality range 275–295 mOsm/kg), and urine sodium of 40 mmol/L (normal urine sodium range 20–40 mmol/l). Which of the following best explains the pathophysiology behind his presentation?
   A. Osmotic demyelination due to rapid correction of chronic hyponatremia
   B. Central diabetes insipidus triggered by serotonergic overstimulation
   C. Syndrome of inappropriate antidiuretic hormone secretion
   D. Dehydration-induced hypovolemia with secondary hyperaldosteronism
   E. Salt-wasting nephropathy due to renal tubular injury
   Correct answer: C

Explanation

This patient's presentation is due to an acute symptomatic seizure in the setting of hyponatremia. His serum and urine studies suggest the syndrome of inappropriate antidiuretic hormone (SIADH) as the cause. Given this information, he most likely took 3,4-methylenedioxymethamphetamine (also known as MDMA, "ecstasy," and "molly"), a psychostimulant structurally similar to serotonin that gives users a feeling of disinhibition, warmth, and interpersonal connection. Important effects of MDMA toxicity include SIADH and polydipsia which can lead to encephalopathy and seizures (as in this patient), serotonin syndrome, acute dystonic reactions, and rarely a toxic leukoencephalopathy. The other options listed are not the proposed mechanism behind MDMA and hyponatremia.

Reference

Shannon M. Methylenedioxymethamphetamine (MDMA, "Ecstasy"). Pediatr Emerg Care. 2000;16(5):377–80. https://doi.org/10.1097/00006565-200010000-00022

Linked questions: 11–12

11. An 8-year-old boy who recently arrived from Tanzania presents to the emergency room with 4 days of acute lower extremity weakness and difficulty walking. Neurologic exam is notable for symmetric lower limb spasticity, weakness, hyperreflexia with bilateral ankle clonus, and bilateral extensor plantar responses. Mental status, cranial nerve, and sensory exam is normal. He is afebrile, his upper extremities are unaffected, and there is no evidence of bowel or bladder dysfunction. Further history reveals significant consumption of cassava. Serum B12, folate, and HIV are normal. Suspecting a myelopathy, you obtain an MRI spine which is normal. What is the most likely etiology?

A. Spinal cord infarct
B. Konzo
C. Lathyrism
D. HTLV1-associated myelopathy
E. Hereditary spastic paraplegia
Correct answer: B

Explanation

This child is likely presenting with konzo, a nonprogressive acute onset myelopathy that is seen in regions where cassava is a staple food. It typically occurs following physical exertion and nadirs in hours to days with initial deficits remaining static for decades. It predominantly affects the corticospinal tracts, thus presenting with spastic paraparesis with preserved sensory, sexual, and sphincter function. MRI and CSF testing is typically normal, though advanced testing is often unavailable in endemic regions. Lathyrism (C) is another cause of myelopathy but is caused by chronic ingestion of grass pea and typically occurs in adult men. The patient does not have significant risk factors or mention of a triggered event to suspect a spinal cord infarct (A), and the acuity of presentation and the consumption of cassava make the other options less likely (D, E).

Reference

Baguma M, Nzabara F, Maheshe Balemba G, Malembaka EB, Migabo C, Mudumbi G, et al. Konzo risk factors, determinants and etiopathogenesis: What is new? A systematic review. Neurotoxicology. 2021;85:54–67. https://doi.org/10.1016/j.neuro.2021.05.001

Linked question

12. What is the proposed mechanism underlying his condition?
    A. Cyanide toxicity leading to mitochondrial dysfunction
    B. Nutritional deficiency leading to impaired myelin synthesis
    C. Viral infection of predominantly CD4+ T lymphocytes leading to an inflammatory response effecting the spinal cord
    D. Toxicity of β-N-oxalylamino-l-alanine to spinal neurons leading to cell death
    E. Disruption of blood flow to the spinal cord leading to cell death
    Correct answer: A

Explanation

Konzo is caused by cyanide toxicity in the setting of ingestion of the cassava root, which is a dietary staple in parts of Africa and Southeast Asia. It contains linamarin, which is converted to cyanide by gut flora that then leads to mitochon-

drial dysfunction. The other options listed are mechanisms of other causes of myelopathy—vitamin B12 deficiency (B), HTLV1 infection (C), lathyrism (D), and spinal cord infarct (E).

Reference

Tylleskar T, Howlett WP, Rwiza HT, Aquilonius SM, Stalberg E, Linden B, et al. Konzo: a distinct disease entity with selective upper motor neuron damage. J Neurol Neurosurg Psychiatry. 1993;56(6):638–43. https://doi.org/10.1136/jnnp.56.6.638

13. A 35-year-old previously healthy woman presents with a several-month history of unsteadiness and increased frequency of falls, particularly in the dark. More recently, she's noted worsening blurry vision. Neurologic exam reveals decreased vibration sense in the lower extremities, absent Achilles reflexes, positive Romberg testing, wide-based gait, and decreased visual acuity bilaterally. Strength and mental status exams are normal. Fundoscopic exam is consistent with pigmentary retinopathy. Serum testing will most likely reveal low levels of which of the following vitamins?
    A. Copper
    B. Vitamin B12
    C. Vitamin A
    D. Vitamin E
    E. Vitamin B1
    Correct answer: D

Explanation

Vitamin E deficiency causes a subacute to chronic myelopathy that predominantly affects the dorsal columns. It can also affect the spinocerebellar tracts and peripheral nerves, leading to the signs and symptoms observed in this patient. Of the options listed, it is the only vitamin deficiency that can lead to retinopathy. Vitamin A deficiency leads to nyctalopia (night blindness) and xerophthalmia (dryness of the cornea and conjunctiva) but not retinopathy. Vitamin B1 deficiency can cause changes in mental status, oculomotor abnormalities (ophthalmoplegia, nystagmus), and ataxia, a triad known as Wernicke's encephalopathy, as well as peripheral neuropathy. Deficiencies in vitamin B12 and copper can lead to myelopathy, myeloneuropathy, and more rarely optic neuropathy and peripheral neuropathy.

Reference

Tanyel MC, Mancano LD. Neurologic findings in vitamin E deficiency. Am Fam Physician. 1997;55(1):197–201.

14. A 54-year-old male welder presents with progressive slowness of movement, resting tremor, and frequent muscle stiffness. He reports working in enclosed spaces

with poor ventilation for over 25 years, where he was regularly exposed to welding fumes without consistent use of respiratory protection. Neurological examination reveals hypomimia, rigidity, and postural instability. MRI of the brain shows hyperintensities in bilateral basal ganglia and thalami. Dopaminergic therapy yields limited improvement. Routine labs, including liver and renal function, are unremarkable. Which of the following is the most likely cause of his Parkinsonian symptoms?

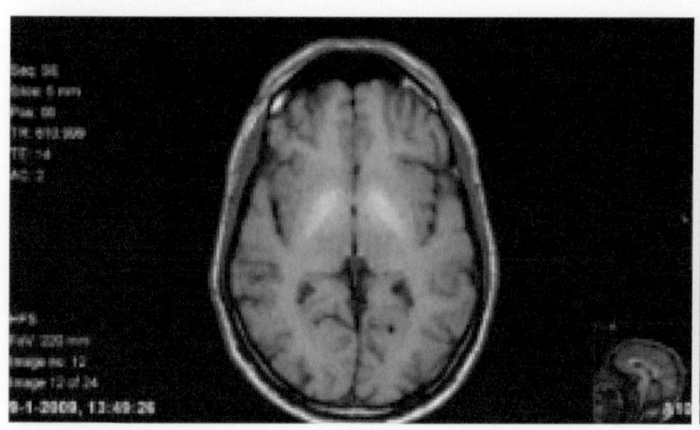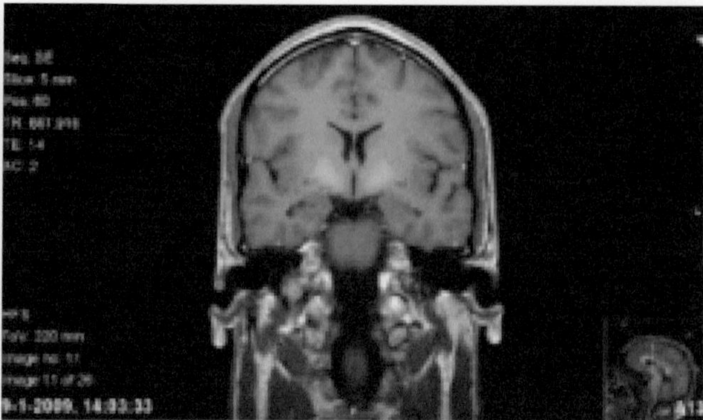

MRI scan of the brain with bilateral high T1 signal intensity in the globus pallidus is shown. Left, transversal view; right, coronal view. (Source: Verhoeven WM, Egger JI, Kuijpers HJ. via Journal of Medical Case Reports. CC BY 2.0 (https://creativecommons.org/licenses/by/2.0/). Images were not modified from original. Please see full attribution with citation below in references section for this question.)

A. Idiopathic Parkinson's disease
B. Chronic lead exposure
C. Manganese neurotoxicity
D. Huntington's disease
E. Wilson's disease
Correct answer: C

Explanation

Manganese is an essential trace element, but chronic inhalation exposure, particularly in occupational settings such as welding, can lead to toxic accumulation in the brain—especially in the basal ganglia. This condition, known as manganism, results in Parkinson-like symptoms including bradykinesia, rigidity, and tremor. However, unlike idiopathic Parkinson's disease (A), manganism typically does not respond well to dopaminergic therapy and may show distinct imaging findings, such as T1 hyperintensities in the globus pallidus. Pathophysiology likely involves oxidative stress and mitochondrial dysfunction. Chronic lead exposure (B) has been associated with neuropathy, muscle and joint pain, memory impairment, and, in extreme cases, coma and seizure.

References

Dobson AW, Erikson KM, Aschner M. Manganese neurotoxicity. Ann N Y Acad Sci. 2004 Mar;1012:115–28. https://doi.org/10.1196/annals.1306.009. PMID: 15105259

Verhoeven WM, Egger JI, Kuijpers HJ. Manganese and acute paranoid psychosis: a case report. J Med Case Rep. 2011;5:146. Published 2011 Apr 12. https://doi.org/10.1186/1752-1947-5-146

15. A 67-year-old woman with a history of chronic insomnia, anxiety, and mild cognitive impairment presents to the clinic with worsening memory loss, daytime confusion, and frequent falls over the past 6 months. Her daughter reports that she has become increasingly forgetful, appears drowsy during the day, and struggles to find words. A review of her medications reveals long-term nightly use of zolpidem and lorazepam. Neurological examination shows mild disorientation and impaired short-term memory. MRI of the brain is notable for mild global atrophy with no acute findings. Which of the following best explains this patient's clinical presentation?

A. Normal aging-related cognitive decline
B. Neurodegeneration due to idiopathic Alzheimer's disease
C. Cumulative neurotoxic effects of chronic sedative-hypnotic use
D. Depression-related pseudodementia
E. Benzodiazepine withdrawal syndrome
Correct answer: C

Explanation

Chronic use of sedative-hypnotics—especially benzodiazepines and Z-drugs (e.g., zolpidem)—has been associated with adverse cognitive effects, including memory impairment, executive dysfunction, increased fall risk, and potentially accelerated neurodegeneration in older adults. These agents act on GABA-A receptors and can impair synaptic plasticity and neurogenesis with long-term use. There are studies that suggest that prolonged exposure, particularly in the elderly, can mimic or worsen dementia-like symptoms.

Reference

Ettcheto M, Olloquequi J, Sánchez-López E, Busquets O, Cano A, Manzine PR, Beas-Zarate C, Castro-Torres RD, García ML, Bulló M, Auladell C, Folch J, Camins A. Benzodiazepines and Related Drugs as a Risk Factor in Alzheimer's Disease Dementia. Front Aging Neurosci. 2020 Jan 8;11:344. https://doi.org/10.3389/fnagi.2019.00344. PMID: 31969812; PMCID: PMC6960222.

16. A 38-year-old man is brought to the emergency department by his roommate, who found him confused and vomiting. The patient had been drinking heavily the night before. On arrival, he is disoriented and tachypneic with poor visual acuity. Labs show a high anion gap metabolic acidosis and an elevated osmolar gap. Fundoscopic exam reveals bilateral optic disc hyperemia. CT scan of the head is initially normal. Fomepizole is administered and he is started on hemodialysis. Over the next 24 hours, his vision deteriorates further and he becomes comatose. Which of the following best explains the patient's acute neurological deterioration?
    A. Hepatic encephalopathy
    B. Thiamine deficiency
    C. Methanol-induced neurotoxicity
    D. Ethylene glycol crystal nephropathy
    E. Wernicke's encephalopathy
    Correct answer: C

Explanation

Methanol (methyl alcohol) is a toxic alcohol found in industrial products and sometimes illicit liquors. After ingestion, methanol is metabolized by alcohol dehydrogenase into formic acid, which causes severe neurotoxicity—most notably optic nerve damage, leading to vision loss, as well as basal ganglia necrosis and coma in severe cases. The hallmark lab findings are a high anion gap metabolic acidosis and elevated osmolar gap. Early treatment with fomepizole or ethanol (to inhibit alcohol dehydrogenase) and hemodialysis is critical to prevent irreversible CNS injury. In contrast, ethylene glycol (D) toxicity primarily affects the kidneys (via oxalate crystal deposition) and also causes CNS depression, but it is methanol that is classically associated with optic neuropathy and basal ganglia damage. Thiamine deficiency can manifest in two different ways neurologically: dry beri-beri and Wernicke's encephalopathy. Dry beri-beri can lead to muscle weakness and peripheral neuropathy. Wernicke's encephalopathy primarily affects the central nervous system and is characterized by the classic triad of ophthalmoplegia, ataxia, and confusion. Hepatic encephalopathy (A) is a reversible neuropsychiatric syndrome caused by liver dysfunction, leading to accumulation of neurotoxins—especially ammonia—that impair brain function and cause symptoms ranging from confusion to coma.

Reference

Kraut JA, Mullins ME. Toxic Alcohols. N Engl J Med. 2018 Jan 18;378(3):270–280. https://doi.org/10.1056/NEJMra1615295. Erratum in: N Engl J Med. 2019 Jan 10;380(2):202. https://doi.org/10.1056/NEJMx180046. PMID: 29342392.

17. A 9-year-old boy with a history of medulloblastoma treated 1 year ago with surgical resection, craniospinal radiation, and chemotherapy is brought to the neurology clinic for evaluation of new-onset academic difficulties, decreased attention span, and frequent forgetfulness. His teacher notes a decline in school performance and difficulty with new learning. Physical exam is unremarkable, and there are no signs of tumor recurrence on follow-up MRI. Neuropsychological testing confirms impaired working memory and reduced processing speed. What is the most likely explanation for this patient's cognitive decline?
    A. Chemotherapy-induced peripheral neuropathy
    B. Tumor recurrence
    C. Radiation-induced white matter damage
    D. Postsurgical hydrocephalus
    E. Steroid-related mood changes
    Correct answer: C

Explanation

Pediatric patients are especially vulnerable to the neurotoxic effects of ionizing radiation, particularly to the developing white matter of the brain. Cranial radiation, often used in treating medulloblastoma, can impair neurogenesis and myelination, leading to progressive cognitive decline, especially in attention, processing speed, and working memory. Possible mechanisms include hippocampal neurogenesis reduction and neuroinflammation. These effects may emerge months to years after treatment, even in the absence of tumor recurrence. Early identification and cognitive rehabilitation are important for improving long-term outcomes. Other dose-dependent neurological complications of ionizing radiation include plexopathy and myelopathy.

Reference

Greene-Schloesser D, Robbins ME. Radiation-induced cognitive impairment--from bench to bedside. Neuro Oncol. 2012 Sep;14 Suppl 4(Suppl 4):iv37–44. https://doi.org/10.1093/neuonc/nos196. PMID: 23095829; PMCID: PMC3480242.

18. A 68-year-old man with a history of alcohol use disorder is found unconscious on a park bench during winter. On arrival to the ED, his temperature is 28 °C (82.4 °F). He is unresponsive, with bradycardia, hypotension, and dilated pupils that are sluggishly reactive. Neurological exam is limited due to his comatose state. Labs show mild hypokalemia and hypophosphatemia. ECG reveals J (Osborn) waves. CT head is unremarkable. EEG shows markedly decreased activity. Passive rewarming is started. Which of the following best explains the patient's current neurological condition?
    A. Irreversible brain death due to cerebral anoxia
    B. Alcohol withdrawal delirium
    C. Pontine hemorrhage
    D. Reversible suppression of CNS activity due to hypothermia
    E. Nonconvulsive status epilepticus

    Correct answer: D. Reversible suppression of CNS activity due to hypothermia

Explanation

This patient has severe hypothermia (<28 °C), which can mimic brain death with coma—with fixed pupils and flat EEG—but is potentially reversible with rewarming. It's critical not to misdiagnose such cases as irreversible until normothermia is restored. Classic findings like Osborn (J) waves on ECG support the diagnosis of hypothermia. Neurological recovery is possible, especially if core functions like circulation and oxygenation are supported.

Reference

Mattu A, Brady WJ, Perron AD. Electrocardiographic manifestations of hypothermia. The American journal of emergency medicine. 2002 Jul 1;20(4):314–26.

19. A 34-year-old man presents to the emergency department 45 min after eating a traditional fugu (puffer fish) dish while vacationing in Japan. He reports numbness around his lips and tongue, followed by tingling in his hands and feet. On exam, his vitals are stable, but he has mild dysarthria, ataxia, and symmetrical muscle weakness. He is fully alert and oriented. The emergency team anticipates the need for airway support. Which of the following best explains this patient's neurological symptoms?
    A. Inhibition of acetylcholinesterase
    B. Excess release of glutamate at NMDA receptors
    C. Autoimmune attack on voltage-gated calcium channels
    D. Blockade of voltage-gated sodium channels
    E. Demyelination of peripheral nerves

    Correct answer: D

Explanation

This patient has classic signs of tetrodotoxin (TTX) poisoning, caused by ingestion of improperly prepared puffer fish. TTX selectively blocks voltage-gated sodium channels in nerves and muscles, preventing action potentials and leading to flaccid paralysis. Mental status remains preserved in early stages, and perioral numbness and descending paralysis can be seen. In severe cases, paralysis progresses to respiratory failure. There are no antidotes and supportive care is provided.

Reference

Isbister GK, Kiernan MC. Neurotoxic marine poisoning. Lancet Neurol. 2005 Apr;4(4):219–28. https://doi.org/10.1016/S1474-4422(05)70041-7. PMID: 15778101.

20. A 56-year-old man with a long history of alcohol use disorder is brought to the hospital by his family due to progressive confusion, apathy, and unsteady gait. They report he has been increasingly withdrawn and forgetful over the past week. On examination, he is disoriented, with dysarthria, gait ataxia, and hyperreflexia. His bloodwork reveals macrocytic anemia and low thiamine levels. Brain MRI shows symmetric T2 hyperintensity and restricted diffusion involving the splenium of the corpus callosum. Which of the following is the most likely diagnosis?

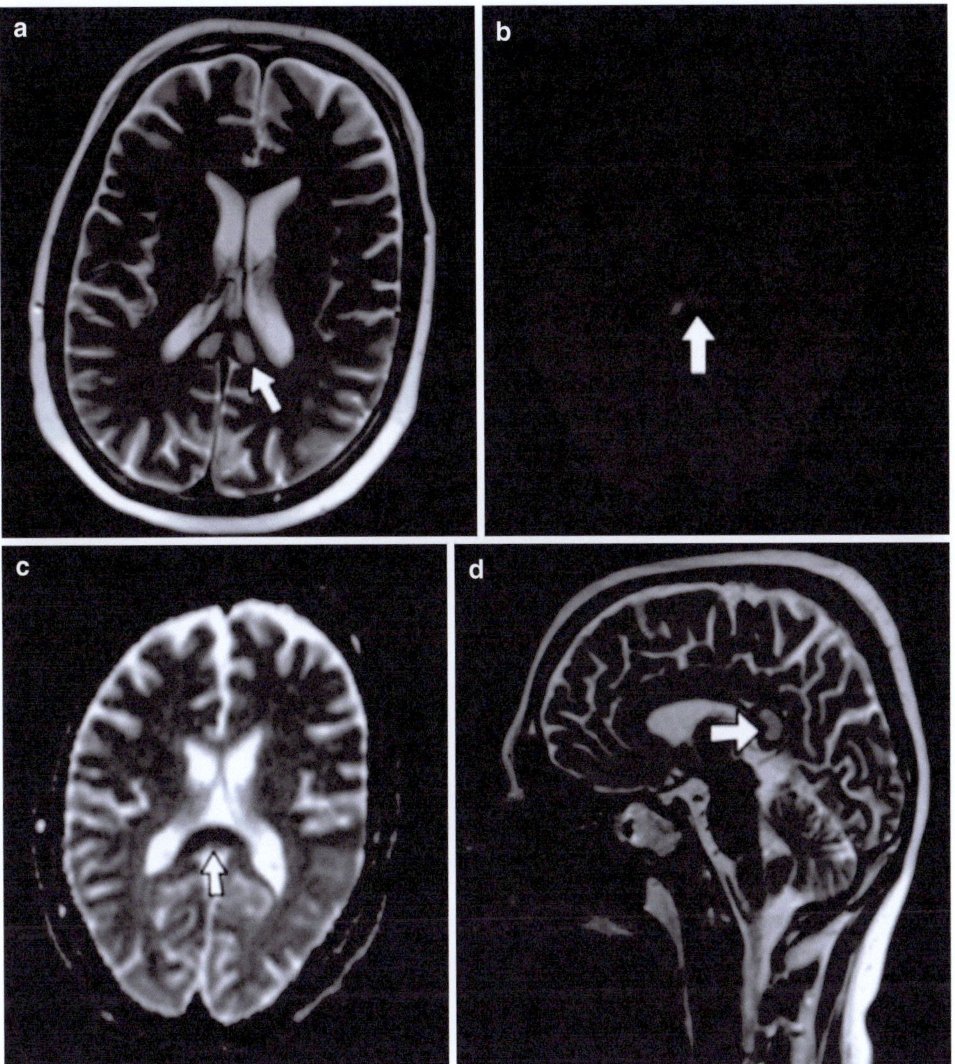

Images: Axial (a-c) and sagittal (d) MRI brain. (Source: Boloursaz S, Nekooei S, Seilanian Toosi F, et al. via Case Reports in Neurological Medicine. CC-BY 4.0 (https://creativecommons.org/licenses/by/4.0/). Image has not been modified from original. Please see full attribution with citation below in references section for this question.)

A. Wernicke's encephalopathy
B. Marchiafava-Bignami disease
C. Central pontine myelinolysis
D. Progressive multifocal leukoencephalopathy
E. Korsakoff syndrome

Correct answer: B

Explanation

Marchiafava-Bignami disease is a rare demyelinating disorder of the corpus callosum, almost exclusively seen in chronic alcoholics, often associated with malnutrition (especially vitamin B deficiency). MRI is key for diagnosis and typically shows symmetric lesions in the corpus callosum, often affecting the splenium, with T2/FLAIR hyperintensity and restricted diffusion. Clinical features include cognitive impairment or confusion, gait ataxia, dysarthria, and disconnection syndrome (if callosal involvement is severe). While Wernicke's encephalopathy is also associated with chronic alcohol use and thiamine deficiency, it primarily affects the mammillary bodies and medial thalami on MRI and presents acutely with confusion, ataxia, and ophthalmoplegia—unlike the corpus callosum lesions seen in Marchiafava-Bignami disease. Central pontine myelinolysis typically results from rapid correction of hyponatremia and involves demyelination of the central pons, leading to symptoms like quadriparesis or locked-in syndrome, not the cognitive and gait disturbances seen here. Progressive multifocal leukoencephalopathy is caused by JC virus reactivation in immunocompromised individuals and shows multifocal white matter lesions without selective callosal involvement. Korsakoff syndrome, a chronic complication of Wernicke's, presents with profound memory deficits and confabulation but lacks the distinctive MRI findings of symmetric corpus callosum involvement seen in Marchiafava-Bignami disease.

References

Boloursaz S, Nekooei S, Seilanian Toosi F, et al. Marchiafava-Bignami and Alcohol Related Acute Polyneuropathy: The Cooccurrence of Two Rare Entities. Case Rep Neurol Med. 2016;2016:5848572. https://doi.org/10.1155/2016/5848572

Tian TY, Pescador Ruschel MA, Park S, Liang JW. Marchiafava-Bignami Disease. 2023 Jul 24. In: StatPearls [Internet]. Treasure Island (FL): StatPearls Publishing; 2025 Jan. PMID: 30252263.

Tozakidou M, Stippich C, Fischmann A. Teaching neuroimages: radiologic findings in Marchiafava-Bignami disease. Neurology. 2011 Sep 13;77(11):e67. https://doi.org/10.1212/WNL.0b013e31822e144b. PMID: 21911733.

Neuro-oncology

Marissa Barbaro and Alexandra Gewirtz

1. A 32-year-old man is referred to neurology after experiencing several months of worsening headache, nausea, and intermittent blurry vision. He reports occasional imbalance when walking long distances. His past medical history is notable for a retinal lesion of unclear etiology resected at age 24. His father died of complications from kidney cancer in his 40 s. On examination, he has mild gait ataxia but no other focal deficits. MRI of the brain below reveals a cystic lesion with an enhancing mural nodule in the cerebellum. Systemic imaging shows multiple renal cysts and a small enhancing mass in the left kidney. Which of the following is the most likely underlying diagnosis?

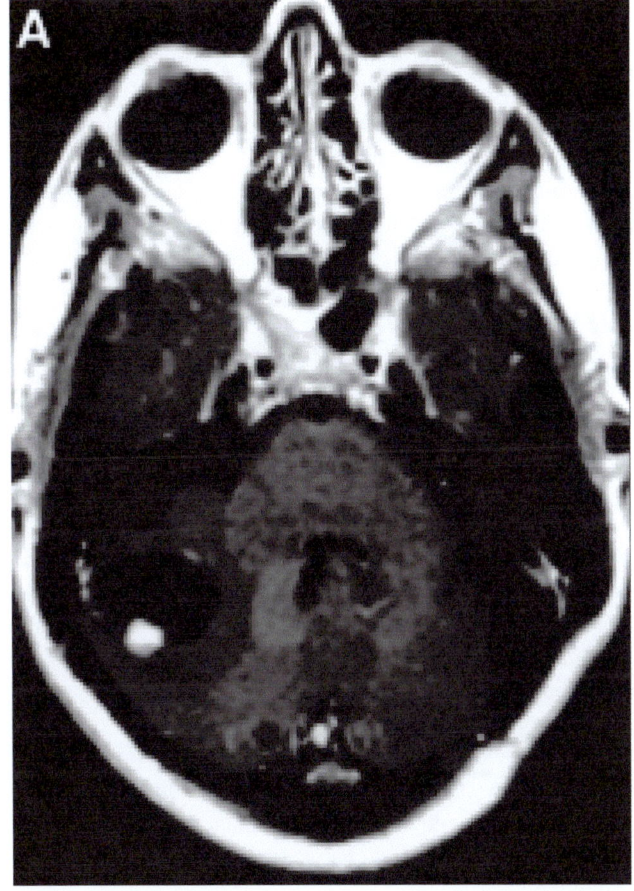

Axial brain MRI. (Source: Schunemann, V., Huntoon, K., Lonser, R. R. CC-BY 4.0 (https://creativecommons.org/licenses/by/4.0/) via *Frontiers in Surgery*. Image has been cropped from source. Please see full attribution with citation below in references section for this question)

M. Barbaro (✉) · A. Gewirtz
Brain and Spine Tumor Center, Laura and Isaac Perlmutter Cancer Center at NYU Langone Health, New York, NY, USA
e-mail: marissa.barbaro@nyulangone.org;
alexandra.gewirtz@nyulangone.org

A. von Hippel-Lindau disease
B. Neurofibromatosis type 2
C. Tuberous sclerosis complex
D. Li-Fraumeni syndrome
E. Sturge-Weber syndrome

Correct answer: A

Explanation

This young adult presents with a symptomatic cerebellar hemangioblastoma, history of retinal hemangioblastoma, and a renal mass, all of which are cardinal features of von Hippel-Lindau disease (VHL). Family history of early onset kidney cancer further supports this diagnosis. VHL is a highly penetrant autosomal dominant tumor predisposition syndrome caused by a pathogenic variant in the VHL tumor suppressor gene on chromosome 3p25. It commonly includes central nervous system (CNS) involvement of hemangioblastomas (the cerebellar and spinal cord), retinal hemangioblastomas, pheochromocytomas, pancreatic cysts and neuroendocrine tumors, renal cell carcinoma, and cystadenomas of the adnexal ligament. CNS hemangioblastomas are often multiple and are composed of abundant capillary vessels and stromal cells. Within the brain, the vast majority are infratentorial.

Neurofibromatosis type 2 (NF2) is another hereditary syndrome which typically presents with bilateral vestibular schwannomas, ependymomas, meningiomas, gliomas, and juvenile posterior lenticular opacities. Hemangioblastomas and renal cell carcinoma are not characteristic. The National Institutes of Health (NIH) criteria designate patients with bilateral vestibular schwannomas or a first-degree family relative with NF2 and either unilateral vestibular schwannoma or two of the following, meningioma, schwannoma, glioma, neurofibroma, and juvenile posterior subcapsular lens opacities, as having the diagnosis.

Tuberous sclerosis complex is another inherited condition associated with cortical tubers, renal angiomyolipomas, characteristic skin involvement (hypomelanotic macules, angiofibromas), and subependymal giant cell astrocytomas. There is an association between tuberous sclerosis and pathogenic variants in *TSC1* and *TSC2* genes.

Li-Fraumeni syndrome is a familial cancer predisposition syndrome caused by germline mutations in the TP53 tumor suppressor gene. There is a significantly increased risk of developing various malignancies such as breast cancer, leukemia, sarcomas, and gliomas but not hemangioblastomas or renal cell carcinoma.

Sturge-Weber syndrome is characterized by the classic facial port-wine stain, leptomeningeal angiomas, and seizures. It is not hereditary and does not involve renal or cerebellar tumors.

References

Mrugala, Maciej M., and others, *Neuro-Oncology Compendium for the Boards and Clinical Practice* (New York, 2023; online edn, Oxford Academic, 1 June 2023), https://doi.org/10.1093/med/9780197573778.001.0001, accessed 22 June 2025.

Neurofibromatosis. Conference statement. National Institutes of Health Consensus Development Conference. Arch Neurol. 1988;45(5):575–8.

Schunemann V, Huntoon K, Lonser RR. Personalized Medicine for Nervous System Manifestations of von Hippel-Lindau Disease. Front Surg. 2016;3:39. https://doi.org/10.3389/fsurg.2016.00039.

2. A 25-year-old woman presents to clinic with a recent history of intermittent numbness and tingling in the right arm. On review of systems, she endorses multiple soft and painless nodules under her skin and café au lait spots since childhood. On examination, she has several mobile subcutaneous nodules along her extremities and decreased sensation along the right C6 dermatome. MRI of the cervical spine with and without contrast shows an enhancing mass along the C5–C6 nerve root. On brain MRI, she has areas of T2 signal hyperintensity in the cerebellum and brain stem. Family history is significant for an older sister who had similar skin findings and underwent surgery for a spinal tumor in her 30 s. Which of the following is the most likely diagnosis?
A. Neurofibromatosis type 1
B. Neurofibromatosis type 2
C. Schwannomatosis
D. Noonan syndrome
E. McCune-Albright syndrome

Correct answer: A

Explanation

This patient presents with classic features of neurofibromatosis type 1 (NF1), an autosomal dominant disorder caused by mutations in the NF1 gene on chromosome 17. The NF1 gene product is neurofibromin, a cytoplasmic protein that functions as a tumor suppressor and a negative regulator of the RAS oncogene, an important controller of cellular proliferation. Based on the National Institutes of Health (NIH) criteria, patients require at least two of the following: six or more café au lait macules, two or more neurofibromas or one plexiform neurofibroma, axillary or inguinal freckling, optic pathway glioma, two or more Lisch nodules, a distinctive osseous lesion (such as sphenoid wing dysplasia), or a first-degree relative with NF1. Patients with NF1 are at increased risk for both low- and high-grade gliomas. The most common intracranial tumor seen in these patients is an optic pathway glioma. Plexiform neurofibromas carry a risk of transformation into malignant peripheral nerve sheath tumors (MPNST). Concerning features that warrant urgent evaluation include rapid increase in size, change in texture, persistent nocturnal pain, or the development of new neurologic deficits. On imaging, many patients with NF1 demonstrate areas of T2 signal hyperintensity, known as NF-associated bright spots. These are common but are not included in the diagnostic criteria and are believed to represent dysplastic glial proliferation. The presence of multiple café au lait spots, subcutaneous neurofibromas, nonspecific areas of T2 hyperintensity on brain MRI, and a nerve root mass in a young adult with a suggestive family history makes NF1 the most likely diagnosis.

Neurofibromatosis type 2 (NF2) is a separate condition characterized by bilateral vestibular schwannomas, meningiomas, and spinal ependymomas. Cutaneous neurofibromas and café au lait spots are not salient features. It is less common than NF1 and is also autosomal dominant, characterized by a pathogenic variant on chromosome 22. The product of the NF2 gene is merlin, which acts as a tumor suppressor. It is estimated that approximately 95% of patients with NF2 exhibit vestibular schwannomas.

Schwannomatosis is an uncommon disorder which is associated with multiple non-vestibular and painful schwannomas. It occurs in both familial and sporadic fashion in 15% and 85% of patients, respectively. In the familial version, there is an association with the SMARCB1 mutation in approximately half of patients. Pathogenic variants in the LZTR1 gene have also been associated with schwannomatosis. This condition lacks café au lait spots and cutaneous neurofibromas and rarely can include meningiomas.

Noonan syndrome is a condition caused by mutations in the PTPN11 gene that has some overlapping features with NF1 such as café au lait spots but does not have the presence of neurofibromas or gliomas. The hallmark features of Noonan syndrome include distinctive facial features, short stature, and congenital heart defects such as pulmonary valve stenosis.

McCune-Albright syndrome is caused by a mutation in the GNAS gene and is defined by the classic triad of precocious puberty, café au lait macules, and polyostotic fibrous dysplasia. It does not have an association with central nervous system tumors.

Reference

Legius E, Messiaen L, Wolkenstein P, Pancza P, Avery RA, Berman Y, et al. Revised diagnostic criteria for neurofibromatosis type 1 and Legius syndrome: an international consensus recommendation. Genet Med. 2021;23(8):1506–13. https://doi.org/10.1038/s41436-021-01170-5.

3. A 40-year-old man presents with progressive headaches and occasional blurry vision with nausea over the past several weeks. Brain MRI reveals a well-circumscribed, lobulated intraventricular mass centered near the foramen of Monro, with mild hydrocephalus. The lesion is T1 isointense and T2 hyperintense and demonstrates heterogeneous contrast enhancement. MRI with and without contrast is featured below, and surgical resection is performed. Histology shows uniform round cells with neuronal differentiation and pseudorosettes, positive synaptophysin staining, and low proliferative index. What is the most likely diagnosis?

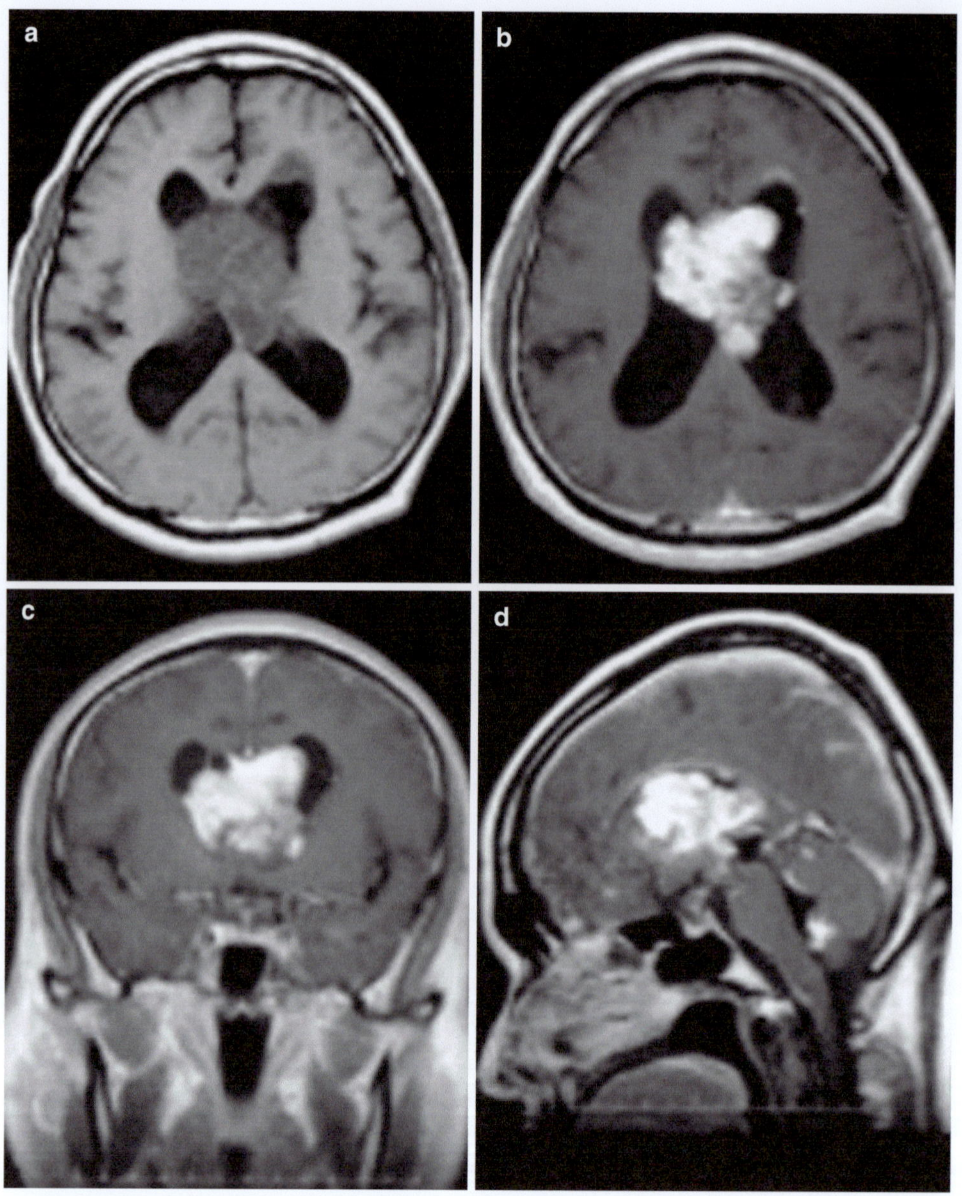

Axial (**a** and **b**), coronal (**c**), and sagittal (**d**) MRI brain sections. (Source: Yano, H., Nakayama, N., Hirose, Y., Ohe, N., Shinoda, J., Yoshimura, S-I., Iwama, T. CC-BY 2.0 (https://creativecommons.org/licenses/by/2.0/) via *Diagnostic Pathology*. Image has not been modified from original. Please see full attribution with citation below in references section for this question.)

A. Subependymoma
B. Central neurocytoma
C. Ependymoma
D. Choroid plexus papilloma
E. Oligodendroglioma

Correct answer: B

Explanation

Central neurocytomas are rare, typically benign, neuronal tumors that arise in the lateral ventricles, most commonly near the foramen of Monro. The median age at presentation is around 34 years old. At diagnosis, patients often have symptoms of obstructive hydrocephalus. Imaging often shows a well-demarcated and heterogeneously enhancing intraventricular mass with a multicystic appearance and occasional calcifications. These tumors arise from the cells of the septum pellucidum and are histologically composed of many well-differentiated small round cells with occasional exhibition of pseudorosettes. All central neurocytomas are WHO grade 2. The Ki-67, a cellular proliferation index, is an important indicator of recurrence if elevated. On staining, these tumors express synaptophysin. The backbone of treatment includes surgical resection; most central neurocytomas are gross totally resected. In cases of subtotal resection or recurrence, fractionated radiation is often employed.

Subependymomas are rare intraventricular tumors that typically occur along the walls of the lateral and fourth ventricles. These lesions are more common in middle aged to older adults. On MRI, subependymomas are typically non-enhancing or minimally enhancing.

Ependymomas arise from ependymal cells lining the ventricles and central canal of the spinal cord. On pathology, these tumors exhibit perivascular rosettes and GFAP positivity with increased cellularly and mitotic activity as compared to central neurocytomas. Ependymomas show avid enhancement on imaging. The 2021 WHO Classification of CNS Tumors categorizes ependymomas based on a combination of histopathologic, molecular, and anatomic features. Tumors are classified by location into supratentorial, posterior fossa, and spinal groups. Supratentorial ependymomas express either the ZFTA (formerly RELA) fusion or YAP1 fusion. Posterior fossa ependymomas are divided into group A and group B based on separate DNA methylation profiles, which have prognostic significance. Spinal ependymomas may show MYCN amplification, particularly in aggressive cases. Additional subtypes include myxopapillary ependymoma and subependymoma. In pediatric populations, ependymomas account for approximately 5% of all brain tumors and 22% of spinal cord tumors.

Choroid plexus papillomas are WHO grade 1 tumors that usually occur in children, often in the lateral ventricles. These lesions are strongly enhancing on MRI with a characteristic lobulated or "cauliflower" appearance. They histologically show an architecture similar to normal choroid plexus, with palm frond-like papillary structures and low mitotic activity. In adults, these tumors are seen more commonly in the fourth ventricle. They can present with obstructive hydrocephalus and associated increased intracranial pressure.

Oligodendrogliomas are slow-growing, cortically based tumors that most commonly arise in the frontal lobes. They are defined by the presence of an IDH mutation and 1p/19q codeletion; histology classically shows a "fried egg" appearance. On imaging, they typically involve the cortex and subcortical white matter as T2 hyperintense lesions and may be non-enhancing or only minimally enhancing on MRI. Calcifications are a common radiographic feature. These tumors are often diagnosed in young to middle-aged adults and most frequently present with seizures due to their cortical location. Other symptoms can include headache, personality changes, or focal neurologic deficits, rather than symptoms of hydrocephalus.

References

Mu W, Dahmoush H. Classification and neuroimaging of ependymal tumors. Front Pediatr. 2023;11:1181211. https://doi.org/10.3389/fped.2023.1181211.

Yano H, Nakayama N, Hirose Y, Ohe N, Shinoda J, Yoshimura S, et al. Intraventricular glioneuronal tumor with disseminated lesions at diagnosis--a case report. Diagn Pathol. 2011;6:119. https://doi.org/10.1186/1746-1596-6-119.

4. A 48-year-old woman presents with amenorrhea and galactorrhea. She reports chronic fatigue and intermittent headaches. On exam, she has bitemporal hemianopsia. Laboratory evaluation shows elevated prolactin level and normal thyroid, cortisol, and growth hormone levels. Brain MRI reveals a 2.2-cm enhancing sellar mass with suprasellar extension compressing the optic chiasm. What is the most likely diagnosis?
   A. Craniopharyngioma
   B. Pituitary macroadenoma
   C. Rathke's cleft cyst
   D. Null cell adenoma
   E. Pituitary carcinoma
   Correct answer: B

Explanation

This patient presents with classic features of a prolactin-secreting pituitary macroadenoma, otherwise known as a prolactinoma or a lactotroph adenoma. Prolactinomas are the most common functioning pituitary macroadenomas, otherwise defined as a mass >1 cm. Associated symptoms include galactorrhea and classic bitemporal hemianopsia due to compression of the optic chiasm. There is often a secondary suppression of gonadotropin-releasing hormone with resultant hypogonadism and amenorrhea. Of note, nonprolactin-secreting tumors can also elevate prolactin levels via distortion or compression of the pituitary stalk, which reduces dopaminergic inhibition of prolactin release. This is called the stalk effect which typically causes a mild to moderate elevation of serum prolactin levels, usually not in excess of 150 μg/L, in contrast to a prolactinoma with levels often exceeding 200 μg/L. First-line treatment for prolactinomas is medical therapy with dopamine agonists, most commonly cabergoline, which is preferred over bromocriptine due to its higher efficacy and better side effect profile. Surgical removal is typically reserved for those patients who have failed medical therapy, intolerability of treatment, or persistent mass effect. Surgery normalizes prolactin levels in most microadenomas and approximately 40–60% of macroadenomas. If surgery is contraindicated or unsuccessful, radiation therapy may be considered. However, radiation carries risks of pituitary hormone deficiency and further visual impairment.

Craniopharyngiomas are rare and histologically benign tumors arising from the remnants of Rathke's pouch. These tumors often appear in the suprasellar region, among other structures associated with the craniopharyngeal duct, and can cause mass effect symptoms such as visual changes and hypopituitarism. They do not secrete hormones, including prolactin. There are two variants of craniopharyngioma, including the adamantinomatous and papillary subtypes. The adamantinomatous version is often characterized by a CTNNB1 mutation, while the papillary tumors often have a BRAFV600E mutation. On imaging, the adamantinomatous subtype typically exhibits cystic components with frequent calcifications, as opposed to the papillary subtype which typically shows a more solid shape. Management of these tumors include a total resection or a subtotal resection with adjuvant radiation therapy. There is ongoing interest in utilizing BRAF inhibitors in the papillary subtype.

Rathke's cleft cysts are benign, nonneoplastic cysts that also arise from embryonic remnants of Rathke's pouch. They may cause pituitary compression and hypopituitarism but do not produce hormones. Imaging reveals a well-circumscribed non-enhancing cystic lesion in the sella, which is distinct from the solid, enhancing appearance of adenomas.

Null cell adenomas are adenomas that do not show evidence of hypersecretion, unlike the case presented here, and exhibit an absence of specific cell-type differentiation based on immunohistochemistry. Null cells are found in the normal pituitary gland with an incompletely understood role. Like other adenomas, they can cause mass effect and effects on the pituitary. They are the second most common type of pituitary adenoma.

Pituitary carcinomas are rare tumors defined by the spread to a site that is discontiguous with the sellar region or with distant metastases. They represent less than 0.1% of pituitary tumors. Treatment includes a combination of surgery, radiation, and chemotherapies such as temozolomide.

Reference

Melmed S. Pituitary-Tumor Endocrinopathies. N Engl J Med. 2020;382(10):937–50. https://doi.org/10.1056/NEJMra1810772.

5. A 40-year-old man presents with new-onset focal seizures involving the right arm. Brain MRI reveals a left frontal lobe lesion that is T2 hyperintense, non-enhancing, and shows minimal mass effect with associated calcifications in the periphery of the mass. There is no associated restricted diffusion. Surgical resection is performed. Which of the following pathologic findings is incorrect?
   A. 1p19q codeletion
   B. IDH mutation
   C. Perinuclear clearing with "fried egg" appearance
   D. Rosenthal fibers
   E. Delicate branching vasculature, otherwise known as "chicken wire appearance"

Correct answer: D

Explanation

Oligodendrogliomas are diffuse infiltrative gliomas of oligodendroglial origin. Median age is between 40 and 50 years old. These tumors tend to be slow-growing, and patients often have prolonged survival with appropriate therapy. Oligodendrogliomas can be graded as CNS WHO grade 2 or 3, with distinct histologic features. Definitive diagnosis requires both an IDH mutation and a 1p/19q codeletion, per WHO criteria. During formalin fixation and paraffin embedding, the tumor cell cytoplasm retracts from the nucleus, which causes the appearance of a clear halo around a centrally located nucleus or a "fried egg" appearance. Oligodendrogliomas are highly vascular tumors with thin-walled and branching capillaries, appearing mesh-like and resembling "chicken wire" on H&E staining. Rosenthal fibers are seen in pilocytic astrocytomas.

Reference

Wesseling P, van den Bent M, Perry A. Oligodendroglioma: pathology, molecular mechanisms and markers. Acta Neuropathol. 2015;129(6):809–27. https://doi.org/10.1007/s00401-015-1424-1.

6. A 56-year-old woman with metastatic triple-negative breast cancer presents with progressive headache, nausea, and gait imbalance. She also reports double vision and intermittent urinary incontinence. Brain MRI with contrast below reveals enhancement along the cerebellar folia. CSF analysis shows elevated opening pressure, lymphocytic pleocytosis, elevated protein, and positive cytology for malignant cells. What is the most appropriate next step in management?

Axial MRI brain sections (**c** and **d**). (Source: Pan, Z., Yang, G., Yuan, T., Wang, Y., Pang, X., Gao, Y., Dong, L. CC-BY 4.0 (https://creativecommons.org/licenses/by/4.0/) via *World Journal of Surgical Oncology.*

Image has been cropped from original. Please see full attribution with citation below in references section for this question.)

A. Start dexamethasone and obtain a brain biopsy.
B. Monitor symptoms closely with repeat imaging in 4 weeks.
C. Refer for radiation and initiate intrathecal chemotherapy via Ommaya reservoir.
D. Begin high-dose methotrexate intravenously.
E. Repeat lumbar puncture for confirmatory cytology.

Correct answer: C

Explanation

Leptomeningeal disease (LMD) is defined as the dissemination of malignant cells within the cerebrospinal fluid and leptomeninges, most often arising in the setting of metastatic solid tumors, hematologic malignancies, or primary CNS tumors. The most common underlying primaries include the breast, melanoma, and lung. It is typically confirmed by the presence of malignant cells on CSF cytology and/or supportive findings on contrast-enhanced MRI. Radiographic patterns include ependymal and leptomeningeal enhancement along the neuroaxis; there is a predilection for the cranial nerves, cauda equina, and cerebellar folia. Cytology is the gold standard for diagnosis which has a high specificity of >95% and only 50% sensitivity with the first lumbar puncture. If the clinical suspicion is high, lumbar punctures can be repeated with sensitivity increasing to 90% with the third test. The standard approach to treatment includes a combination of focal or craniospinal radiation and intrathecal chemotherapy, most commonly delivered via a ventriculoperitoneal device such as an Ommaya reservoir, which allows for safer circulation. The prognosis of leptomeningeal disease remains historically poor, with survival often measured in weeks to months; however, there is growing interest in novel treatments, including targeted agents and proton-based radiation, which have shown promise in improving outcomes for select patients.

In certain cases of leptomeningeal disease when the underlying malignancy harbors a targetable mutation, systemic therapy with a CNS penetrant targeted agent may be prioritized before radiation or intrathecal chemotherapy. In EGFR mutant non-small cell lung cancer, osimertinib (a third-generation EGFR tyrosine kinase inhibitor with excellent CNS penetration) is often used as first-line treatment for LMD, given its ability to achieve meaningful intracranial and leptomeningeal responses. In such cases, radiation and intrathecal therapy may be deferred or reserved for symptomatic or refractory disease. This highlights the evolving standard in LMD management, where treatment is increasingly individualized based on underlying tumor biology, molecular profile, and disease distribution, rather than a uniform stepwise approach.

Steroids may provide temporary symptom relief in vasogenic edema or mass effect but are not dedicated treatment for the underlying disease. Biopsy is not needed, as diagnosis is already established by positive CSF cytology and MRI.

IV methotrexate can penetrate the CSF at high doses and may be used in certain cases. However, intrathecal delivery of methotrexate is more direct and standard for LMD.

While sometimes multiple LPs are needed to confirm diagnosis, this patient already has positive cytology. Additional LPs are unnecessary in this particular case and will delay therapy.

References

Pan Z, Yang G, Yuan T, Wang Y, Pang X, Gao Y, et al. 'Hot cross bun' sign with leptomeningeal metastases of breast cancer: a case report and review of the literature. World J Surg Oncol. 2015;13:43. https://doi.org/10.1186/s12957-015-0483-z.

Wilcox JA, Li MJ, Boire AA. Leptomeningeal Metastases: New Opportunities in the Modern Era. Neurotherapeutics. 2022;19(6):1782–98. https://doi.org/10.1007/s13311-022-01261-4.

7. A 65-year-old man with metastatic melanoma on nivolumab started 1 month prior to evaluation presents with 4 days of progressive bilateral ptosis, dysphagia, and generalized weakness. Neurologic exam reveals symmetric proximal weakness and diminished deep tendon reflexes. Brain and spine MRI are unremarkable. Labs show normal CK and mild transaminitis. EMG reveals a decremental response with repetitive stimulation. What is the most appropriate next step?
   A. Start intravenous immunoglobulin.
   B. Discontinue immunotherapy and observe closely.
   C. Start high-dose corticosteroids and resume immunotherapy.
   D. Request brain biopsy to rule out CNS metastasis.
   E. Administer pyridostigmine only.

   Correct answer: A

Explanation

This patient likely has immune checkpoint inhibitor-associated myasthenia gravis, a serious but known neurologic complication of immunotherapy. This is further supported by the EMG findings and clinical picture. Management requires immunotherapy discontinuation and prompt initiation of immunosuppressive treatment, such as IVIG or plasmapheresis, often combined with corticosteroids. Early and aggressive treatment is essential due to the risk of respiratory failure. Immune checkpoint inhibitors induce the immune system via blockade of the co-inhibitory T-cell signals, thereby unleashing the immune response. Despite their effectiveness, they have been associated with immune-related adverse events and can affect many organ systems. Neurological immune-related adverse events are rare, occurring in 7.2% of cases, and can include a wide range of presentations involving the entire neuroaxis. Among

neuromuscular complications, myasthenia gravis represents the adverse event associated with the highest mortality and morbidity.

Observation alone is not appropriate in a patient with progressive neurologic weakness, especially involving bulbar function. Prompt treatment is essential, as this condition may progress rapidly. Close monitoring of respiratory status and occasionally a higher level of care are needed.

While steroids are often part of treatment for immunotherapy-related myasthenia, resuming immunotherapy is contraindicated during active immune-related neurotoxicity. It may be considered only after full resolution and in selected cases. Steroids are given cautiously given the potential for transient worsening of symptoms early in the course of myasthenia gravis.

This patient's symptoms and negative MRI make CNS metastasis unlikely. Additionally, his EMG findings support a peripheral neuromuscular junction disorder, not a structural brain lesion.

Pyridostigmine may be helpful as an adjunct, but it is not sufficient alone in immunotherapy-related myasthenia, which typically requires immunosuppression due to rapid progression and severity.

References

Marco C, Simó M, Alemany M, Casasnovas C, Domínguez R, Vilariño N, et al. Myasthenia Gravis Induced by Immune Checkpoint Inhibitors: An Emerging Neurotoxicity in Neuro-Oncology Practice: Case Series. J Clin Med. 2022;12(1). https://doi.org/10.3390/jcm12010130.

Schneider BJ, Naidoo J, Santomasso BD, Lacchetti C, Adkins S, Anadkat M, et al. Management of Immune-Related Adverse Events in Patients Treated With Immune Checkpoint Inhibitor Therapy: ASCO Guideline Update. J Clin Oncol. 2021;39(36):4073–126. https://doi.org/10.1200/jco.21.01440.

8. A 5-month-old girl is brought to clinic due to episodes of sudden, repetitive arm and leg stiffening that occur in clusters, particularly after waking. Her parents are concerned about her poor eye contact and minimal social interaction for her age. On physical examination, she is noted to have three hypopigmented macules measuring 1–2 cm on her trunk and thigh. A soft cardiac murmur is also appreciated. Brain MRI reveals multiple subependymal nodules along the lateral ventricles, causing irregularity of the ventricular wall contour. What is the most likely diagnosis?

A. Ataxia telangiectasia
B. Neurofibromatosis type 1
C. Neurofibromatosis type 2
D. Turcot syndrome
E. Tuberous sclerosis
Correct answer: E

Explanation

This presentation is consistent with tuberous sclerosis complex (TSC), a multisystem genetic disorder caused by pathogenic variants in the *TSC1* or *TSC2* genes. The combination of infantile spasms, hypomelanotic macules (ash leaf spots), and subependymal nodules seen on MRI is characteristic. The presence of a cardiac murmur raises concern for a cardiac rhabdomyoma, which is the most common cardiac tumor seen in TSC and often detected in infancy.

TSC is associated with a wide spectrum of neurologic and systemic manifestations, including epilepsy, developmental delay, autism spectrum disorder, renal angiomyolipomas, lung involvement (particularly lymphangioleiomyomatosis in females), and cutaneous findings such as shagreen patches and facial angiofibromas. Treatment of infantile spasms in TSC often involves vigabatrin as first-line therapy, which has shown better efficacy in this population than other antiepileptic drugs. Early developmental screening and ongoing neurodevelopmental follow-up are crucial, as cognitive outcomes vary widely and early intervention services can significantly impact long-term function.

Ataxia telangiectasia is a rare autosomal recessive disorder that presents with progressive cerebellar ataxia, oculocutaneous telangiectasias, and immunodeficiency, typically after infancy. It is not associated with hypomelanotic macules, subependymal nodules, or infantile spasms.

Neurofibromatosis type 1 (NF1) typically presents later in childhood with café au lait macules, axillary freckling, and neurofibromas. It is not associated with subependymal nodules or infantile spasms.

Neurofibromatosis type 2 (NF2) is characterized by bilateral vestibular schwannomas, typically presenting in adolescence or early adulthood with hearing loss. NF2 does not present with early onset seizures, hypopigmented skin lesions, or cardiac tumors.

Turcot syndrome is a familial cancer syndrome involving colorectal adenomas or cancer and primary brain tumors, especially glioblastomas and medulloblastomas. It does not present in infancy and is not associated with hypopigmented skin findings or ventricular lesions.

Reference

Mrugala, Maciej M., and others, *Neuro-Oncology Compendium for the Boards and Clinical Practice* (New York, 2023; online edn, Oxford Academic, 1 June 2023), https://doi.org/10.1093/med/9780197573778.001.0001, accessed 22 June 2025.

9. A 62-year-old man with a 30-pack-year smoking history presents with progressive unsteadiness, slurred speech, and difficulty coordinating his limbs over the past 4 weeks. Neurologic examination reveals gait ataxia, limb dysmetria, and nystagmus. Brain MRI is unremarkable. Lumbar puncture shows mild lymphocytic pleocytosis and elevated protein but no evidence of infection or malignancy. A CT chest shows a right hilar mass concerning for small cell lung carcinoma. A paraneoplastic antibody panel is sent. Which of the following antibodies is most likely to be positive?
A. Anti-Ma2
B. Anti-recoverin
C. Anti-Hu
D. Anti-GAD65
E. Anti-NMDA receptor
Correct answer: C

Explanation

This patient presents with subacute cerebellar degeneration in the setting of suspected small cell lung cancer (SCLC), classic for a paraneoplastic neurologic syndrome (PNS). Anti-Hu antibodies (also known as ANNA-1) are highly associated with SCLC and are associated with paraneoplastic cerebellar degeneration, encephalomyelitis, or sensory neuropathy. These antibodies target intracellular neuronal antigens, triggering a T-cell-mediated immune response that causes damage to the central nervous system. Importantly, paraneoplastic syndromes can precede, coincide with, or follow a cancer diagnosis. In many cases, the neurologic syndrome heralds the discovery of the underlying tumor by months to a year or more. When patients present with suggestive neurologic findings and positive paraneoplastic antibodies, a cancer workup should be initiated even if imaging is initially negative. Diagnosis relies on a combination of clinical findings, CSF, MRI imaging, and serum/CSF paraneoplastic antibody panels. Some patients may not have detectable antibodies but can still meet clinical criteria for PNS based on the syndrome itself and association with an underlying malignancy.

Anti-Ma2 is usually found in younger men with testicular germ cell tumors and causes diencephalic and limbic encephalitis, including symptoms like hypersomnolence, memory loss, and vertical gaze palsy. This clinical picture does not match the patient's isolated cerebellar findings.

Anti-recoverin is associated with paraneoplastic retinopathy, typically seen in small cell lung cancer or breast cancer. It causes painless vision loss due to retinal degeneration, not cerebellar dysfunction.

Anti-GAD65 is commonly associated with stiff-person syndrome, autoimmune epilepsy, and non-paraneoplastic cerebellar ataxia, especially in individuals with autoimmune diseases like type 1 diabetes. It is not strongly associated with malignancy, and its syndromes often develop more gradually.

Anti-NMDA receptor encephalitis presents in young women, often with ovarian teratomas, and includes psychiatric symptoms, seizures, and autonomic instability. It does not cause isolated cerebellar dysfunction and is unrelated to small cell lung cancer.

Reference

Mrugala, Maciej M., and others, *Neuro-Oncology Compendium for the Boards and Clinical Practice* (New York, 2023; online edn, Oxford Academic, 1 June 2023), https://doi.org/10.1093/med/9780197573778.001.0001, accessed 22 June 2025.

10. A 39-year-old woman is undergoing treatment on the inpatient oncology service for a high-grade soft tissue sarcoma. She recently received ifosfamide as part of her chemotherapy regimen. Within 24 h of the infusion, she becomes acutely confused, agitated, and develops a generalized tonic-clonic seizure. On exam, she is disoriented with intermittent myoclonus. No focal neurologic deficits are noted. Basic metabolic panel, glucose, and head CT are unremarkable. EEG shows continuous slowing with periodic triphasic waves. Which of the following chemotherapeutic agents is most likely responsible for this patient's neurologic presentation?
    A. Ifosfamide
    B. Bevacizumab
    C. Temozolomide
    D. Bortezomib
    E. Cisplatin
    Correct answer: A

The clinical presentation is characteristic of ifosfamide-induced encephalopathy, a well-recognized complication that can occur in up to 30% of patients receiving this alkylating agent. Symptoms typically begin within hours to a few days of administration and range from mild confusion to seizures, hallucinations, somnolence, or even coma. The mechanism is believed to involve the accumulation of neurotoxic ifosfamide metabolites, particularly chloroacetaldehyde, which can cross the blood-brain barrier and interfere with mitochondrial function and neuronal metabolism. In addition, the inert metabolite of ifosfamide, S-carboxymethylcysteine, has been theorized to play a role

in neurotoxicity. Risk factors include low serum albumin, renal dysfunction, pretreatment with cisplatin, the presence of abdominopelvic tumor, high doses of ifosfamide, and prior CNS disease.

Early recognition of the syndrome and immediate cessation of drug are the most important initial step. The most widely employed antidote is methylene blue, although studies have shown mixed results in regard to efficacy. Other interventions include thiamine, dexmedetomidine, and hemodialysis. Most patients recover within days, but encephalopathy can be fatal in severe cases.

Bevacizumab is a monoclonal antibody targeting vascular endothelial growth factor and is associated with hypertension, proteinuria, venous and arterial thromboemboli, delayed wound healing, and bowel perforation. While it can cause posterior reversible encephalopathy syndrome, this usually presents with visual disturbances, focal neurologic deficits, and seizures in the setting of severe blood pressure elevation or renal dysfunction. This patient's acute confusion and agitation immediately post-infusion are more characteristic of ifosfamide neurotoxicity.

Temozolomide is an oral alkylating agent commonly used in glioblastoma and other CNS tumors. It functions by damaging cancer cells by adding a methyl group to the O6 position of guanine, thereby interfering with its ability to replicate and leading to cell death. It can be myelosuppressive and increase the risk for opportunistic infections, particularly in combination with radiation or corticosteroids. It is not associated with acute neurotoxicity or seizures.

Bortezomib is a proteasome inhibitor used in the treatment of multiple myeloma. Its most common neurotoxicity is peripheral neuropathy, which can be painful and dose-limiting. It is not typically associated with central neurotoxicity, encephalopathy, or seizures. Acute mental status changes would be very atypical for this agent.

Cisplatin is a platinum-based chemotherapy agent which binds to DNA, forming cross-links between guanine bases and distorting the DNA structure. It is well known for nephrotoxicity, ototoxicity, peripheral neuropathy, and nausea but does not commonly cause acute encephalopathy. High-dose cisplatin can occasionally lead to electrolyte abnormalities (such as hypomagnesemia) which could predispose to seizures, but these are generally delayed and metabolically mediated, not temporally related to infusion as in this case.

Reference

Ajithkumar T, Parkinson C, Shamshad F, Murray P. Ifosfamide encephalopathy. Clin Oncol (R Coll Radiol). 2007;19(2):108–14. https://doi.org/10.1016/j.clon.2006.11.003.

11. A 67-year-old man with recently diagnosed colorectal cancer complains of numbness and tingling in his hands and feet as well as perioral numbness. He feels that his symptoms are worse when it is cold outside. He also complaints of shock-like sensations down his back when he bends his neck in the shower. Neurologic exam reveals decreased sensation to vibration at the first toes bilaterally, impaired proprioception at the first toes bilaterally, and absent deep tendon reflexes, as well as delayed relaxation of finger extensors. Sensation to pinprick and temperature in the feet is largely intact. Which chemotherapeutic agent is most likely to be responsible for these symptoms?
    A. Bortezomib
    B. Oxaliplatin
    C. Vincristine
    D. Methotrexate
    E. Paclitaxel
    Correct answer: B

Explanation

Oxaliplatin is a platinum-based chemotherapy typically used in treatment of colorectal cancer and can cause both acute and chronic sensory polyneuropathy. Neuropathy from oxaliplatin is typically large-fiber neuropathy, with sensation to pinprick and temperature often spared. Symptoms are often exacerbated by cold and can include perioral and throat paresthesias. Lhermitte's sign can be seen. Neurologic exam can reveal delayed relaxation of finger extensors. Similar symptoms (large-fiber neuropathy with Lhermitte sign) can also be seen with cisplatin, but cold-induced symptoms, perioral symptoms, and delayed relaxation of finger extensors are suggestive of oxaliplatin toxicity specifically.

Bortezomib is a proteasome inhibitor commonly used in treatment of multiple myeloma. Bortezomib typically causes a small-fiber axonal sensory neuropathy primarily characterized by painful paresthesias in the distal limbs.

Vincristine is an anti-microtubule agent used in treatment of multiple types of malignancies, including systemic lymphomas and certain pediatric and adult brain tumors. Neuropathy from vincristine is typically sensorimotor, favoring small sensory fibers and motor fibers. Patients can have painful paresthesias as well as motor weakness that most commonly affects dorsiflexion of the feet (i.e., foot drop) and extension of the wrists. Focal mononeuropathies and cranial neuropathies can occur, as can autonomic neuropathy often characterized by abdominal pain and constipation.

Paclitaxel and docetaxel (taxanes) are anti-microtubule agents used in treatment of breast, ovarian, and lung cancers. Peripheral neuropathy is a common side effect of taxanes and is typically mixed large- and small-fiber sensorimotor neuropathy affecting the feet more than the hands. Painful paresthesias are common, with motor weakness less common. Patients can get a phenomenon known as coasting, in which neuropathy symptoms worsen for several months after stopping therapy.

Methotrexate is an antimetabolite commonly used to treat leukemias and lymphomas and can be given intravenously and/or intrathecally. Methotrexate can cause a wide range of neurological toxicities, though peripheral neuropathy is not the most common. Methotrexate can cause acute, subacute, and chronic encephalopathy. Acute encephalopathy is characterized by altered mental status and sometimes seizures and typically occurs within 24–48 h of treatment; this acute encephalopathy is often transient and self-limited. Transverse myelopathy is also possible. Subacute encephalopathy can be characterized by stroke-like episodes with altered mental status and fluctuating focal neurological deficits such as aphasia or focal motor weakness. Chronic leukoencephalopathy can occur months to years after treatment and is characterized by personality changes, behavioral changes, gait impairment, and urinary incontinence; having had whole brain radiation therapy increases the risk of chronic leukoencephalopathy from methotrexate.

Reference

DeAngelis, L. M., Posner, J. B. (2009). Neurologic Complications of Cancer. United Kingdom: Oxford University Press, USA.

Linked questions: 12–13

12. An 8-year-old girl presents with headaches, nausea, vomiting, and imbalance. A brain MRI with and without contrast reveals the following. What is the most likely diagnosis?

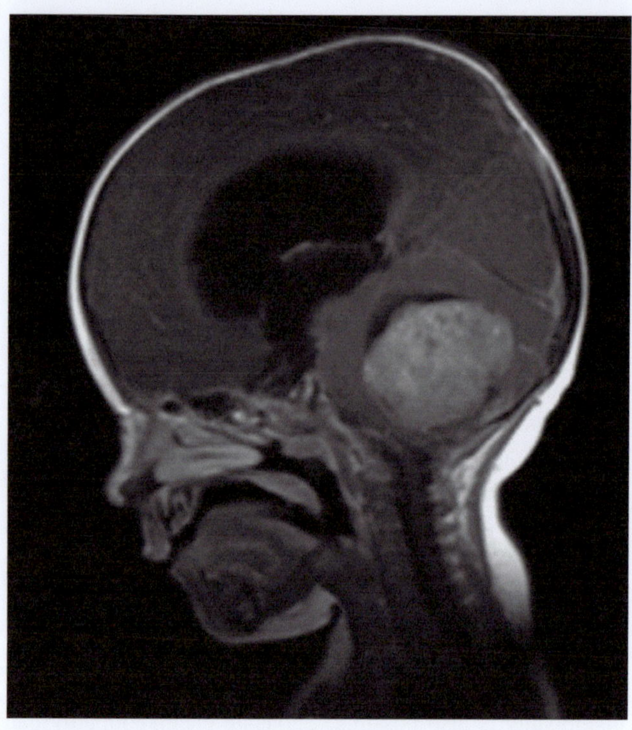

Sagittal brain MRI. (Source: DeSouza, R.-M., Jones, B. R. T., Lowis S. P., Kurian K. M. CC-BY 3.0 (https://creativecommons.org/licenses/by/3.0/) via *Frontiers in Oncology*. Image has been cropped from original. Please see full attribution with citation below in references section for this question.)

A. Glioblastoma
B. Pilocytic astrocytoma
C. Medulloblastoma
D. Chordoma
E. Metastasis from a systemic cancer

Correct answer: C

Explanation

Medulloblastoma is a Central Nervous System World Health Organization (CNS WHO) grade 4 embryonal tumor of the cerebellum most common in children and young adults (median age at diagnosis 9 years). Medulloblastoma is the second most common malignant brain tumor in children. Medulloblastomas are contrast-enhancing cerebellar masses that can exhibit restricted diffusion on MRI due to their hypercellularity.

Glioblastoma is a CNS WHO grade 4 astrocytoma. Glioblastoma typically appears as a heterogeneously enhancing mass lesion with associated T2/FLAIR signal abnormality. While glioblastomas can occur in the posterior fossa and are typically contrast-enhancing, they are uncommon in children and are most commonly supratentorial in location. Glioblastomas are typically diagnosed in the fifth to seventh decades of life and are the most common malignant brain tumors in adults.

Pilocytic astrocytoma is a CNS WHO grade 1 glioma and is the most common glioma seen in children, most often occurring in the first two decades of life. They are most commonly located in the cerebellum but can also be seen in the hypothalamus, third ventricle, optic nerves/optic pathways, brain stem, and spinal cord. Radiographically, pilocytic astrocytomas most often present as a cyst with an enhancing mural nodule, rather than the non-cystic, heterogeneously enhancing mass shown in the image provided.

Chordoma is an aggressive sarcoma of the bone that typically affects the skull base (resulting in cranial neuropathies) or spine (including the cervical spine and lumbosacral spine). They typically appear as expansile T2 hyperintense destructive osseous lesions.

Metastases from systemic malignancies typically appear on imaging as single or multiple contrast-enhancing lesions at the grey-white junction, often with associated vasogenic edema. While brain metastases are the most common brain tumors in adults, they are uncommon in children.

Linked question

13. Which of the following is incorrect regarding the tumor referred to in Question 12?
    A. Small round blue cells and Homer-Wright rosettes are pathologic features of this tumor.
    B. Staging with MRI spine and CSF examination must be done to evaluate for disseminated disease in all patients with this diagnosis.
    C. Extent of resection is a positive prognostic factor.
    D. Postoperative treatment includes a combination of craniospinal irradiation and chemotherapy.
    E. Among molecular subgroups of this tumor, group 3 has the best prognosis

Correct answer: E

Explanation

Medulloblastoma is a CNS WHO grade 4 embryonal tumor of the cerebellum most common in children and young adults (median age at diagnosis 9 years). Medulloblastoma is the second most common malignant brain tumor in children and accounts for approximately 20% of brain tumors in children. Up to 25% of medulloblastomas occur in adults. Medulloblastomas can be seen in the setting of certain inherited cancer syndromes—such as Gorlin syndrome (germline PTCH1, SUFU, or ELP1 mutation), Li-Fraumeni syndrome (germline TP53 mutation), and familial adenomatous polyposis (germline APC mutation). Because medulloblastomas contact the CSF space, they have the potential to disseminate into the spine and CSF. All patients should undergo MRI total spine with and without contrast and spinal fluid sampling with CSF cytology as part of staging workup.

Disseminated/metastatic disease into the spine/CSF is a poor prognosis factor.

On MRI, medulloblastomas are contrast-enhancing cerebellar masses that can exhibit restricted diffusion on MRI due to their hypercellularity.

Medulloblastoma is an embryonal tumor, and small round blue cells with high nuclear-to-cytoplasm ratio are a typical pathologic feature. Homer-Wright rosettes are dedifferentiated tumor cells grouped around a central region and are nearly pathognomonic for medulloblastoma.

Medulloblastomas are classified according to a combination of molecular and histologic features. Medulloblastomas are divided into molecular subgroups based on DNA methylation profiling, which are prognostically and therapeutically relevant. Molecular subgroups for medulloblastoma are as follows: WNT-activated, Sonic hedgehog (SHH)-activated, and non-WNT/non-SHH (further divided into group 3 and group 4). Histologic subgroups include classic, desmoplastic/nodular, or large cell/anaplastic histologies.

WNT-activated medulloblastomas contain beta-catenin (CTNNB1) mutations and have the most favorable prognosis. WNT-activated medulloblastomas typically occur in childhood (most commonly ages 7–14 years) and are predominantly associated with the classic histology. They can occur in patients with germline APC mutations.

SHH-activated medulloblastomas have an intermediate prognosis, with TP53-wildtype variants having a better prognosis and TP53-mutant variants having a poor prognosis. SHH-activated TP53-wildtype variants typically have desmoplastic/nodular histology and can have mutations in PTCH1, SMO, and SUFU; TP53-mutant variants typically have anaplastic/large cell histology. SHH-activated medulloblastomas have a bimodal age distribution (children and young adults) and are the most common medulloblastoma in adults. The TP53-wildtype variants can be seen in patients with germline PTCH1, SUFU, or ELP1 mutations, while the TP53-mutant variants can be seen in patients with germline TP53 mutations.

Group 3 medulloblastomas have a poor prognosis and tend to occur in infants and young children. They are often associated with MYC and MYCN amplification and well as classic histology. Group 4 medulloblastomas have an intermediate prognosis and can occur in all age groups. They are often associated with MYCN amplification as well as classic histology.

Positive prognostic factors for medulloblastoma include WNT-activated subgroup, desmoplastic/nodular histology, age greater than or equal to 3 years at diagnosis, gross total resection, and no disseminated/metastatic disease. Poorer prognostic factors include certain molecular subgroups (group 3, SHH-activated TP53-mutant), presence of MYC or MYCN amplification, large cell/anaplastic histology, age less than 3 years at diagnosis, incomplete resection, brain stem invasion, and disseminated/metastatic disease.

Surgical resection is the first step in treatment of a medulloblastoma, and prognosis is improved with increased extent of resection. Following resection, treatment typically includes craniospinal irradiation (radiation to the whole brain and whole spine) followed by multi-agent chemotherapy. For infants (less than 3 years of age), radiation is typically deferred given the propensity to lead to developmental delay, and multi-agent chemotherapy is given to delay radiation until the child is old enough. While medulloblastomas are aggressive, malignant tumors, survival for medulloblastoma can be up to 80% at 5 years.

References

DeSouza RM, Jones BR, Lowis SP, Kurian KM. Pediatric medulloblastoma - update on molecular classification driving targeted therapies. Front Oncol. 2014;4:176. https://doi.org/10.3389/fonc.2014.00176.

WHO Classification of Tumors. Central Nervous System Tumours. 5th ed. Geneva: World Health Organization; 2021.

Linked questions: 15–17

14. A 10-year-old boy presents with a seizure and is found on brain MRI with and without contrast to have a "bubbly"-appearing T2 hyperintense left mesial temporal lesion. The lesion is resected, and floating neurons are seen on pathology. What is the correct diagnosis?
    A. Dysembryoplastic neuroepithelial tumor (DNET)
    B. Pilocytic astrocytoma
    C. Ganglioglioma
    D. Central neurocytoma
    E. Gangliocytoma
    Correct answer: A

Explanation

Dysembryoplastic neuroepithelial tumor (DNET) is a CNS WHO grade 1 glioneuronal tumor most common in children and young adults (median age at diagnosis approximately 9 years). DNETs are typically located in the temporal lobe and present with seizures. They can be associated with cortical dysplasia. On MRI, DNETs can have mixed signal intensity on FLAIR with T2 hyperintense "bubbles" ("soap bubble" or "bubbly" appearance), with a cystic or multicystic appearance. On pathology, these are glioneuronal tumors positive for both synaptophysin (neuronal element) and GFAP (glial element) that can have oligodendroglia-like cells in the glial component. DNETs contain "floating neurons" on histology, which are neurons with normal cytology that seem to float in a mucoid matrix. DNETs can have

FGFR1 or BRAF mutations. DNETs can be observed if they are radiographically stable and minimally symptomatic/asymptomatic. Surgical resection is the treatment of choice for growing and/or symptomatic lesions.

Pilocytic astrocytoma is a CNS WHO grade 1 glioma and is the most common glioma seen in children, accounting for 17.6% of all childhood primary brain tumors. Pilocytic astrocytomas most commonly occur during the first two decades of life. They are most commonly located in the cerebellum but can also be seen in the hypothalamus, third ventricle, optic nerves/optic pathways, brain stem, and spinal cord. These are well-circumscribed tumors that typically do not invade the brain parenchyma. The optic pathway gliomas seen in neurofibromatosis type 1 are pilocytic astrocytomas. On MRI, they commonly present as a cyst with an enhancing mural nodule. Pathology is characterized by bipolar hairlike astrocytes, and pilocytic astrocytomas can have Rosenthal fibers and eosinophilic granular bodies. Multinucleated cells with horseshoe-shaped nuclear clusters ("pennies on a plate" pattern) can also be seen. Approximately 60–80% of pilocytic astrocytomas have KIAA1549-BRAF fusion gene, and they can have other alterations in the MAPK pathway as well. A small percentage (approximately 5%) can have BRAF V600E mutation. Surgical resection is the mainstay of treatment, and these tumors can be surgically cured. For residual/recurrent disease, targeted therapy with MEK inhibitors (such as trametinib) or RAF inhibitors (such as tovorafenib) can be considered for patients with BRAF fusion mutations. Of note, BRAF inhibitors (such as dabrafenib, encorafenib) should not be used with BRAF fusion mutations because they can increase tumor growth by paradoxically activating the MAPK pathway; such BRAF inhibitors should only be used when BRAF V600E mutation is present, in combination with a MEK inhibitor. Radiation therapy can also be considered for patients old enough to undergo radiation without significant risk of developmental delay (typically adults). Chemotherapy with carboplatin/vincristine has been used for residual/recurrent disease in children, but targeted therapies are favored nowadays when possible.

Ganglioglioma is a CNS WHO grade 1 glioneuronal tumor most common in children and young adults. They are typically located in the temporal lobe and present with seizures, and they are well-circumscribed. Most gangliogliomas present in the first or second decade of life, and the median age at diagnosis is 12 years. Gangliogliomas can have mixed solid and cystic components on MRI and can present as a cyst with an enhancing mural nodule in some cases. On histology, tumor cells exhibit mixed glial and neuronal components, with the glial components positive for GFAP and the neuronal components positive for synaptophysin, chromogranin, and neurofilament. The neuronal component is made up of dysmorphic ganglion cells, and the glial component can resemble astrocytoma or oligodendroglioma. Tumors can have eosinophilic granular bodies on pathology. Approximately 20–60% of gangliogliomas can have BRAF V600E mutations. Surgical resection is the mainstay of treatment. BRAF/MEK inhibitors and/or radiation can be considered for residual or recurrent disease.

Central neurocytoma is a CNS WHO grade 2 intraventricular neuroepithelial tumor. The majority of patients are diagnosed between ages 20 and 40 years. Central neurocytomas are typically located in the supratentorial compartment in the lateral ventricles and/or third ventricle; they are most commonly attached to the septum pellucidum near the foramen of Monro. On MRI, central neurocytomas exhibit a multicystic appearance on T2-weighted images and can have heterogeneous enhancement with gadolinium contrast. On pathology, central neurocytomas are composed of uniform round cells with a neuronal immunophenotype and typically with a low proliferation index. They are positive for synaptophysin, indicating their neuronal origin, and are most often negative for GFAP. Surgical resection is the mainstay of treatment, though radiation therapy can be considered for residual and/or recurrent tumors. The prognosis is typically favorable.

Gangliocytoma is a CNS WHO grade 1 glioneuronal tumor typically located in the temporal lobe. They are primarily seen in children. Dysplastic cerebellar gangliocytoma can be seen in Lhermitte-Duclos disease. Surgical resection is the treatment of choice.

Reference

WHO Classification of Tumors. Central Nervous System Tumours. 5th ed. Geneva: World Health Organization; 2021.

15. A 70-year-old man presents with a several-week history of headaches and vision changes. An brain MRI with and without contrast is shown below. What is the most likely diagnosis?

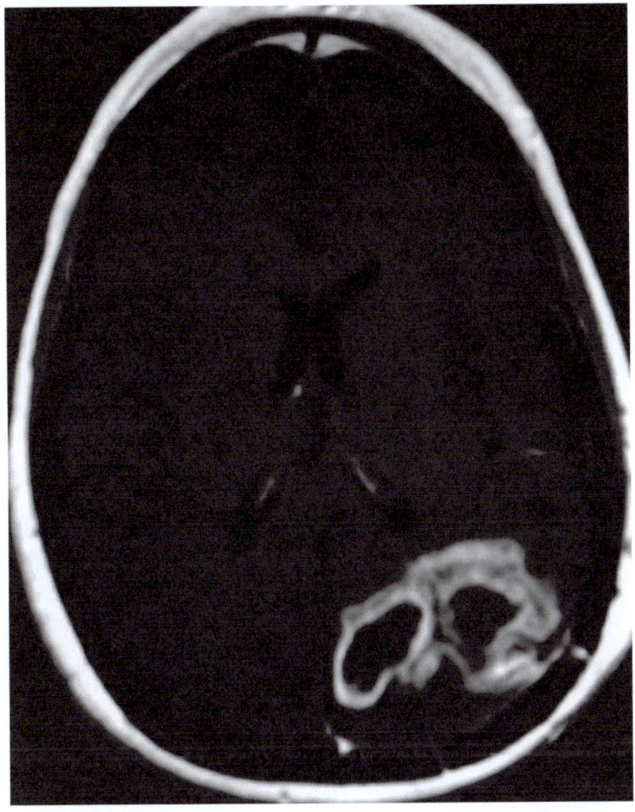

Axial brain MRI. (Source: Huang, R.Y., Neagu, M.R., Reardon, D. A., Wen, P. Y. CC-BY 4.0 (https://creativecommons.org/licenses/by/4.0/) via *Frontiers in Neurology*. Image has been cropped from original. Please see full attribution with citation below in references section for this question.)

A. Oligodendroglioma CNS WHO grade 2
B. Hemangioblastoma CNS WHO grade 1
C. Astrocytoma IDH-mutant CNS WHO grade 2
D. Pleomorphic xanthoastrocytoma CNS WHO grade 2
E. Glioblastoma CNS WHO grade 4

Correct answer: E

Explanation

Glioblastoma CNS WHO grade 4 is an aggressive, malignant, infiltrative high-grade astrocytoma and is the most common malignant brain tumor in adults. Glioblastoma is IDH-wildtype and H3-wildtype by definition. Glioblastoma accounts for approximately 15% of all intracranial neoplasms and 45–50% of all malignant primary brain tumors. Glioblastoma increases in incidence with increasing age and most commonly occurs in patients ages 55–85 years; glio-

blastomas are uncommon in children and comprise only 3% of CNS tumors in children. The prognosis for glioblastoma is poor, with median survival on the order of 18 months even with treatment. Typical features of a glioblastoma on brain MRI with and without contrast include heterogeneous enhancement with administration of gadolinium contrast, areas of central necrosis, and surrounding vasogenic edema. The image shown here depicts a heterogeneously enhancing mass in the left parietal lobe.

Oligodendrogliomas are diffuse gliomas of oligodendroglial origin that can be graded as CNS WHO grade 2 or 3 depending on their histologic features. Diffuse gliomas are gliomas that diffusely infiltrate the CNS parenchyma. These tumors are most common in young adults with a median age at diagnosis of 41 years for CNS WHO grade 2 tumors and 47 years for CNS WHO grade 3 tumors. They often present with seizures. Prognosis is more favorable for oligodendrogliomas than for astrocytomas. On MRI, oligodendrogliomas are expansile, T2/FLAIR hyperintense lesions that can contain calcifications. Grade 2 oligodendrogliomas are typically non-enhancing, whereas grade 3 oligodendrogliomas can exhibit contrast enhancement. The patient in the question stem is older than expected for a newly diagnosed oligodendroglioma, and a CNS WHO grade 2 oligodendroglioma would typically be non-enhancing, whereas the image provided depicts a heterogeneously enhancing mass more indicative of a high-grade tumor. Of note, prior to the fifth edition of the WHO Classification of Tumors of the Central Nervous System (WHO CNS5), grade 2 oligodendrogliomas were referred to as "oligodendroglioma" and grade 3 as "anaplastic oligodendroglioma"; however, as of the WHO CNS 5, they are simply referred to as oligodendroglioma CNS WHO grade 2 or 3.

Astrocytomas are diffuse gliomas of astrocytic origin and are stratified by the presence or absence of mutations in the isocitrate dehydrogenase (IDH) gene. The majority of IDH-wildtype astrocytomas in adults are glioblastoma, CNS WHO grade 4; glioblastoma is an IDH-wildtype tumor by definition. While IDH-wildtype astrocytomas such as glioblastoma are most common in adults in the fifth to seventh decades of life, ¬IDH-mutant astrocytomas occur in younger patients, most commonly in their 30 s–40 s. IDH¬-mutant astrocytomas can be CNS WHO grade 2, 3, or 4 depending on their histologic features. Importantly, IDH-mutant astrocytomas have a notably better prognosis than IDH-wildtype glioblastoma. On MRI, IDH mutant grade 2 astrocytomas typically present as non-enhancing expansile T2 hyperintense lesions. ¬IDH-mutant grade 4 astrocytomas can exhibit heterogeneous contrast enhancement, central necrosis, and vasogenic edema and can be indistinguishable on imaging from an IDH-wildtype glioblastoma. IDH-mutant grade 3 astrocytomas are T2 hyperintense masses that can exhibit contrast enhancement but do not always. The patient in the question stem is older than expected for a newly diagnosed IDH-mutant astrocytoma, and a grade 2 tumor would not typically exhibit the heterogeneous enhancement and central necrosis seen on this image. Of note, prior to the fifth edition of the WHO Classification of Tumors of the Central Nervous System (WHO CNS5), grade 2 astrocytomas were referred to as "diffuse astrocytoma," grade 3 as "anaplastic astrocytoma," and grade 4 as "glioblastoma." However, as of the WHO CNS5, "glioblastoma" is an IDH¬-wildtype tumor by definition, and IDH-mutant tumors are referred to as "astrocytoma, IDH-mutant, CNS WHO grade 2, 3, or 4" based on their histologic features.

Hemangioblastomas are vascular tumors that comprise <2% of all CNS tumors; they are not gliomas. Hemangioblastomas most commonly occur in the cerebellum but can also occur in the brain stem, spinal cord, and retina. Hemangioblastomas can occur sporadically or in association with von Hippel-Lindau (VHL) syndrome. Sporadic hemangioblastomas are more common in adults but can occur at a younger age in patients with VHL syndrome. Radiographically, hemangioblastomas typically present on MRI as a cystic lesion with an associated solidly enhancing nodule, rather than the heterogeneously enhancing mass shown here.

Pleomorphic xanthoastrocytoma (PXA) is a type of astrocytoma most commonly seen in children and young adults, with mean age at diagnosis 26.3 years. They are most commonly superficial and supratentorial in location and often present with seizures. PXAs are typically well-demarcated tumors. PXAs can be graded as CNS WHO grade 2 or 3. On MRI, PXA typically appears as a cystic lesion, often with a solidly enhancing component, rather than the heterogeneously enhancing mass seen in the question stem. The patient in the question stem is also older than would be expected for a patient with a newly diagnosed PXA.

References

Huang RY, Neagu MR, Reardon DA, Wen PY. Pitfalls in the neuroimaging of glioblastoma in the era of antiangiogenic and immuno/targeted therapy - detecting illusive disease, defining response. Front Neurol. 2015;6:33. https://doi.org/10.3389/fneur.2015.00033.

WHO Classification of Tumors. Central Nervous System Tumours. 5th ed. Geneva: World Health Organization; 2021.

Linked question

16. The tumor in Question 15 is resected, and histology is shown below. Which combination of histologic and molecular features is expected with this diagnosis?

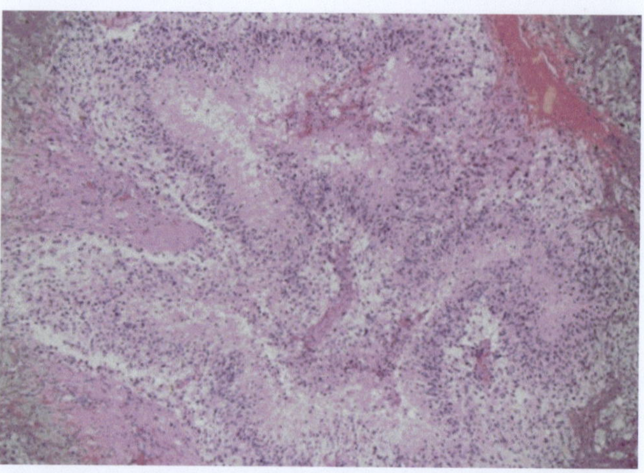

Micrograph. (Source: Mazur, M. D., Nguyen, V., Fults, D.W. CC-BY 3.0 (https://creativecommons.org/licenses/by/3.0/) via *Case Reports in Neurological Medicine*. Image has been cropped from original. Please see full attribution with citation below in references section for this question.)

A. Microvascular proliferation and palisading necrosis; EGFR amplification, TERT promoter mutation, +7/−10

B. "Fried egg" appearance; IDH1 or IDH2 mutation, 1p/19q codeletion

C. Multinucleated astrocytes filled with lipid droplets; BRAF V600E mutation

D. Lipidized stromal cells with rich capillary network; VHL gene loss or inactivation

E. Well-differentiated fibrillary glial cells; IDH1 or IDH2 mutation, p53 mutation, ATRX mutation

Correct answer: A

Explanation

Diffuse gliomas are gliomas that diffusely infiltrate the CNS parenchyma. Adult diffuse gliomas are categorized into two main group: astrocytomas (of astrocytic origin) and oligodendrogliomas (of oligodendroglial origin). Astrocytomas are further divided by the presence or absence of mutation in the isocitrate dehydrogenase (IDH) gene into IDH¬-mutant vs. IDH-wildtype astrocytomas. IDH mutation is prognostically important because it is associated with improved overall survival, and IDH-wildtype astrocytomas have a better prognosis than their IDH-wildtype counterparts.

The majority of IDH-wildtype diffuse gliomas seen in adults are glioblastoma, CNS WHO grade 4. Glioblastoma is an aggressive, malignant, high-grade astrocytoma with a poor prognosis (overall survival on the order of 18 months even with treatment). A glioblastoma can be diagnosed by either histologic or molecular criteria and, as of the WHO CNS 5, is IDH-wildtype by definition. Histologic features that are diagnostic of a glioblastoma include microvascular proliferation (rapid blood vessel growth characterized by multilayered small-caliber blood vessels) and palisading necrosis (shown in the question stem), which are required to make a diagnosis of glioblastoma by histologic criteria. Other histologic features that can be seen in glioblastoma include high-grade features such as high mitotic activity, nuclear atypia, and hypercellularity. A diagnosis of glioblastoma can also be made by molecular criteria in the absence of microvascular proliferation and necrosis; an IDH-wildtype astrocytoma that harbors either EGFR amplification, TERT promoter mutation, or whole chromosome 7 gain with whole chromosome 10 loss (+7/−10) can be called a glioblastoma by molecular criteria as these molecular features portend aggressive tumor behavior akin to that of a histologic glioblastoma despite having the histologic features of a lower-grade tumor. IDH-wildtype astrocytomas that do not meet histologic or molecular criteria for glioblastoma, and which do not harbor histone mutations, are known as "diffuse pediatric-type high-grade glioma, H3-wildtype and IDH-wildtype."

IDH-mutant astrocytomas can have either IDH1 or IDH2 mutations, with the most common mutation being IDH1 R132H. There are three grades of IDH-mutant astrocytoma: astrocytoma, IDH-mutant CNS WHO grade 2, 3, or 4. CNS WHO grade 2 tumors are composed of well-differentiated fibrillary glial cells that diffusely infiltrate the CNS parenchyma and exhibit low mitotic activity. CNS WHO grade 3 tumors exhibit increased mitotic activity and histological anaplasia as well as nuclear atypia but not microvascular proliferation or necrosis. CNS WHO grade 4 tumors exhibit microvascular proliferation and/or necrosis, in addition to high-grade histologic features such as high mitotic activity, hypercellularity, and nuclear atypia. Of note, microvascular proliferation and necrosis can be seen in both glioblastoma and astrocytoma IDH-mutant CNS WHO grade 4, the difference between the two being that glioblastoma is an IDH-wildtype tumor whereas astrocytoma IDH-mutant CNS WHO grade 4 is IDH-mutant. While the median overall survival for a glioblastoma even with treatment is approximately 18 months, the median overall survival for astrocytoma IDH-mutant CNS WHO grade 4 is on the order of 31+ months, showcasing the prognostic importance of IDH mutation. Unlike their IDH-wildtype counterparts, IDH-mutant astrocytomas typically harbor mutations in p53 and ATRX. Importantly, a diagnosis of astrocytoma IDH mutant CNS WHO grade 4 can also be made by molecular criteria, and IDH-mutant astrocytoma that harbors homozygous deletion of CDKN2A or CDKN2B is automatically considered grade 4 regardless of histology, as these molecular alterations portend a more aggressive clinical course.

Oligodendrogliomas are diffusely infiltrative gliomas of oligodendroglial origin. Oligodendrogliomas are character-

ized by uniformly round nuclei slightly larger than those of normal oligodendrocytes. In formalin-fixed, paraffin-embedded tissues, tumor cells can appear as rounded cells with well-defined cell membranes and clear cytoplasm, which produces the characteristic "fried egg" appearance. Oligodendrogliomas also exhibit a dense network of branching capillaries resembling chicken wire ("chicken-wire capillaries"). Oligodendrogliomas can be graded as CNS WHO grade 2 or 3. Grade 2 tumors are well-differentiated and have low or absent mitotic activity. Grade 3 tumors have more aggressive histologic features including high cellularity, marked cytological atypia, and brisk mitotic activity, and microvascular proliferation can be seen. Importantly, oligodendrogliomas are defined by two molecular criteria: IDH mutation (either IDH1 or IDH2 mutation) and whole-arm losses of chromosomes 1p and 19q (1p/19q codeletion). All oligodendrogliomas must have both IDH mutation and 1p/19q codeletion in order to be diagnosed as an oligodendroglioma; if a tumor has only IDH mutation and not 1p/19q codeletion, then the tumor is an astrocytoma. IDH mutation and 1p/19q codeletion are both associated with improved overall survival, and 1p/19q codeletion is also associated with improved response to treatment. Thus, the prognosis for oligodendrogliomas is better than that of astrocytomas, with median overall survival approximately 14–17 years with treatment for oligodendrogliomas (whereas the median overall survival for an IDH-mutant grade 2 astrocytoma is approximately 10–12 years)

Please see the table below for a summary of key molecular features associated with adult diffuse gliomas.

Tumor type	WHO grade	Molecular alterations
Glioblastoma, *IDH*-wildtype	4	*IDH*-wildtype; *TERT* promoter mutation, *EGFR* amplification, +7/−10
Astrocytoma, *IDH*-mutant	2, 3, 4	*IDH1, IDH2*; *ATRX, TP53*. Homozygous deletion of *CDKN2A/B* for grade 4
Oligodendroglioma	2, 3	*IDH1, IDH2*, 1p/19q codeletion

Lipidized stromal cells with a rich capillary network are the main histologic features of hemangioblastomas, which typically exhibit alterations in the *VHL* gene.

Pleomorphic xanthoastrocytomas (PXAs) are characterized histologically by a mixture of spindled, epithelioid, pleomorphic, and multinucleated astrocytes that are sometimes filled with lipid droplets (xanthomatous cells). Eosinophilic granular bodies and Rosenthal fibers can be seen as well. Approximately 60–80% of PXAs will have BRAF V600E mutations, and those without BRAF V600E mutations will contain other MAPK pathway alterations such as BRAF fusions or NTRK alterations. Treatment for

PXA includes maximal safe surgical resection. Targeted therapy with BRAF and MEK inhibitors can be considered for residual or recurrent disease if BRAF V600E mutation is present. Radiation therapy can also be considered for residual/recurrent disease.

References

Mazur MD, Nguyen V, Fults DW. Glioblastoma presenting with steroid-induced pseudoregression of contrast enhancement on magnetic resonance imaging. Case Rep Neurol Med. 2012;2012:816873. https://doi.org/10.1155/2012/816873.

WHO Classification of Tumors. Central Nervous System Tumours. 5th ed. Geneva: World Health Organization; 2021.

Linked question

17. Following surgical tissue sampling for confirmation of the pathologic diagnosis, what would be the most appropriate treatment regimen for the diagnosis from Question 15?
    A. Bevacizumab
    B. Radiation followed by PCV (procarbazine, CCNU, and vincristine)
    C. Radiation + temozolomide followed by adjuvant temozolomide
    D. Lomustine monotherapy
    E. Vorasidenib

Correct answer: C

Explanation

Initial treatment for adult diffuse gliomas, including glioblastoma, should be maximal safe resection when possible. Maximal safe surgical resection is associated with an overall survival benefit in retrospective studies, with increasing extent of resection corresponding with increasing overall survival. Maximal safe resection is also beneficial with respect to reducing mass effect and improving neurological symptoms caused by such mass effect. However, certain tumors are not amenable to surgical resection based on their location (e.g., tumors in the corpus callosum, eloquent areas including Broca's and Wernicke's areas and primary motor cortex, and deeper structures such as the brain stem), in which case a surgical biopsy to establish a tissue diagnosis must be pursued.

Following maximal safe resection or biopsy, standard treatment for a newly diagnosed glioblastoma includes concurrent radiation and oral chemotherapy with temozolomide for 6 weeks, followed by adjuvant temozolomide in 28-day cycles (5 days on, 23 days off) for 6–12 cycles; this is known as the Stupp protocol. Stupp et al. (2005) demonstrated that the combination of radiation + temozolomide followed by adjuvant temozolomide significantly improved overall survival compared with radiation therapy alone in patients with newly diagnosed glioblastoma, with median survival 14.6 months in the radiation + temozolomide group and 12.1 months in the radiation alone group. Temozolomide is an oral alkylating chemotherapy. Radiation therapy is given to a dose of 60 Gy in 30 fractions with a technique known as intensity-modulated radiation therapy (IMRT).

Bevacizumab, a humanized monoclonal antibody that binds to vascular endothelial growth factor A (VEGF-A), is an FDA-approved treatment for recurrent glioblastoma. Bevacizumab is given intravenously. Bevacizumab is an important palliative treatment for glioblastoma because it can reduce peritumoral edema and improve associated neurological symptoms and in turn can decrease patients' need for corticosteroids which have long-term adverse effects. However, while bevacizumab improves progression-free survival in recurrent glioblastoma, it does not improve overall survival. Bevacizumab is typically used for recurrent, rather than newly diagnosed, glioblastoma.

Lomustine (CCNU) is an oral nitrosourea (carmustine/BCNU is the intravenous counterpart) and is an FDA-approved treatment for recurrent glioblastoma.

Radiation followed by PCV (procarbazine, CCNU/lomustine, and vincristine) is the standard treatment for newly diagnosed oligodendroglioma following surgery. The combination of radiation and PCV has been shown to significantly increase overall survival compared with radiation alone in IDH-mutant, 1p/19q codeleted oligodendrogliomas.

Vorasidenib is an oral IDH inhibitor that was recently FDA-approved for treatment of residual or recurrent IDH-mutant grade 2 gliomas (either astrocytomas or oligodendrogliomas) following surgical resection. The phase 3 INDIGO trial demonstrated that treatment with vorasidenib for residual or recurrent IDH-mutant grade 2 gliomas following surgery significantly improved progression-free survival and time to next intervention compared with placebo. Vorasidenib is used in an effort to delay the need for radiation and chemotherapy, as IDH-mutant gliomas tend to occur in younger adults, and such patients can have long-term cognitive sequelae from undergoing radiation at a young age.

References

Buckner, J. C., Shaw, E. G., Pugh, S. L., Chakravarti, A., Gilbert, M. R., Barger, G. R., Coons, S., Ricci, P., Bullard, D., Brown, P. D., Stelzer, K., Brachman, D., Suh, J. H., Schultz, C. J., Bahary, J. P., Fisher, B. J., Kim, H., Murtha, A. D., Bell, E. H., Won, M., … Curran, W. J., Jr. (2016).

Radiation plus Procarbazine, CCNU, and Vincristine in Low-Grade Glioma. The New England journal of medicine, 374(14), 1344–1355. https://doi.org/10.1056/NEJMoa1500925

Cairncross, G., Wang, M., Shaw, E., Jenkins, R., Brachman, D., Buckner, J., Fink, K., Souhami, L., Laperriere, N., Curran, W., & Mehta, M. (2013). Phase III trial of chemoradiotherapy for anaplastic oligodendroglioma: long-term results of RTOG 9402. Journal of clinical oncology: official journal of the American Society of Clinical Oncology, 31(3), 337–343. https://doi.org/10.1200/JCO.2012.43.2674

Mellinghoff, I. K., van den Bent, M. J., Blumenthal, D. T., Touat, M., Peters, K. B., Clarke, J., Mendez, J., Yust-Katz, S., Welsh, L., Mason, W. P., Ducray, F., Umemura, Y., Nabors, B., Holdhoff, M., Hottinger, A. F., Arakawa, Y., Sepulveda, J. M., Wick, W., Soffietti, R., Perry, J. R., … INDIGO Trial Investigators (2023). Vorasidenib in IDH1- or IDH2-Mutant Low-Grade Glioma. The New England journal of medicine, 389(7), 589–601. https://doi.org/10.1056/NEJMoa2304194

Stupp, R., Mason, W. P., van den Bent, M. J., Weller, M., Fisher, B., Taphoorn, M. J., Belanger, K., Brandes, A. A., Marosi, C., Bogdahn, U., Curschmann, J., Janzer, R. C., Ludwin, S. K., Gorlia, T., Allgeier, A., Lacombe, D., Cairncross, J. G., Eisenhauer, E., Mirimanoff, R. O., European Organisation for Research and Treatment of Cancer Brain Tumor and Radiotherapy Groups, … National Cancer Institute of Canada Clinical Trials Group (2005). Radiotherapy plus concomitant and adjuvant temozolomide for glioblastoma. The New England journal of medicine, 352(10), 987–996. https://doi.org/10.1056/NEJMoa043330

Wick, W., Gorlia, T., Bendszus, M., Taphoorn, M., Sahm, F., Harting, I., Brandes, A. A., Taal, W., Domont, J., Idbaih, A., Campone, M., Clement, P. M., Stupp, R., Fabbro, M., Le Rhun, E., Dubois, F., Weller, M., von Deimling, A., Golfinopoulos, V., Bromberg, J. C., … van den Bent, M. J. (2017). Lomustine and Bevacizumab in Progressive Glioblastoma. The New England journal of medicine, 377(20), 1954–1963. https://doi.org/10.1056/NEJMoa1707358

18. Which of the following is a negative prognostic factor in glioblastoma?
    A. MGMT promoter methylation
    B. Older age
    C. Increased extent of resection
    D. Higher performance status
    E. Elevated Ki67 proliferation index
    Correct answer: B

Explanation

Older age is a worse prognostic factor in glioblastoma; younger patients have an improved overall survival compared with older patients. Increasing extent of resection is associated with increasing overall survival in glioblastoma in retrospective studies. Patients with higher neurological performance status have a better prognosis than those with poorer performance status. Performance status is often measured by the Karnofsky Performance Status (KPS) scale.

O6-methylguanine-DNA methyltransferase (MGMT) is a DNA repair enzyme that antagonizes the effects of alkylating chemotherapy, such as temozolomide or lomustine. When MGMT is methylated, it becomes inactive and cannot oppose the effect of alkylating chemotherapy, thus making alkylating chemotherapy more effective. Treatment with temozolomide is significantly more effective in MGMT promoter methylated glioblastomas, and MGMT promoter methylation is associated with improved overall survival. Approximately 1/3 of glioblastomas are MGMT promoter methylated.

High-grade gliomas tend to exhibit an elevated Ki67 proliferation index on histology, but on its own, an elevated Ki67 is not a specific prognostic factor in glioblastoma.

19. A 71-year-old woman presents with a seizure. Her brain MRI is shown below. Upon resection, pathology reveals psammoma bodies.

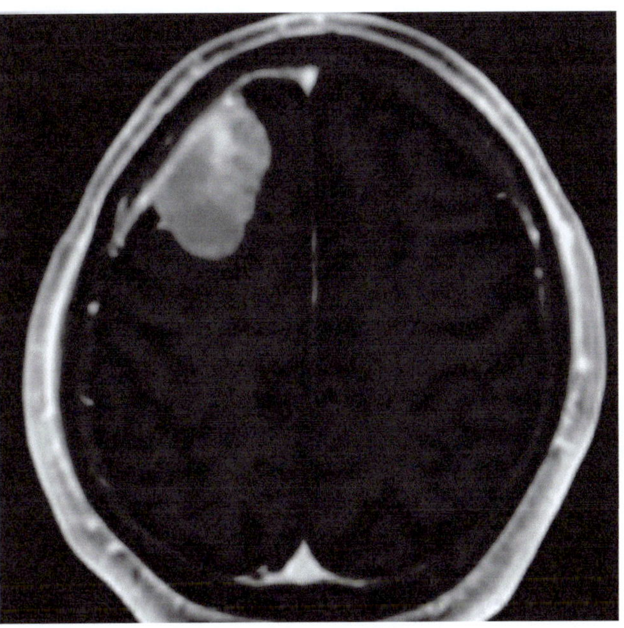

Axial brain MRI. (Source: Okuchi, S., Okada, T., Yamamoto, A., Kanagaki, M., Fushimi, Y., Okada, T., Yamauchi, M., Kataoka, M., Arakawa, Y., Takahashi, J. C., Minamiguchi, S., Miyamoto, S., Togashi, K. CC-BY 4.0 (https://creativecommons.org/licenses/by/4.0/) via *Medicine*. Image has been cropped from original. Please see full attribution with citation below in references section for this question.)

Which of the following is incorrect regarding this tumor type?

A. TERT promoter mutation and CDKN2A/B deletion are indicative of more aggressive behavior.

B. Multiple of these can be seen in neurofibromatosis type 1.

C. It is the most common primary brain tumor in adults.

D. Surgical resection and radiation therapy are the mainstays of treatment.

E. These tumors typically compress rather than invade the brain.

Correct answer: B

Explanation

The tumor shown on this MRI is a meningioma. Meningiomas are dural-based, extra-axial tumors that arise from meningothelial cells of the arachnoid mater. Meningiomas are the most common primary brain tumors in adults, and their incidence increases with age, with median age at diagnosis 66 years. Meningiomas are more common in women than in men, with the incidence 2.32 times higher in women than in men. Meningiomas are most commonly located along the cerebral convexities, falx cerebri/parasagittal regions, olfactory grooves, sphenoid wings, suprasellar/parasellar region, optic pathways, tentorium, and the spinal cord. Exposure to ionizing radiation (e.g., via nuclear disasters or treatment of childhood cancers such as leukemia or medulloblastoma with cranial radiation) is a risk factor for developing meningiomas. Breast cancer is also a risk factor for developing meningiomas. Multiple meningiomas can be seen with certain genetic syndromes, such as neurofibromatosis type 2 (NF2) and Gorlin syndrome. Meningiomas typically compress rather than invade the brain, though brain invasion can be seen with higher-grade tumors.

On MRI, meningiomas typically appear as homogeneously enhancing dural-based masses which can have associated vasogenic edema but do not always. A dural tail is indicative of an extra-axial mass. A CSF cleft (rim of T2 hyperintensity surrounding the mass on T2-weighted image) is also a radiographic indicator of an extra-axial mass.

On pathology, meningiomas are graded as CNS WHO grade 1, 2, or 3. CNS WHO grade 1 meningiomas are typically slow-growing and indolent in behavior, whereas CNS WHO grade 3 meningiomas are aggressive, malignant tumors. CNS WHO grade 2 meningiomas vary in clinical behavior, with some closer to grade 3 and some closer to grade 1 in behavior. There are many morphologic subtypes of meningiomas on histology, with the most common including meningothelial, transitional, and fibrous meningiomas. Calcifications are common. Psammoma bodies (calcified, concentric, lamellated structures) can be seen on histology. Loss of chromosome 22 is common in meningiomas. CNS WHO grade 1 tumors have fewer than 4 mitoses in 10 high-powered fields (HPF). CNS WHO grade 2 tumors meet at least one of the following criteria: (1) 4–19 mitotic figures in 10 HPF, (2) unequivocal brain invasion, (3) clear cell or chordoid morphologic subtype, or (4) at least three of the following: increased cellularity, small cells with high nuclear-to-cytoplasm ratio, prominent nucleoli, sheeting, or foci of spontaneous (non-iatrogenic) necrosis. CNS WHO grade 3 tumors meet at least one of the following criteria: (1) 20 or more mitotic figures in 10 HPF, (2) frank anaplasia (sarcoma-like, carcinoma-like, or melanoma-like appearance), (3) TERT promoter mutation, or (4) homozygous deletion of CDKN2A and/or CDKN2B. Of note, TERT promoter mutation and homozygous deletion of CDKN2A and/or CDKN2B are indicators of more aggressive behavior and automatically make a tumor in which they are present CNS WHO grade 3. Tumors referred to as "atypical meningioma" must meet criteria for CNS WHO grade 2 meningioma, and tumors referred to as "anaplastic (malignant) meningioma" must meet criteria for CNS WHO grade 3 meningioma.

Surgical resection and radiation therapy are the mainstays of treatment for meningiomas, and there are no approved systemic therapies for meningioma. Extent of resection is inversely correlated with the risk of recurrence, with recurrence risk decreasing with increasing extent of resection. CNS WHO grade 1 tumors are typically observed after surgery, with radiation therapy (either fractionated radiation therapy or stereotactic radiosurgery depending on the size and location of the tumor) pursued if there is recurrence after surgery, though radiation therapy can also be considered if there is residual disease after surgery. Radiation therapy is indicated after resection of CNS WHO grade 3 meningiomas given their aggressive behavior. Radiation therapy is pursued for subtotally resected CNS WHO grade 2 meningiomas. However, the role of up-front radiation therapy for gross totally resected CNS WHO grade 2 meningiomas is less clear, as an overall survival benefit has not been clearly demonstrated for up-front radiation therapy after gross total resection of a CNS WHO grade 2 meningioma. Thus, gross totally resected CNS WHO grade 2 meningiomas can be observed with radiation therapy pursued at recurrence, though up-front radiation therapy can also be considered.

References

Okuchi S, Okada T, Yamamoto A, Kanagaki M, Fushimi Y, Okada T, et al. Grading meningioma: a comparative study of thallium-SPECT and FDG-PET. Medicine (Baltimore). 2015;94(6):e549. https://doi.org/10.1097/md.0000000000000549.

WHO Classification of Tumors. Central Nervous System Tumours. 5th ed. Geneva: World Health Organization; 2021.

20. A 16-year-old boy presents with nausea, vomiting, and imbalance and is found to have a contrast-enhancing intraventricular mass in the fourth ventricle causing obstructive hydrocephalus. Pathology from surgical resection is shown below, and a diagnosis of ependymoma is made. Which of the following is correct regarding this diagnosis?

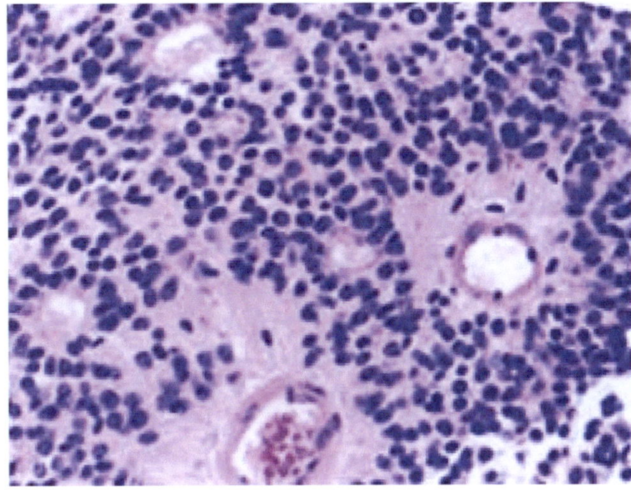

Micrograph. (Source: Ahmed, M. U. CC-BY 4.0 (https://creativecommons.org/licenses/by/4.0/) via *Journal of Enam Medical College.* Image has not been modified from original. Please see full attribution with citation below in references section for this question.)

A. Posterior fossa group A ependymomas are more common in adults.
B. ZFTA fusion is seen in posterior fossa ependymomas.
C. Chemotherapy is the mainstay of treatment for intracranial ependymomas.
D. Perivascular pseudorosettes are a common histologic feature.
E. YAP1 fusion is associated with a less favorable prognosis.

Correct answer: D

Explanation

Ependymomas are ependymal gliomas which, unlike diffuse gliomas, are typically well-circumscribed and compress rather than infiltrate the brain. Ependymomas can be located supratentorially, infratentorially, or in the spinal cord. Supratentorial ependymomas can be seen in adults but are

more common in children, and their incidence decreases with increasing age; the proportion of ependymomas arising from the supratentorial compartment is 41% in children, 27% in adolescents, 12% in young adults, and 11% in adults age >45 years. Posterior fossa ependymomas can develop in any age group but are more common in children. All intracranial ependymomas can have drop metastases/CSF dissemination due to contact with the CSF space and thus require staging with MRI total spine with and without contrast and lumbar puncture with CSF cytology. Prognosis is worse if there are drop metastases/CSF dissemination at diagnosis. Prognosis is also worse for patients younger than 3 years of age at diagnosis.

On MRI, ependymomas exhibit irregular contrast enhancement and can contain cysts or calcifications.

On pathology, intracranial ependymomas can be CNS WHO grade 2 or 3; CNS WHO grade 3 ependymomas were previously referred to as "anaplastic ependymoma" prior to the WHO CNS5. WHO grade 3 tumors can exhibit brisk mitotic activity and microvascular proliferation. Perivascular pseudorosettes and true ependymal rosettes can be seen on histology in ependymomas. Perivascular pseudorosettes (seen in the micrograph provided in the question stem) are tumor cells arranged in a radial fashion around blood vessels. True ependymal rosettes are composed of columnar or cuboidal cells surrounding an empty lumen.

Ependymomas are categorized by their anatomic location (supratentorial, infratentorial, or spinal) and further subcategorized based on molecular criteria. Supratentorial ependymomas have two molecular categories: supratentorial ependymoma, ZFTA fusion-positive, and supratentorial ependymoma, YAP1 fusion-positive. Supratentorial ependymoma, ZFTA fusion-positive, can be seen in both children and adults and has a poorer prognosis. Supratentorial ependymoma, YAP1 fusion-positive, is more common in young children and has a favorable prognosis. Posterior fossa ependymomas are divided into posterior fossa group A (PFA) and posterior fossa group B (PFB) ependymomas based on methylation profiling. PFA ependymomas occur predominantly in infants and young children with a median age at diagnosis of 3 years and have a poor prognosis compared with PFB ependymomas. PFB ependymomas occur in children and adults with median age at diagnosis 30 years and have a favorable prognosis.

Treatment for intracranial ependymomas involves maximal safe resection followed by radiation therapy. Maximal safe resection is prognostically important, as outcomes are more favorable with increasing extent of resection. Focal radiation therapy is typically pursued after surgery for intracranial ependymomas. Ependymomas with drop metastases/

CSF dissemination at diagnosis are treated with craniospinal irradiation. The role of chemotherapy in treatment of ependymomas is less clear and is not typically part of the standard of care outside the context of clinical trials or recurrent disease that does not have safe surgical or radiation options. Most often, chemotherapy is used in infants and young children to try to delay radiation therapy, as radiation in this age group can lead to adverse developmental and cognitive consequences.

Subependymomas are CNS WHO grade 1 tumors characterized by clustering of uniform to mildly pleomorphic tumor cell nuclei in abundant fibrillary matrix. They are typically found in adults (peak incidence age 40–84 years) and are most commonly seen in the fourth ventricle or lateral ventricles, though they can be seen in the third ventricle and spinal cord more rarely. Subependymomas are often asymptomatic and found incidentally, but when symptomatic, they can cause obstructive hydrocephalus and associated signs and symptoms. Subependymomas are managed with surveillance imaging if they are small and incidentally discovered. On MRI, subependymomas are well-demarcated intraventricular lesions that are typically non-contrast-enhancing or minimally contrast-enhancing. If large and/or symptomatic, surgical resection is the mainstay of treatment, and these tumors can be surgically cured. Radiation therapy is reserved for recurrent disease or tumors that are not surgically resectable.

References

Ahmed MU. Rosettes and Pseudorosettes and Their Significance. Journal of Enam Medical College. 2017;7(2):101–6. https://doi.org/10.3329/jemc.v7i2.32656. (https://commons.wikimedia.org/wiki/File:Micrograph_of_perivascular_pseudorosettes.jpg).

WHO Classification of Tumors. Central Nervous System Tumours. 5th ed. Geneva: World Health Organization; 2021.

21. A 45-year-old man presents with low back pain and is found to have the following on MRI lumbar spine with and without contrast. Which of the following is correct about this diagnosis?

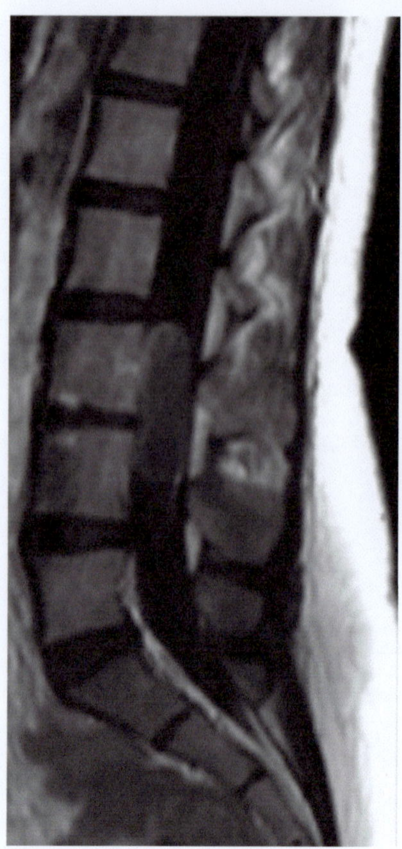

Sagittal MRI lumbar spine. (Source: Roma, D., Palma, P., Capolino, R., Figà-Talamanca, L., Diomedi-Camassei, F., Lepri, F. R., Digilio, M. C., Marras, C. E., Messina, R., Carai, A., Randi, F., Mastronuzzi, A. CC-BY 4.0 (https://creativecommons.org/licenses/by/4.0/) via *BMC Medical Genetics*. Image has been cropped from original. Please see full attribution with citation below in references section for this question.)

A. This is a CNS WHO grade 1 tumor.
B. These tumors are more common in children.
C. They are called myxopapillary ependymoma when located at the filum terminale.
D. Radiation therapy is always indicated after surgical resection.
E. MYCN amplification is a positive prognostic factor.

Correct answer: C

Explanation

Spinal ependymomas are intramedullary spinal cord tumors most commonly seen in adults, with median age at diagnosis 45 years. Spinal ependymomas can be CNS WHO grade 2 or 3. When located at the filum terminale, they are referred to as myxopapillary ependymomas, which are CNS WHO grade 2 tumors. On MRI, spinal ependymomas appear as contrast-enhancing intramedullary masses that can be associated with syringomyelia. NF2 mutations are common in spinal ependymomas. The prognosis for spinal ependymomas is generally favorable. However, the presence of MYCN amplification is a poorer prognostic factor; "spinal ependymoma, ¬MYCN-amplified," is a diagnostic entity without a specific CNS WHO grade which is typically associated with high-grade histology and which has poorer progression-free survival and overall survival compared with other spinal ependymomas. Spinal ependymomas are treated with surgical resection. If a gross total resection is achieved, up-front radiation therapy is not always indicated, and observation can be considered. However, radiation therapy should be pursued if there is a subtotal resection after surgery or for recurrent disease after surgery.

References

Roma D, Palma P, Capolino R, Figà-Talamanca L, Diomedi-Camassei F, Lepri FR, et al. Spinal ependymoma in a patient with Kabuki syndrome: a case report. BMC Med Genet. 2015;16:80. https://doi.org/10.1186/s12881-015-0228-4.

WHO Classification of Tumors. Central Nervous System Tumours. 5th ed. Geneva: World Health Organization; 2021.

22. A 2-year-old girl is found on routine wellness check to have leukocoria on exam and is ultimately diagnosed with retinoblastoma. Which of the following is incorrect regarding retinoblastoma?
    A. Retinoblastoma is the most common primary intra-ocular tumor worldwide.
    B. Familial retinoblastomas arise at an earlier age than sporadic retinoblastomas.
    C. Trilateral retinoblastoma is characterized by a combination of bilateral retinoblastoma and a histologically similar intracranial tumor.
    D. Retinoblastoma is a small round blue cell tumor.
    E. Familial retinoblastoma is characterized by mutations in the PTCH1 gene.

    Correct answer: E

Explanation

Retinoblastoma is a malignant pediatric retinal neoplasm and is the most common primary intraocular tumor in infants worldwide. The mean age at diagnosis is 18 months (younger for bilateral retinoblastoma), and most cases are diagnosed before age 3. Patients often present with leukocoria (white pupillary light reflex) and strabismus. Retinoblastomas can be sporadic or familial and are caused by germline or somatic mutations in the RB1 tumor suppressor gene on chromosome 13. Familial retinoblastoma is caused by germline pathogenic mutation in the RB1 gene and is inherited in an autosomal dominant fashion. Familial retinoblastoma tends to arise at an earlier age (approximately 12 months) than sporadic retinoblastoma (approximately 24 months). Approximately 60% of patients with germline RB1 pathogenic variants develop bilateral tumors, and germline mutation carriers are at higher risk of secondary non-ocular neoplasms, including sarcomas and pineoblastoma. The combination of bilateral retinoblastoma and a histologically similar tumor, most often in the pineal gland (pineoblastoma) or suprasellar region, is known as trilateral retinoblastoma and has a poor prognosis. Histologically, retinoblastoma is a small round blue cell tumor composed of primitive neuroblastic cells. Flexner-Wintersteiner rosettes are a characteristic pathologic feature of retinoblastoma but can occur in other neoplasms such as pineoblastoma. Retinoblastoma is fatal if untreated. Treatment options include ophthalmic artery chemosurgery (OAC), radioactive plaques such as I-125 brachytherapy, and enucleation as well as cryotherapy, laser photoablation, intravitreal chemotherapy, and systemic chemotherapy depending on the tumor size, location, and laterality as well as the presence or absence of vitreous or sub-retinal seeds, presence of absence of metastatic disease, the patient's age, and the patient's visual prognosis.

Mutations in the PTCH1 gene can lead to Gorlin syndrome (nevoid basal cell carcinoma syndrome), an autosomal dominant tumor predisposition syndrome characterized by pathogenic mutations in the PTCH1 or SUFU genes which can lead to developmental anomalies, multiple basal cell carcinomas, odontogenic keratocysts of the jaw, intracranial ectopic calcifications, palmar and/or plantar pits, increased risk of medulloblastoma, multiple meningiomas, and skeletal abnormalities, among others.

Reference

WHO Classification of Tumors. Central Nervous System Tumours. 5th ed. Geneva: World Health Organization; 2021.

23. A 6-year-old girl presents with headaches and lethargy and is found to have a contrast-enhancing cauliflower-like lesion in the left lateral ventricle with obstructive hydrocephalus. Surgical resection is performed, and histology reveals fibrovascular fronds covered by a single layer of epithelial cells. Which is the correct diagnosis?
   A. Central neurocytoma
   B. Pilocytic astrocytoma
   C. Craniopharyngioma
   D. Choroid plexus papilloma
   E. Intraventricular meningioma

Correct answer: D

Explanation

The tumor referred to in the question stem is a choroid plexus papilloma. Choroid plexus papilloma is an intraventricular papillary neoplasm derived from choroid plexus epithelium and is a CNS WHO grade 1 tumor. They are most commonly located in the lateral ventricles, followed by the fourth ventricle and third ventricle. Choroid plexus papillomas are more common in children, accounting for 2–4% of brain tumors occurring in children age <15 years and 10–20% of brain tumors occurring in children in the first year of life. Choroid plexus papillomas often present with obstructive hydrocephalus and associated increased intracranial pressure. It has been debated whether overproduction of CSF contributes to hydrocephalus in choroid plexus papillomas. On CT and MRI, choroid plexus papillomas typically appear as an isodense or hyperdense, T2 hyperintense, and irregularly contrast-enhancing "cauliflower-like" intraventricular mass. CSF spread and drop metastases are rare but possible. On histology, choroid plexus papillomas are characterized by a well-developed papillary pattern of fibrovascular fronds covered by a single layer of cuboidal to columnar epithelial cells. Mitotic activity is typically absent or very low (<2 mitoses/10 HPF). Surgical resection is the mainstay of treatment, and prognosis is favorable particularly with gross total resection.

Atypical choroid plexus papilloma is a choroid plexus papilloma with increased mitotic activity but which does not fulfill criteria for choroid plexus carcinoma and is a CNS WHO grade 2 tumor. Atypical choroid plexus papillomas are more common in the lateral ventricles. Atypical choroid plexus papillomas have higher mitotic activity (two or more mitoses/ten HPF) than CNS WHO grade 1 choroid plexus papillomas and may have one to two of the following four features: increased cellularity, nuclear pleomorphism, blurring of the papillary pattern (solid growth), and areas of necrosis, though these features are not required for diagnosis. Surgical resection is the mainstay of treatment.

Choroid plexus carcinoma is a malignant epithelial neoplasm of the choroid plexus and is CNS WHO grade 3 by definition. Approximately 80% of choroid plexus carcino-mas occur in children. Most choroid plexus carcinomas occur sporadically, but approximately 40% occur in the setting of Li-Fraumeni syndrome with germline TP53 mutation; choroid plexus carcinomas can also be seen in Aicardi syndrome. Metastases are present in approximately 21% of cases at diagnosis. On MRI, choroid plexus carcinomas are typically large contrast-enhancing intraventricular masses with heterogeneous signal on T1- and T2-weighted images and associated edema. Choroid plexus carcinoma must have at least four of the following histologic features: frequent mitoses (usually >5 mitoses/10 HPF), increased cellular density, nuclear pleomorphism, blurring of the papillary pattern with poorly structured sheets of tumor cells, and necrotic areas. Treatment involves surgical resection followed by radiation therapy, though multi-agent chemotherapy with deferred radiation can be considered in young children. Prognosis is poor, with 5-year progression-free survival 38% and 5-year overall survival 62%. TP53 mutations are associated with a less favorable prognosis.

Central neurocytoma most commonly appears on MRI as a mixed solid and cystic intraventricular mass attached to the septum pellucidum and is typically seen in older patients than the patient in the question stem (most are diagnosed between ages 20 and 40 years). Pilocytic astrocytoma most commonly appears on MRI as a mixed solid and cystic lesion in the cerebellum, with a cyst associated with a more solidly enhancing mural nodule. Craniopharyngiomas are typically seen on MRI as sellar/parasellar masses which can have solid and cystic components. Meningiomas can be seen intraventricularly and are typically homogeneously enhancing dural-based masses on MRI, but meningioma would be uncommon in this age group.

Reference

WHO Classification of Tumors. Central Nervous System Tumours. 5th ed. Geneva: World Health Organization; 2021.

Linked questions: 24–25

24. A 75-year-old man presents with confusion and left-sided weakness and is found to have a homogeneously enhancing right periventricular mass. He is ultimately diagnosed with primary CNS lymphoma. Which of the following is incorrect regarding primary CNS lymphoma?
   A. Primary CNS lymphoma is associated with Epstein-Barr virus (EBV) in immunocompromised but not immunocompetent patients.
   B. Whole-brain radiation therapy is the preferred treatment.
   C. Maximal safe resection is not recommended.

D. Most primary CNS lymphomas are diffuse large B-cell lymphoma.

E. Lesions can exhibit restricted diffusion on MRI

Correct answer: B

Linked question

25. For the patient in question 24, which of the following is not required as part of the staging evaluation?
    A. MRI total spine with and without contrast
    B. Lumbar puncture with CSF cytology and flow cytometry
    C. Slit lamp exam
    D. Peripheral blood flow cytometry
    E. CT chest, abdomen, and pelvis with contrast or systemic FDG PET CT

Correct answer: D

Explanation for Questions 24 and 25

Primary CNS lymphoma is a rare extranodal non-Hodgkin lymphoma arising solely from the brain, spinal cord, leptomeninges, and/or eyes without evidence of systemic disease. The majority of primary CNS lymphomas are diffuse large B-cell lymphomas (DLBCL), and primary CNS T-cell lymphomas are exceedingly rare. Primary CNS DLBCL accounts for 2.4–3% of all brain tumors and 4–6% of all extranodal lymphomas. Primary CNS lymphoma can occur in both immunocompetent and immunocompromised patients, and the incidence of primary CNS lymphoma increases with age in immunocompetent patients. Primary CNS DLBCL has a peak incidence during the fifth to seventh decades of life, and the median age at diagnosis is 66 years. Primary CNS lymphoma is associated with Epstein-Barr virus (EBV) in immunocompromised patients but not in immunocompetent patients. Immunocompromised states associated with increased risk of primary CNS lymphoma include poorly controlled HIV/AIDS and iatrogenic chronic immunosuppression (e.g., in patients with solid organ transplants or rheumatologic conditions treated with chronic immunosuppressive medications).

Radiographically, primary CNS lymphoma can appear as a single lesion or as multifocal lesions. Tumors are most often located in the cerebral hemispheres (38%), thalamus and basal ganglia (16%), corpus callosum (14%), and periventricular region (12%). Lesions are most commonly homogeneously enhancing on MRI and can have associated restricted diffusion. Ring enhancement is typically seen in immunocompromised patients. On pathology, a lymphocytic infiltrate can be seen along the perivascular spaces.

All patients with primary CNS lymphoma require staging workup to determine the extent of disease and assess whether there is systemic disease present. Systemic imaging with a CT chest, abdomen, and pelvis with contrast or systemic FDG PET CT is indicated to evaluate for systemic disease, and testicular ultrasound is advised in patients with testes, as testicular lymphoma can spread to the CNS. Bone marrow biopsy can also be considered as part of systemic staging. Lumbar puncture with CSF examination, including CSF cytology and flow cytometry, is indicated to evaluate for CSF spread/leptomeningeal disease. MRI total spine and without contrast is indicated to assess for spinal/leptomeningeal involvement, but peripheral blood flow cytometry is not part of the standard staging evaluation. All patients should have an ophthalmologic exam, including a slit lamp exam, to evaluate for vitreal involvement.

Surgical resection is not considered part of standard treatment for primary CNS lymphoma, and only biopsy is required to establish a tissue diagnosis. Corticosteroids should be avoided prior to biopsy if possible, as steroids are lymphotoxic and can result in a false-negative biopsy result. Multi-agent chemotherapy with high-dose IV methotrexate as the backbone is the mainstay of treatment for primary CNS lymphoma, with complete radiographic response (i.e., resolution of all contrast-enhancing disease) as the treatment goal. Whole-brain radiation therapy is an effective treatment for primary CNS lymphoma but is not favored as up-front treatment given the high risk of cognitive side effects and given that response with whole-brain radiation therapy is often not durable; whole-brain radiation therapy is thus typically reserved as salvage therapy for relapsed or refractory disease. Prognosis for primary CNS lymphoma unfortunately remains poor overall, with median overall survival less than 2 years. Age >65 years at diagnosis and poor performance status are poor prognostic factors.

Reference

WHO Classification of Tumors. Central Nervous System Tumours. 5th ed. Geneva: World Health Organization; 2021.

26. A 5-year-old girl presents with headaches and vomiting and is found to have the enhancing pineal mass shown below (left). Biopsy reveals the pathologic image on the right. What is the most likely diagnosis?

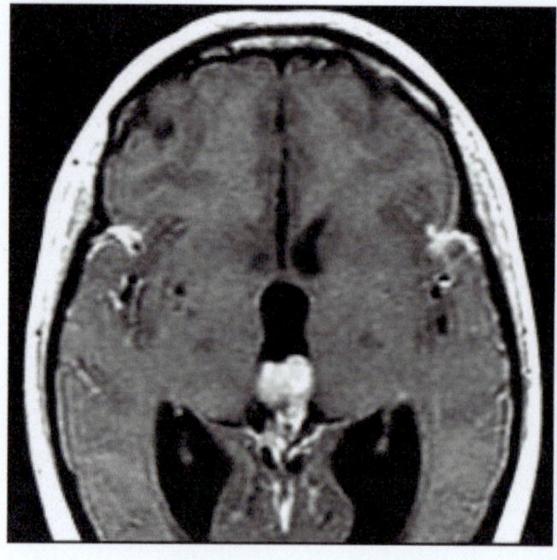 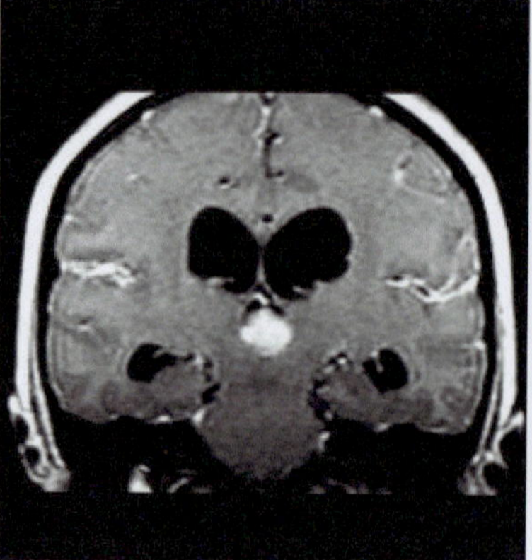 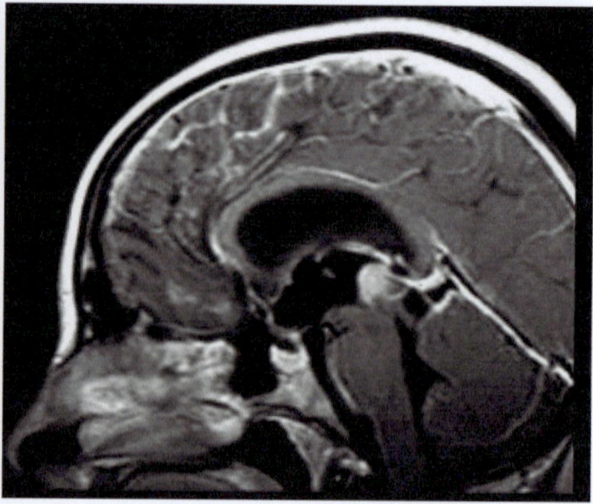

Axial, coronal, and sagittal MRI brain sections. (Source: Golbin, D., Nikitin, K. V., Konovalov, A. N., Pitskhelauri, D. I., Shishkina, L. V., Golanov, A. V., Cherekaev, V. A., Kobiakov, G. L., Absalyamova, O. V., Lasunin, N., Antipina, N. CC-BY 3.0 (https://creativecommons.org/licenses/by/3.0/) via *Cureus*. Image has not been modified from original. Please see full attribution with citation below in references section for this question.)

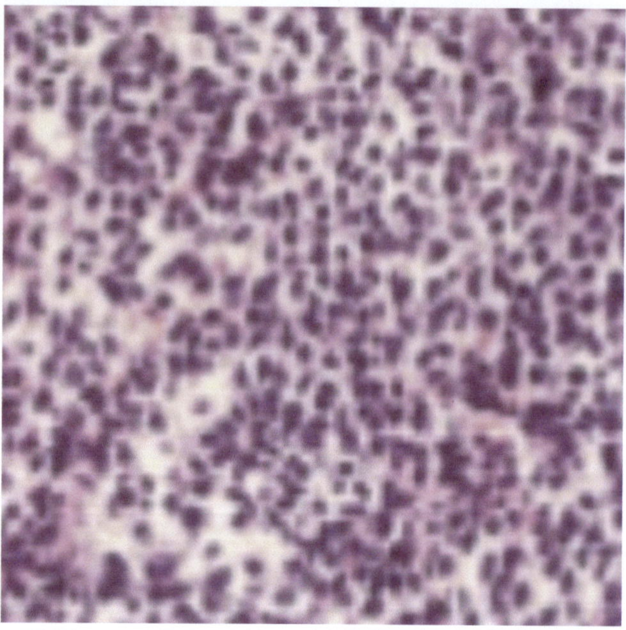

Micrograph. (Source: Golbin, D., Nikitin, K. V., Konovalov, A. N., Pitskhelauri, D. I., Shishkina, L. V., Golanov, A. V., Cherekaev, V. A., Kobiakov, G. L., Absalyamova, O. V., Lasunin, N., Antipina, N. CC-BY 3.0 (https://creativecommons.org/licenses/by/3.0/) via Cureus. Image has been cropped from original. Please see full attribution with citation below in references section for this question.)

A. Pineoblastoma

B. Pineocytoma

C. Pineal parenchymal tumor of intermediate differentiation

D. Papillary tumor of the pineal region

E. Mature teratoma

Correct answer: A

Explanation

Pineal region tumors are rare, accounting for <1% of all intracranial neoplasms. Approximately 27% of pineal region tumors are pineal parenchymal tumors. The tumor depicted in the question stem is a pineoblastoma. Pineoblastoma is a poorly differentiated embryonal tumor arising from the pineal parenchyma and is a CNS WHO grade 4 tumor by definition. Pineoblastomas account for approximately 35% of all pineal parenchymal tumors. Pineoblastomas are more common in children, with a median age at diagnosis of 6 years. Disseminated disease into the spine and/or CSF is observed in 25–33% of patients, and staging evaluation with MRI total spine and lumbar puncture with CSF cytology is therefore needed for all patients. Radiographically, pineoblastomas appear as heterogeneously contrast-enhancing pineal masses that often cause obstructive hydrocephalus. On pathology, pineoblastomas are small round blue cell tumors, exhibiting cells with high nuclear-to-cytoplasm ratio (as depicted in the question stem) and high mitotic activity. Homer-Wright rosettes and Flexner-Wintersteiner rosettes may be seen, with Flexner-Wintersteiner rosettes indicating retinoblastic differentiation. Pineoblastomas with RB1 alteration arise in infants and show similarities with retinoblastoma; the combination of bilateral retinoblastoma and a histologically similar tumor, most often pineoblastoma or a suprasellar tumor, is known as trilateral retinoblastoma. Treatment for pineoblastoma includes maximal safe resection followed by craniospinal irradiation and multi-agent chemotherapy. Pineoblastoma is the most aggressive pineal parenchymal tumor, with median overall survival 4.1–8.7 years.

Pineocytoma is a well-differentiated CNS WHO grade 1 pineal parenchymal tumor. Pineocytomas can occur at any age but are most commonly seen in adults, with a median age at diagnosis of 44 years; they can be incidental findings. On

MRI, pineocytomas appear as well-demarcated contrast-enhancing lesions that can have cystic components. On pathology, pineocytomas are composed of uniform cells forming large pineocytomatous rosettes and/or pleomorphic cells showing gangliocytic differentiation; these tumors are well-differentiated and contain mature cells resembling pinealocytes, with mitotic figures rare or absent. When needed, maximal safe resection is the treatment of choice, though surveillance can be pursued for small, asymptomatic lesions. Prognosis is favorable with 5-year survival 86–91%. The patient in the question stem is younger than would be expected for a pineocytoma, and the small round blue cells seen in the question stem are not characteristic of pineocytoma.

Pineal parenchymal tumor of intermediate differentiation (PPTID) is a pineal parenchymal tumor intermediate in malignancy/aggressiveness between a pineocytoma and a pineoblastoma and can be CNS WHO grade 2 or 3. PPTIDs account for approximately 45% of all pineal parenchymal tumors with median age at diagnosis 33 years. On imaging, PPTIDs appear as heterogeneously enhancing pineal masses. On histology, PPTID is composed of diffuse sheets or large lobules of monomorphic round cells that appear more differentiated than those observed in a pineoblastoma. Low-grade (CNS WHO grade 2) PPTIDs have a more favorable prognosis with 5-year overall survival 74%. High-grade (CNS WHO grade 3) PPTIDs are more aggressive, with higher likelihood of recurrence and spinal dissemination, and 5-year overall survival approximately 39%. Initial treatment for PPTID includes maximal safe resection, but there is not a clear consensus regarding the optimal adjuvant therapy. High-grade PPTIDs are often treated with craniospinal irradiation and multi-agent chemotherapy, similar to pineoblastomas. The patient in the question stem is younger than would be expected for a new diagnosis of PPTID.

Papillary tumor of the pineal region is a neuroepithelial tumor characterized by a combination of papillary and solid areas with epithelial-like cells and immunohistochemistry positive for cytokeratins. Papillary tumor of the pineal region is a rare tumor and can occur in both children and adults, with median age at diagnosis 35 years. On imaging, they are typically well-circumscribed masses with cystic and solid components and heterogeneous enhancement. On histology, these tumors are epithelial in appearance with papillary features and often with ependymal-like differentiation. Five-year overall survival is approximately 73%. Treatment involves maximal safe resection, and radiation therapy can be considered. The patient in the question stem is younger than would be expected for new diagnosis of papillary tumor of the pineal region, and the small round blue cells seen in the picture in the question stem are not expected for this diagnosis.

Mature teratoma is a type of germ cell tumor that contains only fully differentiated adult-type somatic tissue elements. CNS germ cell tumors are most common in children and account for 2–3% of all primary intracranial neoplasms; they are more prevalent in Asia than in the United States or Europe. Mature teratomas contain components exhibiting differentiation along at least two of the three somatic tissue lines (ectoderm, mesoderm, and endoderm), such as the skin, CNS tissue, muscle, cartilage, and bone. These tumors are treated with maximal safe resection. The small round blue cells seen in the picture in the question stem are not expected for mature teratoma, which would be expected to exhibit fully differentiated tissue components.

References

Golbin D, Nikitin KV, Konovalov AN, Pitskhelauri DI, Shishkina LV, Golanov AV, et al. Intraosseous Metastasizing of Pineoblastoma into the Anterior Skull Base, Calvarial Bones, and Vertebrae. Cureus. 2015;7(12):e437. https://doi.org/10.7759/cureus.437.

WHO Classification of Tumors. Central Nervous System Tumours. 5th ed. Geneva: World Health Organization; 2021.

27. A 40-year-old man presents with headaches, dysphagia, and rightward tongue deviation. Brain MRI with and without contrast reveals a destructive bony lesion in the clivus. Pathology ultimately reveals a chordoma. Which of the following is correct regarding chordomas?
    A. Chordomas are malignant soft tissue sarcomas.
    B. Chordomas are most commonly found in the cervical and thoracic spine.
    C. Physaliphorous cells are an uncommon histologic feature.
    D. Chordomas are most common in children.
    E. Chemotherapy is the mainstay of treatment for chordomas.

    Correct answer: A

Explanation

Chordomas are malignant, osteodestructive soft tissue sarcomas of the bone of notochordal differentiation which primarily occur in adults. They typically occur in the skull base (often in the clivus) and in the sacrococcygeal region. Skull base chordomas often cause headaches and cranial neuropathies. On MRI, chordomas appear as contrast-enhancing, T2 hyperintense destructive bony lytic lesions. On pathology, tumor cells are arranged in cords or ribbons separated by a myxoid matrix, and physaliphorous cells (large tumor cells with clear to eosinophilic cytoplasm with vacuolated or bubbly cytoplasm) are seen. Tumor cells are positive for brachyury on immunohistochemistry. Standard treatment for chordoma involves maximal safe resection followed by radiation therapy; chemotherapy is not typically used except in tumors that recur/progress after initial treatment.

Reference

WHO Classification of Tumors. Central Nervous System Tumours. 5th ed. Geneva: World Health Organization; 2021.

Linked questions: 28–29

28. A 4-year-old boy presents with headaches, vomiting, and ataxia. A brain MRI with and without contrast reveals the following. What is the most likely diagnosis?

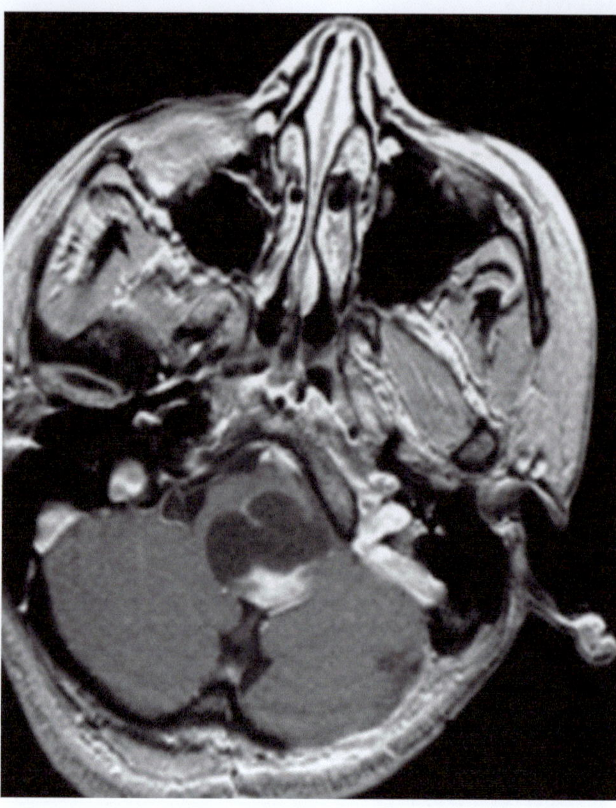

Axial brain MRI. (Source: Hafez, R. F. CC-BY 2.0 (https://creative-commons.org/licenses/by/2.0/) via *World Journal of Surgical Oncology.* Image has been cropped from original. Please see full attribution with citation below in references section for this question.)

A. Pilocytic astrocytoma
B. Medulloblastoma
C. Glioblastoma
D. Pleomorphic xanthoastrocytoma
E. Ganglioglioma

Correct answer: A

Linked question

29. Which of the following is incorrect regarding pathologic features of the tumor in question 28?
    A. KIAA1549:BRAF fusion is the most common molecular alteration.
    B. Bipolar hairlike astrocytes are seen on histology.
    C. Eosinophilic granular bodies can be seen on histology.
    D. Rosenthal fibers can be seen on histology.
    E. MAPK pathway alterations are uncommon.

Correct answer: E

Explanation for Questions 28 and 29

The tumor referred to in questions 28 and 29 is a pilocytic astrocytoma. Pilocytic astrocytoma is a CNS WHO grade 1 astrocytoma and is the most common glioma in children. Pilocytic astrocytomas are most common in the first two decades of life and account for 17.6% of all pediatric primary brain tumors. Pilocytic astrocytomas are most commonly located in the cerebellum but can also occur along the optic pathways (including the optic nerve sheaths), hypothalamus, brain stem, and spinal cord. The optic pathway gliomas seen in neurofibromatosis type 1 are pilocytic astrocytomas.

On MRI, pilocytic astrocytomas often (approximately 2/3 of the time) appear as a cyst with a solidly enhancing mural nodule, as seen in the question stem. Regarding question 18, medulloblastomas are also cerebellar tumors most common in children, but they are typically more heterogeneously enhancing and do not have the cyst with enhancing mural nodule characteristic of pilocytic astrocytomas. Glioblastomas typically appear as heterogeneously enhancing mass lesions and are typically seen in adults (most commonly in the fifth to seventh decades of life). Pleomorphic xanthoastrocytomas and gangliogliomas can also appear as cysts with an enhancing mural nodule but are most commonly supratentorial in location.

On pathology, the tumor cells of pilocytic astrocytomas vary in their morphology. Bipolar cells with elongated nuclei and hairlike processes (i.e., bipolar, hairlike astrocytes) can be seen, as can oligodendrocyte-like cells. Multinucleated cells with horseshoe-shaped nuclear clusters (known as "pennies-on-a-plate" pattern) can also be seen. Mitoses are rare. Eosinophilic granular bodies and Rosenthal fibers are common. Molecularly, pilocytic astrocytomas are associated with MAPK pathway gene alterations, the most common of which is the KIAA1549:BRAF fusion gene (seen in >60% of pilocytic astrocytomas). BRAF point mutations, including BRAF V600E mutation, are less common and only occur in 5–10% of pilocytic astrocytomas.

Maximal safe resection is the mainstay of treatment for pilocytic astrocytomas, and often no adjuvant treatment is required if a gross total resection is achieved. For tumors that cannot be gross totally resected, o those that recur after initial resection, chemotherapy with carboplatin + vincristine can be considered. If BRAF fusion is present, targeted therapy with a MEK inhibitor such as trametinib can be considered. Radiation therapy is typically avoided in children given the potential to cause developmental issues but can be considered in adults for recurrent tumors.

References

Hafez *RF*. Stereotaxic gamma knife surgery in treatment of critically located pilocytic astrocytoma: preliminary result. World J Surg Oncol. 2007;5:39. https://doi.org/10.1186/1477-7819-5-39.

WHO Classification of Tumors. Central Nervous System Tumours. 5th ed. Geneva: World Health Organization; 2021.

30. A 20-year-old man presents with seizures. Brain MRI with and without contrast reveals a mixed cystic and solid right temporal mass. Resection reveals a tumor with multinucleated astrocytes filled with lipid droplets as well as eosinophilic granular bodies. Molecular analysis reveals BRAF V600E mutation. Which is the most likely diagnosis?
    A. Pleomorphic xanthoastrocytoma
    B. Dysembryoplastic neuroepithelial tumor
    C. Gangliocytoma
    D. Pilocytic astrocytoma
    E. Astrocytoma IDH-mutant CNS WHO grade 2
    Correct answer: A

Explanation

Pleomorphic xanthoastrocytoma (PXA) is a type of astrocytoma most commonly seen in children and young adults, with median age at diagnosis 20.5 years. PXA can be graded as CNS WHO grade 2 or 3. They are most commonly superficial and supratentorial in location and often present with seizures. PXAs are typically well-demarcated rather than invasive tumors. On MRI, PXAs typically appear as mixed solid and cystic lesions, with cystic components and solidly enhancing components; they can take on the appearance of a cyst with an enhancing mural nodule. On histology, PXAs contain large pleomorphic often multinucleated cells that can be filled with lipid droplets (xanthomatous cells) as well as spindled cells and eosinophilic granular bodies. CNS WHO grade 3 tumors exhibit higher mitotic activity and pro-

liferation index. BRAF V600E mutation is the most common molecular feature and can be seen in as many as 80% of PXAs; homozygous deletions of CDKN2A or CDKN2B can also be seen. Surgical resection is the mainstay of treatment for PXAs. For residual disease after surgery or tumors that recur after surgery, treatment with targeted therapy (combined BRAF and MEK inhibitors) if BRAF V600E mutation is present, and/or radiation therapy, can be considered.

Dysembryoplastic neuroepithelial tumor (DNET) can present as a cystic lesion causing seizures, and BRAF V600E mutations can be seen, but eosinophilic granular bodies and xanthomatous cells are not typical. The pathologic and molecular features described in the question stem are not typically seen in gangliocytoma. Pilocytic astrocytomas can appear as mixed solid and cystic lesions with eosinophilic granular bodies but are more common in the posterior fossa and more commonly contain KIAA1549-BRAF fusion, whereas BRAF V600E mutation is less common. While IDH-mutant astrocytomas can be seen in this age group, the expected radiographic appearance would be a T2 hyperintense non-enhancing expansile lesion rather than the mixed solid and cystic lesion here, and eosinophilic granular bodies and BRAF V600E mutation would not be expected.

Reference

WHO Classification of Tumors. Central Nervous System Tumours. 5th ed. Geneva: World Health Organization; 2021.

31. An 18-year-old girl presents with a seizure. Brain MRI reveals a cystic lesion in the right temporal lobe. Pathology from the resection reveals a ganglioglioma. Which of the following is incorrect regarding gangliogliomas?
    A. They contain both glial and neuronal elements.
    B. BRAF V600E mutations are uncommon.
    C. They are CNS WHO grade 1 tumors.
    D. Eosinophilic granular bodies are uncommon.
    E. They have a favorable prognosis.
    Correct answer: D

Explanation

Ganglioglioma is a CNS WHO grade 1 glioneuronal tumor most common in children and young adults. Most gangliogliomas present in the first or second decades of life (median age at diagnosis 12 years) but can present at essentially any age. Gangliogliomas can have mixed solid and cystic components on MRI and can present as a cyst with an enhancing mural nodule in some cases. They are typically located in the temporal lobe and present with seizures and are well-circumscribed. On histology, tumor cells exhibit mixed glial and neuronal components, with the glial components positive for GFAP and the neuronal components positive for synaptophysin, chromogranin, and neurofilament. The neuronal component is made up of dysmorphic ganglion cells, and the glial component can resemble astrocytoma or oligodendroglioma. Tumors can have eosinophilic granular bodies on histology. Approximately 20–60% of gangliogliomas have BRAF V600E mutations. Surgical resection is the mainstay of treatment. Targeted therapy with BRAF/MEK inhibitors (if BRAF V600E mutation is present) and/or radiation therapy can be considered for residual or recurrent tumors. These tumors are typically slow-growing with a favorable prognosis, and surgery can be curative.

Reference

WHO Classification of Tumors. Central Nervous System Tumours. 5th ed. Geneva: World Health Organization; 2021.

Joel Salinas

Case 1

A 67-year-old woman presents for evaluation of progressive forgetfulness over the past 2 years. Her daughter reports increasing difficulty remembering recent conversations and misplacing items. The patient has trouble managing finances and recently forgot to attend her grandson's birthday. She has no history of stroke, head trauma, or psychiatric illness. Family history is notable for her mother having dementia in her 80s. Neurologic exam is notable for mild word-finding pauses but no focal deficits. Montreal Cognitive Assessment (MoCA) score is 21/30.

1. What is the most likely clinical diagnosis?
    A. Amnestic mild cognitive impairment
    B. Alzheimer's disease dementia
    C. Vascular dementia
    D. Dementia with Lewy bodies
    E. Frontotemporal dementia
    Correct answer: B

Explanation

The patient meets criteria for major neurocognitive disorder (dementia) due to progressive memory impairment and functional decline. The gradual onset and prominent episodic memory loss are characteristic of Alzheimer's disease dementia.

- A: She meets criteria for at least mild dementia given impairment in instrumental activities of daily living.
- C: There is no evidence of stepwise decline or focal neurologic findings that is more typical of vascular dementia.

J. Salinas (✉)
Department of Neurology (J.S.), Center for Cognitive Neurology, New York University Grossman School of Medicine, New York, NY, USA
e-mail: joel.salinas@nyulangone.org

- D: No early visual hallucinations, REM sleep behavior disorder, or parkinsonism to suggest Lewy body dementia.
- E: No prominent disinhibition, apathy, or language-predominant deficits typical of frontotemporal dementia.

Reference

Jack CR Jr, Bennett DA, Blennow K, et al. NIA-AA research framework: Toward a biological definition of Alzheimer's disease. *Alzheimers Dement*. 2018;14(4):535–62. https://doi.org/10.1016/j.jalz.2018.02.018

2. A lumbar puncture is performed and cerebrospinal fluid (CSF) results show the following:
    Aβ42: 380 pg/mL (normal reference, >600 pg/mL)
    Total tau: 600 pg/mL (normal reference, <350 pg/mL)
    Phosphorylated tau (p-tau181): 75 pg/mL (normal reference, <61 pg/mL)
    Amyloid tau index (ATI): 0.32 (normal reference, ≥1.0)
    How should this CSF profile be interpreted?
    A. Normal CSF profile
    B. Suggestive of non-AD pathology
    C. Consistent with Alzheimer's disease
    D. Diagnostic of Creutzfeldt-Jakob disease
    E. Suggestive of frontotemporal lobar degeneration
    Correct answer: C

Explanation

Decreased Aβ42 and ATI, along with elevated total tau and phosphorylated tau, reflect Alzheimer's pathology—amyloid deposition and tau-related neurodegeneration. This profile is typical of Alzheimer's disease.

- A: These values are abnormal.
- B: This pattern is not suggestive of non-AD dementias.
- D: CJD typically shows very high tau levels (>1200 pg/mL) and positive 14-3-3 protein.
- E: FTLD often lacks amyloid changes.

Reference

Shaw LM, Arias J, Blennow K, et al. Appropriate use criteria for lumbar puncture and CSF testing in the diagnosis of Alzheimer's disease. *Alzheimers Dement.* 2018;14(11):1505–21. https://doi.org/10.1016/j.jalz.2018.07.220

3. Given the patient's diagnosis of mild Alzheimer's disease dementia, confirmed amyloid pathology by CSF, and planned APOE genotyping with counseling on amyloid-related imaging abnormalities (ARIA), which of the following is the most appropriate disease-modifying treatment?
   A. Amyloid-targeting monoclonal antibody therapy (e.g., lecanemab or donanemab)
   B. Memantine
   C. Rivastigmine
   D. Donepezil
   E. Vitamin E

   Correct answer: A

Explanation

Lecanemab and donanemab are FDA-approved for early-stage Alzheimer's disease with biomarker confirmation of amyloid pathology. These therapies are disease-modifying and require ARIA risk counseling, and APOE genotyping is strongly encouraged prior to treatment initiation.

- B: Memantine is used in later stages and is not disease-modifying.
- C: Rivastigmine is a symptomatic treatment and not disease-modifying.
- D: Donepezil is a first-line symptomatic therapy and not disease-modifying.
- E: Vitamin E is not routinely recommended and not disease-modifying.

References

Sims JR, Zimmer JA, Evans CD, Lu M, Ardayfio P, Sparks J, et al. Donanemab in early symptomatic Alzheimer disease: the TRAILBLAZER-ALZ 2 randomized clinical trial. *JAMA.* 2023;330(6):512–27. https://doi.org/10.1001/jama.2023.13239

van Dyck CH, Swanson CJ, Aisen P, et al. Lecanemab in early Alzheimer's disease. *N Engl J Med.* 2023;388(1):9–21. https://doi.org/10.1056/NEJMoa2212948

4. A 59-year-old woman is brought in by her partner because of personality changes over the past 18 months. She has become impulsive, makes inappropriate comments, and has developed a sweet tooth despite a prior history of strict dieting. Her speech is fluent but lacks depth. Neurologic examination is non-focal. MoCA score is 25/30, with errors in abstraction and delayed recall. MRI shows frontal and anterior temporal lobe atrophy.

   What is the most likely diagnosis?
   A. Alzheimer's disease
   B. Frontotemporal dementia, behavioral variant
   C. Primary progressive aphasia
   D. Pseudobulbar affect
   E. Delirium

   Correct answer: B

Explanation

This presentation—early disinhibition, changes in eating habits, preserved language fluency, and focal frontal/anterior temporal atrophy—is classic for behavioral variant frontotemporal dementia (bvFTD). Early personality changes, compulsive behavior, and dietary shifts are hallmark features.

- A: AD more commonly presents with memory impairment and medial temporal atrophy.
- C: PPA presents with language dysfunction as the primary symptom, not behavioral disinhibition.
- D: Pseudobulbar affect causes inappropriate laughter or crying, not a progressive behavioral syndrome.
- E: Delirium presents acutely and fluctuates; this patient has an insidious, progressive course.

Reference

Rascovsky K, Hodges JR, Knopman D, Mendez MF, Kramer JH, Neuhaus J, et al. Sensitivity of revised diagnostic criteria for the behavioural variant of frontotemporal dementia. *Brain.* 2011;134(Pt 9):2456–77. https://doi.org/10.1093/brain/awr179

5. A 72-year-old man is hospitalized for pneumonia. On day 2, the nurse notes that he is confused, disoriented to time and place, and having trouble staying awake during conversations. He believes he is at home and tries to climb out of bed to "feed the chickens." There is no known prior history of cognitive impairment. His temperature is 101.8°F (38.8°C), and laboratory studies reveal a normal glucose and sodium level.

   What is the most likely diagnosis?
   A. Delirium
   B. Alzheimer's disease
   C. Dementia with Lewy bodies
   D. Primary progressive aphasia
   E. Vascular dementia

   Correct answer: A

Explanation

The patient's acute onset of fluctuating attention, disorientation, and hallucinations in the context of infection strongly supports delirium, also called encephalopathy. It is a clinical diagnosis characterized by rapid onset and inattention, often with altered arousal.

- B: Alzheimer's disease presents gradually, not acutely.
- C: Lewy body dementia includes hallucinations but progresses chronically and often includes parkinsonism.
- D: PPA involves progressive language difficulty, not global confusion or disorientation.
- E: Vascular dementia may present with stepwise decline but not acute confusion over hours to days.

Reference

Inouye SK, Westendorp RGJ, Saczynski JS. Delirium in elderly people. *Lancet.* 2014;383(9920):911–22. https://doi.org/10.1016/S0140-6736(13)60688-1

6. A 64-year-old woman with multiple sclerosis presents for evaluation of sudden, brief episodes of uncontrollable crying that occur several times a day. She says the episodes are not triggered by any particular emotion and are distressing and socially embarrassing. Neurologic exam is unchanged from baseline. She is cognitively intact and reports no signs of depression.
   What is the most likely diagnosis?
   A. Depression
   B. Frontotemporal dementia
   C. Pseudobulbar affect
   D. Cataplexy
   E. Panic disorder
   Correct answer: C

Explanation

This is classic pseudobulbar affect (PBA)—sudden, involuntary episodes of laughing or crying that are incongruent or disproportionate to the emotional context. It often occurs in patients with neurologic disease such as MS, ALS, or stroke.

- A: Depression is more persistent, and emotional expression would match mood; this patient denies feeling depressed.
- B: FTD could involve inappropriate affect but would not present with brief, stereotyped emotional outbursts.
- D: Cataplexy involves sudden loss of muscle tone, often in response to laughter, not emotional outbursts themselves.

- E: Panic attacks involve fear, autonomic symptoms, and anxiety, not crying spells without internal distress.

Reference

Brooks BR, Crumpacker D, Fellus J, Kantor D, Kaye RE. PRISM: a novel research tool to assess the prevalence of pseudobulbar affect symptoms across neurological conditions. *PLoS One.* 2013;8(8):e72232. https://doi.org/10.1371/journal.pone.0072232

7. A 75-year-old man presents with progressive memory impairment and visual hallucinations. His wife reports that he sometimes acts out his dreams during sleep and has episodes of confusion that vary day to day. On examination, he has mild cogwheel rigidity and a slow shuffling gait. MoCA score is 20/30.
   Which of the following is the most likely diagnosis?
   A. Parkinson's disease dementia
   B. Alzheimer's disease
   C. Dementia with Lewy bodies
   D. Vascular dementia
   E. Normal pressure hydrocephalus
   Correct answer: C

Explanation

This patient has core features of dementia with Lewy bodies (DLB): visual hallucinations, parkinsonism, REM sleep behavior disorder, and fluctuating cognition. These support the diagnosis of DLB.

- A: Parkinson's disease dementia is diagnosed when dementia appears after at least 1 year of motor symptoms; here, cognitive and motor features overlap.
- B: Alzheimer's typically lacks visual hallucinations or REM sleep behavior disorder.
- D: Vascular dementia usually presents with stepwise decline or focal deficits.
- E: NPH classically presents with gait disturbance, urinary incontinence, and cognitive slowing but not hallucinations or REM sleep behavior disorder.

Reference

McKeith IG, Boeve BF, Dickson DW, et al. Diagnosis and management of dementia with Lewy bodies. *Neurology.* 2017;89(1):88–100. https://doi.org/10.1212/WNL.0000000000004058

8. A 68-year-old former professor presents with progressive difficulty naming objects and understanding conversations over the past year. His speech is fluent but filled with vague terms like "thing" and "it." He frequently misunderstands complex instructions and struggles with word meaning. MRI shows asymmetric atrophy in the anterior left temporal lobe.

Which subtype of primary progressive aphasia is most likely?
   A. Nonfluent/agrammatic variant
   B. Semantic variant
   C. Logopenic variant
   D. Broca (expressive/nonfluent) aphasia
   E. Wernicke (receptive/fluent) aphasia
   Correct answer: B

Explanation

The semantic variant primary progressive aphasia (svPPA) is characterized by fluent but empty speech, impaired single-word comprehension, and naming difficulty. It's associated with left anterior temporal atrophy.

- A: The nonfluent/agrammatic variant involves effortful, halting speech and grammatical errors.
- C: The logopenic variant features word-finding pauses and impaired repetition but intact word meaning.
- D: Broca aphasia is acquired (usually poststroke), not progressive, and shows nonfluent output.
- E: Wernicke aphasia also presents with fluent but nonsensical speech, but it is due to acute lesions in the posterior superior temporal gyrus, not progressive degeneration.

Reference

Gorno-Tempini ML, Hillis AE, Weintraub S, et al. Classification of primary progressive aphasia and its variants. *Neurology*. 2011;76(11):1006–14. https://doi.org/10.1212/WNL.0b013e31821103e6

9. A 70-year-old woman presents for evaluation of apathy. Her daughter reports that she is no longer initiating conversations, socializing, or engaging in previously enjoyed hobbies. She spends most of the day sitting quietly. She does not appear sad, anxious, or tearful. When asked directly, she says she feels "fine" and denies low mood. Neurologic examination is unremarkable. MRI shows moderate white matter hyperintensities.

Which of the following syndromes best describes her presentation?
   A. Major depressive disorder
   B. Akinetic mutism
   C. Apathy
   D. Executive dysfunction
   E. Anosognosia
   Correct answer: C

Explanation

This is apathy, defined by diminished motivation, initiation, and goal-directed behavior—often mistaken for depression. The lack of subjective sadness or negative affect distinguishes it from depression. It is commonly seen in neurodegenerative diseases and with frontal-subcortical circuit disruptions (e.g., white matter disease).

- A: Depression typically includes subjective low mood, anhedonia, or emotional distress.
- B: Akinetic mutism is a more severe syndrome marked by profound lack of movement and speech, often after medial frontal lesions.
- D: Executive dysfunction may contribute to apathy but more commonly manifests as disorganization, impaired planning, or abstraction.
- E: Anosognosia is impaired awareness of one's own deficits; this patient appears aware but indifferent.

Reference

Levy R, Dubois B. Apathy and the functional anatomy of the prefrontal cortex–basal ganglia circuits. *Cereb Cortex*. 2006;16(7):916–28. https://doi.org/10.1093/cercor/bhj043

10. A 77-year-old man is referred for cognitive evaluation. He lives alone and independently manages his medications, finances, cooking, and transportation. On cognitive testing, his Montreal Cognitive Assessment (MoCA) score is 23/30, with deficits in delayed recall and clock drawing. His insight is preserved, and neurologic examination is normal.

Which of the following best describes his clinical status?
   A. Alzheimer's disease dementia
   B. Vascular dementia
   C. Mild cognitive impairment
   D. Subjective cognitive decline
   E. Normal cognition
   Correct answer: C

Explanation

This patient meets criteria for mild cognitive impairment (MCI): objective cognitive deficits (MoCA 23/30) and preserved independence in daily function with no major impact on social or occupational life.

- A: AD dementia requires functional decline; he remains fully independent.
- B: No evidence of cerebrovascular risk, stepwise decline, or focal neurologic signs.

- D: Subjective cognitive decline involves self-reported concerns without objective impairment.
- E: His cognitive testing shows deficits.

Reference

Albert MS, DeKosky ST, Dickson D, et al. The diagnosis of mild cognitive impairment due to Alzheimer's disease: recommendations from the National Institute on Aging-Alzheimer's Association workgroups. *Alzheimers Dement.* 2011;7(3):270–9. https://doi.org/10.1016/j.jalz.2011.03.008

Case 2

A 28-year-old man presents for evaluation of long-standing difficulties with focus and social interactions. He reports being easily distracted at work, frequently interrupting others, and struggling to complete tasks. Since childhood, he has had difficulty understanding sarcasm or social nuance, and he dislikes changes to his routine. He was never formally diagnosed but recently saw a social media post about adult ADHD that prompted this visit.

He has no history of substance use, mood or psychotic symptoms, or head trauma. His medical history is unremarkable. Family history is notable for a brother with ADHD.

11. Which of the following features best supports a diagnosis of autism spectrum disorder (ASD) in this patient?
    A. Frequent task-switching and difficulty sustaining attention
    B. Impulsivity and emotional reactivity
    C. Inflexibility with routines and difficulty interpreting social cues
    D. Restlessness and distractibility
    E. Poor academic performance
    Correct answer: C

Explanation

Core features of ASD in adults include deficits in social communication and restricted/repetitive behaviors, including rigid routines and difficulty with nonverbal or nuanced social interaction.

- A, B, D: These are more characteristic of ADHD.
- E: Nonspecific, can occur in many cognitive/psychiatric conditions.

12. Which of the following is most accurate regarding the co-occurrence of ASD and ADHD?
    A. The conditions are mutually exclusive.
    B. ADHD must be excluded before diagnosing ASD.
    C. Co-occurrence is common and diagnostic criteria can overlap.
    D. ADHD symptoms are explained entirely by ASD.
    E. The co-occurrence is rare in adults.
    Correct answer: C

Explanation

ADHD and ASD frequently co-occur, and DSM-5 allows dual diagnosis. Shared features include executive dysfunction, sensory sensitivities, and emotional regulation challenges.

- A, B: Outdated concepts, no longer part of DSM-5.
- D: ADHD symptoms can be independent and clinically significant.
- E: Co-occurrence is not rare, especially in adults evaluated retrospectively.

13. Which neuropsychological domain is most likely to be affected in both ASD and ADHD?
    A. Language comprehension
    B. Episodic memory encoding
    C. Visuospatial construction
    D. Executive functioning
    E. Long-term memory retrieval
    Correct answer: D

Explanation

Executive dysfunction, including working memory, inhibition, and planning, is common in both ADHD and ASD.

- A: May be impaired in ASD, but not a core overlap
- B, E: Not prominently affected in either disorder
- C: More common in nonverbal learning disabilities or posterior cortical syndromes

References

American Psychiatric Association. *Diagnostic and statistical manual of mental disorders (DSM-5®).* 5th ed. Arlington (VA): American Psychiatric Publishing; 2013.

Antshel KM, Russo N. Autism spectrum disorders and ADHD: overlapping phenomenology, diagnostic issues, and treatment considerations. *Curr Psychiatry Rep.* 2019;21(5):34. https://doi.org/10.1007/s11920-019-1020-5

Case 3

A 74-year-old woman is brought to clinic by her daughter for worsening memory and apathy over 6 months. The patient says "I just don't care anymore" and notes difficulty concentrating and keeping up with conversations. Her daughter reports that the patient has become more withdrawn, has lost interest in hobbies, and is sleeping most of the day. She denies hallucinations or delusions. Past medical history includes type 2 diabetes and osteoarthritis.

On examination, she appears disheveled, maintains minimal eye contact, and answers in monosyllables. Neurologic exam is non-focal. Her Montreal Cognitive Assessment (MoCA) score is 18/30, with impairments in attention, delayed recall, and executive function. Her MRI brain shows mild periventricular white matter changes without cortical atrophy.

14. Which of the following is the most likely diagnosis?
    A. Alzheimer's disease
    B. Functional cognitive disorder
    C. Frontotemporal dementia
    D. Dementia with Lewy bodies
    E. Vascular dementia
    Correct answer: B

Explanation

This patient exhibits reversible cognitive impairment due to depression, also referred to as a functional cognitive disorder or "pseudodementia." Suggestive features include apathy, psychomotor slowing, and sleep changes, disproportionate emotional blunting, subjective cognitive complaints more prominent than objective findings, preserved insight, and minimal cortical atrophy.

- A: AD usually presents with more insidious memory loss and early atrophy.
- C: FTD often shows disinhibition or compulsions, not withdrawal and flat affect.
- D: No visual hallucinations, REM sleep behavior disorder, or parkinsonism.
- E: No focal deficits or stepwise decline.

15. What is the most appropriate next step in management?
    A. Start cholinesterase inhibitor therapy.
    B. Refer for inpatient psychiatric hospitalization.
    C. Begin a trial of antidepressant treatment.
    D. Schedule a neuropsychological evaluation.
    E. Obtain lumbar puncture to assess biomarkers.
    Correct answer: C

Explanation

Initiating treatment for suspected late-life depression is appropriate. Response to treatment is often diagnostic: cognitive impairment due to depression frequently improves with mood treatment, either with psychotropic medication or psychotherapy (e.g., cognitive behavioral therapy).

- A: Cholinesterase inhibitors are not first-line for depression-related cognitive symptoms.
- B: There is no indication of suicidal ideation or psychosis requiring inpatient care.
- D: Helpful but treatment trial should not be delayed.
- E: CSF biomarkers may not clarify etiology and are unnecessary unless initial treatment fails.

16. Which feature most reliably differentiates depression-related cognitive impairment from neurodegenerative dementia?
    A. Presence of white matter changes on MRI
    B. Onset of symptoms over months
    C. Marked impairments in delayed recall
    D. Poor effort during cognitive testing
    E. Apathy and sleep disruption
    Correct answer: D

Explanation

Patients with a functional cognitive disorder (or "pseudodementia") often show variable performance and poor effort—particularly on memory recall tasks—with rapid forgetting not typical of true dementia. Improvement with prompting may be a helpful clue.

- A: White matter changes are nonspecific and common in older adults.
- B: Subacute onset can be seen in both.
- C: Impaired delayed recall is common in both groups.
- E: Apathy and sleep changes are nonspecific and present in both.

Reference

Ball HA, McWhirter L, Ballard C, Bhome R, Blackburn DJ, Edwards MJ, et al. Functional cognitive disorder: dementia's blind spot. *Brain*. 2020;143(10):2895–903. https://doi.org/10.1093/brain/awaa224

Case 4

A 74-year-old man is brought to clinic by his partner due to fluctuating cognition and recent visual hallucinations. He often sees children playing in the living room or insects crawling on the wall. He was diagnosed with Parkinson's disease 2 years ago and started on levodopa, but his cognitive issues have become more prominent in the last 6 months. His MoCA score is 21/30, with notable deficits in visuospatial and executive domains. Neurologic examination reveals bradykinesia and mild rigidity. MRI brain shows mild global atrophy; DAT-SPECT imaging reveals decreased dopamine transporter uptake in the striatum.

17. Which of the following clinical features is most characteristic of dementia with Lewy bodies?
    A. Rapid progression of memory loss
    B. Early language dysfunction
    C. Prominent visuospatial deficits
    D. Prominent motor neuron signs
    E. Predominantly anterograde amnesia
    Correct answer: C

Explanation

Visuospatial dysfunction is a hallmark early feature of DLB, often more prominent than memory impairment in early stages.

- A: DLB tends to have a fluctuating course rather than rapid decline.
- B: Early language dysfunction suggests primary progressive aphasia, not DLB.
- D: Motor neuron signs suggest ALS or related disorders, not DLB.
- E: Prominent anterograde memory loss is typical of Alzheimer's disease.

18. Which of the following clinical features, if present early in the course, supports the diagnosis of probable dementia with Lewy bodies over Alzheimer's disease?
    A. Apathy
    B. Hyposmia
    C. REM sleep behavior disorder
    D. Aphasia
    E. Myoclonus
    Correct answer: C

Explanation

REM sleep behavior disorder (RBD) is a strong supportive feature of DLB, often preceding other symptoms by years.

- A: Apathy is nonspecific and seen in many neurodegenerative conditions.
- B: Hyposmia may occur in both AD and DLB.

- D: Aphasia is more suggestive of primary progressive aphasia.
- E: Myoclonus is more typical in rapidly progressive dementias like CJD.

19. Which treatment strategy is most appropriate for managing hallucinations in this patient?
    A. Increase levodopa dosage.
    B. Add quetiapine.
    C. Initiate donepezil.
    D. Begin high-dose haloperidol.
    E. Add valproic acid.
    Correct answer: C

Explanation

Cholinesterase inhibitors (e.g., donepezil) are first-line treatments for visual hallucinations in DLB and may improve cognitive and neuropsychiatric symptoms.

- A: Increasing dopaminergic therapy can worsen hallucinations.
- B: Quetiapine may be used cautiously but is not first-line; antipsychotics carry high risk of worsening parkinsonism and death in DLB.
- D: Haloperidol is contraindicated in DLB due to severe neuroleptic sensitivity.
- E: Valproic acid is used for agitation or mood stabilization but is not first-line for hallucinations.

Reference

McKeith IG, Boeve BF, Dickson DW, Halliday G, Taylor JP, Weintraub D, et al. Diagnosis and management of dementia with Lewy bodies: fourth consensus report of the DLB Consortium. *Neurology*. 2017;89(1):88–100. https://doi.org/10.1212/WNL.0000000000004058

Case 5

A 61-year-old woman is brought in by her wife due to a 1.5-year history of behavioral changes. She has become socially inappropriate, emotionally blunt, and recently shoplifted without remorse. She compulsively eats sweets and repeatedly taps on the kitchen counter. She was a corporate executive but has struggled with decision-making and organizing tasks. There is no significant past psychiatric history. Family history is positive for a paternal uncle with early-onset dementia. Neurologic exam is unremarkable except for a flat affect.

MoCA score is 24/30, with deficits in abstraction and executive function. MRI brain shows atrophy of the bilateral frontal lobes, greater on the right.

20. Which feature best supports the diagnosis of behavioral variant frontotemporal dementia (bvFTD)?
    A. Word-finding difficulty
    B. REM sleep behavior disorder
    C. Decline in social conduct with preserved memory
    D. Stepwise deterioration
    E. Visual hallucinations and parkinsonism
    Correct answer: C

Explanation

bvFTD often presents with early changes in personality, social conduct, empathy, and impulse control, rather than memory loss.

- A: Suggests a speech/language variant (primary progressive aphasia) or Alzheimer's disease
- B: Associated with Lewy body spectrum disorders
- D: Suggests vascular dementia
- E: Suggests dementia with Lewy bodies

21. Which of the following findings is most supportive of FTD over Alzheimer's disease?
    A. Poor delayed recall
    B. Medial temporal lobe atrophy
    C. Poor insight and emotional blunting early in disease
    D. Logopenic speech
    E. Progressive visuospatial dysfunction
    Correct answer: C

Explanation

In bvFTD, early loss of insight, impaired empathy, apathy, disinhibition, and compulsive behaviors are core diagnostic features.

- A: Suggests Alzheimer's.
- B: Seen in AD.
- D: Logopenic variant primary progressive aphasia is usually AD-related.
- E: Visuospatial deficits suggest posterior cortical atrophy or DLB.

22. Which of the following is the most evidence-based pharmacologic approach to manage behavioral symptoms in bvFTD?
    A. Cholinesterase inhibitors
    B. Levodopa
    C. SSRIs
    D. Antipsychotics
    E. Memantine
    Correct answer: C

Explanation

SSRIs (e.g., sertraline, fluoxetine) can reduce compulsive behaviors, irritability, and disinhibition in FTD. There is no proven disease-modifying therapy, but SSRIs are supported by limited evidence and clinical consensus.

- A: Cholinesterase inhibitors are not effective and may worsen symptoms in FTD.
- B: Not indicated.
- D: Antipsychotics should be used cautiously and only when necessary.
- E: Memantine shows minimal benefit in FTD.

Reference

Rascovsky K, Hodges JR, Knopman D, et al. Sensitivity of revised diagnostic criteria for the behavioral variant of frontotemporal dementia. *Brain*. 2011;134(9):2456–77. https://doi.org/10.1093/brain/awr179

Case 6

An 84-year-old woman presents for evaluation of progressive memory loss over the past 5 years. Her daughter reports increasing difficulty with word-finding, naming familiar people, and remembering recent conversations. On exam, she is alert and oriented but shows impaired delayed recall and confrontational naming. There is no parkinsonism, hallucinations, or cortical visual impairment. MRI reveals bilateral hippocampal atrophy greater than expected for age, but no significant vascular burden or posterior cortical atrophy.

23. Which of the following best characterizes this patient's likely underlying neuropathology?
    A. Amyloid-beta plaques and neurofibrillary tangles
    B. Alpha-synuclein inclusions in the neocortex
    C. TDP-43 pathology in the medial temporal lobe
    D. Tau-positive astrocytic plaques in the motor cortex
    E. Beta-amyloid angiopathy
    Correct answer: C

Explanation

This presentation is characteristic of LATE (limbic-predominant age-related TDP-43 encephalopathy), which mimics Alzheimer's disease but is instead driven by TDP-43 pathology, especially in the amygdala and hippocampus.

- A: Amyloid plaques and tangles define Alzheimer's pathology. While clinically similar, this patient's features and advanced age raise concern for LATE, which lacks AD pathology.

- B: Alpha-synuclein deposition in the neocortex typifies dementia with Lewy bodies, often with visual hallucinations and parkinsonism, which are absent here.
- D: Astrocytic plaques are associated with corticobasal degeneration and progressive supranuclear palsy, neither of which fit this case.
- E: Cerebral amyloid angiopathy can coexist with AD but does not cause this isolated amnestic syndrome.

24. The same 84-year-old woman undergoes biomarker evaluation. Her amyloid PET is negative, and her CSF shows normal Aβ42 and tau levels. However, her cognitive decline continues to progress, predominantly affecting episodic memory and naming.

    Which of the following best explains why her biomarker profile does not match her clinical syndrome?

    A. She has an atypical presentation of Alzheimer's disease with false-negative biomarkers.

    B. Her symptoms are likely due to hippocampal sclerosis from TDP-43 pathology.

    C. She has comorbid frontotemporal lobar degeneration with tau pathology.

    D. The biomarkers are falsely normal due to CSF contamination.

    E. The findings suggest subclinical vascular cognitive impairment.

    Correct answer: B

Explanation

LATE is associated with TDP-43-driven hippocampal sclerosis and, unlike Alzheimer's disease, does not involve amyloid or tau pathology. Hence, CSF and PET biomarkers for AD will be negative or normal, even in the presence of progressive amnestic decline.

- A: Atypical Alzheimer's usually has positive amyloid or tau biomarkers despite unusual presentations.
- C: FTLD with tau pathology typically presents earlier and with behavioral or language symptoms, not isolated memory decline.
- D: There is no indication of lab error or contamination in this case.
- E: Vascular cognitive impairment often presents with executive dysfunction or subcortical features and is associated with white matter changes, not isolated hippocampal atrophy.

25. Which of the following is a known clinical or radiographic feature that helps distinguish LATE from Alzheimer's disease?

    A. Earlier age of onset (<65 years).

    B. Prominent visuospatial deficits.

C. Focal medial temporal lobe atrophy with relative cortical sparing.

D. ApoE ε4 genotype is strongly associated.

E. Rapid progression over 1–2 years

Correct answer: C

Explanation

LATE is characterized by medial temporal lobe atrophy, especially the hippocampus, often greater than expected for age. Unlike AD, neocortical areas may be relatively preserved, and visuospatial and executive functions may remain intact longer.

- A: LATE is associated with advanced age, typically over 80, unlike young-onset AD.
- B: Prominent visuospatial deficits are more typical of posterior cortical atrophy or Lewy body dementia.
- D: ApoE ε4 is associated with AD, not LATE. LATE is not known to have a strong genetic marker.
- E: LATE tends to progress slowly, often over several years.

Reference

Nelson PT, Dickson DW, Trojanowski JQ, et al. Limbic-predominant age-related TDP-43 encephalopathy (LATE): consensus working group report. Brain. 2019;142(6):1503–27. https://doi.org/10.1093/brain/awz099

Case 7

A 76-year-old man with a history of hypertension and mild cognitive impairment is brought to the emergency department by his daughter due to sudden-onset confusion, visual hallucinations, and agitation that began earlier that morning. He had recently started nitrofurantoin for a urinary tract infection. On exam, he is disoriented to time and place, has poor attention, and fluctuates between drowsiness and agitation.

26. Which of the following features most strongly supports a diagnosis of delirium over dementia?

    A. Gradual worsening of memory over the past year

    B. Prominent visual hallucinations

    C. Acute onset and fluctuating course

    D. Mini-Mental State Examination score of 18/30

    E. Presence of urinary tract infection

    Correct answer: C

Explanation

Acute onset and fluctuating course is the hallmark of delirium. It typically develops over hours to days and can wax and wane throughout the day. This is the most important feature distinguishing it from dementia, which is insidious in onset.

- A: More characteristic of dementia (e.g., Alzheimer's disease)
- B: Can be seen in both conditions but are common in delirium
- D: Suggests moderate impairment but does not distinguish between acute and chronic processes
- E: Common precipitant for delirium in older adults but not diagnostic on its own

Reference

Inouye SK, Westendorp RGJ, Saczynski JS. Delirium in elderly people. *Lancet*. 2014;383(9920):911–22. https://doi.org/10.1016/S0140-6736(13)60688-1

27. This 76-year-old man undergoes further evaluation. Labs reveal mild leukocytosis and a positive urinalysis. Head CT shows mild age-related atrophy but no acute findings. The physician suspects delirium and wants to confirm the diagnosis and identify reversible contributors.

    Which of the following is the most appropriate next step in the diagnostic workup?
    A. Order a positron emission tomography (PET) scan to assess cortical metabolism.
    B. Administer the Montreal Cognitive Assessment (MoCA).
    C. Perform a Confusion Assessment Method (CAM) evaluation.
    D. Refer for outpatient neuropsychological testing.
    E. Repeat CT head with contrast to assess for occult malignancy.
    Correct answer: C

Explanation

CAM is a validated bedside tool for the diagnosis of delirium. It evaluates four core features: acute onset and fluctuating course, inattention, disorganized thinking, and altered level of consciousness. It is widely used in both hospital and emergency settings.

- A: Not useful in acute settings
- B: Better suited for MCI or dementia, not ideal in delirious patients
- D: Not feasible or appropriate during an acute confusional state
- E: Unwarranted unless focal neurologic signs or cancer history are present

Reference

Inouye SK, et al. Clarifying confusion: the Confusion Assessment Method. *Ann Intern Med*. 1990;113(12):941–8. https://doi.org/10.7326/0003-4819-113-12-941

28. The patient's delirium is confirmed by CAM assessment. She is started on empiric antibiotics for a urinary tract infection and moved to a room with a visible clock and natural lighting. Over the next 48 hours, her confusion improves.

    Which of the following is the best next step to reduce risk of recurrence and optimize long-term outcomes?
    A. Begin donepezil to prevent further cognitive decline.
    B. Schedule a comprehensive outpatient dementia evaluation.
    C. Start low-dose quetiapine for agitation prophylaxis.
    D. Order a repeat head CT in 72 hours.
    E. Discharge with hospice services.
    Correct answer: B

Explanation

Delirium often unmasks underlying cognitive disorders. Given this patient's age and history of progressive cognitive symptoms over months, an outpatient dementia evaluation is important for diagnostic clarity, functional assessment, and care planning.

- A: Should not be started without a confirmed diagnosis of Alzheimer's disease
- C: Not recommended prophylactically, carries risks in older adults
- D: No indication unless new neurological deficits emerge
- E: Inappropriate at this stage, patient improved with treatment

Reference

Marcantonio ER. Delirium in hospitalized older adults. *N Engl J Med*. 2017;377(15):1456–66. https://doi.org/10.1056/NEJMcp1605501

Case 8

A 62-year-old man is referred for evaluation of suspected dementia. His wife reports that over the past 6 months, he has become withdrawn, forgetful, and has trouble concentrating. He frequently says he feels "foggy" and has lost interest in reading or watching TV. He has no pertinent medical history but recently retired. On exam, he is alert and oriented, and his neurologic exam is normal. On the Montreal Cognitive Assessment (MoCA), he scores 21/30, with deficits in attention and recall. Brain MRI is unremarkable.

29. Which of the following findings would be most suggestive of a primary psychiatric condition rather than a neurodegenerative process?
    A. Gradual worsening of cognitive symptoms over 1–2 years
    B. Deficits on delayed recall with relatively preserved recognition

C. Word-finding difficulty and phonemic paraphasias
D. Family history of dementia and late-life depression
E. Visuospatial construction errors and executive dysfunction

Correct answer: B

Explanation

This recall-recognition dissociation is typical in depression-related cognitive impairment (functional cognitive disorder, or pseudodementia). It reflects retrieval deficits due to poor attention or motivation, rather than encoding deficits seen in Alzheimer's disease.

- A: Suggests a neurodegenerative course, particularly Alzheimer's disease
- C: Suggests primary progressive aphasia or early Alzheimer's disease
- D: Adds weight to a true neurocognitive disorder despite relevance of depression
- E: More characteristic of organic cognitive impairment, particularly AD or vascular dementia

Reference

Ball HA, McWhirter L, Ballard C, Bhome R, Blackburn DJ, Edwards MJ, et al. Functional cognitive disorder: dementia's blind spot. *Brain*. 2020;143(10):2895–903. https://doi.org/10.1093/brain/awaa224

30. Which of the following next steps would be most appropriate to clarify the diagnosis?
    A. Prescribe a cholinesterase inhibitor and reassess in 6 weeks.
    B. Order a positron emission tomography (PET) scan for amyloid.
    C. Refer for comprehensive neuropsychological testing.
    D. Repeat MoCA in 1 week to assess for consistency.
    E. Perform lumbar puncture to assess Alzheimer's biomarkers.

    Correct answer: C

Explanation

Neuropsychological testing is the gold standard to distinguish depression-related cognitive impairment from neurodegenerative disease, especially when cognitive screening is ambiguous. It provides a detailed profile of encoding vs. retrieval deficits and effort testing.

- A: Empiric cholinesterase use is not recommended in unclear cases.
- B: Amyloid PET is costly, not first-line, and unlikely to help here.
- D: May show variability but insufficient for differential diagnosis.

- E: CSF biomarkers are useful but not first-line for distinguishing pseudodementia.

Reference

Ball HA, McWhirter L, Ballard C, Bhome R, Blackburn DJ, Edwards MJ, et al. Functional cognitive disorder: dementia's blind spot. *Brain*. 2020;143(10):2895–903. https://doi.org/10.1093/brain/awaa224

31. Which of the following statements is most accurate regarding his treatment and prognosis?
    A. Cognitive symptoms will resolve fully with antidepressant treatment in most patients.
    B. Cholinesterase inhibitors are effective adjuncts to antidepressants in pseudodementia.
    C. This presentation is predictive of rapid conversion to Alzheimer's disease.
    D. Behavioral activation and psychotherapy are often beneficial alongside pharmacotherapy.
    E. Electroconvulsive therapy (ECT) is contraindicated in older adults with cognitive symptoms.

    Correct answer: D

Explanation

Nonpharmacologic treatments, especially behavioral activation and cognitive behavioral therapy, are evidence-based and can improve both mood and cognitive symptoms. Psychosocial interventions often augment pharmacologic therapy in late-life depression with cognitive features.

- A: Many improve, but full resolution is not guaranteed.
- B: Not recommended and may cause unnecessary side effects.
- C: Does not necessarily predict conversion to Alzheimer's.
- E: ECT is not contraindicated, may be highly effective in treatment-resistant cases.

Reference

Ball HA, McWhirter L, Ballard C, Bhome R, Blackburn DJ, Edwards MJ, et al. Functional cognitive disorder: dementia's blind spot. *Brain*. 2020;143(10):2895–903. https://doi.org/10.1093/brain/awaa224

Case 9

A 59 year-old man is brought by his wife for evaluation of personality changes over the past year. He has become socially inappropriate, indifferent to others' emotions, and increasingly impulsive. He eats excessively, often stuffing large amounts of food into his mouth, and has developed compulsive behaviors such as pacing and repetitive humming. His speech is fluent and grammatically correct, though occasionally tangential. Neurologic examination is otherwise unremarkable.

32. Which of the following is the most likely diagnosis?
    A. Alzheimer's disease
    B. Dementia with Lewy bodies
    C. Semantic variant primary progressive aphasia
    D. Behavioral variant frontotemporal dementia
    E. Functional cognitive disorder due to major depression

Correct answer: D

Explanation

This case is classic for behavioral variant frontotemporal dementia (bvFTD), prominent changes in personality, disinhibition, hyperorality, loss of empathy, and stereotyped behaviors, with relative preservation of memory and language structure early on.

- A: Alzheimer's typically presents with episodic memory deficits and lacks early behavioral changes.
- B: DLB includes hallucinations, parkinsonism, and fluctuating cognition, which are absent here.
- C: Semantic variant PPA involves loss of word meaning, not behavioral changes or compulsions.
- E: Depression-related cognitive symptoms usually involve low motivation, not impulsivity or hyperorality.

Reference

Rascovsky K, Hodges JR, Knopman D, et al. Sensitivity of revised diagnostic criteria for the behavioral variant of frontotemporal dementia. *Brain*. 2011;134(9):2456–77. https://doi.org/10.1093/brain/awr179

33. You order a brain MRI to support your clinical impression.

    Which of the following findings would be most supportive of the diagnosis?
    A. Symmetric hippocampal atrophy
    B. Diffuse cerebral atrophy
    C. Parietal-predominant atrophy
    D. Anterior temporal and frontal lobe atrophy
    E. Occipital lobe hypometabolism

Correct answer: D

Explanation

MRI or FDG-PET imaging in behavioral variant FTD typically shows frontal and anterior temporal lobe atrophy or hypometabolism, which correlates with behavioral symptoms and loss of social cognition.

- A: Suggests Alzheimer's disease
- B: Nonspecific, may reflect aging or late-stage disease
- C: Characteristic of posterior cortical atrophy or AD with visuospatial deficits
- E: Suggests dementia with Lewy bodies

Reference

Rascovsky K, Hodges JR, Knopman D, et al. Sensitivity of revised diagnostic criteria for the behavioral variant of frontotemporal dementia. *Brain*. 2011;134(9):2456–77. https://doi.org/10.1093/brain/awr179

34. Which of the following is most appropriate in the management of this patient?
    A. Initiate donepezil 5 mg daily.
    B. Recommend cholinesterase inhibitors and memantine.
    C. Start a selective serotonin reuptake inhibitor (SSRI).
    D. Refer for deep brain stimulation evaluation.
    E. Avoid psychiatric medication due to the risk of worsening cognition.

Correct answer: C

Explanation

SSRIs are often helpful in FTD for treating compulsive behaviors, disinhibition, and emotional blunting. Though not disease-modifying, they may reduce distress and improve quality of life.

- A, B: Cholinesterase inhibitors and memantine are generally ineffective and may worsen symptoms.
- D: Deep brain stimulation is used in movement disorders, not FTD.
- E: Psychiatric medications can be beneficial when used judiciously.

Reference

Huey ED, et al. *A systematic review of pharmacologic treatments for frontotemporal dementia. Am J Psychiatry.* 2006;163(6):1009–1015. doi:10.1176/ajp.2006.163.6.1009

35. A 72-year-old woman with a history of vascular dementia presents with episodes of uncontrollable crying that occur several times per day. The crying is often out of proportion to her emotions and occurs without a clear trigger. She is aware of the episodes and finds them embarrassing. Her mood between episodes is generally stable. She is not suicidal, and her PHQ-9 score is 3.

Which of the following is the most likely diagnosis?
A. Major depressive disorder
B. Generalized anxiety disorder
C. Pseudobulbar affect
D. Apathy
E. Agitation
Correct answer: C

Explanation

Pseudobulbar affect is characterized by involuntary, inappropriate emotional expression (laughing or crying) that is disconnected from internal mood. It is commonly seen in conditions like vascular dementia, ALS, multiple sclerosis, and TBI. The emotional episodes are brief, stereotyped, and socially distressing.

- A: Major depression involves sustained mood changes and vegetative symptoms, which are absent here.
- B: Anxiety would present with worry, restlessness, and somatic symptoms, not isolated crying spells.
- D: Apathy involves lack of motivation or emotional expression, not uncontrollable emotions.
- E: Agitation can occur in patients living with dementia during frustration or overstimulation, not spontaneously.

Reference

Brooks BR, et al. PRISM: a novel research tool to assess the prevalence of pseudobulbar affect symptoms across neurological conditions. *PLoS One*. 2013;8(8):e72232. https://doi.org/10.1371/journal.pone.0072232

36. A 72-year-old right-handed man is referred for progressive difficulty using household tools. He cannot properly use a screwdriver despite knowing what it is and being physically capable. His examination is notable for preserved strength and coordination. Neuropsychological testing shows impaired constructional praxis but intact memory and language.
   What is the most likely diagnosis?
   A. Ideational apraxia
   B. Ideomotor apraxia
   C. Alien limb phenomenon
   D. Constructional apraxia
   E. Anosognosia
   Correct answer: B

Explanation

Ideomotor apraxia refers to impaired ability to imitate gestures or perform purposeful motor tasks on command, despite intact strength and comprehension. It is often due to lesions of the left inferior parietal or premotor cortex and is common in corticobasal syndrome and other neurodegenerative disorders.

- A: In ideational apraxia, there is difficulty sequencing tasks or using tools appropriately due to conceptual deficits, not just motor execution issues.
- C: Alien limb phenomenon involves involuntary movements of a limb, typically accompanied by a sense of foreignness or lack of control, which is not described here.
- D: Constructional apraxia involves problems with spatial tasks such as drawing or assembling objects but does not typically affect tool use or gesture imitation.
- E: Anosognosia is a lack of awareness of one's deficits, not a motor planning disorder.

Reference

Gross RG, Grossman M. Update on apraxia. *Curr Neurol Neurosci Rep*. 2008;8(6):490–6. https://doi.org/10.1007/s11910-008-0078-y

37. A 58-year-old man presents with 2 years of progressive disinhibition, impulsive spending, and compulsive behaviors. His partner reports apathy, inappropriate jokes, and a loss of empathy. MMSE is 29/30. MRI shows frontal-predominant atrophy.
   What is the most likely diagnosis?
   A. Major depressive disorder with psychosis
   B. Behavioral variant frontotemporal dementia
   C. Alzheimer's disease
   D. Normal pressure hydrocephalus
   E. Schizoaffective disorder
   Correct answer: B

Explanation

Behavioral variant FTD often begins with social disinhibition, compulsions, and emotional blunting, with relative sparing of memory and visuospatial skills early. Frontal or anterior temporal atrophy is characteristic.

- A: Depressive disorders rarely present with disinhibition or compulsive behaviors and typically involve more pervasive mood symptoms.
- C: Alzheimer's disease primarily affects memory and is usually associated with temporoparietal atrophy.
- D: Normal pressure hydrocephalus involves gait disturbance, urinary incontinence, and dementia, not disinhibition.
- E: Schizoaffective disorder typically involves mood symptoms with psychosis, not prominent compulsions or early behavioral changes.

Reference

Rascovsky K, Hodges JR, Knopman D, et al. Sensitivity of revised diagnostic criteria for the behavioral variant of frontotemporal dementia. *Brain*. 2011;134(9):2456–2477. https://doi.org/10.1093/brain/awr179

38. A 65-year-old woman presents with word-finding pauses and impaired sentence repetition. Naming is moderately impaired. MRI shows left temporoparietal atrophy.
    What is the most likely diagnosis?
    A. Semantic variant primary progressive aphasia
    B. Logopenic variant primary progressive aphasia
    C. Nonfluent/agrammatic variant primary progressive aphasia
    D. Anomic aphasia
    E. Wernicke aphasia
    Correct answer: B

Explanation

The logopenic variant of PPA is associated with impaired repetition and word-finding and is linked to Alzheimer's pathology. Imaging often shows left temporoparietal atrophy.

- A: The semantic variant is characterized by loss of word meaning and fluent speech, typically with anterior temporal lobe atrophy.
- C: Nonfluent/agrammatic variant includes effortful, halting speech and grammatical errors, with left posterior fronto-insular atrophy.
- D: Anomic aphasia has naming deficits without repetition issues or temporoparietal atrophy.
- E: Wernicke aphasia involves fluent but nonsensical speech and poor comprehension, often with posterior temporal damage.

Reference

Gorno-Tempini ML, Hillis AE, Weintraub S, et al. Classification of primary progressive aphasia and its variants. *Neurology*. 2011;76(11):1006–1014. https://doi.org/10.1212/WNL.0b013e31821103e6

39. A 76-year-old woman with multiple sclerosis experiences sudden crying spells unlinked to her emotions. These episodes are stereotyped and disruptive. What is the most appropriate treatment?
    A. Haloperidol
    B. Dextromethorphan-quinidine
    C. Amitriptyline
    D. Sertraline
    E. Risperidone
    Correct answer: B

Explanation

Pseudobulbar affect (PBA) involves pathologic emotional expression, such as involuntary crying or laughing. Dextromethorphan-quinidine is the only FDA-approved treatment and is well studied in MS and ALS.

- A: Antipsychotics are not first-line and can have significant side effects.
- C: Amitriptyline is not FDA-approved for PBA and has anticholinergic side effects.
- D: SSRIs may help mood symptoms but are less effective than dextromethorphan-quinidine in PBA.
- E: Risperidone, an antipsychotic, is not indicated for PBA and carries risk of extrapyramidal symptoms.

Reference

Brooks BR, Crumpacker D, Fellus J, Kantor D, Kaye RE. PRISM: a novel research tool to assess the prevalence of pseudobulbar affect symptoms across neurological conditions. *PLoS One*. 2013;8(8):e72232. https://doi.org/10.1371/journal.pone.0072232

40. A 69-year-old man reports difficulty recognizing faces, even those of close relatives, though he can describe facial features. Language and memory are intact.
    What is the most likely lesion location?
    A. Right anterior temporal lobe
    B. Left fusiform gyrus
    C. Right fusiform gyrus
    D. Bilateral dorsolateral prefrontal cortex
    E. Left parietal lobe
    Correct answer: C

Explanation

Prosopagnosia, or facial recognition deficit, is linked to dysfunction of the right fusiform face area. It may occur as an isolated deficit or in the context of posterior cortical atrophy or other neurodegenerative diseases.

- A: The right anterior temporal lobe is involved in semantic memory and social processing, not specifically face recognition.
- B: The left fusiform gyrus is more involved in word recognition than face processing.
- D: The dorsolateral prefrontal cortex affects executive function, not visual processing.
- E: The left parietal lobe is more associated with spatial awareness and language, not face recognition.

Reference

Barton JJS. Disorders of face perception and recognition. *Neurol Clin.* 2003;21(2):521–548. https://doi.org/10.1016/S0733-8619(02)00106-2

41. A 76-year-old woman is brought in by her daughter for evaluation of memory problems. Over the past 6 months, she has become increasingly forgetful, often misplacing items and repeating questions. She also has difficulty finding words but maintains fluent speech. She can still drive and manage her finances. On cognitive testing, she scores 23/30 on the Montreal Cognitive Assessment (MoCA), losing points in memory recall and language.

Which of the following is the most likely diagnosis?
   A. Mild cognitive impairment due to Alzheimer's disease
   B. Semantic variant primary progressive aphasia
   C. Typical aging
   D. Frontotemporal dementia, behavioral variant
   E. Vascular cognitive impairment

   Correct answer: A

Explanation

This case presents an early amnestic syndrome with mild language deficits but preserved functional abilities, characteristic of mild cognitive impairment (MCI) due to Alzheimer's disease. Fluent speech with word-finding difficulty aligns with early Alzheimer's pathology.

- B: Semantic variant PPA is nonfluent, with profound word comprehension loss and anomia, not seen here.
- C: Normal aging typically does not involve objective test impairment or repetitive questions.
- D: Behavioral changes and executive dysfunction predominate in bvFTD.
- E: Vascular cognitive impairment typically presents with stepwise decline and more executive dysfunction than language/memory deficits.

Reference

Albert MS, DeKosky ST, Dickson D, Dubois B, Feldman HH, Fox NC, et al. The diagnosis of mild cognitive impairment due to Alzheimer's disease: recommendations from the National Institute on Aging–Alzheimer's Association workgroups on diagnostic guidelines for Alzheimer's disease. *Alzheimers Dement.* 2011;7(3):270–9. https://doi.org/10.1016/j.jalz.2011.03.008

42. A 58-year-old man presents with difficulty recognizing familiar faces, including those of close family members. He can describe individual facial features but cannot identify people unless they speak. His memory, language, and executive function are otherwise preserved.

What is the most likely neuroanatomical localization?
   A. Left temporoparietal junction
   B. Bilateral hippocampi
   C. Right fusiform gyrus
   D. Dorsolateral prefrontal cortex
   E. Precuneus

   Correct answer: C

Explanation

This is classic prosopagnosia (face blindness), often due to lesions in the right fusiform face area within the inferior temporal cortex.

- A: The left TPJ is more associated with language and reading.
- B: Bilateral hippocampi cause anterograde amnesia, not facial recognition deficits.
- D: The DLPFC is linked to executive function.
- E: The precuneus is implicated in visuospatial imagery and self-referential processing, not face recognition.

Reference

Barton JJS. Disorders of face perception and recognition. *Neurol Clin.* 2003;21(2):521–548. https://doi.org/10.1016/S0733-8619(02)00106-2

43. A 62-year-old woman with a history of recurrent depression presents with subjective memory concerns. She reports difficulty concentrating, slowed thinking, and forgetfulness, particularly under stress. On cognitive testing, she scores 29/30 on the MoCA, missing one item on delayed recall.

Which feature most reliably distinguishes a functional cognitive disorder from dementia?
   A. Low cognitive test scores
   B. Poor insight into deficits
   C. Presence of language impairment
   D. Rapid onset and inconsistent performance
   E. Hippocampal atrophy on MRI

   Correct answer: D

Explanation

Functional cognitive disorder (or pseudodementia, depression-related cognitive impairment) often features fluctuating attention, inconsistent effort, and rapid onset.

- A: True dementia may have low scores, but so can pseudodementia.

- B: Pseudodementia usually involves heightened awareness.
- C: Language impairment is less characteristic.
- E: Hippocampal atrophy supports a neurodegenerative process.

Reference

Ball HA, McWhirter L, Ballard C, Bhome R, Blackburn DJ, Edwards MJ, et al. Functional cognitive disorder: dementia's blind spot. *Brain*. 2020;143(10):2895–903. https://doi.org/10.1093/brain/awaa224

44. A 66-year-old woman is evaluated for progressive difficulty using her right hand. She reports trouble using keys and utensils, despite preserved strength and sensation. On examination, she has normal motor and sensory function but is unable to demonstrate how to brush her hair with a comb placed in her hand.
    Which diagnosis best explains her symptoms?
    A. Corticobasal syndrome
    B. Alzheimer's disease
    C. Parkinson's disease
    D. Apraxia of speech
    E. Posterior cortical atrophy
    Correct answer: A

Explanation

This is classic ideomotor apraxia with asymmetric motor planning dysfunction and alien limb signs, most often due to corticobasal degeneration.

- B: AD can involve apraxia late but not typically in isolation.
- C: Parkinson's disease primarily affects motor speed and rigidity.
- D: Apraxia of speech affects verbal articulation, not limb praxis.
- E: PCA affects visual-spatial skills, not limb praxis.

Reference

Armstrong MJ, Litvan I, Lang AE, et al. Criteria for the diagnosis of corticobasal degeneration. *Neurology*. 2013;80(5):496–503. https://doi.org/10.1212/WNL.0b013e31827f0fd1

45. A 69-year-old retired teacher presents with insidious decline in judgment, social withdrawal, and inappropriate behaviors, including making lewd comments to strangers. His speech is fluent, and memory testing is largely intact.

Which neuropsychological deficit is most likely to be observed?
A. Poor delayed recall
B. Agrammatic speech
C. Visuospatial deficits
D. Loss of theory of mind
E. Prosopagnosia
Correct answer: D

Explanation

Behavioral variant frontotemporal dementia (bvFTD) commonly impairs social cognition, especially theory of mind, the ability to infer others' emotions, intentions, or perspectives.

- A: Memory is relatively preserved early in bvFTD.
- B: Agrammatic speech is more typical of nonfluent PPA.
- C: Visuospatial deficits are more characteristic of Alzheimer's or PCA.
- E: Prosopagnosia relates to occipitotemporal cortex damage, not frontal pathology.

Reference

Gregory C, Lough S, Stone V, et al. Theory of mind in patients with frontal variant frontotemporal dementia and Alzheimer's disease: theoretical and practical implications. *Brain*. 2002;125(Pt 4):752–764. https://doi.org/10.1093/brain/awf079

46. A 71-year-old man presents with gradual difficulty understanding speech over the past year. He often answers inappropriately and appears frustrated during conversations. Neurologic exam is unremarkable. Neuropsychological testing shows preserved fluency but impaired auditory comprehension and repetition. Brain MRI reveals atrophy in the left posterior temporal lobe.
    What is the most likely diagnosis?
    A. Logopenic variant primary progressive aphasia
    B. Semantic variant primary progressive aphasia
    C. Nonfluent/agrammatic variant primary progressive aphasia
    D. Wernicke aphasia
    E. Alzheimer's disease
    Correct answer: A

Explanation

Logopenic variant primary progressive aphasia (lvPPA) typically presents with impaired repetition and word-finding difficulty, often progressing from impaired auditory comprehension. It is associated with left posterior perisylvian or parietal atrophy and is often due to Alzheimer's pathology.

- B: Impaired single-word comprehension and object naming, anterior temporal atrophy
- C: Effortful speech, grammar errors, left frontal atrophy
- D: Sudden onset, typically from stroke
- E: Global memory impairment more prominent early

Reference

Gorno-Tempini ML, et al. Classification of primary progressive aphasia and its variants. *Neurology*. 2011;76(11):1006–1014. https://doi.org/10.1212/WNL.0b013e31821103e6

47. A 65-year-old woman with a history of poorly controlled diabetes presents with subacute confusion, visual hallucinations, and fluctuating attention. On exam, she is inattentive, with prominent asterixis and myoclonus. EEG shows triphasic waves.

    What is the most likely diagnosis?
    A. Creutzfeldt-Jakob disease
    B. Lewy body dementia
    C. Diabetic encephalopathy
    D. Hepatic encephalopathy
    E. Uremic encephalopathy
    Correct answer: E

Explanation

Uremic encephalopathy often presents with altered mental status, asterixis, myoclonus, and triphasic waves on EEG. It is common in patients with diabetes and renal dysfunction.

- A: Rapid progression, but less likely given context.
- B: Insidious onset, not subacute.
- C: Rare term; uremia is more specific.
- D: Requires liver disease context.

Reference

Achanti A, Szerlip HM. Acid-base disorders in the critically ill patient. *Clin J Am Soc Nephrol*. 2023;18(1):102–12. https://doi.org/10.2215/CJN.04500422

48. A 58-year-old man is brought by his wife due to changes in behavior. He has become socially inappropriate, overeats sweets, and shows loss of empathy. He denies problems and performs normally on memory testing. MRI shows frontal and anterior temporal lobe atrophy.

    What is the most likely diagnosis?
    A. Behavioral variant frontotemporal dementia
    B. Alzheimer's disease
    C. Korsakoff syndrome
    D. Normal pressure hydrocephalus
    E. Depression with cognitive impairment
    Correct answer: A

Explanation

bvFTD presents with early personality and behavioral changes, such as disinhibition, compulsions, and dietary changes.

- B: Memory loss usually first.
- C: Associated with thiamine deficiency.
- D: Classic triad includes gait and incontinence.
- E: Insight often preserved in depression.

Reference

Rascovsky K, et al. Sensitivity of revised diagnostic criteria for the behavioral variant of frontotemporal dementia. *Brain*. 2011;134(Pt 9):2456–2477. https://doi.org/10.1093/brain/awr179

49. A 79-year-old woman with hypertension presents with sudden-onset inability to speak fluently and difficulty writing. She can comprehend speech and follow commands. Exam reveals right facial weakness and hemiparesis.

    What is the most likely lesion location?
    A. Left inferior frontal gyrus
    B. Left superior temporal gyrus
    C. Left occipital cortex
    D. Right parietal cortex
    E. Right frontal operculum
    Correct answer: A

Explanation

Broca's area (left inferior frontal gyrus) governs speech production. Lesions cause expressive aphasia with preserved comprehension.

- B: Associated with Wernicke's aphasia
- C: Involved in vision
- D: Causes neglect
- E: Less relevant unless left-handed

50. A 60-year-old retired teacher complains of recent memory difficulty. MoCA score is 25/30 with deficits in delayed recall and abstraction. She remains independent in ADLs. MRI shows mild hippocampal atrophy.

    What is the most likely diagnosis?
    A. Mild cognitive impairment due to Alzheimer's disease
    B. Alzheimer's disease dementia
    C. Depression
    D. Normal aging
    E. Limbic encephalitis
    Correct answer: A

Explanation

MCI due to AD features early memory loss with preserved function and mild hippocampal atrophy.

- B: AD dementia involves functional decline.
- C: Depression has variable attention and effort.
- D: Would not show MoCA impairment.
- E: Rapid onset and often seizures/psychiatric features.

Reference

Albert MS, DeKosky ST, Dickson D, et al. The diagnosis of mild cognitive impairment due to Alzheimer's disease: recommendations from the National Institute on Aging-Alzheimer's Association workgroups. *Alzheimers Dement*. 2011;7(3):270–9. https://doi.org/10.1016/j.jalz.2011.03.008

Case 10

A 58-year-old man is brought by his wife due to increasingly inappropriate behavior over the past year. He has been making impulsive financial decisions, making crude jokes at work, and recently attempted to hug a stranger in a grocery store. He denies any memory issues. On cognitive testing, he performs poorly on measures of social cognition and executive function but scores normally on orientation and short-term recall. MRI reveals focal atrophy of the bilateral frontal lobes, greater on the right.

51. What is the most likely diagnosis?
    A. Alzheimer's disease
    B. Behavioral variant frontotemporal dementia
    C. Major depressive disorder
    D. Vascular dementia
    E. Primary progressive aphasia
    Correct answer: B

Explanation

bvFTD often presents with disinhibition, apathy, loss of empathy, compulsive behaviors, or dietary changes. Memory and visuospatial function are often preserved early. The frontal atrophy, social-emotional dysregulation, and executive dysfunction are characteristic.

- A: Alzheimer's presents with early amnestic features and parietal atrophy.
- C: MDD may mimic apathy but lacks disinhibition and frontal atrophy.
- D: Vascular dementia tends to have stepwise decline and focal neurologic signs.
- E: PPA presents with early language deficits, not behavioral symptoms.

Reference

Rascovsky K, Hodges JR, Knopman D, et al. Sensitivity of revised diagnostic criteria for the behavioral variant of frontotemporal dementia. *Brain*. 2011;134(9):2456–77. https://doi.org/10.1093/brain/awr179

52. Which of the following biomarkers or clinical features would most support the diagnosis in this patient?
    A. Low cerebrospinal fluid (CSF) beta-amyloid and high tau
    B. Positive amyloid PET scan
    C. Negative Alzheimer's biomarkers and presence of compulsive rituals
    D. Elevated neurofilament light chain (NfL) in plasma
    E. Generalized cerebral atrophy on MRI
    Correct answer: C

Explanation

Supportive features of bvFTD include negative Alzheimer's disease biomarkers, focal frontal/temporal atrophy, and specific behavioral signs such as compulsive or ritualistic behaviors. Amyloid PET and CSF studies can help rule out AD.

- A and B: Consistent with Alzheimer's.
- D: Elevated NfL may be seen but is nonspecific.
- E: Generalized atrophy lacks diagnostic specificity.

Reference

Rascovsky K, Hodges JR, Knopman D, et al. Sensitivity of revised diagnostic criteria for the behavioral variant of frontotemporal dementia. *Brain*. 2011;134(9):2456–77. https://doi.org/10.1093/brain/awr179

53. Which of the following medications has shown some benefit in managing behavioral symptoms in this patient's condition?
    A. Donepezil
    B. Haloperidol
    C. Sertraline
    D. Levodopa
    E. Memantine
    Correct answer: C

Explanation

Selective serotonin reuptake inhibitors (SSRIs) like sertraline or citalopram can modestly reduce disinhibition, compulsive behavior, and irritability in bvFTD. No medications are FDA-approved for disease modification in FTD.

- A and E: Not effective and may worsen behavior
- B: Reserved for severe agitation due to side effects
- D: No role in bvFTD

Reference

Rascovsky K, Hodges JR, Knopman D, et al. Sensitivity of revised diagnostic criteria for the behavioral variant of frontotemporal dementia. *Brain*. 2011;134(9):2456–77. https://doi.org/10.1093/brain/awr179

Case 11

A 59-year-old man presents for evaluation of cognitive changes. He has a history of moderate traumatic brain injury (TBI) after a motor vehicle accident 18 months ago. He was comatose for 2 weeks, followed by a prolonged inpatient rehabilitation stay. Since discharge, his family reports increasing forgetfulness, distractibility, and emotional outbursts. He recently became lost while walking to a familiar store. MRI shows moderate frontotemporal volume loss with periventricular white matter changes.

54. Which of the following most accurately describes the expected cognitive profile in this patient?
    A. Severe anterograde amnesia with spared executive function
    B. Executive dysfunction with impaired attention and processing speed
    C. Fluent aphasia with impaired repetition
    D. Isolated visuospatial dysfunction
    E. Semantic memory impairment with spared episodic recall

    Correct answer: B

Explanation

Cognitive deficits after moderate or severe TBI often involve executive dysfunction, impaired attention, slowed processing speed, and difficulty with memory encoding or retrieval. The frontal and temporal lobe volume loss seen on imaging supports these deficits. Behavioral changes (e.g., emotional outbursts, impulsivity) also commonly result from frontal lobe injury.

- A: While memory issues are common, executive dysfunction and attention deficits are more characteristic.
- C: Fluent aphasia with impaired repetition suggests Wernicke or conduction aphasia, not TBI.
- D: Isolated visuospatial deficits are more typical of posterior cortical syndromes (e.g., PCA).
- E: Semantic memory impairment with spared episodic recall is suggestive of semantic variant PPA, not post-TBI.

Reference

Rabinowitz AR, Levin HS. Cognitive sequelae of traumatic brain injury. *Psychiatr Clin North Am*. 2014;37(1):1–11. https://doi.org/10.1016/j.psc.2013.11.004

55. The same 59-year-old man is referred for neuropsychological testing following moderate TBI. His exam reveals impulsivity, variable attention, impaired short-term memory, and difficulties with planning. He asks the examiner to repeat instructions frequently, and his responses slow with increasing task complexity.

    Which neuropsychological finding is most consistent with frontal-subcortical dysfunction?
    A. Poor confrontation naming with semantic paraphasias
    B. Impaired delayed recall with intact encoding and cueing
    C. Perseveration on set-shifting tasks
    D. Constructional apraxia with neglect
    E. Fluent speech with impaired single-word comprehension

    Correct answer: C

Explanation

Perseveration, repeating a response despite changing task demands, is a hallmark of executive dysfunction, commonly due to frontal lobe injury, particularly affecting the dorsolateral prefrontal cortex. Set-shifting (e.g., switching between number and letter sequences) is often impaired after TBI, reflecting deficits in cognitive flexibility and control.

- A: Suggests semantic variant PPA, not typical of TBI.
- B: Pattern seen in depression or subcortical dementia, but TBI-related memory issues often include encoding and retrieval.
- D: Suggestive of right parietal injury, often from stroke or PCA.
- E: Fluent speech with impaired comprehension occurs in Wernicke aphasia, not from TBI.

Reference

Dikmen SS, Machamer JE, Powell JM, Temkin NR. Outcome 3 to 5 years after moderate to severe traumatic brain injury. *Arch Phys Med Rehabil*. 2003;84(10):1449–57. https://doi.org/10.1016/s0003-9993(03)00287-9

56. The patient and his spouse return 6 months later. Although he is physically independent, his wife notes personality changes—he is more irritable, socially inappropriate, and prone to outbursts. He also seems indifferent to these behaviors. Cognitive testing shows mild executive dysfunction but no clear dementia.

    Which of the following is the most appropriate next step in management?
    A. Start cholinesterase inhibitor therapy.
    B. Refer for inpatient cognitive rehabilitation.
    C. Begin a selective serotonin reuptake inhibitor (SSRI).

D. Order a PET scan to evaluate for frontotemporal dementia.

E. Recommend return to work with no restrictions.

Correct answer: C

Explanation

SSRIs are frequently used in TBI to address post-injury mood lability, irritability, impulsivity, and emotional dysregulation. They are often first-line treatments for behavioral disturbances, even when cognitive testing is relatively preserved.

- A: Not effective for behavioral symptoms post-TBI and not indicated without dementia.
- B: Inappropriate for someone with high independence and mild deficits.
- D: No evidence supports FTD; time course and context (post-TBI) suggest nondegenerative etiology.
- E: Premature given persistent behavioral symptoms.

Reference

Silver JM, McAllister TW, Arciniegas DB. Depression and cognitive complaints following mild traumatic brain injury. *Am J Psychiatry*. 2009;166(6):653–61. https://doi.org/10.1176/appi.ajp.2009.08111676

57. A 76-year-old woman with mild Alzheimer's disease presents for a follow-up visit. Her family reports that while her memory has remained stable, she has recently begun exhibiting increased apathy, loss of interest in activities she previously enjoyed, and social withdrawal. She denies sadness or suicidal ideation. Her cognitive testing is unchanged from 6 months ago, and physical exam is unremarkable.

    Which of the following behavioral symptoms is most commonly associated with Alzheimer's disease and is present in this case?

    A. Delusions
    B. Hallucinations
    C. Apathy
    D. Elation
    E. Disinhibition

    Correct answer: C

Explanation

Apathy is the most common neuropsychiatric symptom in Alzheimer's disease, particularly in the early to moderate stages. It is characterized by diminished motivation, reduced goal-directed behavior, and emotional indifference. It can occur independently of depression and is often underrecognized despite its significant impact on quality of life and caregiver burden.

- A: Delusions may occur later but are less common in early AD.
- B: Hallucinations are more typical of dementia with Lewy bodies.
- D: Elated mood is rare in AD and more suggestive of mania.
- E: Disinhibition is more characteristic of frontotemporal dementia.

Reference

Cummings JL, Mega M, Gray K, Rosenberg-Thompson S, Carusi DA, Gornbein J. The Neuropsychiatric Inventory: comprehensive assessment of psychopathology in dementia. *Neurology*. 1994;44(12):2308–2314. https://doi.org/10.1212/WNL.44.12.2308

58. A 68-year-old man with Parkinson's disease undergoes bilateral subthalamic nucleus deep brain stimulation (STN-DBS) to manage his motor fluctuations. Postoperatively, his tremor and rigidity improve significantly. However, within weeks, his family reports that he has become unusually cheerful, is sleeping less, makes impulsive financial decisions, and expresses grandiose ideas. He has no prior psychiatric history.

    Which of the following is the most likely explanation for his behavioral change?

    A. Dopaminergic overdose syndrome
    B. Normal psychological adjustment after motor improvement
    C. STN-DBS-induced hypomania
    D. Postoperative delirium
    E. Serotonin syndrome

    Correct answer: C

Explanation

STN-DBS can lead to mood and behavioral changes, including hypomania and mania, particularly in the early postoperative period. These effects are thought to be related to spread of stimulation to limbic regions or altered dopaminergic tone. Hypomania may manifest as euphoria, decreased sleep, impulsivity, and grandiosity.

- A: Dopaminergic overdose syndrome involves medication-induced behavioral changes but is less likely here given recent DBS.
- B: Adjustment to motor improvement would not cause hypomania.
- D: Postoperative delirium presents with inattention and fluctuating mental status, not mood elevation.
- E: Serotonin syndrome includes neuromuscular and autonomic findings, not purely mood changes.

Reference

Temel Y, Kessels A, Tan S, Topdag A, Boon P, Visser-Vandewalle V. Behavioural changes after bilateral subthalamic stimulation in advanced Parkinson disease: a systematic review. *Parkinsonism Relat Disord.* 2006;12(5):265–272. https://doi.org/10.1016/j.parkreldis.2006.01.004

59. A 24-year-old woman with drug-resistant temporal lobe epilepsy is being evaluated for surgical treatment. She has frequent focal impaired awareness seizures and reports persistent memory problems. Her neuropsychological testing shows deficits in verbal memory and executive function. She also endorses anhedonia, fatigue, and feelings of worthlessness. MRI shows left hippocampal sclerosis.

    Which of the following statements best reflects the neuropsychiatric and cognitive comorbidities of epilepsy?
    A. Depression in epilepsy is rare and usually secondary to medication side effects.
    B. Memory impairment is unrelated to the seizure focus.
    C. Cognitive and psychiatric comorbidities are common and may impact surgical candidacy.
    D. Executive dysfunction is only seen with generalized epilepsy.
    E. Psychiatric symptoms in epilepsy always resolve after surgery.

Correct answer: C

Explanation

Cognitive and psychiatric comorbidities, particularly depression, anxiety, and memory deficits, are common in epilepsy, especially temporal lobe epilepsy. These comorbidities can impact quality of life and must be carefully evaluated before epilepsy surgery. Psychiatric conditions may persist or even worsen postoperatively, especially if unaddressed preoperatively.

- A: Depression is common in epilepsy and not merely a medication side effect.
- B: Verbal memory impairment is associated with left temporal lobe foci.
- D: Executive dysfunction is not exclusive to generalized epilepsy and can be seen in focal epilepsy.
- E: Psychiatric symptoms may persist or emerge even after surgery.

Reference

Kanner AM. Psychiatric comorbidities in epilepsy: should they be considered in the classification of epileptic disorders? *Epilepsy Behav.* 2016;64(Pt B):306–8. https://doi.org/10.1016/j.yebeh.2016.06.040

60. A 68-year-old man is admitted for pneumonia and develops confusion, fluctuating attention, and episodes of mutism and posturing. Neurologic exam reveals rigidity, negativism, and staring. He does not follow commands consistently. EEG shows diffuse slowing without epileptiform activity. Routine labs are unremarkable.

    Which of the following is the most accurate interpretation of this presentation?
    A. The patient has nonconvulsive status epilepticus.
    B. The patient meets criteria for hypoactive delirium only.
    C. Catatonia and delirium are mutually exclusive diagnoses.
    D. Delirium and catatonia can co-occur and are associated with worse outcomes.
    E. The EEG confirms a diagnosis of catatonia.

Correct answer: D

Explanation

Catatonia and delirium are increasingly recognized to coexist, especially in older adults and medically ill populations. When present together, outcomes are poorer, and careful evaluation is required, as treatments differ. Benzodiazepines, typically avoided in delirium, may be indicated when catatonia is present. Diagnosis requires recognition of overlapping features and tailored management.

- A: EEG does not show epileptiform discharges, ruling out nonconvulsive status epilepticus.
- B: Hypoactive delirium does not account for the catatonic signs like posturing and mutism.
- C: They are not mutually exclusive; they often co-occur.
- E: EEG is nonspecific for catatonia and primarily used to exclude seizures.

Reference

Wilson JE, Carlson R, Duggan MC, et al. Delirium and catatonia in critically ill patients: the Delirium and Catatonia Prospective Cohort Investigation. *Crit Care Med.* 2017;45(11):1837–1844. https://doi.org/10.1097/CCM.0000000000002642

61. A 51-year-old woman with bipolar disorder is brought to the emergency department for immobility, refusal to eat, mutism, and waxy flexibility. She is afebrile and hemodynamically stable. Laboratory workup, urinalysis, and head CT are unremarkable. Bush-Francis Catatonia Rating Scale score is 10. Lorazepam 1 mg IV is administered, and 30 min later, she becomes more responsive and begins following commands.

What is the next best step in management?
A. Begin high-dose antipsychotic therapy.
B. Discharge home with outpatient psychiatric follow-up.
C. Initiate a scheduled lorazepam trial.
D. Administer electroconvulsive therapy (ECT) immediately.
E. Order a lumbar puncture to rule out autoimmune encephalitis.

Correct answer: C

Explanation

The patient's positive response to the lorazepam challenge is diagnostic of catatonia. The next appropriate step is to initiate scheduled lorazepam, typically 1–2 mg every 8 h, with close monitoring and dose adjustment. Benzodiazepines are the first-line treatment for catatonia. ECT is reserved for refractory or severe cases (e.g., malignant catatonia).

- A: High-dose antipsychotics can worsen catatonia or precipitate malignant catatonia.
- B: Discharge is unsafe; continued inpatient treatment is required.
- D: ECT is not the immediate next step after a positive lorazepam response unless refractory.
- E: Lumbar puncture is not necessary in the absence of atypical features.

Reference

Francis A. Catatonia: diagnosis, classification, and treatment. *Curr Psychiatry Rep*. 2010;12(3):180–5. https://doi.org/10.1007/s11920-010-0113-y

62. A 19-year-old collegiate soccer player presents 2 days after sustaining a concussion during a game. He did not lose consciousness but reports persistent headache, difficulty concentrating, slowed thinking, and increased sensitivity to noise. Neurological examination is normal. MRI of the brain is unremarkable.

    Which of the following cognitive symptoms is most commonly associated with concussion?
    A. Aphasia
    B. Hemispatial neglect
    C. Impaired working memory and attention
    D. Anterograde amnesia lasting more than 24 hours
    E. Visual agnosia
    Correct answer: C

Explanation

The most common cognitive symptoms of concussion include impaired attention, working memory, and processing speed. These symptoms often resolve over days to weeks but in some individuals may persist longer as part of post-concussive syndrome. Diagnosis is clinical, and neuroimaging is typically normal.

- A: Aphasia suggests focal cortical lesion, not typical of uncomplicated concussion.
- B: Hemispatial neglect is associated with parietal lobe damage, not concussion.
- D: Anterograde amnesia >24 hours is uncommon and would suggest more severe TBI.
- E: Visual agnosia points to posterior cortical damage, not a typical concussion finding.

Reference

McCrory P, Meeuwisse W, Dvorak J, et al. Consensus statement on concussion in sport—the 5th international conference on concussion in sport held in Berlin, October 2016. *Br J Sports Med*. 2017;51(11):838–847. https://doi.org/10.1136/bjsports-2017-097699

63. A 67-year-old woman with mild cognitive impairment (MCI) presents for follow-up. She is independent in daily activities but complains of increasing difficulty remembering recent conversations and managing her medications. She is interested in nonpharmacologic options to preserve her cognition.

    Which of the following is the most evidence-based component of cognitive rehabilitation in MCI?
    A. Psychoanalysis
    B. Mindfulness-based stress reduction
    C. Global cognitive stimulation without strategy training
    D. Task-specific cognitive training with compensation strategies
    E. Transcranial magnetic stimulation (TMS)
    Correct answer: D

Explanation

Cognitive rehabilitation in MCI is most effective when it includes structured, task-specific cognitive training paired with real-world compensation strategies, such as using calendars or to-do lists. These approaches aim to enhance function in targeted cognitive domains and support independence.

- A: Psychoanalysis is not indicated or supported for cognitive rehabilitation.
- B: Mindfulness-based stress reduction may improve quality of life but has limited evidence for direct cognitive improvement in MCI.
- C: Global stimulation without strategy lacks specific benefit for functional outcomes.
- E: TMS remains investigational in MCI and is not a standard component of rehabilitation.

Reference

Clare L, Kudlicka A, Oyebode JR, et al. Individual goal-oriented cognitive rehabilitation to improve everyday functioning for people with early-stage dementia: A multicentre randomised controlled trial (GREAT). *Int J Geriatr Psychiatry*. 2019;34(5):709–721. https://doi.org/10.1002/gps.5076

64. A 23-year-old woman is brought to the emergency department by her roommate for bizarre behavior and confusion. Over the past few days, she has become increasingly paranoid, talking to herself, and had a generalized tonic-clonic seizure earlier today. On exam, she is agitated and unable to follow commands. CT head is unremarkable. CSF shows lymphocytic pleocytosis and elevated protein. EEG reveals diffuse slowing with extreme delta brush pattern.

What is the most likely diagnosis?
A. Herpes simplex virus encephalitis
B. Anti-NMDA receptor encephalitis
C. Schizophrenia
D. Hashimoto encephalopathy
E. Temporal lobe epilepsy
Correct answer: B

Explanation

Anti-NMDA receptor encephalitis typically affects young women and presents with a subacute onset of psychiatric symptoms (e.g., paranoia, hallucinations), seizures, dyskinesias, autonomic instability, and cognitive dysfunction. The extreme delta brush pattern on EEG is highly suggestive. Diagnosis is confirmed via CSF NMDA receptor antibody testing. Underlying ovarian teratomas should be ruled out.

- A: HSV encephalitis may present similarly, but EEG often shows focal temporal abnormalities; PCR is key for diagnosis.
- C: Schizophrenia typically lacks seizures, CSF abnormalities, and EEG findings.
- D: Hashimoto encephalopathy is rare, associated with thyroid antibodies, but lacks extreme delta brush.
- E: Temporal lobe epilepsy can cause psychiatric symptoms but would not explain the global encephalopathy, CSF findings, or EEG pattern.

Reference

Dalmau J, Lancaster E, Martinez-Hernandez E, et al. Clinical experience and laboratory investigations in patients with anti-NMDAR encephalitis. *Lancet Neurol*. 2011;10(1):63–74. https://doi.org/10.1016/S1474-4422(10)70253-2

65. An 82-year-old man with moderate Alzheimer's disease is brought in by his daughter for increasing agitation, especially in the late afternoon. He has started yelling and pacing and occasionally becomes physically aggressive. He has no signs of infection or pain, and recent labs and brain imaging are unremarkable. His daughter reports that the behavior worsens when he is overstimulated.

What is the most appropriate initial management approach?
A. Initiate low-dose risperidone.
B. Refer for inpatient psychiatric hospitalization.
C. Begin scheduled haloperidol.
D. Implement nonpharmacologic behavioral interventions.
E. Start prazosin for agitation.
Correct answer: D

Explanation

The first-line approach to managing agitation in dementia involves nonpharmacologic strategies. These include environmental modifications, ensuring comfort, optimizing routine, caregiver education, and reducing triggers such as overstimulation or unmet needs. Pharmacologic treatments are reserved for severe, dangerous, or refractory symptoms.

- A: Risperidone carries black box warnings for increased mortality in dementia patients and should only be used for severe or dangerous agitation.
- B: Psychiatric hospitalization is not appropriate for mild to moderate agitation without danger to self or others.
- C: Haloperidol has a high risk of extrapyramidal symptoms and should be avoided unless necessary and under close supervision.
- E: Prazosin may be useful in PTSD-related agitation or in specific cases but not first-line for dementia-related agitation.

Reference

Kales HC, Gitlin LN, Lyketsos CG. Assessment and management of behavioral and psychological symptoms of dementia. *BMJ*. 2015;350:h369. https://doi.org/10.1136/bmj.h369

66. A 29-year-old man presents to clinic 3 months after a mild traumatic brain injury sustained in a motor vehicle collision. He reports poor concentration, irritability, depressed mood, and insomnia. He is working part-time but finds it difficult to focus or stay motivated. He denies suicidal ideation. His medical history is unremarkable, and his neurologic examination is normal.

Which of the following psychiatric conditions is most commonly associated with mild to moderate TBI?

A. Generalized anxiety disorder

B. Bipolar disorder

C. Major depressive disorder

D. Schizophrenia

E. Obsessive-compulsive disorder

Correct answer: C

Explanation

Major depressive disorder (MDD) is the most commonly diagnosed psychiatric disorder following mild to moderate TBI. Risk is elevated due to injury-related disruption of frontolimbic circuits, psychosocial stressors, and adjustment to functional limitations. Post-TBI depression often emerges within the first year and significantly affects recovery and quality of life.

- A: Anxiety may occur post-TBI, but MDD is more prevalent and has stronger evidence.
- B: Bipolar disorder is rarely a direct consequence of TBI.
- D: Schizophrenia is not commonly precipitated by TBI.
- E: OCD is less commonly reported after TBI compared to mood disorders.

Reference

Bombardier CH, Fann JR, Temkin NR, Esselman PC, Barber J, Dikmen SS. Rates of major depressive disorder and clinical outcomes following traumatic brain injury. *JAMA*. 2010;303(19):1938–1945. https://doi.org/10.1001/jama.2010.599

67. A 56-year-old woman is admitted after cardiac arrest with prolonged resuscitation. She remains unresponsive. Neurology is consulted on hospital day 5. She opens her eyes spontaneously but does not follow commands. She does not speak, track with her eyes, or show purposeful movement, though she occasionally withdraws to pain. MRI reveals diffuse anoxic injury. Her family asks about prognosis and current level of consciousness.

    Which of the following best describes her current state?

    A. Brain death

    B. Minimally conscious state

    C. Vegetative state (unresponsive wakefulness syndrome)

    D. Locked-in syndrome

    E. Psychogenic unresponsiveness

    Correct answer: C

Explanation

This patient demonstrates wakefulness without awareness, a hallmark of the vegetative state (also called unresponsive wakefulness syndrome). These patients may have preserved sleep-wake cycles and eye-opening but lack any evidence of conscious awareness, language comprehension, or purposeful behavior.

- A: Brain death: Patients do not open eyes or breathe spontaneously and lack all brain stem reflexes.
- B: Minimally conscious state: Requires reproducible signs of awareness such as visual pursuit or command following, which are not present.
- D: Locked-in syndrome: Characterized by intact awareness with quadriplegia and preserved vertical eye movements, not seen here.
- E: Psychogenic unresponsiveness: Usually lacks structural brain injury and may involve resistance to eye opening or inconsistent behaviors.

Reference

Giacino JT, Kalmar K, Whyte J. The JFK Coma Recovery Scale-Revised: measurement characteristics and diagnostic utility. *Arch Phys Med Rehabil.* 2004;85(12):2020–2029. https://doi.org/10.1016/j.apmr.2004.02.033

68. A 33-year-old woman presents with episodes of right arm weakness and tremors that began 6 months ago. The episodes occur unpredictably, are more frequent under stress, and resolve spontaneously. Neurologic examination is notable for give-way weakness of the right upper limb and variable tremor suppression with distraction. Brain MRI and EMG/NCS are unremarkable. She reports a prior history of childhood trauma and current psychosocial stressors.

    Which of the following features most strongly supports a diagnosis of functional neurologic disorder?

    A. Negative MRI of the brain

    B. Presence of childhood trauma

    C. Inconsistency of symptoms during examination

    D. Absence of medical comorbidities

    E. Symptoms triggered by emotional distress

    Correct answer: C

Explanation

Positive clinical signs (e.g., Hoover's sign, entrainment of tremor, variability with distraction) are the most reliable and specific indicators of functional neurologic disorder (FND).

Diagnosis relies on identifiable internal inconsistencies in symptom presentation that are not consistent with known neurologic disease.

- A: Negative MRI of the brain: While supportive, a normal MRI alone is not diagnostic.
- B: Presence of childhood trauma: Increases risk but lacks diagnostic specificity.
- D: Absence of medical comorbidities: FND can occur with or without comorbidities.
- E: Symptoms triggered by emotional distress: Nonspecific, not exclusive to FND.

Reference

Espay AJ, Aybek S, Carson A, et al. Current concepts in diagnosis and treatment of functional neurological disorders. *JAMA Neurol.* 2018;75(9):1132–1141. https://doi.org/10.1001/jamaneurol.2018.1264

69. A 27-year-old man is referred for evaluation of episodic behavioral outbursts during sleep. His partner reports sudden episodes of thrashing, pelvic thrusting, and loud vocalizations, often occurring within 30 min of falling asleep. The events last less than a minute and are followed by amnesia. He denies daytime sleepiness or mood symptoms. Neurologic examination is normal. A routine EEG is unrevealing.

What is the most likely diagnosis?
A. REM sleep behavior disorder
B. Nocturnal panic attacks
C. Frontal lobe epilepsy
D. Psychogenic non-epileptic seizures
E. Narcolepsy with cataplexy
Correct answer: C

Explanation

Nocturnal frontal lobe epilepsy (NFLE) typically presents with brief, stereotyped, hypermotor events during non-REM sleep, often with pelvic thrusting, vocalizations, and sudden arousals. The events are typically amnesic and cluster during early sleep cycles. Routine EEG may be unrevealing due to deep epileptogenic foci, and video-EEG monitoring is often needed.

- A: REM sleep behavior disorder: Occurs in later sleep stages with dream enactment and lacks hypermotor features
- B: Nocturnal panic attacks: Involve autonomic symptoms and fear, not stereotyped motor outbursts
- D: Psychogenic non-epileptic seizures: Lack stereotypy and often present with psychosocial stressors

- E: Narcolepsy with cataplexy: Involves daytime sleepiness and atonia, not sleep-onset hypermotor behaviors

Reference

Provini F, Plazzi G, Tinuper P, et al. Nocturnal frontal lobe epilepsy: a clinical and polygraphic overview of 100 consecutive cases. *Brain.* 1999;122(6):1017–1031. https://doi.org/10.1093/brain/122.6.1017

70. A 68-year-old woman with mild cognitive impairment due to Alzheimer's disease is being evaluated for disease-modifying therapy. Her amyloid PET scan is positive, and tau PET imaging shows intermediate levels of cortical tau deposition. She is otherwise healthy, with normal renal and hepatic function and no history of stroke. Her family is interested in new treatment options.

Which of the following statements about donanemab is most accurate?
A. It targets tau aggregates and is approved for advanced Alzheimer's disease.
B. It is administered orally once daily for 12 months.
C. It removes amyloid plaques but has no effect on tau burden.
D. It showed slowed clinical decline in early AD but was possibly less effective in high tau PET burden.
E. It is contraindicated in patients with intermediate tau burden on PET.
Correct answer: D

Explanation

Donanemab is a monoclonal antibody that targets N3pG-modified amyloid-β and was shown to slow cognitive and functional decline in patients with early symptomatic Alzheimer's disease, particularly those with low or intermediate tau burden. In the TRAILBLAZER-ALZ 2 trial, efficacy was reduced in patients with high tau PET burden, suggesting earlier-stage patients may benefit more.

- A: Donanemab targets amyloid, not tau, and is not indicated for advanced AD.
- B: It is administered intravenously, not orally.
- C: Donanemab has been associated with reduced tau progression in early stages.
- E: Intermediate tau levels are not a contraindication; reduced efficacy, not safety, is the concern with high tau.

Reference

Sims JR, Zimmer JA, Evans CD, Lu M, Ardayfio P, Sparks J, et al. Donanemab in early symptomatic Alzheimer disease: the TRAILBLAZER-ALZ 2 randomized clinical trial. *JAMA*. 2023;330(6):512–27. https://doi.org/10.1001/jama.2023.13239

71. A 71-year-old man with progressive memory impairment over 2 years presents for evaluation. His neurologic exam is normal aside from impaired delayed recall. MRI reveals mild medial temporal atrophy. His MoCA score is 22/30. He is otherwise in good health. His daughter asks if he should undergo amyloid PET imaging.

Which of the following best reflects current appropriate use criteria for ordering amyloid PET imaging?

A. It is recommended for routine dementia screening in all patients over 65.

B. It is appropriate in patients with typical Alzheimer's disease presentation and supportive MRI findings.

C. It is inappropriate in patients with suspected frontotemporal dementia.

D. It may be appropriate when clinical diagnosis is uncertain despite a thorough evaluation.

E. It is only used to monitor treatment response in patients receiving amyloid-lowering therapy.

Correct answer: D

Explanation

Amyloid PET imaging is considered appropriate in certain clinical scenarios, particularly when diagnostic uncertainty remains after a comprehensive evaluation. According to the Amyloid Imaging Task Force (AIT), Society of Nuclear Medicine and Molecular Imaging (SNMMI), and Alzheimer's Association guidelines, it is useful in patients with unexplained cognitive decline, atypical presentations, or early-onset dementia.

- A: Amyloid PET is not recommended for routine screening or in asymptomatic individuals.
- B: It is not typically indicated when the clinical picture already strongly supports Alzheimer's disease.
- C: It may still be useful in atypical cases or mixed presentations, including suspected FTD where differentiation from AD is unclear.
- E: PET is not currently approved or routinely used for monitoring treatment response.

Reference

Johnson KA, Minoshima S, Bohnen NI, et al. Appropriate use criteria for amyloid PET: A report of the Amyloid Imaging Task Force. *Alzheimers Dement*. 2013;9(1):e1–e16. https://doi.org/10.1016/j.jalz.2013.01.002

72. A 73-year-old woman with mild cognitive impairment due to Alzheimer's disease is being considered for lecanemab therapy. She has no significant medical comorbidities, and her MRI shows no evidence of microhemorrhages. APOE genotyping is pending. Her family asks about benefits and risks of lecanemab.

Which of the following is a key finding from the CLARITY-AD trial of lecanemab?

A. Lecanemab halts progression of Alzheimer's disease in all patients.

B. Lecanemab was associated with cognitive benefit but increased risk of ARIA.

C. Lecanemab showed benefit only in patients without APOE ε4 alleles.

D. Lecanemab is an oral medication approved for advanced dementia.

E. Lecanemab is not effective in patients with MCI due to Alzheimer's disease.

Correct answer: B

Explanation

In the CLARITY-AD trial, lecanemab, a monoclonal antibody targeting soluble amyloid protofibrils, significantly slowed clinical decline in patients with early symptomatic Alzheimer's disease (MCI or mild dementia). However, it was also associated with amyloid-related imaging abnormalities (ARIA), especially in APOE ε4 carriers.

- A: Lecanemab slows but does not halt, disease progression.
- C: APOE ε4 carriers also benefited but had higher risk of ARIA.
- D: Lecanemab is administered intravenously, not orally, and is indicated for early AD, not advanced stages.
- E: The trial specifically included MCI due to AD, showing benefit in this group.

Reference

van Dyck CH, Swanson CJ, Aisen P, et al. Lecanemab in early Alzheimer's disease. *N Engl J Med*. 2023;388(1):9–21. https://doi.org/10.1056/NEJMoa2212948

73. A 66-year-old retired accountant is referred for evaluation of difficulty managing finances and following multistep tasks. His wife reports increasing disorganization, impulsivity, and inability to plan activities over the past year. He scores 27/30 on the Montreal Cognitive Assessment (MoCA), with impairments in trail-making and verbal fluency. MRI reveals mild frontal lobe atrophy. There is no history of stroke, substance use, or head trauma.

Which of the following best characterizes executive dysfunction?

A. Inability to recall previously learned information

B. Impaired visuospatial processing and spatial neglect

C. Difficulty with motor programming and apraxia

D. Impairment in planning, organizing, and goal-directed behavior

E. Loss of language fluency and grammatical structure

Correct answer: D

Explanation

Executive dysfunction refers to impairments in the control and regulation of cognitive processes, particularly those involving planning, sequencing, inhibition, working memory, and flexible thinking. It is commonly associated with frontal lobe pathology and can present subtly even when global cognitive scores remain relatively intact.

- A: Describes episodic memory impairment, often due to medial temporal lobe dysfunction
- B: Reflects visuospatial dysfunction, seen in parietal lesions or neglect syndromes
- C: Suggests apraxia, a motor planning disorder often due to parietal damage
- E: Suggests agrammatic aphasia, a language disorder involving left perisylvian structures

Reference

Stuss DT, Levine B. Adult clinical neuropsychology: lessons from studies of the frontal lobes. *Annu Rev Psychol.* 2002;53:401–433. https://doi.org/10.1146/annurev.psych.53.100901.135220

74. A 38-year-old woman with relapsing-remitting multiple sclerosis (RRMS) presents for a routine follow-up. She reports doing well physically but has recently noticed increased forgetfulness, difficulty concentrating at work, and trouble organizing tasks. Her Expanded Disability Status Scale (EDSS) score remains unchanged. On neuropsychological testing, she demonstrates slowed processing speed and impaired working memory, with preserved language and visuospatial abilities.

    Which of the following best describes the typical pattern of cognitive dysfunction in multiple sclerosis?

    A. Rapidly progressive global dementia with early aphasia and apraxia

    B. Prominent memory loss with hippocampal atrophy on MRI

    C. Selective impairment in language and verbal fluency

    D. Deficits in processing speed, attention, and working memory

    E. Frontal behavioral syndrome with marked disinhibition

Correct answer: D

Explanation

Cognitive dysfunction in MS is common and may affect up to 65% of patients, even in the absence of significant physical disability. The most frequent deficits are in processing speed, attention, and working memory, often referred to as subcortical cognitive impairment. Executive dysfunction may also be seen, but language, general intelligence, and long-term memory are usually spared, especially in the early stages.

- A: Describes a cortical dementia such as Alzheimer's disease, not the subcortical pattern seen in MS.
- B: Hippocampal atrophy is associated with Alzheimer's disease, not MS.
- C: Language is generally preserved in MS; verbal fluency may decline due to executive dysfunction, not primary language impairment.
- E: Frontal behavioral syndromes suggest frontotemporal dementia, not MS.

Reference

Benedict RHB, Zivadinov R. Risk factors for and management of cognitive dysfunction in multiple sclerosis. *Nat Rev Neurol.* 2011;7(6):332–342. https://doi.org/10.1038/nrneurol.2011.61

75. A 76-year-old man admitted with community-acquired pneumonia becomes acutely disoriented and agitated on hospital day 3. He is pulling out his IV and cannot sustain attention. Vitals: T 100.6°F, HR 96 bpm, BP 132/78 mm Hg, O_2 sat 94% on 2L. There is no prior psychiatric history.

    What is the most likely diagnosis?

    A. Delirium due to a primary psychiatric disorder

    B. Delirium due to a general medical condition

    C. Dementia with behavioral disturbance

    D. Alcohol withdrawal delirium

    E. Schizophrenia, late-onset type

Correct answer: B

Explanation

The patient displays hallmark features of delirium: acute onset, inattention, fluctuating course, and altered consciousness. Pneumonia is a common precipitant, especially in older adults. The most appropriate DSM-5 diagnosis is delirium due to another medical condition.

- A: Delirium is not typically due to primary psychiatric illness.

- C: Dementia presents more insidiously and lacks fluctuations in attention.
- D: No alcohol history or withdrawal signs.
- E: Late-onset psychosis is rare and would not present with acute confusion.

Reference

Inouye SK, Westendorp RGJ, Saczynski JS. Delirium in elderly people. *Lancet*. 2014;383(9920):911–922. https://doi.org/10.1016/S0140-6736(13)60688-1

76. A 58-year-old man is found confused and agitated at home. His partner reports he took "a lot of Benadryl and alcohol" to help with sleep. On exam, he has flushed face, dilated pupils, dry mouth, and urinary retention. He is disoriented and incoherent.

    What is the most likely cause?
    A. Alcohol withdrawal delirium
    B. Anticholinergic toxicity causing delirium
    C. Benzodiazepine overdose
    D. Hepatic encephalopathy
    E. Acute psychosis
    Correct answer: B

Explanation

Diphenhydramine and other anticholinergics can cause delirium with peripheral signs: dry mouth, flushed skin, urinary retention, and mydriasis. Central effects include agitation, hallucinations, and confusion, especially when combined with CNS depressants like alcohol.

- A: No history of recent alcohol cessation or withdrawal symptoms.
- C: Benzodiazepines typically cause sedation, not hyperactivity.
- D: No evidence of liver disease.
- E: Psychosis lacks the autonomic and attentional symptoms seen here.

Reference

Tune LE. Anticholinergic effects of medication in elderly patients. *J Clin Psychiatry*. 2001;62(Suppl 21):11–14.

77. A 44-year-old man with alcohol use disorder presents to the emergency department with confusion, agitation, visual hallucinations, and tremulousness. He last drank 3 days ago. Vitals: BP 168/102 mm Hg, HR 120 bpm, T 99.2°F. He is disoriented to time and place and attempts to climb out of bed.

    What is the most likely diagnosis?

A. Alcohol intoxication
B. Alcohol withdrawal delirium
C. Wernicke encephalopathy
D. Schizophreniform disorder
E. Korsakoff syndrome
Correct answer: B

Explanation

This patient presents with delirium tremens, a severe form of alcohol withdrawal that typically occurs 48–96 hours after cessation. Symptoms include disorientation, autonomic instability, hallucinations, and tremor. This is a medical emergency requiring benzodiazepines and supportive care.

- A: Alcohol intoxication does not typically present with tremor or autonomic instability.
- C: Wernicke's presents with ophthalmoplegia, ataxia, and confusion—not tremor and hallucinations.
- D: Psychotic disorders do not cause autonomic instability or acute fluctuating attention.
- E: Korsakoff syndrome presents with amnesia and confabulation—not acute delirium.

Reference

Schuckit MA. Recognition and management of withdrawal delirium (delirium tremens). *N Engl J Med*. 2014;371(22):2109–13. https://doi.org/10.1056/NEJMra1407298

78. A 68-year-old man with metastatic prostate cancer and a history of chronic benzodiazepine use presents with fluctuating confusion, visual hallucinations, and tremulousness. Labs reveal hypercalcemia and mild hyponatremia. CT head is unremarkable. He is alert but unable to focus attention and misidentifies objects.

    What is the most appropriate diagnosis?
    A. Schizophrenia
    B. Delirium due to multiple etiologies
    C. Substance-induced psychotic disorder
    D. Vascular dementia
    E. Alzheimer's disease
    Correct answer: B

Explanation

This case involves multiple contributors to acute delirium: hypercalcemia, hyponatremia, and benzodiazepine withdrawal. The DSM-5 allows for the diagnosis of delirium due to multiple etiologies when more than one plausible cause exists. The acute onset, inattention, and hallucinations point away from a primary psychotic or neurodegenerative condition.

- A: Schizophrenia is not characterized by acute onset or fluctuating attention.
- C: Substance-induced psychosis lacks the inattention and fluctuating course seen here.
- D: Vascular dementia is chronic and usually lacks hallucinations.
- E: Alzheimer's has a gradual onset and does not cause fluctuating consciousness.

Reference

American Psychiatric Association. *Diagnostic and statistical manual of mental disorders, fifth edition, text revision (DSM-5-TR)*. Arlington (VA): American Psychiatric Association; 2022.

79. A 58-year-old man presents with memory difficulties, slowed thinking, and irritability. He has a history of untreated obstructive sleep apnea (OSA) and hypothyroidism. Neurologic exam is normal. MRI shows mild periventricular white matter changes without atrophy. TSH is 11.2 µIU/mL.

    Which diagnosis best accounts for his cognitive symptoms?
    A. Vascular dementia
    B. Alzheimer's disease
    C. Dementia due to a medical condition
    D. Frontotemporal dementia
    E. Depression with functional neurologic disorder
    Correct answer: C

Explanation

This patient has two potentially reversible causes of cognitive impairment: OSA and hypothyroidism. When a known medical condition is capable of producing the observed cognitive symptoms, DSM-5 allows the diagnosis of major neurocognitive disorder due to another medical condition.

- A: No clear evidence of stroke or stepwise decline
- B: Typical features (e.g., early memory loss, hippocampal atrophy) not present
- D: No disinhibition or personality changes suggestive of FTD
- E: No clear signs of major depression on history or exam

Reference

Siddiqi ZA, et al. Reversible and treatable causes of dementia. *Continuum (Minneap Minn)*. 2016;22(2):490–508. https://doi.org/10.1212/CON.0000000000000302

80. A 42-year-old man with untreated HIV presents with several months of worsening apathy, slowed thinking, and difficulty walking. Neurologic exam reveals bradyphrenia, poor coordination, and broad-based gait. MRI of the brain shows diffuse white matter hyperintensities without contrast enhancement or mass effect.

    What is the most likely diagnosis?
    A. Alzheimer's disease
    B. HIV-associated dementia
    C. Normal pressure hydrocephalus
    D. Primary CNS lymphoma
    E. Progressive multifocal leukoencephalopathy (PML)
    Correct answer: B

Explanation

HIV-associated dementia is a subcortical dementia that presents with apathy, bradyphrenia, and motor symptoms such as gait instability. It typically occurs in individuals with advanced, untreated HIV and may show diffuse white matter changes on MRI.

- A: Alzheimer's typically begins with episodic memory loss and cortical atrophy.
- C: NPH includes urinary incontinence and ventriculomegaly, not diffuse white matter changes.
- D: CNS lymphoma presents with focal lesions, mass effect, and usually enhances with contrast.
- E: PML causes focal neurologic deficits and asymmetric white matter lesions.

Reference

Clifford DB, Ances BM. HIV-associated neurocognitive disorder. *Lancet Infect Dis*. 2013;13(11):976–986. https://doi.org/10.1016/S1473-3099(13)70269-X

81. A 70-year-old man with chronic insomnia presents with cognitive slowing, confusion, and recent falls. He has been taking diazepam daily for years. Neurologic exam reveals mild dysmetria and slowed responses. MRI is normal. Lab tests are unremarkable.

    What is the most likely cause of his cognitive symptoms?
    A. Alzheimer's disease
    B. Frontotemporal dementia
    C. Vascular dementia
    D. Substance-/medication-induced dementia
    E. Parkinson's disease dementia
    Correct answer: D

Explanation

Long-term use of benzodiazepines, particularly in older adults, can lead to reversible cognitive impairment without necessarily increasing dementia risk. Symptoms include slowed processing, confusion, and ataxia. A diagnosis of substance-/medication-induced major neurocognitive disorder is appropriate when symptoms correlate with drug exposure.

- A: No early memory impairment or hippocampal findings
- B: No behavioral disinhibition or language dysfunction
- C: No vascular history or focal deficits
- E: No parkinsonism on exam

Reference

Hofe IV, Stricker BH, Vernooij MW, Ikram MK, Ikram MA, Wolters FJ. Benzodiazepine use in relation to long-term dementia risk and imaging markers of neurodegeneration: a population-based study. *BMC Med.* 2024;22(1):266. https://doi.org/10.1186/s12916-024-03437-5

82. A 74-year-old woman presents with gradual memory loss and executive dysfunction. She has type 2 diabetes, hypertension, and a history of breast cancer treated with chemotherapy. MRI shows moderate white matter disease and mild temporal atrophy. Her daughter reports worsening forgetfulness, apathy, and slowed gait.

    Which diagnosis best accounts for her condition?
    A. Alzheimer's disease
    B. Dementia due to multiple etiologies
    C. Vascular dementia
    D. Normal pressure hydrocephalus
    E. Mild cognitive impairment
    Correct answer: B

Explanation

This patient has features of both Alzheimer's disease (e.g., memory loss, apathy) and vascular contributions (white matter changes, executive dysfunction, slowed gait), along with prior chemotherapy exposure. The DSM-5 allows for multiple contributing causes under "dementia due to multiple etiologies."

- A: Doesn't fully explain gait change or white matter disease.
- C: Doesn't explain the amnestic features or apathy.
- D: Ventricular enlargement is absent.
- E: Functional impairment meets criteria for dementia, not MCI.

Reference

American Psychiatric Association. *Diagnostic and statistical manual of mental disorders, fifth edition, text revision (DSM-5-TR)*. Arlington (VA): American Psychiatric Association; 2022.

83. A 63-year-old man is brought to the emergency department after becoming suddenly confused during a walk. He repeatedly asks "Where am I?" and "What day is it?" He is otherwise alert, follows commands, and has no focal deficits. There is no seizure activity or head trauma. Symptoms resolve after 6 h. MRI is normal.

    What is the most likely diagnosis?
    A. Transient ischemic attack (TIA)
    B. Transient global amnesia (TGA)
    C. Complex partial seizure
    D. Delirium
    E. Conversion disorder
    Correct answer: B

Explanation

TGA is characterized by sudden-onset anterograde amnesia lasting <24 h with preserved alertness and no focal deficits. It commonly occurs in middle-aged to older adults and resolves spontaneously. Etiology is unclear but may involve venous congestion or hippocampal dysfunction.

- A: TIA would be expected to cause focal neurologic deficits.
- C: No automatisms or postictal signs.
- D: Delirium causes inattention and clouding of consciousness.
- E: TGA has a characteristic clinical pattern not explained by conversion disorder.

Reference

Ropper AH. Transient global amnesia. *N Engl J Med.* 2023;388(7):635–40. https://doi.org/10.1056/NEJMra2213867

84. A 10-year-old boy struggles with reading and writing despite average intelligence and good classroom attendance. His parents report that he reads slowly and avoids homework. School assessments confirm that his academic performance in reading is significantly below expectations.

    What is the most appropriate diagnosis?
    A. Attention-deficit/hyperactivity disorder (ADHD)
    B. Specific learning disorder
    C. Intellectual disability
    D. Autism spectrum disorder
    E. Oppositional defiant disorder
    Correct answer: B

Explanation

Specific learning disorder is diagnosed when a child has difficulty in academic skills (e.g., reading, writing, math) not explained by intellectual disability, sensory deficits, or poor instruction. This child shows discrepancy between ability and performance, classic for a reading disorder.

- A: No evidence of inattention or hyperactivity.
- C: Performance is impaired in one area, not globally.
- D: No social or communication impairments.
- E: No oppositional behavior is reported.

Reference

American Psychiatric Association. *Diagnostic and Statistical Manual of Mental Disorders, Fifth Edition, Text Revision (DSM-5-TR)*. Arlington, VA: American Psychiatric Association; 2022.

85. A 5-year-old girl is evaluated for language delay. She speaks in simple one to two word phrases and has difficulty understanding longer sentences. Her hearing is normal. She enjoys playing with other children and engages in imaginative play. There are no behavioral problems or motor delays.

    What is the most likely diagnosis?
    A. Childhood-onset fluency disorder
    B. Social (pragmatic) communication disorder
    C. Autism spectrum disorder
    D. Language disorder
    E. Global developmental delay
    Correct answer: D

Explanation

Language disorder involves difficulties in acquisition and use of spoken or written language, including reduced vocabulary and impaired sentence structure. The child has age-inappropriate expressive and receptive language but normal social interaction, ruling out autism spectrum disorder.

- A: No stuttering or fluency issues.
- B: No social communication deficits.
- C: No restricted interests or social deficits.
- E: Other domains (e.g., motor, social) are preserved.

Reference

Bishop DV. Ten questions about terminology for children with unexplained language problems. *Int J Lang Commun Disord.* 2014;49(4):381–415. https://doi.org/10.1111/1460-6984.12101

86. A 4-year-old boy is brought in for concerns about social development. He does not make eye contact, rarely interacts with peers, and becomes distressed when routines are disrupted. He has a fascination with lining up objects. Language is delayed, and he often repeats phrases. Hearing is normal.

    What is the most likely diagnosis?
    A. Social (pragmatic) communication disorder
    B. Autism spectrum disorder
    C. Intellectual disability
    D. Language disorder
    E. Specific learning disorder
    Correct answer: B

Explanation

Autism spectrum disorder (ASD) is characterized by social communication deficits and restricted, repetitive behaviors. This child's limited eye contact, distress with changes in routine, and repetitive interests are core features. Language delay and echolalia are common in ASD.

- A: Does not include repetitive behaviors.
- C: Cognitive delays would be global and not necessarily include the core features of ASD.
- D: Doesn't account for restricted interests or social impairments.
- E: Learning disorders affect academic skills, not social interaction or behavior patterns.

Reference

American Psychiatric Association. *Diagnostic and statistical manual of mental disorders, fifth edition, text revision (DSM-5-TR)*. Arlington (VA): American Psychiatric Association; 2022.

87. A 7-year-old boy is evaluated for behavioral concerns at school. He frequently leaves his seat during class, blurts out answers, and is easily distracted. His grades are below average despite normal intelligence. Similar behavior is reported at home.

    What is the most likely diagnosis?
    A. Oppositional defiant disorder
    B. Attention-deficit/hyperactivity disorder (ADHD), combined type
    C. Conduct disorder
    D. Autism spectrum disorder
    E. Specific learning disorder
    Correct answer: B

Explanation

ADHD combined type involves both inattentive and hyperactive/impulsive symptoms. The child exhibits impulsivity, distractibility, and hyperactivity across settings (school and home), meeting diagnostic criteria.

- A: Would include defiant and argumentative behavior, not just inattention or hyperactivity.
- C: Involves more severe behaviors like aggression and violation of rules.
- D: No evidence of social or communicative impairments.
- E: Academic difficulties here are likely secondary to attention problems.

Reference

Faraone SV, et al. Attention-deficit/hyperactivity disorder. *Nat Rev Dis Primers*. 2015;1:15020. https://doi.org/10.1038/nrdp.2015.20

88. A 3-year-old girl has not yet begun to speak, is unable to feed herself, and cannot follow one-step commands. She was born at term with no complications. Her motor milestones were also delayed. Genetic testing reveals a de novo MECP2 mutation.

   What is the most likely diagnosis?
   A. Specific learning disorder
   B. Language disorder
   C. Autism spectrum disorder
   D. Global developmental delay
   E. Childhood-onset schizophrenia
   Correct answer: D

Explanation

Global developmental delay is diagnosed in children under 5 with significant delay in multiple developmental domains (language, motor, social, etc.). The MECP2 mutation suggests a genetic cause (e.g., Rett syndrome), consistent with global delays.

- A: Learning disorders are diagnosed in school-aged children with specific academic difficulties.
- B: Only affects language, not global development.
- C: May overlap but doesn't explain motor and receptive delay in isolation.
- E: Onset is later; psychosis is not the presenting feature.

Reference

Shevell M, et al. Practice parameter: evaluation of the child with global developmental delay. *Neurology*. 2003;60(3):367–380. https://doi.org/10.1212/01.WNL.0000031431.81555.16

89. A 68-year-old right-handed man presents with poor writing ability and difficulty copying figures after a stroke. He can recognize objects by touch but cannot name them. Neurologic exam shows left visual field neglect and left-sided apraxia. MRI reveals a lesion in the right parietal lobe and splenium of the corpus callosum.

   Which of the following best explains his symptoms?
   A. Balint syndrome
   B. Broca aphasia
   C. Disconnection syndrome
   D. Frontal lobe degeneration
   E. Ideomotor apraxia
   Correct answer: C

Explanation

Disconnection syndromes result from interruption of interhemispheric pathways, such as the corpus callosum, leading to failures in transferring information between hemispheres. This explains the alexia without agraphia, tactile anomia, and apraxia despite preserved basic functions.

- A: Balint syndrome involves simultanagnosia, oculomotor apraxia, and optic ataxia.
- B: Broca aphasia involves nonfluent speech, not the features here.
- D: Would present with executive dysfunction and disinhibition.
- E: A component here but broader deficits point to a disconnection syndrome.

Reference

Geschwind N. Disconnexion syndromes in animals and man. *Brain*. 1965;88(2):237–294. https://doi.org/10.1093/brain/88.2.237

90. A 74-year-old woman presents with progressive memory loss over 3 years, difficulty managing finances, and repeating herself in conversations. Neurologic examination is normal. MRI shows bilateral hippocampal atrophy. Neuropsychological testing reveals deficits in episodic memory with preserved language and visuospatial function.

   What is the most likely underlying pathology?
   A. Hippocampal sclerosis
   B. Cortical microinfarcts
   C. β-amyloid plaques and tau neurofibrillary tangles
   D. Lewy bodies in cortical and subcortical regions
   E. TDP-43 proteinopathy
   Correct answer: C

Explanation

The clinical picture is consistent with Alzheimer's disease (AD), which is characterized by early episodic memory impairment and progressive decline in other cognitive domains. The hallmark pathological findings in AD include extracellular β-amyloid plaques and intracellular tau neurofibrillary tangles, particularly in the medial temporal lobes. Hippocampal atrophy on MRI supports this diagnosis.

- A: More common in older adults but less widespread early on than AD
- B: Suggestive of vascular dementia, which typically causes executive dysfunction
- D: Seen in Lewy body dementia, which usually includes visual hallucinations and parkinsonism
- E: Associated with FTD and LATE, with different progression patterns

Reference

DeTure MA, Dickson DW. The neuropathological diagnosis of Alzheimer's disease. *Mol Neurodegener.* 2019;14(1):32. https://doi.org/10.1186/s13024-019-0333-5

91. A 69-year-old man is brought to the clinic by his family due to rapidly worsening confusion and behavioral changes over the past 8 weeks. He has developed ataxia, startle myoclonus, and difficulty speaking. MRI of the brain (see below) reveals hyperintensities in the caudate nuclei and cortical ribboning on diffusion-weighted imaging. EEG shows periodic sharp wave complexes.

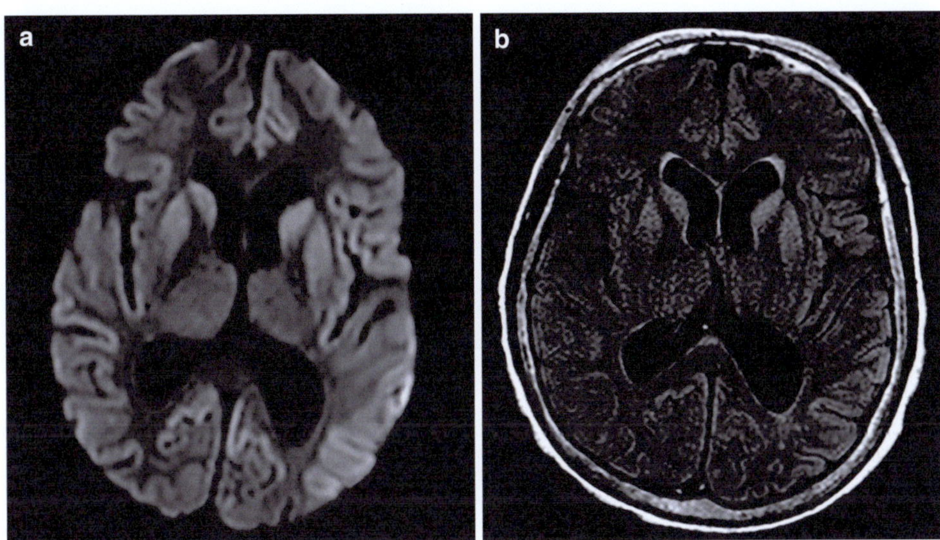

Axial MRI brain, DWI on the left and FLAIR on the right. (Source: Jang JW et al. via BMC Neurology (2014). CC-BY 4.0 (https://creativecommons.org/licenses/by/4.0/deed.en). Image has not been modified. See full attribution below in references.)

What is the most likely diagnosis?

A. Alzheimer's disease
B. Vascular dementia
C. Autoimmune limbic encephalitis
D. Creutzfeldt-Jakob disease
E. Dementia with Lewy bodies

Correct answer: D

Explanation

Creutzfeldt Jakob disease (CJD) is a prion disorder characterized by rapidly progressive dementia, myoclonus, ataxia, and neuropsychiatric symptoms. Cortical ribboning and basal ganglia hyperintensities on MRI and periodic sharp wave complexes on EEG are classic findings.

- A: Alzheimer's typically progresses over years.

- B: Vascular dementia may have stepwise decline, not global rapid progression.
- C: Autoimmune encephalitis may present similarly but often includes seizures and can be subacute; diagnosis requires antibody testing.
- E: Dementia with Lewy bodies usually has a slower progression and visual hallucinations or REM sleep behavior disorder.

Reference

Jang, JW., Park, S.Y., Park, Y.H. et al. Symptomatic aggravation after corticosteroid pulse therapy in definite sporadic Creutzfeldt-Jakob disease with the feature of Hashimoto's encephalopathy. *BMC Neurol* **14**, 179 (2014). https://doi.org/10.1186/s12883-014-0179-y

92. A 61-year-old woman presents with subacute personality changes, anxiety, and memory impairment. Over the next 4 weeks, she develops visual hallucinations, insomnia, and intermittent limb jerking. CSF 14-3-3 protein is positive. MRI shows bilateral caudate and putamen hyperintensities on DWI. EEG is nonspecific. The family asks about prognosis and treatment options.

Which of the following statements is most accurate regarding her condition?

A. High-dose corticosteroids are first-line therapy for this condition.

B. Plasmapheresis is recommended to reduce prion protein burden.

C. Disease-modifying therapy targeting tau pathology is currently under investigation.

D. The condition is rapidly fatal with no proven disease-modifying treatment.

E. Most patients recover spontaneously within 6 months.

Correct answer: D

Explanation

This clinical scenario is consistent with sporadic Creutzfeldt-Jakob disease (CJD), a prion disease marked by rapid neurodegeneration. The presence of 14-3-3 protein in CSF, basal ganglia hyperintensities on DWI, and subacute neurologic decline are characteristic. Unfortunately, CJD is uniformly fatal, with no effective disease-modifying therapy.

- A: Corticosteroids may be used in autoimmune encephalitis, not prion disease.
- B: Plasmapheresis has no role in treating prion diseases.
- C: Tau-targeting therapies are being studied for Alzheimer's and other tauopathies, not prion diseases.
- E: CJD is not self-limiting and progresses inexorably to death, often within months.

Reference

Hermann P, Appleby B, Brandel JP, et al. Biomarkers and diagnostic guidelines for sporadic Creutzfeldt-Jakob disease. *Lancet Neurol*. 2021;20(3):235–246. https://doi.org/10.1016/S1474-4422(20)30477-4

93. A 64-year-old man presents with 6 weeks of progressive confusion, memory loss, and gait instability. Family notes personality changes and startle myoclonus. MRI shows cortical ribboning and DWI hyperintensities in the caudate. CSF is positive for RT-QuIC. The patient's spouse asks whether he may have contracted this from someone else and if they are at risk.

Which of the following statements best reflects the current understanding of disease transmission?

A. Creutzfeldt-Jakob disease is commonly transmitted via close personal contact.

B. The vast majority of cases arise sporadically without identifiable exposure.

C. Most cases are linked to consumption of contaminated beef products.

D. Household members should be screened for subclinical disease.

E. The disease is inherited in most affected individuals.

Correct answer: B

Explanation

Approximately 85–90% of Creutzfeldt-Jakob disease (CJD) cases are sporadic, meaning they occur without identifiable genetic or environmental exposure. While CJD is transmissible through certain medical procedures (e.g., contaminated neurosurgical instruments), person-to-person transmission through casual contact is not a recognized route.

- A: CJD is not spread through casual or household contact.
- C: Variant CJD, linked to bovine spongiform encephalopathy, is extremely rare and geographically limited.
- D: There is no recommendation to screen asymptomatic family members in sporadic cases.
- E: Inherited prion diseases account for only ~10–15% of cases and involve mutations in the PRNP gene.

Reference

Geschwind MD. Rapidly progressive dementia. *Continuum (Minneap Minn)*. 2016;22(2):510–537. https://doi.org/10.1212/con.0000000000000319

94. A 53-year-old man presents with progressive insomnia, difficulty concentrating, and weight loss over several months. Family reports episodes of autonomic instability including tachycardia and hyperhidrosis. Neurologic exam reveals dysarthria and ataxia. His father died in his 50s from a similar illness. Polysomnography shows loss of slow-wave and REM sleep. Genetic testing reveals a D178N mutation in the PRNP gene.

Which of the following neuropathologic findings is most characteristic of this condition?

A. Widespread cortical spongiform changes with astrocytic gliosis

B. Nigral degeneration with Lewy bodies

C. Thalamic degeneration with neuronal loss in the mediodorsal and anterior nuclei

D. Hippocampal sclerosis with TDP-43 inclusions

E. Inflammation of the limbic system with perivascular lymphocytic infiltrates

Correct answer: C

Explanation

Fatal familial insomnia (FFI) is a rare autosomal dominant prion disease caused by a D178N mutation in the PRNP gene when coupled with a methionine at codon 129. It features progressive insomnia, dysautonomia, motor symptoms, and cognitive decline. The most distinctive pathologic hallmark is degeneration of the thalamus—particularly the mediodorsal and anterior nuclei—which are critical in regulating sleep and arousal.

- A: Cortical spongiform changes are seen in sporadic CJD.
- B: Lewy bodies are characteristic of Parkinson's disease and dementia with Lewy bodies.
- D: TDP-43 pathology is typical in frontotemporal lobar degeneration and LATE.
- E: Limbic inflammation is more consistent with autoimmune encephalitis.

Reference

Montagna P, Gambetti P, Cortelli P, Lugaresi E. Familial and sporadic fatal insomnia. *Lancet Neurol.* 2003;2(3):167–176. https://doi.org/10.1016/s1474-4422(03)00323-5

Robert W. Charlson

1. A 53-year-old man with relapsing remitting multiple sclerosis (MS) and a prior diagnosis of recurrent major depressive disorder (MDD) presents to his MS clinic with reports of increasing difficulty with fatigue and low mood. He has a stable neurologic exam, and on further questioning, he endorses a long history of depressive episodes, with marked decrease in mood typically lasting several months. He is frustrated that he has failed several adequate trials of antidepressants including fluoxetine and mirtazapine over the last few years. On further review of symptoms, he also endorses distinct mood periods lasting 5 days of racing thoughts, elevated mood, decreased need for sleep, and impulsivity. He has not had periods of severe impairment at work or in his relationship during these episodes. What is the most likely diagnosis?
   A. Major depressive disorder with anxious features
   B. Bipolar II disorder
   C. Schizoaffective disorder
   D. Borderline personality disorder
   Correct answer: B

Explanation

Bipolar II disorder is a common disorder, which often is initially diagnosed as major depressive disorder (MDD) until the recognition or emergence of hypomanic episodes. Symptoms of hypomania are the same as mania (elevated or irritable mood, increased energy, racing thoughts, decreased need for sleep, impulsive spending or risky sexual behaviors, distractibility), except that the episode does not impair functioning and can last for fewer days than a manic episode. Patients may not respond to traditional antidepressants, and their use in bipolar II disorder is controversial. Mood stabilizers such as lamotrigine or lithium are the most commonly used medication treatments.

R. W. Charlson (✉)
Neurology Residency: Manhattan Track, Department of Neurology, New York University Grossman School of Medicine, New York, NY, USA
e-mail: Erik.Charlson@NYULangone.org

Reference

MacQueen GM, Young LT. Bipolar II disorder: symptoms, course, and response to treatment. Psychiatr Serv. 2001;52(3):358–61. https://doi.org/10.1176/appi.ps.52.3.358.

2. A 37-year-old woman presents to the emergency department (ED) with an acute change in behavior. She has no prior mental health history, but in the last 2 weeks, she has barricaded herself in her bedroom, refusing to leave due to fear of the FBI surveillance. On exam, she is withdrawn and suspicious-appearing and refuses to answer questions. Initial workup in the ED includes a negative urine toxicology and unremarkable CT brain imaging. Further neurologic and medical workup is unrevealing. During her admission for medical workup over the next 5 days, her symptoms remit, and she requests discharge home. The psychiatry consultation service does not feel she meets the criteria for involuntary psychiatric admission, and on follow-up, she is back to her prior baseline, working full-time and declining paranoid ideation. What features of this case distinguish it as Brief Psychotic Disorder as opposed to another psychotic disorder?
   A. Symptoms in brief psychotic disorder are less severe
   B. Paranoid ideation is required to make this diagnosis
   C. A marked stressor is required as an inciting event
   D. Brief psychotic disorder is distinguished from schizophrenia or schizophreniform disorder by the duration of symptoms
   Correct answer: D

Explanation

Brief psychotic disorder is a relatively rare condition, defined as the sudden onset of psychotic symptoms (delusions, hallucinations, disorganized speech, or disorganized or catatonic behaviors) that lasts in all no more than 1 month, with a return to premorbid baseline functioning. Schizophrenia includes a requirement of impaired occupational or social functioning for at least 6 months, as opposed to schizophreniform disorder, which is from 1 month to 6 months. Episodes of brief psychotic disorder do not need an acute stressor to be identified, and they may recur. They should not be diagnosed in the presence of substance use or intoxication or an acute medical condition.

Reference

Castagnini A, Galeazzi GM. Acute and transient psychoses: clinical and nosological issues. BJPsych Advances. 2016;22(5):292–300. https://doi.org/10.1192/apt.bp.115.015198.

3. A 23-year-old woman with a prior history of rheumatoid arthritis presents to the ED with a 6-week change in behavior. She was in her senior year of college when she started to note decreasing need for sleep, racing thoughts, confusion, and irritability. She began to feel that she had discovered a whole new field of study and stayed up days on end drafting a new "manifesto." She stopped attending classes and wrote letters to her professors that alienated her mentors. Eventually, she began to experience auditory hallucinations. On evaluation, she showed pressured speech, flight of ideas, and grandiosity. She was admitted for an acute episode of mania with psychotic features and started on lithium and risperidone. Which clinical feature of her history would change your diagnosis?
   A. She had recently experienced the loss of her father
   B. Her hallucinations did not last more than 1 week
   C. She had a family history of obsessive-compulsive disorder and bipolar disorder
   D. She had been started on a recent course of high-dose oral prednisone and pregabalin by her rheumatologist

Correct answer: D

Explanation

The patient presents with a manic episode (racing thoughts, insomnia, disorganized behaviors, grandiosity), as well as psychotic symptoms of hallucinations. An important consideration in a patient presenting with new-onset psychiatric symptoms is the presence of recent medication changes or medical conditions. Steroids such as prednisone are well known to lead to neuropsychiatric complications, including depression, mania, psychosis, anxiety, and other symptoms. Treatment involves tapering or cessation of steroids, as well as sedating antipsychotics such as olanzapine for psychotic symptoms. Most studies suggest full recovery with treatment.

Reference

Brito-Santana L, Medinas RL, Neves A, Gago J. Steroid-induced psychosis: a spectrum of neuropsychiatric glucocorticoid side effects. BMJ Case Rep. 2024;17(7). https://doi.org/10.1136/bcr-2023-259134.

4. A 45-year-old man presents for evaluation, after being diagnosed with early-onset Parkinson's disease 3 months ago. He is distraught, anxious-appearing, and endorsing several symptoms suggestive of depression. He reports sadness, negative thoughts about the future, and fatigue. He also briefly experienced suicidal thinking, but states this has resolved after talking more with his wife and considering his family. What features of this case suggest adjustment disorder as opposed to major depressive disorder?
   A. The presence of suicidal ideation by definition means that this represents MDD
   B. The time frame of symptoms is inconsistent with adjustment disorder
   C. The relationship of symptoms to an acute stressor as well as the lack of additional findings to meet the criteria for an episode of MDD
   D. Adjustment disorder does not entail the presence of depressive symptoms

Correct answer: C

Explanation

Adjustment disorders are defined as the development of emotional or behavioral symptoms in response to an identifiable stressor. It usually occurs within 3 months of the stressor and leads to marked distress out of proportion to the intensity of the stressor or significant impairment in functioning. It requires that the symptoms are not better explained by another psychiatric disorder—i.e. MDD or another mood disorder. Typically, adjustment disorders will resolve within 6 months of the removal of the stressor, and it may be associated with suicidal thinking at times. Adjustment disorders may have depressed mood, anxiety, or disturbance of conduct.

Reference

Bachem R, Casey P. Adjustment disorder: A diagnosis whose time has come. J Affect Disord. 2018;227:243–53. https://doi.org/10.1016/j.jad.2017.10.034.

5. A 55-year-old woman presents for evaluation. She has been followed by her psychiatrist for several years and

currently reports persistent sadness at least 4 days a week, insomnia, guilty ruminations, lack of energy, poor concentration, and occasional thoughts of suicide. She has been trialed on escitalopram for several months at an adequate dose and then changed to sertraline with some minor improvement in her symptoms. Which of the following is not a generally recommended strategy for dealing with treatment-resistant depression?

A. Continue sertraline but add buproprion as an augmentation strategy
B. Continue sertraline but add fluoxetine as an augmentation strategy
C. Continue sertraline but add aripiprazole
D. Taper off sertraline, and start venlafaxine as monotherapy

Correct answer: B

Explanation

Despite many different medications approved for MDD, and several different classes of medications, treatment-resistant depression (TRD) remains a significant problem in psychiatry. As many as 30% of patients may develop TRD, which is defined (somewhat variably) as an inadequate response to a trial of two different antidepressants at an adequate dose and duration. Strategies include adding an atypical antipsychotic (arirpiprazole, quietiapine), buproprion, buspirone, lithium, or other agents, or switching classes (i.e., from a selective serotonin reuptake inhibitor (SSRI) to a serotonin–norepinephrine reuptake inhibitor (SNRI)). Guidelines do not support treatment with two simultaneous antidepressants from the same SSRI class.

Reference

Nuñez NA, Joseph B, Pahwa M, Kumar R, Resendez MG, Prokop LJ, et al. Augmentation strategies for treatment resistant major depression: A systematic review and network meta-analysis. J Affect Disord. 2022;302:385–400. https://doi.org/10.1016/j.jad.2021.12.134.

6. A 69-year-old woman presents with episodes awakening from sleep. These involve a feeling of her heart racing, shortness of breath, tingling in her hands, feelings of internal restlessness, and feelings of choking. The episodes occur quite quickly and do not have any clear trigger. She worries during the episode that she may be dying. During the last episode, she called 911 and had a full cardiac and medical workup without any underlying etiology identified. She presents to your office stating that she is now dreading further episodes when she falls asleep. She states that her she continues to work, has been stressed recently taking care of her aging parent, and having increasing difficulties at work. What is your diagnosis, and what treatment would you recommend?

A. Generalized anxiety disorder; start long-acting alprazolam daily
B. Restless legs syndrome; start pramipexole
C. Panic disorder; start escitalopram
D. Adjustment disorder; referral to psychotherapy and sleep training

Correct answer: C

Explanation

Panic disorder is a relatively common diagnosis, and panic attacks can occur in up to 5% of the population at some point in their lives. They are typically diagnosed after a patient presents for a concern for a medical event—and palpitations are the most common physical symptom. Their semiology varies however—and the DSM-5 defines panic disorder as recurrent unprovoked panic attacks, with a panic attack being an episode of acute fear or discomfort, marked by four or more of the following symptoms: palpitations, sweating, trembling, shortness of breath, feelings of choking, chest pain, nausea, chills or hot sensations, paresthesias, derealization, fear of losing control, or fear of dying. To meet the criteria for panic disorder, the patient must have had at least one panic attack followed by the fear of further attacks or a change in behavior related to the attacks. It should not occur in response to specific phobias. It also may lead to agoraphobia or fear of leaving one's home. The first-line standard treatment is the initiation of an SSRI medication. Of note, standing benzodiazepines are not recommended as a first-line treatment.

Reference

DeGeorge KC, Grover M, Streeter GS. Generalized Anxiety Disorder and Panic Disorder in Adults. Am Fam Physician. 2022;106(2):157–64.

7. A 42-year-old woman presents with several months of new-onset depression and anxiety. She notes that she does not have a prior history of anxiety, but that recently her worries have been "out of control," and that she is feeling restless, agitated, sleeping less, and exhausted. She is noting other worries, including fear about her hair thinning, altered sweating, heart racing, and shakiness. What medical workup would be the highest yield to diagnose the cause of her new-onset symptoms?

A. CT scan of her head
B. Check urine toxicology for marijuana exposure
C. Check TSH and free T4
D. Abdominal ultrasound

Correct answer: C

Explanation

The patient in this case has a diagnosis of an anxiety disorder in the setting of a medical disorder. Thyroid disease is common in the general population, affecting women especially, and the most common cause of thyroid disease is Grave's disease. Thyrotoxicosis produces symptoms that are identical to anxiety symptoms, including insomnia, palpitations, racing thoughts, abnormal sweating, among other symptoms. Clinicians diagnosing new-onset psychiatric symptoms should be aware of common medical conditions that may present with anxiety, depressive, or other psychiatric symptoms.

References

Fukao A, Takamatsu J, Arishima T, Tanaka M, Kawai T, Okamoto Y, et al. Graves' disease and mental disorders. J Clin Transl Endocrinol. 2020;19:100207. https://doi.org/10.1016/j.jcte.2019.100207.

Lekurwale V, Acharya S, Shukla S, Kumar S. Neuropsychiatric Manifestations of Thyroid Diseases. Cureus. 2023;15(1):e33987. https://doi.org/10.7759/cureus.33987.

8. A 55-year-old man with a prior medical history of multiple sclerosis, hypertension, and diabetes presents for evaluation for worsening anxiety. He notes that over the last year, he has been experiencing a significant increase in anxiety symptoms, including constant inner tension, racing thoughts, difficulty relaxing when he tries to sleep, and occasional jerking of his legs. He currently takes a low dose of sertraline in addition to his MS medication. He notes a high degree of stress at work in the last few months, and that he has been struggling to keep up with his work load. He is worried about how the MS diagnosis is affecting his job as a consultant and has been taking less time to sleep and adding higher and higher doses of amphetamine and dextroamphetamine to his morning meds. Over the next few weeks, he starts to pick out hairs from his head due to his ongoing anxiety, leading to noticeable hair loss. He also has started to notice feelings of his heart racing when he tries to sleep at night. What is the next best intervention?
A. Start high-dose alprazolam 2 mg four times a day for extreme anxiety
B. Add risperidone 0.5 mg twice daily to augment his current dose of sertraline
C. Reduce and try to taper off amphetamine and dextroamphetamine
D. Start melatonin at bedtime and light therapy during the morning

Correct answer: C

Explanation

The patient presents with symptoms significant for severe anxiety, as well as some depressive symptoms. It is important to recognize that anxiety symptoms may be secondary to side effects of medications, especially with various medications that may be commonly prescribed. These include corticosteroids, stimulant medications, thyroid medications, decongestants, inhalers, and even antidepressants. The appropriate step when evaluating new-onset anxiety where a medication (e.g., amphetamine and dextroamphetamine in this case) may be a culprit would be to try to limit or even taper off if possible.

Reference

Childress A. Recent advances in pharmacological management of attention-deficit/hyperactivity disorder: moving beyond stimulants. Expert Opin Pharmacother. 2024;25(7):853–66. https://doi.org/10.1080/14656566.2024.2358987.

9. A 27-year-old woman with no prior medical history presents for evaluation. She notes an increase in difficulty sleeping in the last few months and more difficulty with getting to her new job on time. She notes some frustration and low mood, but denies hopelessness or suicidal ideation. She is most frustrated by her difficulty with intrusive thoughts about safety, and her checking behaviors have started to make it difficult to leave the house. She has to check the locks and count to certain numbers in her head, and frequently returns home to check that the stove has been turned off, and count a certain number of times before walking through the doorway. You discuss with her the intrusive thoughts and her compulsions that are attempts to neutralize those thoughts. You discuss options for her treatment of her diagnosis of obsessive-compulsive disorder (OCD), which include:
A. Risperidone and other antipsychotic medications are first-line therapies
B. Psychotherapies such as exposure therapy have no evidence of effectiveness
C. Medications used most often are SSRIs, and they require higher doses and for longer duration than many other psychiatric disorders
D. It is rare to have another psychiatric comorbidity with OCD

Correct answer: C

Explanation

Obsessive-compulsive disorder (OCD) is defined by both obsessions and compulsions, which lead to significant dysfunction in one's life. Obsessions are long-term recurrent and intrusive thoughts that are usually distressing to the individual and can include ideas of cleanliness, symmetry, perfection, religiosity, or other themes commonly. These thoughts often lead to the build-up of significant internal tension, and the compulsions are attempts to neutralize that tension. For example, with obsessions of cleanliness, one may use hand washing to try to neutralize these worries, which only works briefly and serves to reinforce the obsessive thought. It is very common for patients with OCD to have other psychiatric disorders, including depression, autism, schizophrenia, and others. The treatment of this focuses on medications, typically high-dose SSRIs, and while antipsychotics may be used, they are typically only second-line agents. Psychotherapy can be effective and includes techniques such as exposure therapy and cognitive behavioral therapy.

Reference

Singh A, Anjankar VP, Sapkale B. Obsessive-Compulsive Disorder (OCD): A Comprehensive Review of Diagnosis, Comorbidities, and Treatment Approaches. Cureus. 2023;15(11):e48960. https://doi.org/10.7759/cureus.48960.

10. A 25-year-old woman presents to the emergency department with an inability to walk. The sudden loss of mobility occurred over the last 24 h in the setting of an argument with her family. She was triaged to an urgent spinal cord injury pathway and seen by neurology and neurosurgery. Initial imaging showed normal CT total spine, as well as negative MRI spine. Her brain imaging and CSF studies were also within normal limits. On neurologic exam, she was unable to lift either leg antigravity, but when examined sitting, she was able with encouragement to show near full strength. She had a positive Hoover's sign and prominent "giveway" weakness. Over the next few days, while working with PT and OT, she regained the ability to walk initially with a walker and then without assistance. While the psychiatry consultation service was consulted, she insisted that she had no significant stressors, no depressive symptoms and was not experiencing anxiety. Per collateral information, she had a history of childhood trauma and struggled to graduate from college and find work. What is the most likely diagnosis that led to her hospitalization, and what is the recommended treatment?
    A. MRI-negative spinal cord tumor; a 5-day course of IV steroids; PT
    B. Panic disorder with motor manifestations; standing lorazepam and olanzapine
    C. Catatonia; high-dose lorazepam standing every 4 h
    D. Functional neurologic disorder (FND); cognitive behavioral therapy; PT and rehabilitation; discussion of the diagnosis
    Correct answer: D

Explanation

The patient presents with an initial presentation that suggests an acute neurologic disorder, and the diagnosis of an FND rests not on a set of negative findings (normal MRIs, CSF, etc.), but on the positive findings that make the diagnosis. In this case, the variability of findings in the neurologic exam, as well as the positive exam findings such as a Hoover's sign. FND is common in neurologic settings, and motor weakness and non-epileptic seizures are the most common presentations. Treatment involves making the diagnosis with the patient and explaining the findings in a supportive manner. Patients with FND are not feigning illness, and many patients do not present with agitation nor acute anxiety or depressive symptoms. The most common recommended treatments include cognitive behavioral therapy and physical and occupational therapy.

Reference

Aybek S, Perez DL. Diagnosis and management of functional neurological disorder. Bmj. 2022;376:o64. https://doi.org/10.1136/bmj.o64.

11. A 19-year-old man was brought into the clinic by his mother. He had no prior medical history, and she noted that he had been doing well in school until his senior year when he started to become more withdrawn. For the past 12 months, he was reported to spend most of his days in his room and appeared apathetic and flat. At times, he would appear to be laughing to himself and had "an odd expression." He stopped going out to see friends. He reported at times that he thought he could see messages on a bus that went by each day that related to only himself. On review of symptoms, he endorsed hearing voices at times when alone at home and could feel frightened. After further testing and evaluation, you diagnose him with schizophrenia and start risperidone. Which of the following is NOT true in the evaluation of his diagnosis:
    A. It would be important to evaluate for regular cannabis or other substance use
    B. He should be referred for imaging of the brain
    C. It is rare that the symptom onset occurs at such a young age
    D. CT scans of the brain area unlikely to be abnormal
    Correct answer: C

Explanation

The patient in this vignette presents with symptoms suggestive of new-onset schizophrenia. This diagnosis is considered the most severe of perhaps all psychiatric illness. The rate of diagnosis is about 7.2 per 1,000 adults, with a slightly higher rate in men than in women. This disease usually starts in young adults, with a particular peak around age 20–25 years. The diagnosis requires two or more of the following symptoms be present for at least 1 month: delusions, hallucinations, disorganized speech (frequent derailment or incoherence), grossly disorganized behaviors, and negative symptoms. The signs of the disturbance must persist for more than 6 months, including negative symptoms, and it is important to evaluate for substances such as cannabis that can contribute to psychotic symptoms or unmask them. While imaging is an important part of the workup of first-break psychotic symptoms, it is usually unremarkable. Treatment involves antipsychotic medications, social support, psychotherapy, and other interventions.

Reference

Jauhar S, Johnstone M, McKenna PJ. Schizophrenia. Lancet. 2022;399(10323):473–86. https://doi.org/10.1016/s0140-6736(21)01730-x.

12. A 33-year-old woman is referred for a psychiatric evaluation by an endocrinologist who has been seeing her for fatigue and brain fog, due to the patient's suspicion for "a hormonal imbalance." The woman has seen rheumatology, gastroenterology, neurology, gynecology, and several other specialists as well for ongoing muscle pain, stomach irritation, abdominal bloating and pain, pelvic cramping, muscle weakness, and other complaints. She is worried about having a tumor as well as a possibly undiagnosed neurologic disorder. She finds that each evaluation, rather than relieving her anxiety, leads to an increase in her concern, as she feels dismissed by many specialists. She is reluctant to come to see a psychiatrist but is feeling very frustrated by her search for answers. Which of the following statements is NOT true about her diagnosis—somatic symptom disorder?
    A. Patients with this disorder experience one or more somatic symptoms that are distressing or impair function
    B. Patients with this disorder consciously feign symptoms
    C. This disorder has a female predilection and has an estimated prevalence of 5% of the population
    D. Patients with this disorder are at risk for iatrogenic harm from various tests, procedures, or surgeries that are not indicated

    Correct answer: B

Explanation

Somatic symptom disorder is a relatively common condition, and it depicts individuals who experience significant distress over physical symptoms (frequently but not always pain) without a clear medical explanation or structural pathology. The thoughts or feelings should be excessive or should lead to unusual amounts of time worrying about the health concerns. In general, medications are not indicated in the treatment of these patients, but rather management encourages clear communication between patient and doctor, with frequent visits, and appropriate referrals to mental health providers if there are comorbid anxiety or depression symptoms.

Reference

Dunphy L, Penna M, El-Kafsi J. Somatic symptom disorder: a diagnostic dilemma. BMJ Case Rep. 2019;12(11). https://doi.org/10.1136/bcr-2019-231550.

13. A 23-year-old woman presents for evaluation of worsening symptoms. She was diagnosed recently with multiple sclerosis, and she reports having a difficult time managing her symptoms. She notes being worked up in the setting of a serious car accident, when she sustained significant injury and was hospitalized. During this workup, she had CT and then MRI brain scans, which showed typical demyelinating lesions. Further investigation of her history revealed a prior episode of Lhermitte's sign and an MRI spine showed several demyelinating lesions. Recently, she reports developing intrusive memories of the accident, nightmares, avoidance of driving due to fear, feelings of detachment and negative emotions, as well as hypervigilance and an exaggerated startle response. She is referred for psychotherapy and diagnosed with posttraumatic stress disorder (PTSD). What kind of therapy is recommended first-line for PTSD?
    A. Shared Decision-Making and Collaborative Care
    B. Trauma-Focused Psychotherapy
    C. Eye Movement Desensitization and Restructuring (EMDR)
    D. All of the above

    Correct answer: D

Explanation

In the most recent version of the DSM-5, posttraumatic stress disorder (PTSD) is shifted from the anxiety disorders into the category of trauma-associated disorders. Core symptoms involve at least one intrusive symptom (flashbacks, intrusive memories, nightmares, etc.), one avoidant symptom (avoiding memories or thoughts of the trauma), two negative mood or cognitive symptoms (low mood, feelings of detachment, etc.), and two symptoms of altered arousal (hypervigilance, increased startle, etc.). Treatment strategies include various therapy approaches mentioned above, as well as medications. There is strong evidence for the use of SSRI and SNRI medications in the treatment of PTSD.

Reference

Schrader C, Ross A. A Review of PTSD and Current Treatment Strategies. Mo Med. 2021;118(6):546–51.

14. A 29-year-old woman presents for evaluation. She was recently discharged from the hospital where she was admitted for acute on chronic suicidal ideation. She reports improvement after the hospital stay, but she still feels a high degree of mood lability. Within the period of 1 day, she notes going from feelings of severe depression to stable or even elevated mood. She notes a long-standing pattern of unstable relationships, as well as chronic feelings of emptiness. She has a history of cutting on her wrists and legs with a razor blade at times, often "to relieve stress." She can feel unpredictable anger and rage, often at perceived slights of relationship stressors. You review her discharge diagnosis of borderline personality disorder. What is NOT a core feature of this disorder?

    A. Affective instability with highly reactive mood
    B. A lack of core sense of identity
    C. Self-harming behaviors or impulses
    D. Stable relationships

Correct answer: D

Explanation

Borderline personality disorder is a relatively uncommon but probably underdiagnosed condition, with a prevalence estimated to be around 1.5% of the population. It is marked by a number of core features and represents a chronic and pervasive pattern of maladaptive coping skills. It is likely due to a combination of social, psychological, and genetic factors and is often found in individuals with a history of abuse or trauma. Core features of this disorder include frantic attempts to avoid abandonment, a pattern of unstable relationships ("splitting"), lack of a sense of identity and feelings of emptiness, recurrent suicidal ideation and gestures, mood lability, and intense feelings of rage and anger. Psychotherapy—in particular dialectical behavioral therapy—is the mainstay of treatment. Medications are controversial, but most commonly include SSRIs for depressive symptoms and mood stabilizers for mood lability.

Reference

Mendez-Miller M, Naccarato J, Radico JA. Borderline Personality Disorder. Am Fam Physician. 2022;105(2):156–61.

15. A 21-year-old woman presents for refill of her amphetamine and dextroamphetamine prescription. She notes that she has been using the medication for studying. On review of her psychiatric symptoms, she endorses being concerned about her weight and body shape. She describes quite rigid rules around food intake and an extreme fear about gaining any weight. She finds the amphetamine and dextroamphetamine helpful "to control my appetite," but denies laxative use and denies episodes of binging or purging. Despite a significantly reduced BMI on your exam, she still sees herself as "very overweight." What is the most likely diagnosis?

    A. Bulimia
    B. Avoidant/Restrictive Food Intake Disorder
    C. Anorexia, restricting type
    D. Pica

Correct answer: C

Explanation

This patient presents with symptoms consistent with anorexia nervosa, diagnosed in the DSM-5 as a pattern of behavior marked by severe restriction of food intake, leading to significantly low body weight, along with the intense fear of gaining weight or becoming overweight. This is also marked by a severely distorted sense of one's body image. These patients are typically preoccupied by their weight and spend significant amounts of time developing rules around food intake. Medical complications are many and important to recognize, including cardiac complications, hair thinning, neutropenia, hormonal imbalance, electrolyte disturbances, among others.

Reference

Attia E, Walsh BT. Eating Disorders: A Review. Jama. 2025;333(14):1242–52. https://doi.org/10.1001/jama.2025.0132.

16. A 29-year-old patient presents to the emergency department with acute psychiatric symptoms. He is pacing, agitated, shouting at the staff that he is being followed by the authorities and that there is a conspiracy against him. He presents to the staff a stack of literally hundreds of papers that outline his theories, often with fragmented sentences, illogical passages, and single words repeated over and over again. He notes that he has not slept in weeks and has racing thoughts and pressured speech. The patient and his family note that these episodes have occurred intermittently over the past few years. But they also note that in between them, he has persistent paranoid ideation and even delusions of being "part of a vast conspiracy" that have led him to quit his job and led to difficulties with finding stable housing. He has never presented for psychiatric treatment and has no history of substance use. What is the most likely diagnosis?

    A. Paranoid schizophrenia
    B. Major depressive disorder
    C. Brief psychotic disorder
    D. Schizoaffective disorder, bipolar type

Correct answer: D

Explanation

The diagnosis of schizoaffective disorder in DSM-5 represents a bridge between schizophrenia and the mood disorders. The core of the diagnostic criteria involves patients who experience significant mood episodes (either manic episodes as in this case or major depressive episodes) along with concurrent psychotic symptoms (hallucinations, delusions, and negative symptoms such as apathy, withdrawal, and cognitive impairment). Critically, patients with this condition must also have psychotic symptoms for at least 2 weeks in the absence of any mood episode. The treatment for this typically involves antipsychotic therapies, as well as treatment for the specific mood disorder.

Reference

Malaspina D, Owen MJ, Heckers S, Tandon R, Bustillo J, Schultz S, et al. Schizoaffective Disorder in the DSM-5. Schizophr Res. 2013;150(1):21–5. https://doi.org/10.1016/j.schres.2013.04.026.

17. A 36-year-old woman presents for evaluation. She is accompanied by her husband who expressed concern about the severity of her depression. The patient only nods yes and no at times, speaks very little, and looks mainly down to the floor when speaking, avoiding eye contact. Her husband notes she has been talking about ending her life and has recently written a list of things to give away to friends and family. She has been treated with escitalopram 20 mg and buproprion 300 mg for the past 6 weeks, with good adherence, but no significant response. She denies having a suicidal plan but feels that she is not sure why life is worth living. After reviewing other medication trials in the past, you discuss with her the possibility of a trial of esketamine for acute depression with suicidal features. What side effect would not be expected?
    A. Renal calculi
    B. Elevation in blood pressure
    C. Dissociation
    D. Bladder dysfunction
    Correct answer: A

Explanation

Ketamine is an uncompetitive NMDA antagonist that has recently been approved for use for treatment-resistant depression as well as depression with suicidal ideation. Numerous studies support its use, with notable effects being its extremely rapid onset of action and response. The most common side effects include dissociative symptoms. Other risks include BP elevation and bladder dysfunction. It is approved for use as a nasal spray, but requires monitoring after administration for safe use.

Reference

Jelen LA, Stone JM. Ketamine for depression. Int Rev Psychiatry. 2021;33(3):207–28. https://doi.org/10.1080/09540261.2020.1854194.

18. A 56-year-old woman presents for evaluation, referred by her primary care physician. She and her husband note that she has had increasing periods of sadness over the last few years. These are marked by no longer pursuing activities that she once enjoyed, poor sleep, low energy, negative thoughts about herself and the future, hopelessness, and even thoughts of death. She denies any history of manic episodes. She denies substance use or abuse. She has never been in psychiatric treatment before. What is the most likely diagnosis and a reasonable starting treatment for this patient?
    A. Bipolar disorder, lithium monotherapy
    B. Major depressive disorder, escitalopram, and psychotherapy
    C. Adjustment disorder, olanzapine and fluoxetine
    D. Cyclothymia, cognitive behavioral therapy, and light therapy
    Correct answer: B

Explanation

Depressive disorders are common and account for a significant level of disability and impairment for many patients. In this case, the patient meets the criteria for major depressive disorder, with episodes that last for at least 2 weeks and are marked by at least five core symptoms of depression: depressed mood, loss of interest or pleasure, significant changes in weight, sleep disruptions, psychomotor agitation or retardation, fatigue, feelings of worthlessness or excessive guilt, impaired concentration, or suicidal ideation. Studies of treatment have often shown benefits of combined treatment with medications and psychotherapy. Typical first-line medications include SSRIs given their safety and tolerability profile (e.g. escitalopram, citalopram, sertraline, paroxetine, fluoxetine, among others). Other commonly prescribed medications including buproprion and SNRIs (e.g. venlafaxine and duloxetine). Well-studied psychotherapy approaches to major depression include cognitive behavioral therapy.

Reference

Soleimani L, Lapidus KA, Iosifescu DV. Diagnosis and treatment of major depressive disorder. Neurol Clin. 2011;29(1):177–93, ix. https://doi.org/10.1016/j.ncl.2010.10.010.

19. A 57-year-old woman with a long history of suicidal ideation, mixed manic episodes, and frequent hospitalizations presents for a second opinion about her diagnosis.

She notes severe depression and feels that she would be most helped by starting amphetamine and dextroamphetamine, as she also fears she has attention-deficit/hyperactivity disorder (ADHD). She questions the diagnosis given to her of bipolar disorder, because she notes that she is usually quite depressed, not manic. She has recently had significant side effects to her regimen of quetiapine and lithium. After listening to her symptoms and story, you state that in your opinion, her history is consistent with a diagnosis of bipolar disorder. Which statement is not an accurate description of an aspect of bipolar disorder?

A. Most bipolar patients spend the majority of their mood states in mania
B. Benzodiazepines have some effect on manic symptoms, but less so than traditional mood stabilizers; they can, however, significantly help anxiety
C. Antidepressants are often much less effective and potentially dangerous for patients with bipolar disorder
D. Bipolar disorder can be a dangerous disorder, with high rates of suicide, especially in mixed states

Correct answer: A

Explanation

Bipolar disorder is a relatively common disorder, with roughly 3% of the population affected. It is marked by the presence of at least one manic episode, which is a distinct period of elevated or irritable mood for at least 1 week, along with at least three of the following: grandiosity, decreased need for sleep, pressured speech, flight of ideas or racing thoughts, distractibility, increased goal-directed activity, or involvement in risk-taking activities. As is true of most all psychiatric disorders, the patient must be experiencing significant dysfunction as well. Manic episodes can last a few weeks or months, but many patients with bipolar disorder will spend most of their mood episodes in depressive states. Patients may also experience mixed states, with features of both mania and depression simultaneously. While sometimes prescribed, conventional antidepressants appear to be much less effective in patients with bipolar depression, and they may precipitate a manic episode. The most common medications used include mood stabilizers such as lithium, valproic acid, quetiapine, or cariprazine. Bipolar depressive episodes can be treated with lamotrigine, lithium, or lurasidone. The rate of suicide in bipolar disorder is significantly higher than in the general population and may be as high as 10% or more over the course of a lifetime.

Reference

Tondo L, Vázquez GH, Baldessarini RJ. Depression and Mania in Bipolar Disorder. Curr Neuropharmacol. 2017;15(3):353–8. https://doi.org/10.2174/15701 59x14666160606210811.

20. A 63-year-old woman presents for persistent and disabling anxiety in the setting of her recent diagnosis of multiple sclerosis. She has become frightened of every sensation she feels in her legs and arms, despite being reassured by her neurologist that she has stable disease and is taking a highly effective disease modifying therapy. Her husband is with her and notes frustration with his wife's "spinning out of control" with worries. She is having difficulty sleeping and ongoing muscle cramps. She cannot control these worries and fears she is "going to lose my mind." She is distressed by the anxiety about her health, but then starts to discuss her anxiety about her son's health, her work as a realtor, the health of her husband (who is quite healthy), and the "state of the world." Through tears, she states she is looking for a medication to help her—but then notes she is quite afraid of any possible side effects. You diagnose her with generalized anxiety disorder (GAD) and discuss treatment options. Which of the following statements is NOT true?

A. Difficulty controlling worry is a hallmark of GAD
B. Physical symptoms are common with GAD and include muscle tension, restlessness, poor sleep, and other physical signs of worry
C. GAD is a rare disorder, with a prevalence of less than 1% of the general population
D. GAD cannot be diagnosed unless there is evidence of social, occupational, or other dysfunction

Correct answer: C

Explanation

Generalized anxiety disorder (GAD) is a psychiatric disorder that is marked by excessive, uncontrollable worrying that leads to impairment in the functioning of an individual. It has been linked to certain genes and frequently co-occurs with other anxiety disorders or depression. It is a relatively common disorder affecting 3–5% of the population in most studies. The core concepts of GAD diagnosis include that the worries appear "excessive," and also that the person has difficulty controlling the worries. They are often associated with fatigue, restlessness, fatigue, irritability, or muscle tension. Medications are approved to treat GAD, including SSRIs including fluoxetine, sertraline, paroxetine, and citalopram, as well as SNRIs including venlafaxine and duloxetine. Benzodiazepines can be prescribed but usually for short periods of time. Psychotherapy is also an important treatment, and these include cognitive behavioral therapy as well as supportive therapy.

Reference

Mishra AK, Varma AR. A Comprehensive Review of the Generalized Anxiety Disorder. Cureus. 2023;15(9):e46115. https://doi.org/10.7759/cureus.46115.

21. A 39-year-old man presents for treatment of his anxiety. In particular, he notes that he has developed a near-certain fear that he has developed amyotrophic lateral sclerosis. He is observing his muscles hundreds of times a day, and he has begun to measure his calf every day monitoring for atrophy and feels intense anxiety and dread with every muscle twitch he feels. He had a normal EMG/NCS with a local neurologist, but feels "it's probably because he missed the start of the illness." These thoughts are intrusive and distressing. On reviewing prior history, he notes that in the past he previously had been quite convinced he had developed a sexually transmitted disease, despite not having been sexually active at the time. He had been to many primary care doctors and even specialists seeking reassurance, but this did not seem to resolve his anxiety. Which of the following is the correct diagnosis for his condition?

A. Obsessive-compulsive disorder
B. Generalized anxiety disorder
C. Schizoaffective disorder, bipolar type
D. Illness anxiety disorder

Correct answer: D

Explanation

The patient's symptoms are typical for illness anxiety disorder, a condition that is marked by the preoccupation and recurrent fear of having a serious illness. The fears are often intrusive, unwanted, recurrent, and not particularly responsive to simple reassurance even by health professionals. It is frequently marked by maladaptive behaviors (in this instance, his significant time spent measuring and checking aspects of his body), and these individuals often devote large amounts of time to studying their illness of concern. In general, illness anxiety disorder is not marked by many symptoms—but rather by the excessive worry about having a specific disease. Treatment is centered on psychological therapies, in this case cognitive behavioral therapy focused on reframing certain core beliefs and automatic thoughts.

Reference

Kikas K, Werner-Seidler A, Upton E, Newby J. Illness Anxiety Disorder: A Review of the Current Research and Future Directions. Curr Psychiatry Rep. 2024;26(7):331–9. https://doi.org/10.1007/s11920-024-01507-2.

Autonomic Nervous System Disorders

14

Alejandra Gonzalez-Duarte

Questions

1. A 65-year-old man with a history of bilateral carpal tunnel release presents with progressive pins and needles, pain, and contact allodynia in the feet that have ascended to the distal legs over several months. His medical history is notable for early satiety, alternating diarrhea and constipation, involuntary weight loss of 18 kg (40 pounds) over 6 months, lightheadedness, decreased sweating, urinary retention, and erectile dysfunction. He endorses progressive fatigue and shortness of breath after climbing two flights of stairs. His blood pressure drops from 112/68 mm Hg while sitting to 60/40 mm Hg after 3 min of standing. The EMG shows a length-dependent sensorimotor peripheral neuropathy. His brother and father had similar symptoms. What is the most appropriate next step in the evaluation?
   A. Evaluate with a skin or abdominal fat biopsy, genetic testing, or cardiac PYP scintigraphy to rule out ATTR amyloidosis
   B. Repeat HbA1C and fasting glucose to rule out diabetic neuropathy
   C. Evaluate with cerebral MRI and DaT scan to rule out multiple system atrophy (MSA)
   D. Order serum B12 and methylmalonic acid levels to assess for nutritional neuropathy
   E. Order a paraneoplastic antibody panel
   Correct answer: A

Explanation

This patient has peripheral neuropathy, autonomic dysfunction, unexplained weight loss, cardiac symptoms, and a family history suggestive of a hereditary condition. The combination of bilateral carpal tunnel (a classic red flag), shortness of breath, autonomic symptoms (e.g., orthostatic hypotension, GI dysmotility), and length-dependent sensorimotor neuropathy is highly suggestive of hereditary transthyretin (hATTR) amyloidosis. PYP scintigraphy is used to identify cardiac transthyretin amyloid deposits noninvasively, especially in older men. Genetic testing is essential in suspected hATTR amyloidosis to confirm the diagnosis and subtype. The biopsies can confirm the amyloid deposition. Although diabetes is a common cause of peripheral neuropathy, it does not explain the strong family history. Also, the clinical presentation is more systemic and rapidly progressive than typical diabetic neuropathy, which usually evolves over years rather than months. Multiple system atrophy (MSA) causes autonomic failure, but it primarily presents with central neurodegeneration—parkinsonism or cerebellar signs—which are not described here. Moreover, MSA does not cause sensorimotor peripheral neuropathy or family history. Finally, while B12 deficiency and paraneoplastic syndromes can cause sensorimotor neuropathy with autonomic symptoms, they rarely cause this degree of dysautonomia, and patients do not exhibit the family history or bilateral carpal tunnel syndrome.

Reference

Conceição I, González-Duarte A, Obici L, Schmidt HHJ, Simoneau D, Ong ML, et al. "Red-flag" symptom clusters in transthyretin familial amyloid polyneuropathy. *J Peripher Nerv Syst*. 2016;21(1):5–9. https://doi.org/10.1111/jns.12153.

2. A 57-year-old man with a history of hypertension and squamous cell carcinoma of the tongue treated with radiation therapy 5 years ago presents with labile blood pressure. He reports presyncope symptoms including lightheadedness, "coat-hanger" distribution pain in the neck, and worsening symptoms with standing, walking, or after meals. His blood pressure is 178/98 mm Hg

A. Gonzalez-Duarte (✉)
Department of Neurology, Dysautonomia Center, New York University School of Medicine, New York, NY, USA
e-mail: alejandra.gonzalez-duarte@nyulangone.org

supine with a heart rate of 65 bpm, 132/90 mm Hg sitting, with a heart rate of 68 bpm, and 98/70 mm Hg standing with a heart rate of 70 bpm, indicating orthostatic hypotension with no significant compensatory heart rate increase. During chewing and handgrip, his blood pressure increased by 30 mm Hg. The sweat function testing was normal. What is the most likely diagnosis?

A. Pure autonomic failure (PAF)
B. Vasovagal syncope
C. Afferent baroreflex failure
D. Carcinoid
E. Parkinson's disease

Correct answer: C

Explanation

Labile blood pressure exaggerated by minor stressors such as chewing or handgrip is classic for afferent baroreflex failure. A history of head and neck radiation supports the possibility of damage to the baroreceptor afferents—specifically the glossopharyngeal and vagus nerves—which impairs the transmission of blood pressure signals to the brainstem. This leads to a loss of baroreflex buffering, resulting in exaggerated hypertensive responses and orthostatic hypotension without compensatory tachycardia. PAF involves peripheral autonomic degeneration, often with impaired sweating and low plasma norepinephrine. Vasovagal syncope presents with transient hypotension and bradycardia triggered by emotional stress, pain, or prolonged standing and does not explain the exaggerated hypertensive response with chewing or the supine hypertension. Carcinoid syndrome presents with flushing, diarrhea, wheezing, and serotonin elevation. Parkinson's disease may involve autonomic failure, but it also includes motor features as bradykinesia, rigidity, and tremors.

References

Lamotte G, Coon EA, Suarez MD, Sandroni P, Benarroch EE, Cutsforth-Gregory JK, Mauermann ML, Berini SE, Shouman K, Sletten D, Goodman BP, Low PA, Singer W. Natural History of Afferent Baroreflex Failure in Adults. Neurology. 2021 Jul 13;97(2):e136–e144. https://doi.org/10.1212/WNL.0000000000012149. Epub 2021 May 4. PMID: 33947784; PMCID: PMC8279567.

Norcliffe-Kaufmann LJ, Reynolds HR. Afferent baroreflex failure and tako-tsubo cardiomyopathy. Clin Auton Res. 2011 Feb;21(1):1–2. https://doi.org/10.1007/s10286-010-0113-3. PMID: 21240537.

Linked questions: 3–4

3. A 29-year-old woman presents with recurrent episodes of loss of consciousness. Her most recent episode occurred 2 weeks ago while having blood drawn and was preceded by lightheadedness, blurry vision, palpitations, and cold sweat. She collapsed and recovered spontaneously within 20 seconds, without disorientation. During a tilt table test, her supine blood pressure was 100/84 mm Hg with a heart rate of 69 bpm. At 3 min of head-up tilt, her blood pressure was 96/80 mm Hg with a heart rate of 89 bpm. At 10 min, during blood sampling for catecholamines, her blood pressure dropped to 76/48 mm Hg with a heart rate of 49 bpm. Based on this information, which of the following statements is correct?

A. The blood pressure at 3 min supports orthostatic hypotension as the cause of her episodes
B. The simultaneous fall in blood pressure and heart rate at 10 min while having the blood drawn supports vasovagal syncope as the cause of her episodes
C. The increase in heart rate at 3 min supports postural tachycardia syndrome (POTS) as the cause of her episodes
D. The absence of heart rate increase is suggestive of neurogenic orthostatic hypotension

Correct answer: B

Explanation

The simultaneous fall in blood pressure and heart rate at 10 min supports vasovagal syncope as the cause of her episodes. This pattern is typical of vasovagal syncope, a form of reflex syncope, especially when triggered by emotional stress or pain (such as a blood draw). It involves a delayed drop in blood pressure accompanied by bradycardia, leading to transient cerebral hypoperfusion and brief loss of consciousness. This patient had only a modest drop in blood pressure at 3 min, which does not meet the formal criteria for orthostatic hypotension (OH)—defined as a sustained decrease in systolic BP of ≥20 mm Hg or diastolic BP of ≥10 mm Hg within 3 min of standing or tilt. Her heart rate increased by only 20 bpm, and this occurred alongside a drop in blood pressure, which is not consistent with postural tachycardia syndrome (POTS). The diagnostic criteria for POTS include a heart rate increase of ≥30 bpm (or exceeding 120 bpm) within 10 min of standing or tilt, without orthostatic hypotension. Lastly, neurogenic OH is characterized by sustained hypotension within 3 min of standing or tilt, without appropriate heart rate compensation. In this case, hypotension occurred later (at minute 10) and was preceded by an appropriate initial heart rate increase, which argues against neurogenic OH.

Reference

Freeman, R. et al. (2011). Consensus statement on the definition of orthostatic hypotension, neurally mediated syncope and the postural tachycardia syndrome. *Clinical Autonomic Research*, 21(2), 69–72. https://doi.org/10.1007/s10286-011-0119-5

Linked question

4. Treatment in this case described in the prior question should include:
   A. Increase water and salt intake
   B. Midodrine 5 mg every 8 hours
   C. Fludrocortisone 0.1 mg bid
   D. Reassurance that this is benign condition and can be treated with behavioral therapies
   E. Pacemaker implantation to improve profound bradycardia episodes

   Correct answer: D

Explanation

Vasovagal syncope is benign in most cases, particularly in young, healthy individuals. First-line treatment focuses on patient education, reassurance, and behavioral strategies, including recognizing early warning signs, practicing counterpressure maneuvers (e.g., leg crossing, muscle tensing), and avoiding known triggers such as dehydration, prolonged standing, and blood draws. Although fluid and salt loading may help by increasing plasma volume and reducing susceptibility to hypotension, this intervention typically does not prevent the withdrawal of sympathetic tone, which is the primary mechanism in vasovagal syncope. Similarly, midodrine and fludrocortisone are not effective in preventing the vasodilation and bradycardia characteristic of vasovagal syncope and are not considered first-line treatments in typical presentations. Pacemaker implantation is considered inappropriate and unnecessarily invasive in this context, as the patient has no structural heart disease, and pacing would not prevent reflex-mediated cardioinhibitory responses.

Reference

Johansson M, Fedorowski A. Situational vs vasovagal syncope: one but different? Heart. 2023 Dec 15;110(1):3–4. https://doi.org/10.1136/heartjnl-2023-323180. PMID: 37591689.

Linked questions: 5–6

5. A 32-year-old woman, previously an active runner, presents with chronic fatigue, orthostatic intolerance, and palpitations upon standing. Symptoms began after a respiratory infection that required bed rest for 10 days. She also has a history of joint hypermobility and mild intention tremor. During a tilt table testing, her heart rate increased from 82 bpm to 122 bpm, while her blood pressure rose from 108/70 mm Hg to 128/89 mm Hg, and she reported reproducing her typical symptoms of lightheadedness and palpitations. Which of the following statements is correct?
   A. Any increase in heart rate during tilt with preserved blood pressure is diagnostic of postural orthostatic tachycardia syndrome (POTS)
   B. The patient has orthostatic hypotension, but the heart rate compensates for the fall in blood pressure
   C. The tilt test is normal
   D. The patient meets diagnostic criteria for POTS
   E. The patient meets criteria for vasovagal syncope

   Correct answer: D

Explanation

Postural orthostatic tachycardia syndrome (POTS) is defined as a heart rate increase of ≥30 bpm (or reaching over 120 bpm) within 10 min of standing or head-up tilt, without orthostatic hypotension, and accompanied by symptoms such as palpitations, lightheadedness, or fatigue. This patient meets all diagnostic criteria: her heart rate increased by 40 bpm, there was no drop in blood pressure (in fact, her BP increased slightly), and she reports lightheadedness and palpitations upon standing. In contrast to these specific criteria, not every heart rate increase indicates POTS—the rise must meet the threshold and be associated with symptoms; smaller or asymptomatic increases are not diagnostic. Additionally, there is no drop in blood pressure, ruling out orthostatic hypotension, and no evidence of bradycardia, hypotension, or syncope, which makes vasovagal syncope unlikely.

Reference

Raj SR, Guzman JC, Harvey P, Richer L, Schondorf R, Seifer C, Thibodeau-Jarry N, Sheldon RS. Canadian Cardiovascular Society Position Statement on Postural Orthostatic Tachycardia Syndrome (POTS) and Related Disorders of Chronic Orthostatic Intolerance. Can J Cardiol. 2020 Mar;36(3):357–372. https://doi.org/10.1016/j.cjca.2019.12.024. PMID: 32145864.

Linked question

6. Which of the following statements best explains additional contributing factors to the development of this patient's condition described in the prior question?
   A. POTS is a primary cardiac arrhythmia unrelated to systemic or connective tissue factors
   B. A recent infection requiring bed rest and deconditioning may contribute to impaired autonomic regulation and the development of POTS
   C. Deconditioning after illness typically causes orthostatic hypotension, not postural tachycardia
   D. Long COVID causes only pulmonary symptoms
   E. Hypermobile joints protect against excessive heart rate changes due to enhanced vagal tone

Correct answer: B

Explanation

POTS is not a primary arrhythmia, but rather a form of dysautonomia involving abnormal autonomic cardiovascular reflexes. A recent infection, particularly one requiring bed rest and resulting in deconditioning, may contribute to impaired autonomic regulation and the development of POTS. Post-viral autonomic dysfunction, as increasingly observed in long COVID, is also recognized as a potential trigger. Additionally, joint hypermobility syndromes—such as Ehlers–Danlos syndrome—are frequently associated with POTS, likely due to vascular laxity, which promotes venous pooling in the lower extremities and abdominal vasculature, contributing to orthostatic intolerance.

Reference

Sebastian SA, Co EL, Panthangi V, Jain E, Ishak A, Shah Y, Vasavada A, Padda I. Postural Orthostatic Tachycardia Syndrome (POTS): An Update for Clinical Practice. Curr Probl Cardiol. 2022 Dec;47(12):101384. https://doi.org/10.1016/j.cpcardiol.2022.101384. Epub 2022 Aug 31. PMID: 36055438.

7. A 64-year-old man presents with severe lightheadedness upon standing, resulting in occasional falls, a stooped posture, anterocollis, and a staggering gait. On further questioning, he reports erectile dysfunction, urinary urgency, and nocturia. Neurological examination reveals mildly saccadic pursuit, brisk reflexes, bilateral ataxia, difficulty with finger-to-nose testing, extensor plantar responses, and severe discoloration of the feet. Orthostatic vital signs show:

   - Supine: BP 155/92 mm Hg, HR 62 bpm
   - After 1 min standing: BP 103/80 mm Hg, HR 65 bpm
   - After 3 min standing: BP 89/65 mm Hg, HR 68 bpm

Which is the most likely diagnosis?
   A. Autoimmune autonomic ganglionopathy
   B. Postural tachycardia syndrome (POTS)
   C. Afferent baroreflex failure
   D. Multiple system atrophy (MSA)

Correct answer: D

Explanation

Multiple system atrophy (MSA) is a rare, progressive, adult-onset neurodegenerative disorder characterized by autonomic failure (including orthostatic hypotension (OH), urinary and erectile dysfunction, and gastrointestinal symptoms) and motor dysfunction, which may present as parkinsonism (MSA-P) or cerebellar ataxia (MSA-C). A hallmark of MSA is a lack of compensatory heart rate increase despite profound hypotension, indicating neurogenic OH in contrast to non-neurogenic OH seen in other conditions such as sepsis or hemorrhage. Neurological signs such as saccadic pursuit, brisk reflexes, extensor plantar responses, and ataxia further support a neurodegenerative etiology. In contrast, autoimmune autonomic ganglionopathy typically presents with isolated autonomic failure, normal or elevated norepinephrine levels, and no central signs. Postural tachycardia syndrome (POTS) is defined by an exaggerated heart rate increase (>30 bpm) without hypotension, which this patient does not exhibit. Afferent baroreflex failure usually causes blood pressure lability and lacks the motor and cerebellar findings seen in MSA.

Reference

Poewe W, Stankovic I, Halliday G, Meissner WG, Wenning GK, Pellecchia MT, Seppi K, Palma JA, Kaufmann H. Multiple system atrophy. Nat Rev Dis Primers. 2022 Aug 25;8(1):56. https://doi.org/10.1038/s41572-022-00382-6. PMID: 36008429.

8. Which of the following findings is most consistent with MSA in the early stages of disease?
   A. Low supine norepinephrine levels with mild increase upon standing without loss of smell
   B. Markedly reduced olfaction and reduced cardiac sympathetic innervation
   C. Abnormal MoCA assessment
   D. Severe peripheral anhidrosis
   E. Increased dopamine transporter binding on DaT-SPECT

Correct answer: A

Explanation

The combination of low supine norepinephrine levels with only a mild increase upon standing and preserved olfaction is most consistent with multiple system atrophy (MSA). This reflects central (preganglionic) autonomic failure, where impaired sympathetic output limits the expected rise in norepinephrine during orthostatic stress, but olfactory function typically remains intact, especially in early stages. In contrast, markedly reduced olfaction and reduced cardiac sympathetic innervation are hallmark features of Parkinson's disease and dementia with Lewy bodies (DLB). These conditions are associated with postganglionic (peripheral) autonomic denervation, which often presents early in the disease. An abnormal MoCA assessment suggests early cognitive involvement, which is more characteristic of DLB than MSA, as MSA generally preserves cognition in the early stages. Severe anhidrosis can occur in MSA but is not diagnostic on its own. When accompanied by olfactory loss, it more strongly points toward DLB or advanced Parkinson's disease, where small fiber and postganglionic autonomic involvement is more pronounced. Lastly, increased dopamine transporter binding on DaT-SPECT would be atypical in MSA, Parkinson's disease, or DLB—all of which show reduced dopamine transporter availability due to nigrostriatal degeneration.

Reference

Wenning GK, Fanciulli A, Krismer F, Palma J-A, Stankovic I, Seppi K, et al. Multiple system atrophy: advances in pathophysiology, diagnosis, and treatment. *Lancet Neurol.* 2024;23(3):215–28. https://doi.org/10.1016/S1474-4422(24)00396-X.

9. A 35-year-old man presents with recurrent episodes of headache, facial flushing, hypertension up to 240 mm Hg, bradycardia, dyspnea, and whole-body spasms. He experiences up to three episodes per day, each lasting approximately 10 min, often triggered by rectal manipulation or urinary catheterization. Six months ago, he sustained a traumatic spinal cord injury at the C6–C7 level following a motor vehicle accident, resulting in quadriparesis.

    What is the most likely diagnosis?
    A. Spinal shock
    B. Autonomic dysreflexia
    C. Pheochromocytoma
    D. Mast cell activation
    Correct answer: B

Explanation

This patient exhibits classic features of autonomic dysreflexia (AD), a potentially life-threatening complication that occurs in individuals with spinal cord injuries at or above the T6 level where sympathetic outflow to the splanchnic vascular bed is most affected. AD is characterized by sudden,

severe hypertension, often accompanied by bradycardia due to the baroreflex-mediated vagal response, along with symptoms such as headache, facial flushing, dyspnea, and generalized spasms. These episodes are typically triggered by noxious stimuli below the level of injury, including bladder or bowel distension, urinary catheterization, or rectal manipulation. The sympathetic nervous system becomes hyperactive below the lesion, but descending inhibitory signals from the brainstem cannot reach the spinal sympathetic neurons, resulting in uncontrolled vasoconstriction and elevated blood pressure. Episodes are usually brief and resolve once the triggering stimulus is removed, but prompt recognition and treatment are critical to prevent serious complications such as stroke or cardiac arrhythmia. Spinal shock refers to the acute phase following spinal cord injury, with flaccid paralysis, areflexia, and hypotension—not episodic hypertension months after injury. Pheochromocytoma causes paroxysmal hypertension with palpitations, headache, and diaphoresis, but it is not triggered by procedural stimuli and would not be expected in a young man with a known spinal injury and clear precipitating factors. Mast cell activation may cause flushing, hypotension, urticaria, or anaphylaxis, but not severe hypertension or neurological features like spasms or bradycardia.

Reference

Eldahan KC, Rabchevsky AG. Autonomic dysreflexia after spinal cord injury: Systemic pathophysiology and methods of management. Auton Neurosci. 2018 Jan;209:59–70. https://doi.org/10.1016/j.autneu.2017.05.002. Epub 2017 May 8. PMID: 28506502; PMCID: PMC5677594.

10. A 68-year-old man presents to the neurology clinic with complaints of dizziness, fatigue, and lightheadedness upon standing that began gradually over the past 3 weeks. He reports several near-falls when getting out of bed and describes a "black curtain" coming over his vision when standing quickly. He also notes dry mouth, constipation, and occasional blurred vision, particularly in dim lighting. There is no history of syncope, recent illness, or dietary changes. His medical history includes major depressive disorder, for which he takes amitriptyline, and hypertension, treated with lisinopril. He was recently diagnosed with overactive bladder, for which oxybutynin 5 mg twice daily was initiated. In addition, terazosin, an alpha-1 adrenergic blocker, was prescribed for benign prostatic hyperplasia. Which of the following would be the most appropriate next step in managing this patient's condition?
    A. Increase his fluid and salt intake
    B. Add midodrine to raise his blood pressure

C. Discontinue terazosin, switch oxybutynin to only nightly, and reduce the dose of amitriptyline
D. Refer for autonomic testing
E. Begin fludrocortisone therapy

Correct answer: C

Explanation

The most appropriate first step is to identify and reduce or eliminate offending medications. The combination of terazosin, which can cause orthostatic hypotension, and two medications with strong anticholinergic properties—amitriptyline and oxybutynin—is likely contributing to his symptoms. These drugs impair autonomic reflexes, leading to reduced baroreflex compensation, postural blood pressure drops, and parasympathetic side effects such as dry mouth, blurred vision, and constipation. Non-pharmacologic and pharmacologic interventions can follow if symptoms persist.

Paul Sanmartin

1. A 68-year-old female with history of well-controlled hypertension is admitted to the hospital for an acute episode of altered mental status. The patient works as a housekeeper and was noted to become disoriented, dysarthric, and somnolent. Upon arrival to the hospital, her vital signs were normal. Once admitted, she became intermittently agitated.

   On exam, the patient is somnolent and able to tell her name, occasionally able to follow commands, and intermittently able to name objects. Cranial nerve exam is notable for sluggish pupil reactivity, no tongue bite. There are no motor deficits.

   CT/CTA of the head and neck showed no acute abnormalities, no large vessel occlusions, nor stenosis. Lab workup is unremarkable. Rapid response EEG showed a thetha/alpha background without obvious abnormalities. Urine toxicology was positive for marijuana, for which she reports accidental edible ingestion.

   Which of the following mechanisms of action best explains her symptoms?
   A. Partial agonism of CB1 receptors in the central nervous system
   B. Antagonism of muscarinic acetylcholine receptors
   C. Inhibition of GABA transaminase
   D. NMDA receptor antagonism
   Correct answer: A

Explanation

In older adults, tetrahydrocannabinol (THC) ingestion, particularly through edibles, is increasingly recognized as a cause of reversible encephalopathy, often presenting with confusion, agitation, and fluctuating alertness without focal deficits or abnormal imaging. THC is a partial agonist at CB1 receptors, which are widely expressed in cortical, limbic, and cerebellar regions. Activation leads to disruption in neurotransmitter release, contributing to sedation, altered perception, dysarthria, agitation, and in higher doses or naïve individuals, encephalopathy.

B. Antagonism of muscarinic acetylcholine receptors—This is the mechanism behind anticholinergic toxicity (e.g., diphenhydramine, atropine), which presents with mydriasis, dry skin, tachycardia, and hyperthermia, not consistent with this case.

C. Inhibition of GABA transaminase—This is the mechanism by which vigabatrin works to increase GABA availability. While increased GABA availability can cause sedation, this is not the mechanism by which cannabis exerts its effect. Vigabatrin does not tend to cause episodic confusion as in this vignette.

D. NMDA receptor antagonism—This is the primary mechanism of ketamine, phencyclidine (PCP), and dextromethorphan. These can cause dissociation, hallucinations, and hypertension, but again, not the best match here.

References

Dutta S, Selvam B, Das A, Shukla D. Mechanistic origin of partial agonism of tetrahydrocannabinol for cannabinoid receptors. J Biol Chem. 2022;298(4):101764. https://doi.org/10.1016/j.jbc.2022.101764.

Vučković S, Srebro D, Vujović KS, Vučetić Č, Prostran M. Cannabinoids and Pain: New Insights From Old Molecules. Front Pharmacol. 2018;9:1259. https://doi.org/10.3389/fphar.2018.01259.

2. A 64-year-old male with unknown medical history is brought to the hospital by EMS for confusion, mild agitation, and a recent fall. The patient is not a reliable historian and is disheveled, homeless, and carries several packs of old cigarettes. He reports alcohol use but mentions this is not consistent. When asked about seizures or alcohol withdrawal history, he denies both.

P. Sanmartin (✉)
Department of Neurology, New York University Grossman School of Medicine, New York, NY, USA
e-mail: paul.sanmartin@nyulangone.org

On arrival to the emergency department, he is hypertensive (175/85 mm Hg), HR 88 BPM, and afebrile. Lab workup is significant for mild normocytic normochromic anemia, toxicology positive for fentanyl. He adamantly denies any illicit drug use.

On exam, the patient is awake, alert, and oriented to person and place only. He can name, read, repeat, and is able to follow midline commands, but has difficulties with complex commands. Cranial nerves are remarkable for occasional beats of vertical and horizontal nystagmus. No tremors. Strength is symmetric in all extremities. Truncal and gait ataxia are present.

You decide to start thiamine, what is appropriate dose in this case?

A. Thiamine 100 mg IV
B. Thiamine 200 mg PO once followed by 100 mg daily thereafter
C. Thiamine 500 mg IV 3 times daily for 3 days followed by 200 mg daily thereafter
D. Thiamine 500 mg IV and IV dextrose

Correct Answer: C

Explanation

The correct answer is (C) Thiamine 500 mg IV 3 times daily for 3 days followed by 200 mg daily thereafter is indicated in this case since the presentation is highly suggestive of Wernicke's encephalopathy, a neurologic emergency associated with thiamine deficiency, most often due to chronic alcohol use. Although the patient denies consistent alcohol use and illicit drugs, his presentation—including disorientation, truncal ataxia, horizontal and vertical nystagmus—is classic. Additionally, his disheveled appearance, unreliable history, and homelessness increase the suspicion for malnutrition and thiamine deficiency, regardless of reported alcohol intake. The presence of ophthalmoplegia/nystagmus, ataxia, and confusion constitutes the classic triad of Wernicke's encephalopathy, though all three are not always present in a single individual. Given the high morbidity of untreated Wernicke's encephalopathy and the relative safety of thiamine supplementation, high-dose parenteral thiamine is the recommended approach. The evidence-based regimen in suspected acute Wernicke's encephalopathy is 500 mg IV three times daily for 3 days, followed by 200 mg daily for several days, typically continued orally once stabilized. This regimen is supported by neurological and nutritional guidelines to ensure adequate CNS penetration and reversal of the acute phase. Option A (100 mg IV) and Option B (200 mg orally followed by 100 mg) are insufficient for treating suspected Wernicke's encephalopathy. Oral absorption may be unreliable in malnourished or acutely ill patients, and doses below 500 mg IV are generally considered inadequate for reversing acute symptoms. Option D (thiamine 500 mg IV and IV dextrose) is dangerous: giving dextrose before thiamine in a thiamine-deficient patient can precipitate or worsen Wernicke's enceph-

alopathy due to increased metabolic demand, exacerbating cellular injury in the brain. Thiamine must always be given before glucose in patients at risk of deficiency.

References

Cook CC, Hallwood PM, Thomson AD. B Vitamin deficiency and neuropsychiatric syndromes in alcohol misuse. Alcohol Alcohol. 1998;33(4):317–36. https://doi.org/10.1093/oxfordjournals.alcalc.a008400.

Thomson AD, Cook CC, Touquet R, Henry JA. The Royal College of Physicians report on alcohol: guidelines for managing Wernicke's encephalopathy in the accident and Emergency Department. Alcohol Alcohol. 2002;37(6):513–21. https://doi.org/10.1093/alcalc/37.6.513.

3. A 63-year-old female with no medical history presents to the hospital with a 2-month history of bilateral upper and lower extremity numbness. Symptoms have slowly progressed, and she describes her extremities as "heavy." Approximately 1 month prior to presentation, she developed gait issues, and at this point, she is currently using a walker. She denies urinary/fecal issues, recent infections, diarrhea, diplopia, dysphagia, cancer treatment, or cancer diagnosis.

Neurological exam reveals a normal mental status, normal cranial nerves, but her tongue is noted to be smooth and red, but without typical papillae. Strength is 4+/5 throughout. Sensory exam showed no sensory level. Sensation to light touch and temperature intact throughout. Vibratory and temperature sensations are mildly decreased in both hands and absent from the knees and extending distally. Reflexes are 3+ throughout, 2 beats of ankle clonus, plantar response is downgoing, and a Hoffmann's sign is present bilaterally. Truncal ataxia is noted. Gait is severely ataxic.

Based on the history and exam, what anatomic structure(s) are affected, and what is the most likely diagnosis?

A. Peripheral nerves: Guillain–Barré syndrome (GBS)
B. Peripheral nerves: Chronic inflammatory demyelinating polyradiculoneuropathy (CIDP)
C. Posterior columns and corticospinal tracts: Subacute combined degeneration (SCD)
D. Spinal cord: Transverse myelitis

Correct answer: C

Explanation

The correct answer is (C) Posterior columns and corticospinal tracts: Subacute combined degeneration (SCD). This patient presents with a progressive 2-month history of sensory disturbances, gait ataxia, and signs of both posterior column and corticospinal tract dysfunction. The neurological exam reveals loss of vibration and proprioception, particularly in the lower extremities, which points to posterior column involvement. Additionally, the presence of hyperreflexia, ankle clonus, and a positive Hoffmann's sign—all signs of upper motor neuron dysfunction—indicates corticospinal tract involvement.

The smooth, red tongue without papillae noted on exam is consistent with atrophic glossitis, a classic clue for vitamin B12 deficiency. B12 deficiency is the hallmark cause of subacute combined degeneration (SCD) of the spinal cord. SCD affects the dorsal columns (causing impaired proprioception, vibration sense, and sensory ataxia) and the lateral corticospinal tracts (leading to spasticity, hyperreflexia, and sometimes mild weakness). The lack of a sensory level helps rule out structural cord lesions like transverse myelitis. The relatively preserved motor strength further supports SCD, where motor symptoms tend to lag behind sensory deficits. Option A (Guillain–Barré syndrome, GBS) is incorrect because GBS is typically an acute ascending motor neuropathy that evolves over the course of days to weeks, not months. GBS is also characterized by hyporeflexia or areflexia, not hyperreflexia and clonus. Furthermore, GBS does not produce upper motor neuron signs like a Hoffmann's sign. Option B (CIDP) is also a peripheral demyelinating process, and like GBS, it affects peripheral nerves, not the spinal cord tracts. CIDP leads to distal and proximal weakness, areflexia, and sometimes mild sensory symptoms, but it does not cause hyperreflexia, clonus, nor Hoffmann's sign. This patient's exam is inconsistent with peripheral nerve pathology. Option D (transverse myelitis) is a spinal cord process, but it would typically present with a sensory level, often accompanied by bowel/bladder dysfunction and subacute progression over days to a few weeks. This patient has no sensory level and no autonomic symptoms.

References

Hemmer B, Glocker FX, Schumacher M, Deuschl G, Lücking CH. Subacute combined degeneration: clinical, electrophysiological, and magnetic resonance imaging findings. J Neurol Neurosurg Psychiatry. 1998;65(6):822–7. https://doi.org/10.1136/jnnp.65.6.822.

Saji AM, Lui F, De Jesus O. Spinal Cord Subacute Combined Degeneration. StatPearls. Treasure Island (FL): StatPearls Publishing Copyright © 2025, StatPearls Publishing LLC.; 2025.

4. A 34-year-old female with a history of febrile seizure during childhood, borderline personality disorder, anxiety, depression, and previous suicidal ideations presents to the ED with multiple episodes she describes as tunnel vision followed by an out-of-body sensation followed by dysarthria and confusion. Each episode lasts approximately 2 min and is followed by severe exhaustion. These episodes started about 1 year ago. They were infrequent at first, but over the past 2 weeks, they have been occurring multiple times per day. She was seen multiple times in urgent care or other health facilities, and the episodes were attributed to her borderline personality disorder. She denies family history of epilepsy. Neurological exam is normal. Initial head CT and lab workup are unremarkable. The patient is currently driving.

What is the best next step in management?

A. Seizure precautions and start levetiracetam 500 mg twice a day

B. Seizure precautions and discharge patient and schedule an ambulatory EEG

C. Seizure precautions and start oxcarbazepine 300 mg twice daily

D. Brain MRI with and without contrast

Correct answer: C

Explanation

The correct answer is (C) Seizure precautions and start oxcarbazepine (OXC) 300 mg twice daily. This patient presents with stereotyped episodes with clinical semiology suggestive of focal impaired awareness (FIA) seizures. Her episodes involve tunnel vision, an out-of-body sensation, inability to express herself, and post-ictal exhaustion, all of which are classic for focal seizures with impaired awareness (formerly referred to as complex partial seizures), likely of dominant temporal lobe onset. The recent increase in frequency and daily occurrence further raises concern for undiagnosed focal epilepsy. While her psychiatric history and normal initial workup may have led to prior misattribution of her symptoms, the clinical picture now strongly suggests epileptic seizures, warranting immediate treatment. Oxcarbazepine (OXC) is an appropriate first-line treatment for focal epilepsy. It is a voltage-gated sodium channel blocker, pharmacologically similar to carbamazepine but better tolerated, with a more favorable side effect profile. It is commonly started at 300 mg twice daily, especially in younger patients or those with no prior antiepileptic exposure. Given the patient's psychiatric comorbidities, oxcarbazepine is the most reasonable option as OXC can help with mood stabilization. Option A (levetiracetam 500 mg BID) is a reasonable antiepileptic for focal seizures and widely used; however, given this patient's history of borderline personality disorder, anxiety, and depression, levetiracetam (LEV) is less ideal. LEV is known to cause or exacerbate mood instability, irritability, depression, and suicidality, which could be particularly problematic in this case. Because of this psychiatric side effect profile of LEV, clinicians often choose alternatives when mood disorders are prominent. Option B (ambulatory EEG and discharge) would delay treatment in a patient now having daily events while driving—an immediate safety concern. While EEG can support diagnosis, clinical history is sufficient to initiate treatment in this case given stereotyped events. Ambulatory EEG can follow once seizures are better controlled and driving has been suspended (driving restrictions are typically determined by state law). Option D (MRI with and without contrast) is important in the workup of new-onset focal epilepsy, especially in adults, to rule out structural causes like cortical dysplasia or hippocampal sclerosis. However, it is not the most immediate next step in a patient having frequent daily events while driving. In this case, while the patient is experiencing multiple events per day, along with an unremarkable CT head and normal neurological exam, the best next step is to begin treatment and obtain an MRI afterward. In summary, the correct approach is to initiate oxcarbazepine, which is a first-line treatment for focal seizures, while simultaneously instituting seizure precautions, including driving restrictions. The choice of oxcarbazepine over levetiracetam is driven by pharmacological considerations in the context of her psychiatric comorbidities.

Reference

Kanner AM, Bicchi MM. Antiseizure Medications for Adults With Epilepsy: A Review. Jama. 2022;327(13):1269–81. https://doi.org/10.1001/jama.2022.3880.

5. A 50-year-old right-handed male with a history of anxiety is seen in the emergency department (ED) after an episode of involuntary right arm movement. The patient is a business analyst and was in a meeting when suddenly he noticed a tingling sensation in the right arm, which was later followed by a feeling that he was losing control over his entire right arm, gradually the arm lifted, and he was unable to lower his arm down. This lasted about 45 s and was followed by mild dysarthria, during which time he was able to lower his arm but unable to lift it. The rest of this episode lasted about 2 min after which he was able to move all extremities without difficulty, and his speech was clear.

   On arrival to the ED, BP 136/95 mm Hg, HR 85 BPM, afebrile with normal oxygen saturation. CT head and CTA head and neck are unremarkable. Neurological exam is normal except for agraphesthesia in the right hand.

   The patient is ultimately diagnosed with a stroke, where would you localize the lesion based on the history and physical exam?

   A. Left frontal region
   B. Left temporal region
   C. Left parietal region
   D. Left midbrain

   Correct answer: C

Explanation

The correct answer is (C) Left parietal region. This patient's episode consists of a transient sensorimotor disturbance in the right arm, starting with tingling (positive sensory symptoms) followed by involuntary elevation and inability to control the arm (motor impairment), and a brief post-event weakness or negative motor symptom. Most telling, however, is that on neurological examination, he has agraphesthesia in the right hand, a highly localizing cortical sensory sign. Agraphesthesia—the inability to recognize numbers or letters drawn on the skin—is classically associated with parietal lobe dysfunction, particularly in the dominant hemisphere. It reflects a disturbance in higher-order somatosensory processing, not simple primary sensory or motor function. His course of symptom onset, normal CT imaging, and partial recovery suggest a small cortical infarct (possibly embolic) involving the left parietal cortex, which processes contralateral somatosensory input, including proprioception and graphesthesia. The initial tingling and limb posturing may reflect a sensory-motor dissociation. Option A (Left frontal region) would be more typical for primary motor cortex involvement, causing contralateral weakness (not tingling or agraphesthesia). A frontal stroke might cause Broca's aphasia or grasp reflex, neither of which are described here. Option B (Left temporal region) would more likely cause language symptoms, auditory hallucinations, or memory impairments, depending on the subregion. There are no signs of aphasia, auditory processing, or amnestic symptoms. Option D (Left midbrain) would produce brainstem signs—such as cranial nerve involvement, vertical gaze palsy, or crossed findings. The patient has no such brainstem features, making a midbrain stroke very unlikely.

Reference

Tabi YA, Husain M. Clinical assessment of parietal lobe function. Pract Neurol. 2023;23(5):404–7. https://doi.org/10.1136/pn-2023-003746.

6. An 83-year-old right-handed male with a history of atrial fibrillation on warfarin, right carotid endarterectomy, type 2 diabetes (recent hemoglobin A1c 9.2%), hypertension, and hyperlipidemia is evaluated in the emergency department (ED) for multiple episodes of right-hand numbness associated with perioral paresthesias, which started the day prior. The numbness and paresthesias involve the right corner of his mouth and the entire right hand. Each episode lasts about 2 min and self-resolves. Earlier today, he was evaluated in urgent care, where he had an EKG performed, which was unremarkable, and he was discharged home. His wife advised him to come to the ED. On admission, his BP is 204/115 mm Hg, HR 82 BPM, and afebrile. Lab workup is unremarkable.

Exam is remarkable for subtle numbness in the left upper and lower lip region along with the left side of his chin. Graphesthesia and stereognosis are normal.

MRI demonstrates an acute stroke, which of the following is the most likely localization of the infarct?

A. Left frontal lobe
B. Left parietal lobe
C. Left thalamus
D. Left temporal lobe

Correct answer: C

Explanation

The correct answer is (C) Left thalamus. This patient presents with transient, stereotyped sensory episodes involving the right hand and perioral region, specifically the right corner of the mouth and the entire hand. This presentation is classic for a stuttering "cheiro-oral syndrome." Cheiro-oral syndrome involves sensory disturbances in the fingers and perioral region contralateral to a brainstem or thalamic lesion, which localizes to the ventral posterior nuclei of the thalamus, particularly the ventral posterolateral (VPL) and ventral posteromedial (VPM) nuclei. The VPL nucleus of the thalamus receives sensory input from the body (via the medial lemniscus and spinothalamic tract), while the VPM nucleus receives sensory input from the face (via the trigeminothalamic tract). A small infarct affecting the posterolateral thalamus on the left could easily produce isolated contralateral face and hand sensory disturbances, as both the hand and perioral region are closely represented somatotopically in the thalamus. These symptoms can occur in pure sensory strokes, often due to small vessel disease (common in hypertensive, diabetic patients). The subtle numbness in the right upper and lower lip and chin, along with transient hand paresthesias, all point to disruption of thalamocortical sensory relay pathways. Importantly, the lack of motor weakness, visual field deficits, language disturbance, or cortical sensory signs (e.g., graphesthesia, stereognosis) supports a deep subcortical lesion, rather than a cortical stroke. Option A (left frontal lobe) is incorrect because frontal lesions cause motor deficits, not pure sensory syndromes. There is no evidence of weakness or executive dysfunction in this patient. In conclusion, the pattern of face and hand sensory symptoms—particularly involving the perioral region and hand—is highly localizing to the contralateral VPM/VPL region of the thalamus, making option A the correct answer. Option B (left parietal lobe) would be considered if the patient had cortical sensory loss, such as impaired graphesthesia, stereognosis, or neglect. However, these were preserved. A parietal lesion would also typically not spare the legs unless very focal. Option D (left temporal lobe) is incorrect, as this region is more involved in language, memory, and auditory processing, not in primary somatosensation of the face or extremities.

Reference

Satpute S, Bergquist J, Cole JW. Cheiro-Oral syndrome secondary to thalamic infarction: a case report and literature review. Neurologist. 2013;19(1):22–5. https://doi.org/10.1097/NRL.0b013e31827c6c0e.

7. A 72-year-old male with history of atrial fibrillation on rivaroxaban, hypertension, and hyperlipidemia presents to the emergency department (ED) with right visual loss. Four days prior, the patient underwent cataract surgery, for which he was advised to hold rivaroxaban. Immediately after the procedure, the right eye was covered with a gauze. Today, after he uncovered his eye, he noted severely decreased visual acuity. Vital signs on presentation were normal, lab workup was unremarkable, which included a normal erythrocyte sedimentation rate (ESR) and c-reactive protein (CRP).

On neurological exam, you note his visual acuity on the left is 20/40, while on the right he is only able to perceive light. Fundoscopy demonstrates a pale right retina.

What is the most likely diagnosis?

A. Central retinal vein occlusion (CRVO)
B. Central retinal artery occlusion (CRAO)
C. Non-arteritic ischemic optic neuropathy (NAION)
D. Arteritic ischemic optic neuropathy (AION)

Correct answer: B

Explanation

The correct answer is (B) Central retinal artery occlusion (CRAO). This patient presents with sudden, painless, severe monocular vision loss, which is classic for CRAO. The visual acuity is profoundly reduced in the right eye—only able to perceive light—and fundoscopy reveals a pale retina, which is the hallmark of CRAO due to retinal ischemia. This is an ophthalmologic emergency that results from occlusion of the central retinal artery, most commonly due to embolism, often from cardioembolic sources such as atrial fibrillation (of which this patient has a history). The central retinal artery, a branch of the ophthalmic artery (itself from the internal carotid artery), supplies the inner retinal layers. Occlusion leads to acute ischemia of the retina, manifesting as a pale fundus with a cherry-red spot in the macula (though this cherry red spot is not described in this question, it is often noted on fundoscopy in practice). The patient's recent interruption of anticoagulation (rivaroxaban held for surgery) adds to the embolic risk, and the timeline—vision loss noticed immediately after removing the postoperative dressing—is consistent with delayed recognition of an acute event rather than gradual visual decline. Option A (CRVO) typically presents with subacute vision loss, not sudden and profound. Fundus exam in CRVO shows "blood and thunder" appearance, with retinal hemorrhages, venous dilation, and cotton wool spots, not pallor. CRVO is more commonly seen in elderly females. Options C non-arteritic ischemic optic neuropathy (NAION) and D arteritic ischemic optic neuropathy (AION) both refer to anterior ischemic optic neuropathy. NAION is more common and often seen in patients with small crowded optic discs and vascular risk factors. It can present with sudden monocular vision loss, but vision loss is usually less severe than CRAO, and optic disc edema is typically seen. This patient's pale retina, rather than disc edema, argues against AION/NAION. In arteritic AION (D) due to giant cell arteritis, the vision loss may be severe, but it typically affects older patients (often >75) and is accompanied by systemic symptoms (e.g., jaw claudication, scalp tenderness, fatigue), and would expect ESR and CRP to be elevated, which is not the case here.

References

Mehta S. Central Retinal Artery Occlusion and Branch Retinal Artery Occlusion (Retinal Artery Occlusion). Porter RE. The Merck Manual of Diagnosis and Therapy. Rahway, NJ: Merck & Co Inc.; Reviewed/Revised Apr 2024 | Modified Sept 2024.

Tripathy K, Patel BC. Cherry Red Spot. StatPearls. Treasure Island (FL): StatPearls Publishing Copyright © 2025, StatPearls Publishing LLC.; 2025.

8. A 68-year-old right-handed Hispanic female with a history of uncontrolled hypertension, chronic kidney disease stage IV, anxiety, hyperlipidemia, and polysubstance use disorder is evaluated in the emergency department (ED) with uncontrollable whole-body movements, which started 2 h prior to admission. While these movements are ongoing, the patient is awake and intermittently able to nod yes/no to questions, and is demonstrating dance-like movements affecting the face, limbs, and trunk. These movements are asymmetric and asynchronous. Urine toxicology is positive for the causative agent.

   What is the mechanism of action of the illicit substance causing the patient's symptoms?
   A. Inhibition of GABA transaminase
   B. NMDA receptor antagonism
   C. Dopamine and norepinephrine reuptake inhibition
   D. Serotonin receptor agonism
   E. Direct stimulation of nicotinic acetylcholine receptors
   Correct answer: C

Explanation

The correct answer is (C) Dopamine and norepinephrine reuptake inhibition. The patient's clinical presentation is consistent with cocaine-induced chorea, also known as "crack dancing," characterized by involuntary, purposeless, hyperkinetic movements affecting the face, limbs, and trunk. This may be seen in cocaine intoxication, especially in patients with predisposing vulnerabilities such as renal disease or hypertension. Cocaine exerts its neurologic and cardiovascular effects primarily through blockade of monoamine reuptake transporters, specifically for dopamine, norepinephrine, and serotonin. The choreiform movements are linked to dopamine reuptake inhibition in the basal ganglia, particularly affecting the striatum, leading to a hyperdopaminergic state. This pathophysiologic mechanism closely resembles that seen in conditions like Huntington's disease and levodopa-induced dyskinesias. Option A (Inhibition of GABA transaminase) is the mechanism of vigabatrin, used in epilepsy; GABAergic hyperactivity would more likely suppress movements rather than cause chorea. Option B (NMDA receptor antagonism) is associated with ketamine or PCP. These can cause dissociation and agitation, but not classically choreiform movements. Option D (Serotonin receptor agonism) describes agents like LSD or psilocybin, which can cause perceptual disturbances and agitation but are not typically associated with chorea. Option E (Direct stimulation of nicotinic receptors) is linked to nicotine or organophosphate toxicity, which results in cholinergic crises, not chorea.

Reference

Byroju VV, Rissardo JP, Durante Í, Caprara ALF. Cocaine-induced Movement Disorder: A Literature Review. Prague Med Rep. 2024;125(3):195–219. https://doi.org/10.14712/23362936.2024.19.

9. An 18-year-old female presents to the emergency department (ED) with altered mental status. The patient is awake, but unable to provide any history. She was found on the floor today by her roommate. When her roommate tried to help the patient to stand, she was unable to walk and fell to the floor again. Upon presentation to the ED, vital signs and lab workup are unremarkable.

   By the time you evaluate the patient, she is awake but did not want to provide further information. On exam, she is oriented to person and place only and able to follow both midline and cross-body commands, speech is clear, and there is no aphasia. Cranial nerve exam is normal. Strength is 4+/5 in all extremities with normal muscle tone. Hyperreflexia, bilateral sustained ankle clonus, and Hoffmann's signs are noted. Vibration and proprioception are absent in the hands and feet. Babinski sign is present bilaterally. Gait is severely ataxic.

The patient reports using a recreational substance, what is the mechanism of action of the illicit substance causing the patient's presentation?

A. NMDA receptor antagonism
B. Inactivation of vitamin B12 by oxidation of its cobalt center
C. Inhibition of serotonin reuptake
D. Inhibition of the dopamine transporter (DAT)
E. Agonism of cannabinoid receptors

Correct answer: B

Explanation

The correct answer is (B) Inactivation of vitamin B12 by oxidation of its cobalt center. This patient's constellation of findings—spasticity, hyperreflexia, bilateral Babinski and Hoffmann signs, along with posterior column dysfunction (loss of vibration and proprioception) and ataxic gait—points toward a subacute combined degeneration (SCD)-like picture, which involves the dorsal columns and corticospinal tracts. Recreational use of nitrous oxide (N_2O), or laughing gas (referred to as "whippits"), leads to oxidation of the cobalt ion in vitamin B12, rendering it functionally inactive. This inactivation disrupts methylmalonyl-CoA mutase and methionine synthase, impairing myelin synthesis in the spinal cord. The clinical result is posterior column degeneration (sensory ataxia) and corticospinal tract damage (causing upper motor neuron signs), effectively creating a vitamin B12 deficiency. This may sometimes be misdiagnosed as acute inflammatory demyelinating polyneuropathy (AIDP) when it is associated with a loss or decrease of reflexes. Option A (NMDA receptor antagonism) refers to substances like ketamine or PCP, which cause dissociation, hallucinations, and agitation, but not the combined spinal cord tract signs seen here. Option C (Inhibition of serotonin reuptake) applies to MDMA or SSRIs, typically causing mood elevation or serotonin syndrome, not a myelopathy. Option D (Inhibition of dopamine transporter) describes cocaine or methamphetamine, which leads to sympathetic overdrive, chorea, or seizures, but not B12-inactivation myelopathy. Option E (Agonism of cannabinoid receptors) refers to THC, causing sedation or altered perception, but does not affect the spinal cord.

References

Ménétrier T, Denimal D. Vitamin B12 Status in Recreational Users of Nitrous Oxide: A Systematic Review Focusing on the Prevalence of Laboratory Abnormalities. Antioxidants (Basel). 2023;12(6). https://doi.org/10.3390/antiox12061191.

Singh H, Beriwal N, Minhas JS, Robinson C. Subacute combined degeneration from nitrous oxide abuse. Radiol Case Rep. 2024;19(12):5600–4. https://doi.org/10.1016/j.radcr.2024.08.031.

10. A 28-year-old male without significant past medical history presents to the emergency department (ED) from the airport for an episode of a fall associated with loss of consciousness. The patient was on a cruise to Antarctica, and while he was on the boat deck, he fell backward and lost consciousness for about 5 min. He regained consciousness quickly, but had a holocephalic headache, which was constant and severe. The patient took a plane from Argentina to New York City and came to the ED as soon as he landed.

On presentation, vitals were normal and lab workup was significant for a white blood cell count of $12.4 \times 10^3/\mu L$. Neurological exam is remarkable for normal fundoscopy bilaterally, anosmia, and ageusia. Remainder of exam is normal.

Brain imaging is abnormal; based on the history and exam, what are the most likely imaging abnormalities?

A. Bilateral subdural hematomas
B. Bifrontal contusions
C. Subarachnoid hemorrhage
D. Diffuse axonal injury

Correct answer: B

Explanation

The correct answer is (B) Bifrontal contusions. This young man suffered a backward fall with loss of consciousness and later presented with anosmia and ageusia, as well as a severe global headache. His neurological exam is otherwise normal, including normal fundoscopy, which argues against increased intracranial pressure or large hemorrhage. The key localizing clues are the loss of smell and taste, pointing toward injury to the olfactory pathway, most commonly affected in frontal lobe trauma. The olfactory nerves (CN I) originate in the nasal mucosa, traverse the cribriform plate, and synapse in the olfactory bulbs lying on the orbital surface of the frontal lobes. A posterior-directed fall, especially onto a hard surface (like a ship deck), can cause the brain to rebound forward (a coup-contrecoup mechanism), resulting in bifrontal contusions. These often involve the orbitofrontal cortex, where the olfactory bulbs and tracts are located, leading to anosmia. Option A (Bilateral subdural hematomas) typically presents with progressive mental status changes, not isolated anosmia. Option C (Subarachnoid hemorrhage) often causes sudden thunderclap headache, neck stiffness, or focal deficits; and anosmia is not a common feature of subarachnoid hemorrhage. Option D (Diffuse axonal injury) is more commonly associated with rotational trauma, often leading to coma or persistent deficits, and would not typically present with isolated anosmia or intact consciousness.

Reference

Proskynitopoulos PJ, Stippler M, Kasper EM. Post-traumatic anosmia in patients with mild traumatic brain injury (mTBI): A systematic and illustrated review. Surg Neurol Int. 2016;7(Suppl 10):S263–75. https://doi.org/10.4103/2152-7806.181981.

11. A 68-year-old male with history of uncontrolled hypertension, hyperlipidemia, and type 2 diabetes was initially admitted to the neuro critical care unit with a hypertensive cerebellar bleed. Given a good neurological exam and lack of hydrocephalus, he was successfully treated with medical management. The patient was then sent to the medical floor for hyperglycemia management. Neurology is consulted at this point for altered mental status.

    When speaking to the patient's primary team, they report that he is unable to engage with physical and occupational therapy. He is minimally verbal, but is able to feed himself, take a bath, and clean himself. Initially, it was thought that he was depressed in the setting of hemorrhagic stroke, so he was started on fluoxetine without improvement.

    Neurological exam is notable for minimal verbal output, cranial nerves are intact, strength is symmetric throughout, and reflexes are 2+ throughout. No dysmetria is noted. Decreased voluntary movements are noted throughout the evaluation.

    What is the most likely diagnosis and the next step in management?
    A. Depression, switch antidepressant
    B. Mutism, add bromocriptine
    C. Hydrocephalus, repeat head CT
    D. Ischemic infarct, CTA followed by MRI brain without contrast

Correct answer: B

Explanation

The correct answer is (B) Cerebellar mutism, add bromocriptine. This patient is exhibiting marked reduction in speech (mutism) and voluntary movement following a hypertensive cerebellar hemorrhage, with preserved strength, functional capacity (feeding, bathing), and cranial nerve function. These findings are classic for cerebellar mutism syndrome (CMS)—a condition well-described in children after posterior fossa tumor surgery, but also recognized in adults after cerebellar hemorrhage, infarct, surgery, or trauma. This syndrome is not due to depression, aphasia, or hydrocephalus and is often underrecognized in adult populations. Cerebellar mutism is thought to result

from disruption of cerebello-thalamo-cortical pathways, particularly involving the dentate nucleus, superior cerebellar peduncles, and their projections to the contralateral thalamus and supplementary motor area. The vermis, often injured in hemorrhages or resections, plays a key role in modulating affect and initiation of speech. This explains the apathy, akinesia, and mutism seen in these patients, despite preserved alertness and ability to perform basic motor tasks. Bromocriptine is a dopamine D2 receptor agonist, which stimulates dopamine receptors in the basal ganglia and frontal lobes. It is used in Parkinson's disease, hyperprolactinemia, and neuroleptic malignant syndrome, but also in post-stroke akinetic-mute states and cerebellar mutism syndrome, particularly when features suggest hypodopaminergic cortical activity (e.g., abulia, akinesia, and reduced initiation). In this patient, the use of bromocriptine aims to boost frontal-striatal-cerebellar circuitry, enhancing motivation, initiation of movement, and speech output, which are characteristically reduced in CMS. (A) Depression is unlikely; the patient has minimal verbal output but remains behaviorally engaged. (C) No clinical or radiological signs suggest hydrocephalus. (D) There's no evidence of a new ischemic event.

References

Amor-García M, Fernández-Llamazares CM, Manrique-Rodríguez S, Narrillos-Moraza Á, García-Morín M, Huerta-Aragonés J, et al. Bromocriptine for the treatment of postoperative cerebellar mutism syndrome in pediatric patients: Three case reports. J Oncol Pharm Pract. 2021;27(7):1753–7. https://doi.org/10.1177/1078155220982046.

Fabozzi F, Margoni S, Andreozzi B, Musci MS, Del Baldo G, Boccuto L, et al. Cerebellar mutism syndrome: From pathophysiology to rehabilitation. Front Cell Dev Biol. 2022;10:1082947. https://doi.org/10.3389/fcell.2022.1082947.

12. A 48-year-old right-handed female with no significant medical history presents to the emergency department (ED) with a 3-day history of recurrent brief episodes of retro-orbital pain. Occasionally, the pain is associated with right conjunctival injection and lacrimation. She averages 10–15 episodes per day, each episode lasting about 5 min in duration. The patient has no history of migraines or headaches. She denies any recent fevers, sick contacts, visual changes, new medications, or illicit drug use. Admission vitals are normal, and labs are unremarkable.

    Neurological exam is normal, fundoscopy and visual acuity are normal bilaterally. No tenderness at palpation of the temples. Head CT is unremarkable.

The patient must take a flight later today, what would be a reasonable next step in management?

A. Prescribe as needed acetaminophen, metoclopramide, and magnesium
B. Prescribe as needed sumatriptan 50 mg PO
C. Prescribe indomethacin 50 mg TID
D. Prescribe as needed subcutaneous sumatriptan 6 mg
E. Admit the patient for MRI/MRA of the brain with and without contrast

Correct answer: C

Explanation

The correct answer is (C) Prescribe indomethacin 50 mg. This patient presents with recurrent, brief episodes of severe retro-orbital pain, sometimes associated with conjunctival injection and lacrimation, and no prior headache history. These features are characteristic of a trigeminal autonomic cephalalgia (TAC), a group of primary headache disorders that includes cluster headache, paroxysmal hemicrania, hemicrania continua, short-lasting unilateral neuralgiform headache attacks with conjunctival injection and tearing (SUNCT), and short-lasting unilateral neuralgiform headaches with cranial autonomic symptoms (SUNA). Based on the short duration (~5 min), high frequency (10–15 times/day), and presence of autonomic symptoms, the most likely diagnosis is paroxysmal hemicrania. This TAC subtype is classically completely responsive to indomethacin, making a therapeutic trial of indomethacin both diagnostic and therapeutic. If the headache responds dramatically to indomethacin, the diagnosis is virtually confirmed. The dose can later be adjusted to the lowest effective dose for maintenance, and gastric protection (e.g., with a PPI) is often needed due to GI side effects. (A) Acetaminophen, metoclopramide, magnesium: Appropriate for migraine, not effective in TACs. This patient's headache features (short duration, autonomic signs) are not typical of migraine. (B/D) Sumatriptan (oral or SC): More useful in cluster headaches, but not typically effective in paroxysmal hemicrania, and SC triptans are not ideal for attacks of such short duration. (E) MRI/MRA: Would be recommended, but can be completed in a non-urgent fashion (e.g., at outpatient follow-up) given her normal neurological exam and unremarkable CT head, and does not need to delay initiating a diagnostic indomethacin trial.

References

Bahra A. Paroxysmal hemicrania and hemicrania continua: Review on pathophysiology, clinical features and treatment. Cephalalgia. 2023;43(11):3331024231214239. https://doi.org/10.1177/03331024231214239.

Burish M. Cluster Headache, SUNCT, and SUNA. Continuum (Minneap Minn). 2024;30(2):391–410. https://doi.org/10.1212/con.0000000000001411.

13. A 20-year-old male without significant medical history presents to the ED (emergency department) after a witnessed bilateral tonic–clonic seizure. The patient was in his usual state of health, when he suddenly became disoriented, sat down, and this was followed by bilateral tonic–clonic activity associated with foaming at the mouth and postictal confusion, which persisted approximately 45 min after the tonic–clonic movements had resolved. On admission, his vitals are normal. His labs are notable for mild leukocytosis $10.2 \times 10^3/\mu L$ (neutrophil-predominant—85%) and a mild lactic acidosis (3.6). Toxicology is negative. The patient mentioned a few months ago he woke up once in the morning with dried blood around his pillow and severe muscle pain. Sometimes in the mornings, he has severe tremors involving both hands and sometimes his feet, and he sometimes drops objects. There is no family history of epilepsy. To his knowledge, the patient has never had a seizure before.

Neurological exam is normal. There is no evidence of tongue bite. Deep tendon reflexes are 3+ throughout, bilateral Hoffmann's signs are present, and three beats of ankle clonus are noted bilaterally. Head CT is normal.

Based on the patient's age and history, which antiseizure medications would you avoid?

A. Zonisamide
B. Topiramate
C. Oxcarbazepine
D. Clobazam
E. Levetiracetam
F. Valproic acid

Correct answer: C

Explanation

The correct answer is (C) Oxcarbazepine. This young man likely has juvenile myoclonic epilepsy (JME), a genetic generalized epilepsy syndrome that typically presents in adolescents or young adults with early morning myoclonic jerks (as in his tremors and object dropping), tonic–clonic seizures, and sometimes absence seizures. His history of waking with dried blood on his pillow and muscle pain suggests unrecognized nocturnal generalized seizures, and the bilateral Hoffmann's signs and ankle clonus may reflect transient postictal hyperreflexia or a subtle sign of transient post-ictal cortical irritability. Oxcarbazepine (OXC), like carbamazepine (CBZ) and phenytoin (PHT), is a sodium channel blocker that is effective for focal seizures, but can exacerbate generalized epilepsy, especially JME. These medications can worsen myoclonus and increase the frequency of generalized seizures. This paradoxical worsening occurs because sodium channel blockers suppress focal discharges but may disinhibit thalamocortical pathways that are central to generalized epileptiform activity. (A) Zonisamide: Broad-spectrum antiseizure drug effective for both focal and generalized seizures. (B) Topiramate: Also broad-spectrum, effective in JME, though sometimes limited by cognitive side effects. (D) Clobazam: Benzodiazepine with efficacy in myoclonic and generalized seizures; often used as adjunctive therapy. (E) Levetiracetam: Broad-spectrum, well-tolerated, and commonly used in JME. (F) Valproic acid: is a first-line treatment for JME. Valproic acid is highly effective for all seizure types associated with the syndrome.

References

Fanella M, Egeo G, Fattouch J, Casciato S, Lapenta L, Morano A, et al. Oxcarbazepine-induced myoclonic status epilepticus in juvenile myoclonic epilepsy. Epileptic Disord. 2013;15(2):181–7. https://doi.org/10.1684/epd.2013.0563.

Wolf P, Yacubian EM, Avanzini G, Sander T, Schmitz B, Wandschneider B, et al. Juvenile myoclonic epilepsy: A system disorder of the brain. Epilepsy Res. 2015;114:2–12. https://doi.org/10.1016/j.eplepsyres.2015.04.008.

14. An 85-year-old female with history of hyperlipidemia presents to the emergency department (ED) with memory problems, which began suddenly 4 days prior to presentation. As per the patient's son, the patient is highly functional and takes care of her husband, but 4 days ago, she was in her usual state of health when she suddenly started repeating herself, seemed confused, and kept asking the same questions repeatedly. Her family reports she seems to be forgetful about where she left specific objects. The symptoms did not improve, and although she seemed able to function, her memory issues have persisted. Upon arrival, her vital signs are normal, lab workup is significant for mild leukocytosis with a white blood cell count of $11.2 \times 10^3/\mu L$.

On exam, she is awake, oriented to person and place only, and she is unable to tell you the current date, her date of birth, or who the current president is (all of which is unusual for her). She is able to name, read, and repeat. Occasional perseveration is noted. She is unable to name 0/3 words after 5 min. Cranial nerves are normal, no apraxia, no neglect, strength is symmetric throughout, and coordination is normal.

What is the most likely diagnosis?
A. Transient global amnesia
B. Thalamic amnesia
C. Transient epileptic amnesia.
D. New-onset dementia.
E. Cortical basal degeneration syndrome.
Correct answer: A

Explanation

The correct answer is (B) Thalamic amnesia. This patient presents with sudden-onset profound memory impairment without focal motor deficits or a fluctuating sensorium. The key features include acute anterograde amnesia, repetitive questioning, disorientation to time, and perseveration, all in the setting of preserved naming, reading, and repetition. These findings suggest disruption of memory circuits, particularly involving deep subcortical structures. The thalamus, specifically the anterior nucleus, plays a crucial role in episodic memory as part of the Papez circuit, which connects the hippocampus, mammillary bodies, anterior thalamic nuclei, and cingulate cortex. Lesions in this circuit, especially in the dominant thalamus, can result in a syndrome of anterograde amnesia, confusion, and perseveration, often mimicking limbic encephalitis or mesial temporal pathology. In older adults with vascular risk factors (like this patient with hyperlipidemia), small strokes involving the anterior or medial thalamus can produce acute isolated memory loss—also referred to as thalamic amnesia. Unlike hippocampal or cortical lesions, language and praxis are usually preserved. (A) Transient global amnesia (TGA): While also characterized by acute memory loss, TGA is typically short-lived (resolves within 24 h). This patient's symptoms have persisted for 4 days, which is incompatible with TGA. (C) Transient epileptic amnesia: Usually presents with brief (minutes to hours) episodes of amnesia, often recurring, and sometimes with other signs of seizures. This case lacks the stereotyped, brief, recurrent pattern associated with epileptic activity and has ongoing memory deficits, making transient epileptic amnesia less likely. (D) New-onset dementia: Dementia has a gradual onset and progressive course. This patient's sudden change from baseline is inconsistent with typical neurodegenerative dementia. (E) Corticobasal degeneration: A rare neurodegenerative condition presenting with asymmetric rigidity, apraxia, and cortical signs (e.g., alien limb, myoclonus). The absence of these signs rules it out.

References

Aggleton JP, O'Mara SM. The anterior thalamic nuclei: core components of a tripartite episodic memory system. Nat Rev. Neurosci. 2022;23(8):505–16. https://doi.org/10.1038/s41583-022-00591-8.

Grulich J, Lösken E, Müri RM. Unique amnestic syndrome after isolated left anterolateral thalamic stroke: a case report. BMC Neurol. 2025;25(1):76. https://doi.org/10.1186/s12883-025-04085-9.

15. An 82-year-old male with history of atrial fibrillation on rivaroxaban, depression, anxiety, hypertension, and end-stage renal disease presents to the ED with severe abnormal movements. Symptoms started the night prior to presentation. At onset, these movements were severe. He describes brief, severe loss of muscle tone in arms and legs. When he woke up this morning, he could not sit or stand, and he was unable to walk. He suffers from insomnia for which he was recently prescribed gabapentin 600 mg nightly by his primary care physician.

On admission, he is tachycardic (HR 112 BPM). Labs remarkable for BUN 38 mg/dL, and creatinine 6.1 mg/dL. Electrolytes are normal including calcium, magnesium, and sodium, and ammonia is within normal limits. Initial head CT is normal.

On exam, he appears slightly drowsy, but is otherwise oriented to person and place. Cranial nerves are unremarkable. Strength is symmetric in upper and lower extremities, although he demonstrates negative myoclonus in both upper extremities.

The patient started gabapentin around 6 days prior to presentation. He was initially prescribed 600 mg at night for insomnia but was taking up to 1200 mg per night. Gabapentin (GBP) toxicity diagnosis is made.

In a patient with end-stage renal disease, what is the maximum recommended gabapentin daily dose?

A. Gabapentin 600 mg daily
B. Gabapentin 100 mg daily
C. Gabapentin 300 mg daily
D. Gabapentin 200 mg daily
E. No restriction

Correct answer: C

Explanation

The correct answer is (C) Gabapentin 300 mg daily. This patient presents with gabapentin toxicity in the setting of end-stage renal disease (ESRD). He developed severe myoclonus and gait instability shortly after starting gabapentin at doses significantly above the recommended limit for patients with impaired renal clearance. Gabapentin is excreted entirely unchanged by the kidneys. When kidney function is impaired, gabapentin can reach supratherapeutic levels leading to neurotoxicity, and this may manifest with a range of movement disorders: tremors, myoclonus, ataxia, asterixis, and dyskinesias have been described.

Reference

Raouf M, Atkinson TJ, Crumb MW, Fudin J. Rational dosing of gabapentin and pregabalin in chronic kidney disease. J Pain Res. 2017;10:275–8. https://doi.org/10.2147/jpr. S130942.

Neuroimmunologic and Paraneoplastic CNS Disorders

16

Mirza Omari

1. Autoimmune encephalitis is strongly associated with which of the following:
   A. Cardiac arrhythmias
   B. Underlying tumors
   C. Vitamin deficiencies
   D. Bone fractures
   Correct answer: B

Explanation

Paraneoplastic syndromes occur when substances released by the tumor or an immune response to the cancer disrupt normal functioning of other tissues or organs. This process can lead to an auto-attack of the central nervous system.

Reference

Rosenfeld MR, Titulaer MJ, Dalmau J. Paraneoplastic syndromes and autoimmune encephalitis: Five new things. Neurol Clin Pract. 2012;2(3):215–23. https://doi.org/10.1212/CPJ.0b013e31826af23e.

2. What is most common type of autoimmune encephalitis?
   A. Anti-Leucine-rich glioma-inactivated 1 (LGI-1) limbic encephalitis
   B. Anti-N-methyl-D-aspartate (NMDA) receptor encephalitis
   C. Anti-γ-aminobutyric acid-A (GABA-A) receptor encephalitis
   D. Anti-contactin-associated protein-like 2 (CASPR2) encephalitis
   Correct answer: B

Explanation

Autoimmune causes of encephalitis have been reported to be at least as common as viral causes in Olmsted County, USA. Interestingly, the incidence of autoimmune encephalitis rose in the second 10-year epoch of this study, likely owing to growing awareness of these disorders and more widespread diagnostic capacities.

Reference

Dubey D, Pittock SJ, Kelly CR, McKeon A, Lopez-Chiriboga AS, Lennon VA, et al. Autoimmune encephalitis epidemiology and a comparison to infectious encephalitis. Ann Neurol. 2018;83(1):166–77. https://doi.org/10.1002/ana.25131.

3. Of the following, which category of individuals is most likely to be affected by anti-NMDA receptor encephalitis?
   A. Elderly men
   B. Middle-aged women
   C. Young women and children
   D. Infants under 1 year
   Correct answer: C

Explanation

The California Encephalitis Project found that among persons under 30 years of age, N-methyl-D-aspartate receptor (NMDAR)-antibody encephalitis was more common than any individual infectious cause of encephalitis.

Reference

Gable MS, Sheriff H, Dalmau J, Tilley DH, Glaser CA. The frequency of autoimmune N-methyl-D-aspartate receptor encephalitis surpasses that of individual viral etiologies in young individuals enrolled in the California Encephalitis Project. Clin Infect Dis. 2012;54(7):899–904. https://doi.org/10.1093/cid/cir1038.

M. Omari (✉)
Department of Neurology, New York University Grossman School of Medicine, New York, NY, USA
e-mail: mirza.omari@nyulangone.org

4. The most reliable diagnostic test for NMDA encephalitis requires:
   A. Serum antibody testing alone
   B. Cerebrospinal fluid (CSF) antibody testing
   C. Brain biopsy
   D. Blood glucose levels
   Correct answer: B

Explanation

NMDAR antibodies are consistently detected in the CSF of patients and said to be absent in ~20% of serum samples, even though the immunological response likely begins in the periphery, perhaps most clearly in patients with ovarian teratomas. In addition, serum NMDAR antibodies occur at ~3% of healthy individuals; therefore, antibodies in the CSF will lend supportive, and more specific, evidence of a pathologic process.

Reference

Graus F, Titulaer MJ, Balu R, Benseler S, Bien CG, Cellucci T, et al. A clinical approach to diagnosis of autoimmune encephalitis. Lancet Neurol. 2016;15(4):391–404. https://doi.org/10.1016/s1474-4422(15)00401-9.

5. Which tumor is most commonly associated with NMDA encephalitis?
   A. Lung carcinoma
   B. Ovarian teratoma
   C. Breast carcinoma
   D. Testicular seminoma
   Correct answer: B

Explanation

The frequency of tumor presence varies with age and sex. In NMDAR-encephalitis, ~40% of all cases were found to have cancer with female patients accounting for ~90% of cases. 95% of the tumors detected were ovarian teratomas. Therefore, it is recommended that all female patients be screened with a pelvic ultrasound, transvaginal ultrasound, and/or abdominal-pelvic MRI/CT.

Reference

Nguyen L, Wang C. Anti-NMDA Receptor Autoimmune Encephalitis: Diagnosis and Management Strategies. Int J Gen Med. 2023;16:7–21. https://doi.org/10.2147/ijgm.S397429.

6. First-line immunotherapy typically includes:
   A. Chemotherapy and radiation
   B. IV immunoglobulin (IVIg) and steroids
   C. Antiviral medications
   D. Insulin therapy
   Correct answer: B

Explanation

About 75% of patients recover to baseline of have mild residual symptoms, but unfortunately, the rest can sustain significant disability, and the disease can even cause death. Initial management should focus in treating with corticosteroids and/or intravenous immunoglobulins (IVIg) or plasma exchange while in parallel looking for and removing the teratoma.

Reference

Dalmau J, Lancaster E, Martinez-Hernandez E, Rosenfeld MR, Balice-Gordon R. Clinical experience and laboratory investigations in patients with anti-NMDAR encephalitis. Lancet Neurol. 2011;10(1):63–74. https://doi.org/10.1016/s1474-4422(10)70253-2.

7. A characteristic EEG finding in severe NMDA encephalitis is:
   A. Extreme delta brush pattern
   B. Spike-and-wave discharges
   C. Normal EEG
   D. Bifrontal epileptiform discharges
   Correct answer: A

Explanation

The 2016 diagnostic criteria for probable NMDAR-encephalitis includes:

1. Rapid onset (less than 3 months) of at least four of six major groups of clinical symptoms including: abnormal psychiatric, behavior or cognitive dysfunction; dyskinesias, or rigidity/abnormal postures; decreased level of consciousness; and autonomic dysfunction or central hypoventilation.
2. Abnormal EEG (focal or diffuse slow or disorganized activity, epileptic activity, or extreme delta brush) or CSF pleocytosis/oligoclonal bands.
3. Exclusion of other diagnoses.

"Extreme delta brush" indicates rhythmic delta activity at 1–3 Hz with bursts of rhythmic beta activity superimposed onto each delta wave. Though rarely present, it is suggested to be specific to NMDAR-encephalitis.

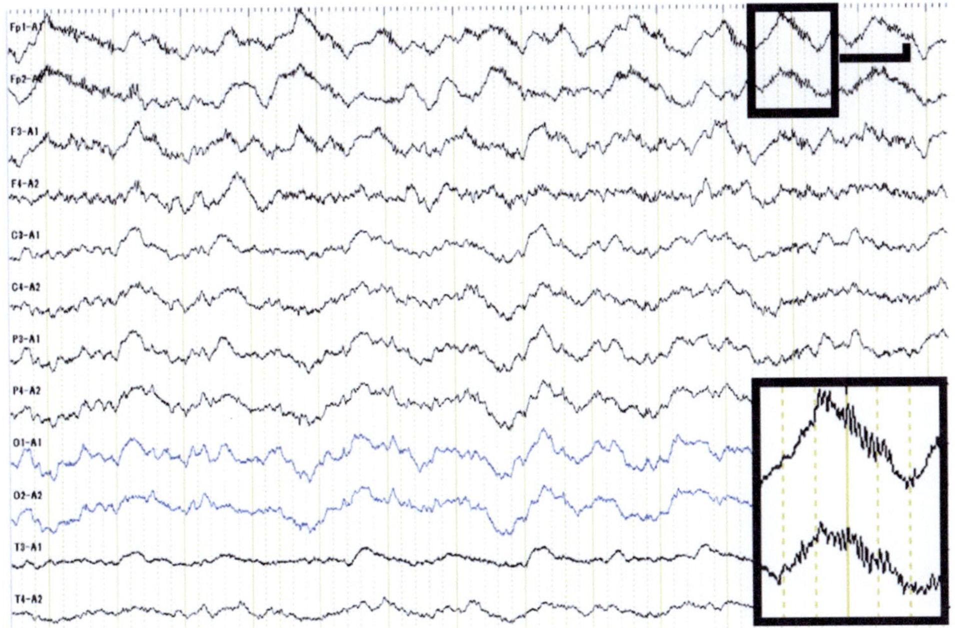

EEG demonstrating extreme delta brush pattern. (Source: Mizoguchi, T., Hara, M., Hirose, S., Nakajima, H. CC-BY 4.0 (https://creativecommons.org/licenses/by/4.0/) via *Frontiers in Immunology*. Image has been cropped from source. Mizoguchi T, Hara M, Hirose S, Nakajima H. Novel qEEG Biomarker to Distinguish Anti-NMDAR Encephalitis From Other Types of Autoimmune Encephalitis. Front Immunol. 2022;13:845272. https://doi.org/10.3389/fimmu.2022.845272)

References

Mizoguchi T, Hara M, Hirose S, Nakajima H. Novel qEEG Biomarker to Distinguish Anti-NMDAR Encephalitis From Other Types of Autoimmune Encephalitis. Front Immunol. 2022;13:845272. https://doi.org/10.3389/fimmu.2022.845272.

Nguyen L, Wang C. Anti-NMDA Receptor Autoimmune Encephalitis: Diagnosis and Management Strategies. Int J Gen Med. 2023;16:7–21. https://doi.org/10.2147/IJGM.S397429

8. Which of the following symptoms is *least* likely in early-stage NMDA encephalitis?
   A. Psychosis
   B. Seizures
   C. Hyperglycemia
   D. Movement disorders
   Correct answer: C

Explanation

All except hyperglycemia can be clinical clued of early stages of NMDAR-encephalitis. New-onset psychosis, dystonia/chorea/rigidity, seizures, and/or status epilepticus can all be seen; however, no systemic effects on glucose levels have been described.

Reference

Lancaster E. The Diagnosis and Treatment of Autoimmune Encephalitis. J Clin Neurol. 2016;12(1):1–13. https://doi.org/10.3988/jcn.2016.12.1.1.

9. Autonomic dysfunction in NMDA encephalitis may manifest as which of the following?
   A. Labile blood pressure
   B. Improved coordination
   C. Weight gain
   D. Hyperactive reflexes
   Correct answer: A

Explanation

Dysautonomia is a common feature of this disorder. Symptoms typically progress through the initial disease course and can even be life-threatening. Particularly in NMDAR-encephalitis, we can see wide fluctuations in blood pressure with tachyarrhythmias and bradyarrhythmias, which prompt collaboration with cardiology. There are cases when pacing is necessary. Other dysautonomic features include orthostatic hypotension, constipation, and abnormal sudomotor function.

Reference

Uy CE, Binks S, Irani SR. Autoimmune encephalitis: clinical spectrum and management. Pract Neurol. 2021;21(5):412–23. https://doi.org/10.1136/practneurol-2020-002567.

10. Which of the following has been identified as a potential trigger of NMDA-encephalitis?
    A. Herpes simplex virus (HSV) encephalitis
    B. Influenza vaccination
    C. Migraine headaches
    D. Diabetes mellitus
    E. Cryptococcal meningitis
    Correct answer: A

Explanation

20–30% of patients with HSV encephalitis go on to develop NMDAR-encephalitis weeks to months after the infectious encephalitis. These tend to have a poorer functional status.

Reference

Dumez P, Villagrán-García M, Bani-Sadr A, Benaiteau M, Peter E, Farina A, et al. Specific clinical and radiological characteristics of anti-NMDA receptor autoimmune encephalitis following herpes encephalitis. J Neurol. 2024;271(10):6692–701. https://doi.org/10.1007/s00415-024-12615-7.

11. LGI-1 limbic encephalitis most commonly presents with:
    A. Sleep disturbances and nerve pain
    B. Memory loss and seizures
    C. Psychosis and facial movements
    D. Movement disorders in children
    Correct answer: B

Explanation

Patients who have involvement of the limbic structures, such as in LGI-1 antibody encephalitis, often experience a dense amnesia affecting anterograde memory and loss of retrograde autobiographical details. In addition, seizures are also common and often trigger neurological attention as disorientation can initially be perceived as delirium.

Reference

Uy CE, Binks S, Irani SR. Autoimmune encephalitis: clinical spectrum and management. Pract Neurol. 2021;21(5):412–23. https://doi.org/10.1136/practneurol-2020-002567.

12. Which of the following symptoms would favor a diagnosis of LGI-1 antibody encephalitis?
    A. Visual loss
    B. Faciobrachial dystonic seizures
    C. Ataxia
    D. Hemiplegia
    Correct answer: B

Explanation

Faciobrachial dystonic seizures are frequent, brief events with posturing of the ipsilateral face and arm that often occur hundreds of times per day. The leg may also be involved, and the sudden leg spasms can precipitate falls. Less often, patients can have piloerection seizures, which are experienced as paroxysmal dizzy spells, again short-lived and frequent. These seizures have been associated with LGI-1 encephalitis.

Reference

Uy CE, Binks S, Irani SR. Autoimmune encephalitis: clinical spectrum and management. Pract Neurol. 2021;21(5):412–23. https://doi.org/10.1136/practneurol-2020-002567.

13. Which electrolyte abnormality is frequently seen in LGI-1 antibody encephalitis?
    A. Hyperkalemia
    B. Hyponatremia
    C. Hypercalcemia
    D. Hypokalemia
    Correct answer: B

Explanation

Patients with LGI-1 encephalitis may have intractable hyponatremia. It is thought that this is caused by improper secretion of ADH and simultaneous LGI-1 expression in the hypothalamus and kidney.

Reference

Wang M, Cao X, Liu Q, Ma W, Guo X, Liu X. Clinical features of limbic encephalitis with LGI1 antibody. Neuropsychiatr Dis Treat. 2017;13:1589–96. https://doi.org/10.2147/ndt.S136723.

14. LGI-1 antibody encephalitis most commonly affects which age and sex group?
    A. Young women
    B. Men over 60
    C. Children under 10
    D. Adolescent girls
    Correct answer: B

Explanation

Men over 60 are at highest risk for LGI-1 encephalitis. In women, it tends to occur at an average age of 45.

Reference

Wang M, Cao X, Liu Q, Ma W, Guo X, Liu X. Clinical features of limbic encephalitis with LGI1 antibody. Neuropsychiatr Dis Treat. 2017;13:1589–96. https://doi.org/10.2147/ndt.S136723.

15. Which brain region is most often affected on MRI in LGI-1 antibody encephalitis?
    A. Frontal cortex
    B. Occipital lobe
    C. Hippocampus/mediotemporal lobe
    D. Cerebellum

Correct answer: C

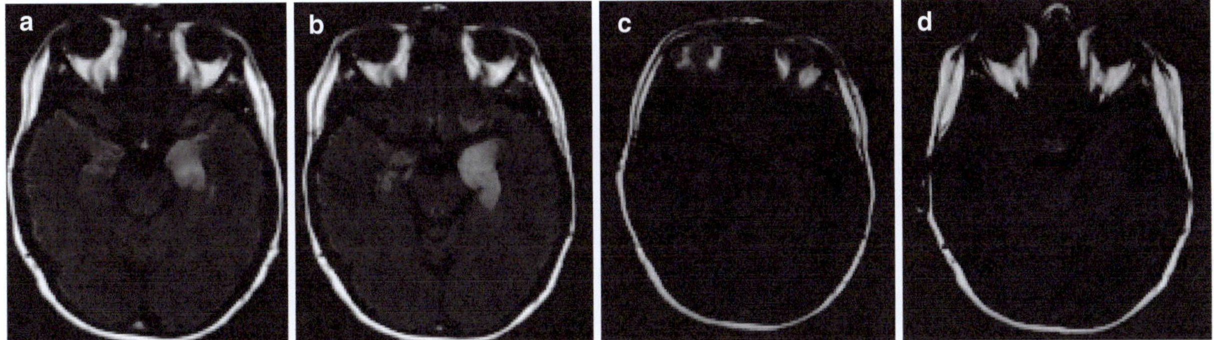

Axial MRI brain sections. The images demonstrate the evolution of T2-hyperintense signal enlarging (**a**. 7 days after admission; **b**. 1 month after discharge) and shrinking (**c**. 1 month after discharge; **d**. 4 months after discharge) over the course of the disease. (Source: McGinley, M., Morals-Vidal, S., Ruland, S. CC-BY 4.0 (https://creativecommons.org/licenses/by/4.0/) via *Frontiers in Neurology*. Image has not been modified from source. McGinley M, Morales-Vidal S, Ruland S. Leucine-Rich Glioma Inactivated-1 and Voltage-Gated Potassium Channel Autoimmune Encephalitis Associated with Ischemic Stroke: A Case Report. Front Neurol. 2016;7:68. https://doi.org/10.3389/fneur.2016.00068)

Explanation

Patients with LGI-1 antibody encephalitis tend to have involvement of bilateral temporal lobes and can demonstrate abnormal signal on MRI in the hippocampus regions. The basal ganglia is often involved. Without any immunotherapy, hippocampus atrophy can develop.

References

McGinley M, Morales-Vidal S, Ruland S. Leucine-Rich Glioma Inactivated-1 and Voltage-Gated Potassium Channel Autoimmune Encephalitis Associated with Ischemic Stroke: A Case Report. Front Neurol. 2016;7:68. https://doi.org/10.3389/fneur.2016.00068.

Wang M, Cao X, Liu Q, Ma W, Guo X, Liu X. Clinical features of limbic encephalitis with LGI1 antibody. Neuropsychiatr Dis Treat. 2017;13:1589–96. https://doi.org/10.2147/ndt.S136723.

16. Which of the following is a common psychiatric manifestation in LGI-1 antibody encephalitis?
    A. Mania
    B. Paranoia, hallucinations, or depression
    C. Obsessive-compulsive disorder
    D. Catatonia

Correct answer: B

Explanation

The emergence of a new psychotic disorder, especially in older patients, warrants workup for autoimmune encephalitis. Involvement of the limbic system can precipitate personality and behavioral changes.

Reference

Wang M, Cao X, Liu Q, Ma W, Guo X, Liu X. Clinical features of limbic encephalitis with LGI1 antibody. Neuropsychiatr Dis Treat. 2017;13:1589–96. https://doi.org/10.2147/ndt.S136723.

17–26. Match the following antibodies with the neoplasm (A–H) with which they are associated:

17. NMDA Receptor
18. ANNA-1 (Hu)
19. ANNA-2 (Ri)
20. CASPR2
21. Ma2
22. Purkinje cell antibody (PCA-1, Yo)
23. Anti-voltage-gaged calcium channel (P/Q type)
24. SOX1
25. Amphiphysin
26. CRMP5
  A. Meningioma
  B. Breast cancer
  C. Small cell lung cancer
  D. Ovarian teratoma
  E. Malignant thymoma
  F. Testicular germinoma
  G. Lymphoma

H. Ovarian cancer

Correct answers (17–26):

17. D
18. C
19. D
20. E
21. F
22. H
23. C
24. C
25. B
26. C

Explanations for Questions 17–26

Although not exclusively, these antibodies are typically associated with the following neoplasms and clinical syndromes.

Question	Antibody	Clinical syndrome	Associated neoplasm
17	NMDA Receptor	Encephalitis (often with a psychiatric prodrome)	Ovarian teratoma
18	ANNA-1 (Hu)	Limbic encephalitis	Small-cell lung cancer
19	ANNA-2 (Ri)	Opsoclonus myoclonus syndrome	Breast adenocarcinoma
20	CASPR2	Morvan's syndrome	Malignant thymoma (higher risk when associated with Morvan's syndrome)
21	Ma2	Limbic encephalitis, narcolepsy/cataplexy	Testicular germinoma
22	Purkinje Cell Antibody (PCA-1, Yo)	Cerebellar ataxia	Ovarian cancer
23	Voltage-gated Calcium Channel (P/Q type)	Lambert Eaton myasthenic syndrome	Small-cell lung cancer
24	SOX1	Lambert Eaton myasthenic syndrome	Small-cell lung cancer
25	Amphiphysin	Stiff person syndrome, axonal neuropathy	Breast cancer, small-cell lung cancer
26	CRMP5	Limbic encephalitis	Small-cell lung cancer

Reference for Questions 17–26

Gilligan M, McGuigan C, McKeon A. Paraneoplastic Neurologic Disorders. Curr Neurol Neurosci Rep. 2023;23(3):67–82. https://doi.org/10.1007/s11910-023-01250-w.

Headache Disorders

17

Nisha Malhotra and Sarah Bobker

Linked questions: 1–2

1. During his summer camp's soccer match, a 7-year-old boy begins to tire. Within 20 min, he can no longer muster the energy to keep running. He begins holding the left side of his head and struggles to track the ball. He starts vomiting and is taken off the field. He has a hard time describing his symptoms to his coach, but, when asked, is able to at least convey that he has never experienced this before. What is the most likely diagnosis?
   A. Tension-type headache
   B. Thunderclap headache
   C. Headache attributed to intracranial astrocytoma
   D. Migraine headache
   Correct answer: D

Explanation

The vignette describes a boy with a gradually progressive and debilitating probable headache, associated with light sensitivity, vomiting, and fatigue on a hot summer day. The most common age of presentation for migraine in boys is best estimated to be 7 years. Children have a limited ability to describe their symptoms, especially when they are new; often just observing changes in the child's behavior or asking them to draw how they feel can be helpful in making a diagnosis.

Tension-type headache is featureless and, hence, would not have accompanying photophobia, vomiting, or disability.

Thunderclap headache, although also potentially disabling and, at times, associated with vomiting or light sensitivity, would reach maximum intensity within *seconds*.

Intracranial astrocytomas, though the most common primary brain tumor in boys and may present with headache, are less common than migraine.

N. Malhotra · S. Bobker (✉)
Department of Neurology, New York University Grossman School of Medicine, New York, NY, USA
e-mail: nisha.malhotra@nyulangone.org;
sarah.bobker@nyulangone.org

References
Raieli V, D'Amico A, Piro E. Migraine in Children Under 7 Years of Age: a Review. Curr Pain Headache Rep. 2020;24(12):79. https://doi.org/10.1007/s11916-020-00912-5.
Szperka C. Headache in Children and Adolescents. Continuum (Minneap Minn). 2021;27(3):703–31. https://doi.org/10.1212/con.0000000000000993.

Linked question

2. The boy in the prior question is taken to a local emergency room given his disability and limited ability to articulate symptoms. In the emergency department, an MRI of the brain is performed. What are the findings you expect to see that would be further supportive of this diagnosis?
   A. Pachymeningeal enhancement
   B. Benign arachnoid cyst
   C. Pilocytic astrocytoma
   D. Subarachnoid hemorrhage
   Correct answer: B

Explanation

Migraine does not lead to any specific findings on brain MRI, so we expect this boy's imaging to be normal. Incidental findings are always possible and must be kept in mind. In this case, an incidental and benign arachnoid cyst is the best answer choice. Not all patients with a first-time migraine require brain imaging. Clinical judgment should be used when deciding whether or not to pursue this.

It is worth noting that persons with migraine are more likely to have nonspecific white matter hyperintensities (WMHs) on MRI imaging than persons without migraine. Although there is this well-described association, the exact relationship between WMHs and migraine is still under research investigation. WMHs are generally less common in children and increase with age.

The other answers offer a secondary, rather than primary, headache etiology. Pachymeningeal enhancement may be seen in inflammatory, infectious, neoplastic, and/or intracranial pressure disorders (specifically cerebrospinal fluid [CSF] leak or spontaneous intracranial hypotension [SIH]).

Pilocytic astrocytoma is the most common brain tumor in children, affecting an estimated 1 in 100,000 children before the age of 20.

Subarachnoid hemorrhage is not common in children. The most common causes are by trauma or ruptured cerebral aneurysm, and studies show that women have a slightly higher lifetime risk than men.

Reference

Zhang W, Cheng Z, Fu F, Zhan Z. Prevalence and clinical characteristics of white matter hyperintensities in Migraine: A meta-analysis. Neuroimage Clin. 2023;37:103312. https://doi.org/10.1016/j.nicl.2023.103312.

3. A 32-year-old woman is 8-weeks pregnant and experiencing an increased frequency of headaches. She endorses a preexisting history of migraine, typically associated with menstrual cycle, occurring about 1 time per month since menarche at baseline. These have historically responded to ibuprofen, but this is her first pregnancy, and she has been reluctant to treat with anything for fear of potential harm to the baby. She is now having 3 headache days per week. Of the following *acute treatment* options, which is "the safest" to offer her a trial of at this time:
   A. Around-the-clock naratriptan
   B. Occipital nerve blocks
   C. Ibuprofen
   D. Ubrogepant
   Correct answer: B

Explanation

Migraine can worsen in pregnancy, particularly in the first trimester when hormonal swings are the most significant. In general, there are no "100% safe" treatments in pregnancy due to a lack of research in this area, but relative safety of occipital nerve blocks has been well-described and is widely used among headache providers. Another favorable option for acute migraine treatment in pregnancy, but not listed here, are the market-available neuromodulation devices.

While historically triptans have been discouraged from use during pregnancy due to limited data, anecdotal evidence over now many years has shown that sumatriptan may be the safest of the seven triptans to use, as no additional risk of birth defects have been found with its use when compared with birth defect incidence in the general population.

The use of NSAIDs, like ibuprofen, is probably low risk with limited use, but use should be discouraged. Studies show that there may be a small to moderate association between NSAIDs and the risk of anophthalmia/microphthalmia, amniotic bands/limb body wall defects, pulmonary valve stenosis, oral clefts, and neural tube defects.

Ubrogepant is a newer, Gepant (anti-calcitonin gene-related peptide [CGRP]) class medication without enough time on the market or any specific safety studies in pregnancy to consider use in pregnant individuals at the time of publication.

References

Bushman ET, Blanchard CT, Cozzi GD, Davis AM, Harper L, Robbins LS, et al. Occipital Nerve Block Compared With Acetaminophen and Caffeine for Headache Treatment in Pregnancy: A Randomized Controlled Trial. Obstet Gynecol. 2023;142(5):1179–88. https://doi.org/10.1097/aog.0000000000005386.

Parikh SK, Delbono MV, Silberstein SD. Managing migraine in pregnancy and breastfeeding. Prog Brain Res. 2020;255:275–309. https://doi.org/10.1016/bs.pbr.2020.07.011.

4. A 24-year-old woman with anxiety (well-controlled with venlafaxine 75 mg daily) and epilepsy (well-controlled with topiramate 50 mg nightly) is experiencing a gradual increase in headache frequency. Her headaches are associated with sensitivities to light, sound, and motion, as well as nausea. She has had to take 3 days off work already just this month due to her symptoms. What is the best next step in a *preventive treatment* plan from the below options?
   A. Switch venlafaxine to duloxetine
   B. Add gabapentin 300 mg nightly
   C. Add galcanezumab
   D. Switch topiramate to valproic acid
   Correct answer: C

Explanation

All of the above plans are acceptable to consider. Duloxetine, gabapentin, and valproic acid all have evidence in migraine prevention. However, given that her comorbid conditions are well-controlled at this time, it is probably best not to alter those treatments, making the addition of galcanezumab the best next step.

Galcanezumab is a newer anti-calcitonin gene-related (CGRP) monoclonal antibody (mAb) treatment. It is targeted to (at least part of) migraine pathophysiology as we understand it today, by blocking CGRP, an inflammatory central nervous system (CNS) protein known to be elevated in migraine. This treatment has no significant drug interactions and very few side effects. The most common adverse effect is topical injection site reactions.

5. A 40-year-old man with episodic migraine with typical visual aura presents to your clinic reporting that his headaches have not been responsive to any previously tried abortive treatments. These include: sumatriptan, naratriptan, and multiple available over-the-counter medications (e.g., naproxen, ibuprofen, and acetaminophen). He asks if there is anything *new* he can try next time he has a breakthrough headache. You choose to prescribe him:
   A. Rizatriptan
   B. Butalbital-acetaminophen-caffeine
   C. Ubrogepant
   D. Metoclopramide
   Correct answer: C

Explanation

Although all of the above options are reasonable acute migraine treatments to consider as they have yet to be tried in this patient, the newest treatment listed is ubrogepant. Ubrogepant is a Gepant class medication, which blocks calcitonin gene-related peptide (CGRP). At the time of publication, there are also two other abortive Gepant class medications in use: rimegepant and zavegepant. Another newer abortive migraine treatment, but not listed here, is lasmiditan, a Ditan class treatment, which binds to and activates the 5-HT1F receptor subtype.

Rizatriptan may be effective for this patient, but the previous failure of sumatriptan and naratriptan makes this choice less favorable for this particular patient.

Butalbital-acetaminophen-caffeine is another effective abortive medication for many patients; however, it is a controlled substance due to its mild-moderate abuse potential and carries the potential to cause "rebound" (or medication overuse) headache.

Metoclopramide is primarily an anti-emetic that blocks dopamine D2 receptors in the chemoreceptor trigger zone (CTZ) in the brainstem to mitigate nausea and vomiting. Metoclopramide does, notably, also have an analgesic benefit for some patients, believed to be due to suppression of pain signals transmitted through this area. However, this analgesic effect is variable, and further, metoclopramide is not a "new" migraine treatment option.

6. A 28-year-old woman presents to your clinic reporting migrainous symptoms on 15 or more days per month for the last 5 years despite several treatment trials. Thus far, she has tried and been failed by nortriptyline, atenolol, and topiramate, as she was not able to tolerate the side effects of these medications. At this point, what is the best next step in a *preventive treatment* plan from the below options to offer her?
   A. OnabotulinumtoxinA
   B. Gabapentin

C. Venlafaxine
D. Valproic acid
Correct answer: A

Explanation

OnabotulinumtoxinA, administered via the PREEMPT Protocol, has been approved by the Food and Drug Administration (FDA) for the treatment of chronic migraine since 2010. It is a 31-site anatomic injection protocol administered every 3 months. This patient meets the criteria for chronic migraine based on the presence of 15 or more headache days per month for at least 3 months. OnabotulinumtoxinA binds locally to nerves and blocks the neuromuscular junction. In chronic migraine treatment, it acts predominantly by inhibiting *sensory, rather than motor*, mechanisms.

Although gabapentin, venlafaxine, and valproic acid may also be effective preventive treatments in chronic migraine, they carry a greater risk of side effects, and this particular patient has exhibited previous sensitivities to other medication trials.

To note, the newer anti-calcitonin gene-related peptide (CGRP) monoclonal antibodies (mAbs) or Gepants may also be potential options for this patient, but they are not listed here. While both anti-CGRP treatments and onabotulinumtoxinA are effective, safe, and typically well-tolerated, onabotulinumtoxinA has been studied for a longer period of time, has fewer systemic side effects, is more cost-efficient, and is easier to use and maintain adherence.

References

Burstein R, Blumenfeld AM, Silberstein SD, Manack Adams A, Brin MF. Mechanism of Action of OnabotulinumtoxinA in Chronic Migraine: A Narrative Review. Headache. 2020;60(7):1259–72. https://doi.org/10.1111/head.13849.

Pallapothu MR, Quintana Mariñez MG, Chakkera M, Ravi N, Ramaraju R, Vats A, et al. Long-Term Management of Migraine With OnabotulinumtoxinA (Botox) vs Calcitonin Gene-Related Peptide Antibodies (Anti-CGRP). Cureus. 2023;15(10):e46696. https://doi.org/10.7759/cureus.46696.

7. Of the following preventive treatments, which has the "most specific" pathophysiology to treating migraine as we know of it at this time?
   A. Topiramate
   B. Amitriptyline
   C. Propranolol
   D. Fremanezumab
   Correct answer: D

Explanation

Fremanezumab is a calcitonin gene-related peptide (CGRP) monoclonal antibody (mAb). CGRP mAbs specifically target CGRP, an inflammatory neuropeptide associated with migraine. CGRP studies over recent years have led to major insights into the pathophysiology of migraine. CGRP is released from nerve endings in the trigeminal system during migraine attacks and plays a role in neuronal central sensitization leading to pain and other migraine symptoms.

The other treatments listed also have demonstrated evidence for migraine prevention, although their exact mechanisms of effect are not fully understood. Topiramate is primarily an antiepileptic drug (AED); it is believed to "calm" hyperexcitable neurons, affecting GABA and glutamate.

Amitriptyline is a tricyclic antidepressant (TCA) and probably works by inhibiting the uptake of various neurotransmitters, particularly serotonin and norepinephrine.

Propranolol is primarily a heart rate medication (a beta blocker [BB]); its mechanism may be vascular or by neurotransmitter mediation, among other theories.

Linked questions: 8–9

8. A 30-year-old woman with chronic migraine has improved to an episodic headache pattern with monthly erenumab injections. She presents to your clinic for follow-up and mentions that she and her partner are actively family planning. You tell her that erenumab is not known to be safe in pregnancy and must be stopped well in advance of conception. She agrees to stop erenumab and will wait to try to conceive for 6 months, at your advice. She asks you what she might more safely be able to take in the meantime, anticipating her headaches will return to a chronic pattern quickly. Which of the following is the best next *preventive treatment* option for this patient?
   A. Valproic acid
   B. Atogepant
   C. Topiramate
   D. Amitriptyline
   Correct answer: B

Explanation

Erenumab is a calcitonin gene-related peptide (CGRP) monoclonal antibody (mAb), which is not known to be safe in pregnancy at the time of publication. Given these drugs are newer to the market, there is a lack of adequate anecdotal (population) data to consider them. There are also no prospective safety studies, as is typically the case for treatments in pregnancy overall. These antibodies have a long half-life (~28 days) and can stay in the body for an extended period even after discontinuation of use, especially when used for several consecutive months. A 5–6-month "wash out" period is currently advised prior to conception.

Atogepant is a newer Gepant class medication. The Gepants also block CGRP, but are orally delivered and have a much shorter half-life (~11 h). It would be reasonable to trial this patient on atogepant during her "wash out" period, as it will hopefully give her some coverage during these months. Given this is also a newer and understudied drug, it should also be discontinued before intended conception; however, ~7–10 days prior is probably reasonable given the shorter half-life.

Valproic acid and topiramate should be avoided at all costs in pregnancy given their potential to contribute to major birth defects and fetal developmental problems.

Amitriptyline is felt to probably be safe in pregnancy; however, it is not the best next step here, as the patient's profound response to anti-CGRP therapy with erenumab can be used (somewhat) as a predictor for possible atogepant response.

Linked question

9. The patient from the prior question returns to see you 6 months later. She reports she has found the above medication choice to be a reasonable alternative to erenumab and is only having 1–2 headache days per month. She wishes to start trying to conceive now. What should you tell her to do next?
   A. Continue the treatment until she receives a positive pregnancy test
   B. Get the "OK" from her Ob/Gyn to continue the treatment
   C. Stop the treatment
   D. Switch to another preventive treatment that is 100% safe in pregnancy
   Correct answer: C

Explanation

Atogepant is a newer drug without enough evidence to support continuing use in pregnancy at the time of publication. She should stop the treatment now, in advance of a positive pregnancy test.

It is often advisable to work alongside an Ob/Gyn or Maternal Fetal Medicine (MFM) specialists when determining which medications to continue during pregnancy, but atogepant lacks any evidence in pregnancy to consider at all.

It is important to note that there are no "100% safe" treatments in pregnancy, due to a lack of well-designed prospective safety trials in this patient population.

10. A 58-year-old man with a history of episodic migraine since youth is referred to you by his cardiologist. The patient recently underwent cardiac stenting for unstable angina and has been adherent with the recommended dual anti-platelet therapy. Which statement best reflects the potential use of lasmiditan as an abortive therapy for this patient?

A. Lasmiditan is contraindicated in patients with vascular disease due to its vasoconstrictive effects

B. Lasmiditan may be considered in patients with vascular disease because it does not cause vasoconstriction and has a similar safety profile in patients with and without vascular risk factors

C. Lasmiditan requires concurrent use of triptans for efficacy

D. Lasmiditan should only be used in patients with vascular disease if there are no other abortive treatment options for the patient, and a complete risk/benefit discussion is had

Correct answer: B

Explanation

Lasmiditan is a newer Ditan class medication, which selectively targets the 5-HT1F receptors on trigeminal neurons. It does not activate 5-HT1B/1D receptors as the triptans do; thus, it avoids vasoconstriction. Pooled trial data support the use of lasmiditan in patients with vascular risk factors with no increased risk of serious vascular events.

Triptans are *contraindicated* in patients with vascular disease due to activation of 5-HT1B/1D receptors leading to vasoconstrictive effects.

Lasmiditan should be used *instead of* triptans in patients with vascular risk.

Lasmiditan use is supported in patients with vascular disease.

References

Krege JH, Lipton RB, Baygani SK, Komori M, Ryan SM, Vincent M. Lasmiditan for Patients with Migraine and Contraindications to Triptans: A Post Hoc Analysis. Pain Ther. 2022;11(2):701–12. https://doi.org/10.1007/s40122-022-00388-8.

Shapiro RE, Hochstetler HM, Dennehy EB, Khanna R, Doty EG, Berg PH, et al. Lasmiditan for acute treatment of migraine in patients with cardiovascular risk factors: posthoc analysis of pooled results from 2 randomized, double-blind, placebo-controlled, phase 3 trials. J Headache Pain. 2019;20(1):90. https://doi.org/10.1186/s10194-019-1044-6.

Linked questions: 11–13

11. A college student is experiencing headaches during her finals week. She is pre-med and has, admittedly, been sacrificing sleep for more time studying in the library. The headaches are bilateral and squeezing. She says they are more "annoying" than anything else. She is still able to go on runs, do her schoolwork, and maintain a social life, but she wonders what is going on with her. The most likely diagnosis is:

A. Migraine
B. Hemicrania continua
C. New daily persistent headache
D. Tension-type headache

Correct answer: D

Explanation

Tension-type headache (TTH) is defined by the International Classification of Headache Disorders-3 (ICHD-3) as a prolonged (hours to days, or unremitting), mild or moderate, often bilateral, and tightening headache. It is featureless; hence, it is not accompanied by other symptoms. It is oftentimes triggered by stress, poor posture, eye strain, and/or sleep disturbances, which is implied in this patient's lifestyle during finals.

Migraine must be accompanied by either photo–/phonophobia or nausea/vomiting and is often disabling. A migraine diagnosis can be made with relative certainty by utilizing the acronym "PIN" (think, "PIN the diagnosis") based on the ID Migraine Screener assessing *"Photo/phono-sensitivity," "Inability to function,"* and *"Nausea."*

Hemicrania continua (HC) is a trigeminal autonomic cephalalgia (TAC) and would, therefore by definition, be 100% unilateral and associated with ipsilateral cranial autonomic symptoms.

New daily persistent headache (NDPH) is a persistent headache that begins with a clearly remembered onset and becomes continuous and unremitting within 24 h. Although it may be featureless, mimicking tension headache, this prompt does not suggest a date/moment of clear onset and, thus, NDPH is not the appropriate answer. NDPH may also be phenotypically similar to migraine.

Linked question

12. In order to improve her headaches, you tell the student from the prior question she should first:

A. Try sumatriptan as needed on no more than 9 days per month

B. Initiate some lifestyle changes and rely on over-the-counter medications on no more than 2–3 days per week

C. Immediately get a brain MRI

D. All of the above

Correct answer: B

Explanation

It is first and foremost important to recommend healthier lifestyle changes, as that is likely to improve her headache frequency. Over-the-counter anti-inflammatories (OTCs) like ibuprofen or acetaminophen can be relied on with decent benefit for tension-type headache (TTH) and should be limited to use on no more than 3 days per week consistently.

Sumatriptan is a migraine-specific abortive, triptan class, medication. Given this is a TTH, it is more likely that OTCs will be effective in her moments of need than sumatriptan.

An immediate brain MRI is not indicated here, as there is no warning or "red flag" features, other than that this patient's headache is new. If/when symptoms do not clinically improve with instated treatment plan and/or newer concerning symptoms develop, it would then be reasonable to obtain a brain MRI at a later date.

Linked question

13. The student from the prior question admits she will not be able to follow your recommendations right now, as she is extremely high achieving and anticipates more long days and nights in the library in order to maintain her top-of-the-class distinction. She wonders, if she were to initiate a daily *preventative medication*, which of the following would be best for her?
    A. Cyclobenzaprine
    B. Topiramate
    C. Propranolol
    D. OnabotulinumtoxinA
    Correct answer: A

Explanation
Cyclobenzaprine is a muscle relaxant medication with tricyclic antidepressant (TCA) properties that has shown some evidence for the prevention of tension-type headache (TTH). Its exact mechanism of action is unknown, but subsequent muscle relaxation and effects on neurotransmitters are postulated to be helpful. The other options listed are used in the prevention of migraine.

Topiramate is an antiepileptic drug (AED) with evidence for the prevention of migraine headache.

Propranolol is a beta blocker (BB) with evidence for the prevention of migraine headache.

OnabotulinumtoxinA, administered via the PREEMPT Protocol, is an FDA-approved treatment only for the prevention of chronic migraine.

14. A 25-year-old man presents with recurrent headaches. These began 3 weeks ago and have become excruciating and more frequent over time. He is now having up to 3 episodes per day or night (noting that they often wake him up ~2–4 AM). The headaches last 15–45 min and are always behind his right eye. His right eye also becomes wet, red, and puffy. You tell him there is a newer treatment you would like to try to get approved by his insurance to improve his condition. This treatment is:
    A. Verapamil
    B. Depakote
    C. Indomethacin
    D. Galcanezumab
    Correct answer: D

Explanation
The vignette is describing cluster headache (CH). Although verapamil and valproic acid are also reasonable treatments for the prevention of CH, galcanezumab is the newest of these to market.

Indomethacin is the treatment of choice for various indomethacin-responsive headaches. Hemicrania continua (HC) and paroxysmal hemicrania (PH) are, by definition, *completely* responsive to indomethacin and are defined by differing headache durations and temporality than cluster headache. Other headache types such as primary stabbing headache, primary cough headache, and hypnic headache may show a response to indomethacin as well.

15. A 36-year-old, healthy woman presents to the emergency room with a constant headache for the last 4 weeks. The headache is only ever on the right side of her head, and she has noticed that her right eye is often watering and that her eyelid on that side droops slightly as well. She shows you a photograph of herself from a week ago, and you agree with this observation. After ruling out a structural lesion with brain MRI and MRA, she is given IV ketorolac, IV magnesium, and IV fluids without any clinical improvement. A neurology consultation is called, and she is discharged home with a treatment that is anticipated to resolve her symptoms in time, called:
    A. Prednisone
    B. Verapamil
    C. Indomethacin
    D. Galcanezumab
    Correct answer: C

Explanation
The vignette describes a unilateral, continuous headache with associated ipsilateral cranial autonomic features. This is most consistent with hemicrania continua (HC), which most commonly onsets in adulthood. HC is an indomethacin-responsive headache, and *complete response* to indomethacin is crucial to the making this diagnosis.

The other treatments are all reasonable treatment choices in cluster headache (CH): Prednisone would be a "transitional preventive" (short-term, rapid-acting treatment used early in a CH cycle to provide immediate relief while preventative medications take time to take effect).

Verapamil remains the first-line and gold standard preventive treatment in CH.

Galcanezumab is a newer calcitonin gene-related peptide (CGRP) monoclonal antibody (mAb) treatment approved for the prevention of episodic CH.

16. A 47-year-old man is experiencing left-sided retro-orbital headaches lasting 5 min and accompanied by ipsilateral facial diaphoresis and nasal congestion. There are 20 attacks per day, and this is intermittently affecting

his ability to work. His current neurologist has tried prednisone courses, verapamil, topiramate, and galcanezumab thus far, with no benefit despite 6 months of treatment trials. He comes to you for a second opinion. What is the best next treatment to offer him?

A. Double the dose of galcanezumab
B. Indomethacin trial
C. Lithium
D. Melatonin

Correct answer: B

Explanation

This patient has a trigeminal autonomic cephalalgia (TAC). The TACs are differentiated from each other by both the duration and the frequency of attacks. This patient has been treated incorrectly for cluster headache (CH), without benefit, for >3 months. Although CH may become chronic and/or be more refractory to treatment, the duration of the described attacks is too short, and the frequency of the described attacks is too high, for CH. This vignette is describing paroxysmal hemicrania (PH), and the patient should be given an indomethacin trial. If headache resolution follows, the diagnosis of PH is confirmed.

Even in CH, it would not be advisable to increase the dose of galcanezumab, a newer calcitonin gene-related peptide (CGRP) monoclonal antibody (mAb), given a lack of efficacy and safety data in this area at the time of publication.

Lithium and melatonin would potentially be reasonable later-line treatment alternatives for a more refractory TAC, but it is not the "best next" step.

Linked questions: 17–19

17. A 36-year-old man comes to your office describing brief, but severe and frequent, headaches on the right side of his forehead and temple. The pain occurs in a series of stabs, lasting anywhere from a few seconds to 10 min at a time. What imaging studies should first be performed?

A. MRI brain without contrast
B. MR angiography Brain without contrast
C. MRI brain with and without contrast
D. A & B
E. B & C

Correct answer: E

Explanation

There is not yet enough historical information here to make a diagnosis. The patient's headache is side-locked to the right and severe and should, therefore, be imaged to ensure no underlying structural etiology. A *contrasted* brain MRI should be performed to take a good look at the skull base. An MR angiography of the brain is advised as well given this could be classical trigeminal neuralgia, wherein there is neu-

rovascular contact between the trigeminal nerve (TN) and a neighboring artery.

Linked question

18. For the patient in the prior question, the imaging studies return normal, without any structural abnormalities. You ask the patient a few more questions about his symptoms. There is no accompanying nausea or vomiting; however, there is some mild light sensitivity during the attacks. He reports that the waves of pain occur spontaneously and are not triggered by chewing or talking or wind blowing on his face. You then happen to witness an episode occur while he is in your office and notice that his right eye is red and tearing. What is the most likely diagnosis?

A. SUNCT
B. Idiopathic trigeminal neuralgia
C. Cluster headache
D. Migraine

Correct answer: A

Explanation

The diagnosis is Short-lasting Unilateral Neuralgiform headache with Conjunctival injection and Tearing (SUNCT). This is a trigeminal autonomic cephalalgia (TAC) wherein attacks of moderate-to-severe unilateral headache, accompanied by cranial autonomic symptoms, last from 1 to 600 s and occur as a series of stabs. As with all TACs, there can be associated photo−/phonophobia ipsilaterally as well (though typically more mild than as seen in migraine).

Trigeminal neuralgia is also a brief (from 1 s to 2 min), unilateral headache or facial pain that occurs as recurrent stabs or electric-like shocks (i.e. lancinations), and although cranial autonomic symptoms *may occur* with trigeminal neuralgia as well, the defining historical feature here is that SUNCT is not precipitated by innocuous stimuli within the affected trigeminal distribution, as is the case with trigeminal neuralgia.

Cluster headache is another TAC, characterized by attacks with a duration of 15 min to 3 h and a frequency of once every other day to up to 8 times per day.

Migraine is more disabling, typically with prominent photo−/phonophobia, nausea or vomiting, and associated disability. Migraine attacks are more prolonged, lasting 4–72 h.

Linked question

19. The patient from the prior question feels validated to have a diagnosis and wonders what can be done to treat his symptoms. You offer:

A. Verapamil
B. Lamotrigine
C. Oxcarbazepine
D. Galcanezumab

Correct answer: B

Explanation

Lamotrigine is currently the first-line treatment for SUNCT/SUNA (Short-lasting Unilateral Neuralgiform headache attacks with Autonomic symptoms).

Verapamil and galcanezumab are reasonable treatment options for cluster headache and/or migraine.

Oxcarbazepine is the first-line pharmaceutical treatment for trigeminal neuralgia.

20. A 72-year-old woman presents with a mild-to-moderate pressure-like sensation over her parietal region. The pain occasionally spikes to a more severe intensity. The region of pain is round and never spreads out beyond a diameter of 4 cm. Contrasted brain imaging is obtained and unremarkable. What is the diagnosis?
    A. Epicrania fugax
    B. Auriculotemporal neuralgia
    C. Nummular headache
    D. Hypnic headache
    Correct answer: C

Explanation

"Nummular" translates to "resembling a coin" in Latin. Nummular headache is characterized by a sharp contour and fixed size (typically 1–6 cm diameter) and is round or elliptical in shape. The pain may be continuous or intermittent. Its most common site is of the parietal scalp. This is a primary headache disorder; hence, contrasted neuroimaging must be obtained to rule out underlying structural or secondary etiology before making the diagnosis.

Epicrania fugax is a brief, paroxysmal and stabbing headache occurring in a linear or zig-zag trajectory across the surface of one hemicranium, commencing and terminating in the distributions of different nerves. This is a rare primary headache disorder that also requires advanced neuroimaging before making a formal diagnosis. It is described in the appendix of the International Classification of Headache Disorders-3 (ICHD-3).

Auriculotemporal neuralgia presents as neuralgiform (i.e., brief recurring shooting, stabbing, or sharp, electric-like or lancinating) pain along the distribution of the auriculotemporal nerve.

"Hypnic" comes from the Greek language, meaning "inclined to sleep." Hypnic headache develops only during sleep and causes wakening. It lasts 15 min and up to 4 h, and there are no characteristic associated symptoms. It typically onsets after age 50, but may occur in younger patients as well. It is also known as "alarm clock" headache.

Linked questions: 21–23

21. A 22-year-old boy with no previous history of headaches presents to your office with a daily and continuous head-

ache for the past 7 months. He remembers that he was sitting on his couch watching TV on July 2nd last year when he first noticed the headache. He recalls that, in the week prior to onset, he was sick with a severe gastrointestinal virus. The headache sometimes causes him to feel nauseous and sensitive to bright lights. You need to obtain some tests to make a formal diagnosis, but what is the *most likely clinical diagnosis* at this time?
    A. New daily persistent headache
    B. Chronic migraine without aura
    C. Chronic tension-type headache
    D. Spontaneous intracranial hypotension
    Correct answer: A

Explanation

The vignette describes a clearly remembered, acute onset of a daily and continuous headache. This is the defining clinical feature of new daily persistent headache (NDPH). Although the pathogenesis is unclear, various factors may play a role in triggering NPDH, most often systemic infections (viral or bacterial) and/or stressful life events (emotional trauma, chronic daily stress).

The phenotype of this patient's headache is indeed consistent with chronic migraine without aura; however, the *acute* and remembered chronic onset makes NDPH the more correct answer here.

It is important to remember that NPDH may also take on a tension-type headache phenotype (be otherwise "featureless," lacking nausea/vomiting and/or hypersensitivities to the environment). This is not the case for the above patient.

Spontaneous intracranial hypotension (SIH) should always be on the differential diagnosis for a new and continuous headache. However, clinically, the history of a preceding viral illness makes NDPH more likely in this case. Although SIH may occur without a clear trigger, some predictors include mild-to-severe trauma, straining/lifting, spinal pathology (bone spurs, calcified disc material), and underlying connective tissue disorders such as Ehlers–Danlos or Marfan syndrome.

Linked question

22. Before settling on this diagnosis for the patient in the prior question, which of the following studies must you obtain?
    A. MRI total spine with and without contrast
    B. MRI brain without contrast
    C. MRI brain with and without contrast
    D. MRI cervical spine with and without contrast
    E. A & C
    F. A & B
    Correct answer: E

Explanation

New daily persistent headache (NDPH) is a diagnosis of exclusion. It may require extensive laboratory testing, advanced neuroimaging, or even some procedures (in some cases, a lumbar puncture, temporomandibular or sinus imaging, and/or CT myelogram) be performed to make the diagnosis. Of the listed choices, a contrasted MRI of neuroaxis (brain and total spine) is the best option.

A non-contrasted MRI brain would potentially miss radiographic stigmata of intracranial hypotension (such as pachymeningeal enhancement), as well as intracranial lesions/tumors.

A contrasted MRI cervical spine would not provide sufficient detail to identify a potential spinal fluid collection, which would collect in the lower spine due to gravity.

Linked question

23. For the patient in the prior question, the requested imaging studies return normal. After further questioning, you learn that the patient does not feel his headache changes with position (it is not meaningfully improved with lying flat, nor improved when he is upright). He has not yet been tried any treatments for his condition. What should you do next?
    A. Treat this patient as you would for chronic migraine
    B. Treat this patient as you would for chronic tension-type headache
    C. Recommend a CT myelogram
    D. Recommend a lumbar puncture
    Correct answer: A

Explanation

New daily persistent headache (NDPH) should be treated like the phenotypic headache it resembles. In this case, the phenotype resembles chronic migraine. The patient is treatment-naive and warrants treatment initiation.

A CT myelogram may be indicated at some point to more definitively rule out intracranial hypotension by a CSF-venous fistula (CVF). However, this is an invasive procedure carrying some risk, CVFs are quite rare, and the clinical history does not support an orthostatic nature to suggest that further investigation is needed at this time. It is best to first try evidence-based headache treatment.

A lumbar puncture would be helpful in diagnosing headaches related to intracranial pressure dysregulation, in particular *high* intracranial pressure. However, as with a CT myelogram, this test is invasive, carries some risk, and the clinical history does not support further investigation at this time.

24. A young woman with localized stabbing pain lasting up to a few seconds at a time presents to your office for treatment. These stabs occur spontaneously and at a random, irregular frequency. The pain is not disabling, and there are no sinus symptoms. The location of the stabs seems to move around to different spots and does not occur along any specific nerve distribution. Brain MRI and MRA are normal. What is the diagnosis?
    A. Short-lasting Unilateral Neuralgiform headache Attacks (SUNA)
    B. Trigeminal neuralgia
    C. Primary stabbing headache
    D. Nummular headache
    Correct answer: C

Explanation

Primary stabbing headache (PSH) is an "other" primary headache disorder as classified by the International Classification of Headache Disorders-3 (ICHD-3). It is characterized by transient (typically <3 s) multifocal stabs of pain that occur spontaneously and not along a specific nerve distribution. This condition is benign and brief, and once getting a diagnosis and reassurance, most patients choose to defer treatment. If treatment is indicated, Indomethacin is the first-line and *potentially* effective. Other treatments to consider for this condition include melatonin, gabapentin, or COX-2 inhibitors.

Short-lasting Unilateral Neuralgiform headache with Autonomic symptoms (SUNA) is a trigeminal autonomic cephalalgia (TAC) wherein attacks of moderate-to-severe pain in a strictly unilateral distribution are accompanied by cranial autonomic symptoms, last from 1 to 600 s, and occur as a series of stabs. The mention of "no sinus symptoms" in this vignette is broadly suggesting that there are no cranial autonomic features.

Trigeminal neuralgia (TN) is also characterized by brief (from 1 s to 2 min), stabbing or electric-like (i.e. lancinating) pain; however, *it distinctly occurs along branches of the trigeminal nerve.*

"Nummular," translating to "resembling a coin" in Latin, is characterized by continuous or intermittent pain that is sharply contoured (round or elliptical in shape) and fixed in size (typically 1–6 cm diameter).

25. A 48-year-old man presents with 6 months of persistent, dull facial pain that does not follow the distribution of any specific nerve. The pain is daily and prolonged, sometimes described as aching or nagging, and is not associated with sensory loss or any other neurological deficits or symptoms. Brain imaging and dental evaluations are unremarkable. Which of the following statements is most accurate regarding the likely diagnosis?
    A. The diagnosis is confirmed by a specific laboratory test
    B. Treatment with oxcarbazepine will effectively treat this condition

C. The best next step is a multimodal treatment approach

D. The condition will likely remit on its own within another few weeks

Correct answer: C

Explanation

The most likely diagnosis is Persistent Idiopathic Facial Pain (PIFP). PIFP has varying presentations but must recur daily for at least 2 h/day for at least 3 months. It can be facial and/or oral but, by definition, is poorly localized (not following the distribution of a specific nerve). PIFP is typically dull, aching, or nagging in quality. Dental and secondary neurological causes must be excluded to make the diagnosis. Treatment can be challenging in this condition and is typically most effective by a multimodal approach, incorporating medication (most often neuropathic or antiepileptic), non-pharmacological therapies (CBT, acupuncture, neuromodulation), and potentially minimally invasive procedures (local nerve blocks, onabotulinumtoxinA).

There is no specific laboratory test to confirm PIFP, or any headache disorder for that matter, at least at the time of publication. It is important to note that labs can sometimes *be helpful* when making a diagnosis (such as elevated erythrocyte sedimentation rate [ESR] and/or C-reactive protein [CRP] being more suggestive of Giant Cell Arteritis [GCA]).

Oxcarbazepine is an antiepileptic drug (AED) that may ultimately be trialed in PIFP; however, alone it is not likely to be effective enough. Oxcarbazepine is, rather, considered a decently effective drug for trigeminal neuralgia (TN).

PIFP is a chronic condition with no readily identifiable cause or cure. It is not likely to remit on its own. Answer D is more descriptive of episodic cluster headache, which cycles with a clear onset and offset.

Linked questions: 26–27

26. A 32-year-old man presents with sudden onset headache, described as the worst headache of his life. Patient reports being in his usual state of health. The headache began while engaging in sexual activity. Of the following, which imaging modality is the most important to first obtain?
    A. MRI brain without contrast
    B. MR venography brain without contrast
    C. CT brain/CT angiogram of the brain and neck
    D. Carotid duplex

Correct answer: C

Explanation

The vignette describes a patient with a "thunderclap" headache, for which secondary causes of headache must be ruled out. Potentially life-threatening vascular causes, such as Reversible Cerebral Vasoconstriction Syndrome (RCVS) and ruptured cerebral aneurysm (leading to subarachnoid hemorrhage [SAH]), must be quickly evaluated for with a CT brain and angiogram.

Other possible causes of thunderclap headache include arterial dissection, elevated intracranial pressure, central venous sinus thrombosis (CVST), spontaneous intracranial hypotension (SIH), and *as diagnoses of exclusion,* primary headache associated with sexual activity or primary thunderclap headache.

Reference

Utku U. Primary headache associated with sexual activity: case report. Med Princ Pract. 2013;22(6):588–9. https://doi.org/10.1159/000350415.

Linked question

27. For the patient in the prior question, a CT angiogram is obtained with the *imaging* shown below. What is the mechanism of action of the medication that can best help to treat this condition?

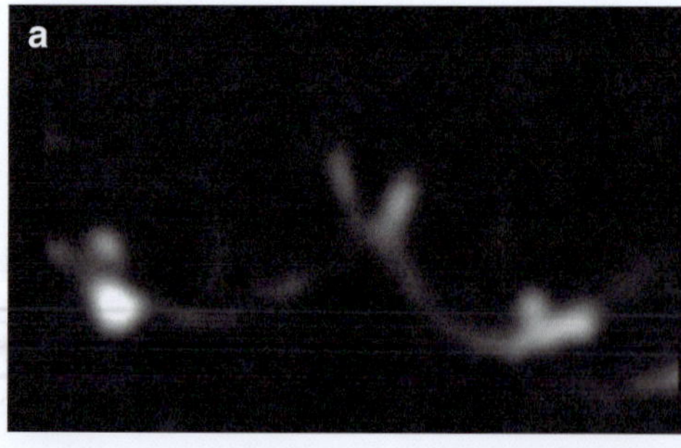
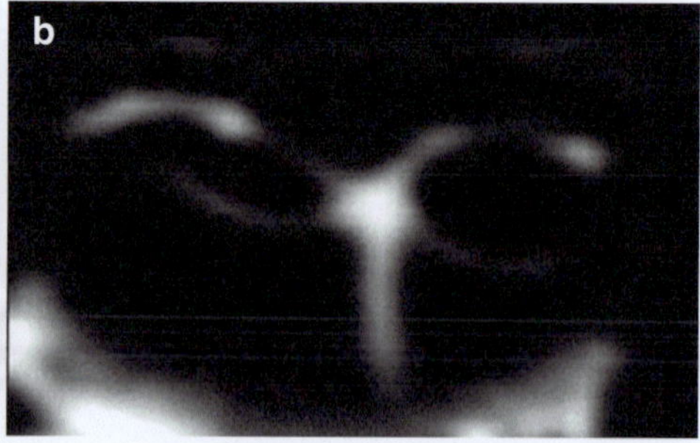
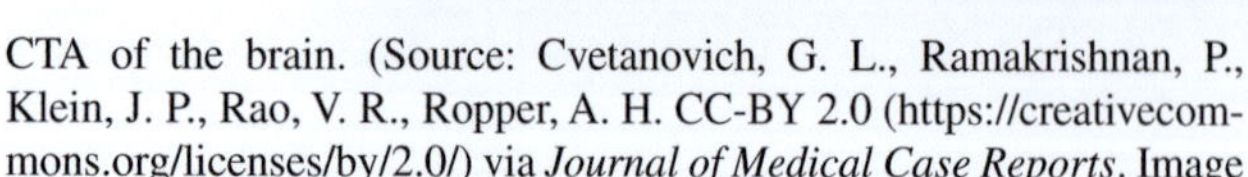

CTA of the brain. (Source: Cvetanovich, G. L., Ramakrishnan, P., Klein, J. P., Rao, V. R., Ropper, A. H. CC-BY 2.0 (https://creativecommons.org/licenses/by/2.0/) via *Journal of Medical Case Reports*. Image has been cropped from source. Please see full attribution with citation below in references section for this question.)

A. 5-HT1B agonist
B. Serotonin and norepinephrine reuptake inhibitor
C. Carbonic Anhydrase inhibitor
D. Calcium channel blocker
E. Alpha-1 antagonist

Correct answer: D

Explanation

The CT angiogram (CTA) reveals focal segments of vascular narrowing of large and medium arteries, with dilated segments following the area of narrowing, consistent with RCVS. If CTA imaging is unrevealing but clinical suspicion is high enough, Digital Subtraction Angiography (DSA) can be considered in the appropriate setting. The primary treatment for RCVS is the removal of triggers (typically vasoactive medications or drugs). Calcium channel blockers (CCBs) like nimodipine and verapamil are used orally and, sometimes, intravascularly to treat RCVS. It is important to note that such treatment does not necessarily prevent potential complications of RCVS like hemorrhage or stroke. Intra-arterial administration of CCBs has been shown to improve vasoconstriction.

Triptans are 5-H1B agonists and, hence, *vasoconstrictive*. These should be avoided at all costs in RCVS.

Serotonin and norepinephrine reuptake inhibitors (SNRIs) are preventive treatment options for migraine and/or tension-type headache.

Carbonic anhydrase inhibitors like acetazolamide would be appropriate in disorders of elevated intracranial pressure.

Alpha-1 antagonists like doxazosin and tamsulosin are often used to treat hypertension and/or benign prostatic hyperplasia.

References

Cvetanovich GL, Ramakrishnan P, Klein JP, Rao VR, Ropper AH. Reversible cerebral vasoconstriction syndrome in a patient taking citalopram and Hydroxycut: a case report. J Med Case Rep. 2011;5:548. https://doi.org/10.1186/1752-1947-5-548.

Miller TR, Shivashankar R, Mossa-Basha M, Gandhi D. Reversible Cerebral Vasoconstriction Syndrome, Part 1: Epidemiology, Pathogenesis, and Clinical Course. AJNR Am J Neuroradiol. 2015;36(8):1392–9. https://doi.org/10.3174/ajnr.A4214.

Miller TR, Shivashankar R, Mossa-Basha M, Gandhi D. Reversible Cerebral Vasoconstriction Syndrome, Part 2: Diagnostic Work-Up, Imaging Evaluation, and Differential Diagnosis. AJNR Am J Neuroradiol. 2015;36(9):1580–8. https://doi.org/10.3174/ajnr.A4215.

Linked questions: 28–29

28. A 26-year-old woman (body mass index [BMI] 34) presents with gradual progressive headache that is worse when laying down and better when sitting upright. She denies any changes to her vision. Her imaging findings are shown below. What is the best next step?

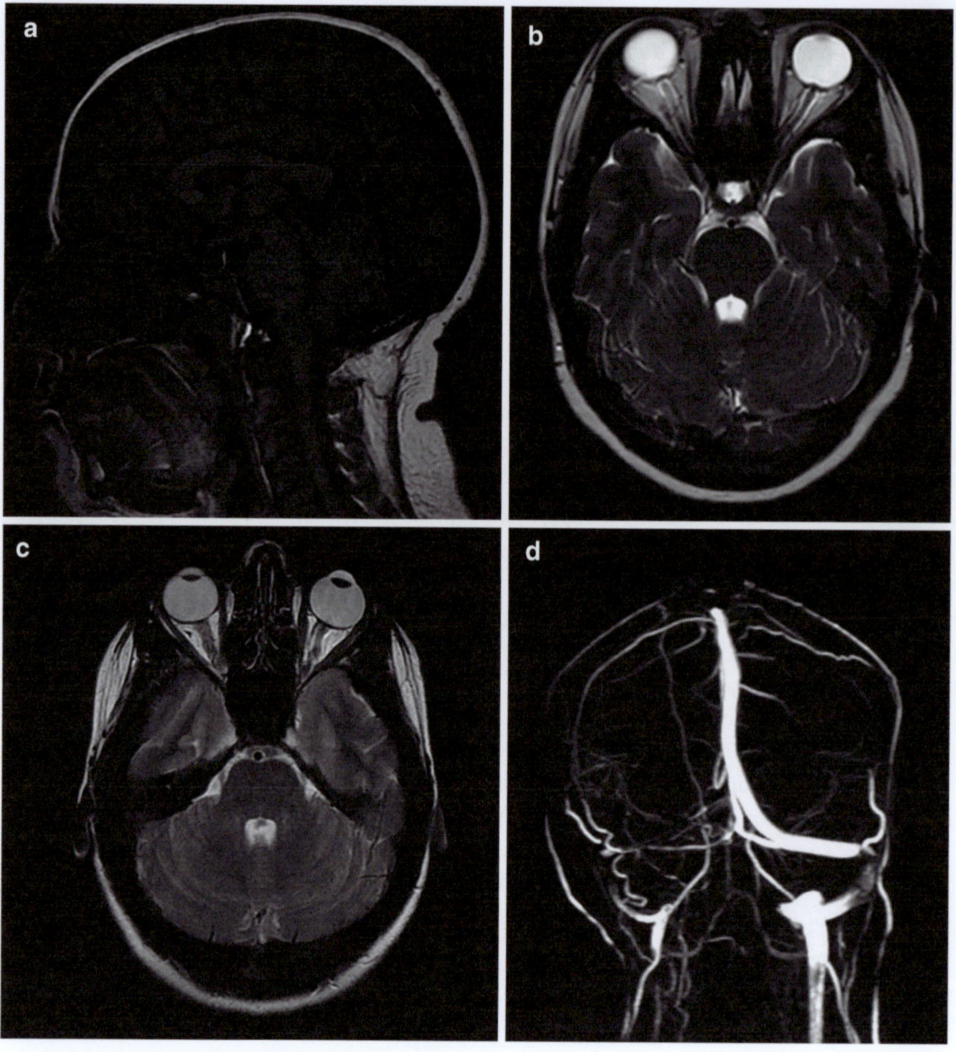

(**a**) Sagittal MRI brain, (**b** and **c**) Axial MRI brain, (**d**) MR venography. (Source: Mollan, S. P., Ali, F., Hassan-Smith, G., Botfield, H., Friedman, D. I., Sinclair, A. J. CC-BY 4.0 (https://creativecommons.org/licenses/by/4.0/) via *Journal of Neurology, Neurosurgery, and Psychiatry*. Image has not been modified from source. Please see full attribution with citation below in references section for this question.)

A. Ask the patient about recent medication changes
B. Obtain a lumbar puncture
C. Start a carbonic anhydrase agonist
D. Both A and B
E. All of the above

Correct answer: D

Explanation

The diagnosis is idiopathic intracranial hypertension (IIH), previously known as "pseudotumor cerebri." Brain MRI findings may include empty sella sign (panel A in image above), flattening of the ocular posterior globe, and protrusion of the optic nerve head (panel B in image above), optic nerve tortuosity (panel C in image above), and venous sinus stenosis (panel D in image above). On fundoscopic exam, patients will often have disc edema; co-management with an ophthalmologist (preferably a neuro-ophthalmologist if available) to evaluate and regularly monitor for changes in disc edema is advised. Clinically, pulsatile tinnitus, diplopia, transient visual obscurations, and a positional headache (worse when lying flat) are often described.

It is prudent to ask about medication changes, as some retinoids, birth controls, tetracyclines, and lithium may increase intracranial pressure (ICP), and discontinuation of these medications may be curative. A lumbar puncture (LP), confirming elevated intracranial pressure (>25 cm H_2O) is done to confirm the diagnosis.

The mainstay of pharmaceutical treatment in IIH is carbonic anhydrase *inhibitors*.Further, if no active visual symptoms, can probably delay initiation until after the diagnostic LP if done swiftly.

References

Barkatullah AF, Leishangthem L, Moss HE. MRI findings as markers of idiopathic intracranial hypertension. Curr Opin Neurol. 2021;34(1):75–83. https://doi.org/10.1097/wco.0000000000000885.

Mollan SP, Ali F, Hassan-Smith G, Botfield H, Friedman DI, Sinclair AJ. Evolving evidence in adult idiopathic intracranial hypertension: pathophysiology and management. J Neurol Neurosurg Psychiatry. 2016;87(9):982–92. https://doi.org/10.1136/jnnp-2015-311302.

Tan MG, Worley B, Kim WB, Ten Hove M, Beecker J. Drug-Induced Intracranial Hypertension: A Systematic Review and Critical Assessment of Drug-Induced Causes. Am J Clin Dermatol. 2020;21(2):163–72. https://doi.org/10.1007/s40257-019-00485-z.

Wang MTM, Bhatti MT, Danesh-Meyer HV. Idiopathic intracranial hypertension: Pathophysiology, diagnosis and management. J Clin Neurosci. 2022;95:172–9. https://doi.org/10.1016/j.jocn.2021.11.029.

Linked question

29. A lumbar puncture is obtained for the patient in the prior question, revealing normal cerebrospinal fluid studies (including cell counts, protein, glucose, infectious panels, cytology) and an opening pressure of 34 cm H_2O. Which of the following is the *most effective* treatment for the patient's condition?
    A. Weight loss
    B. Acetazolamide
    C. Lumbar drain
    D. Optic nerve fenestration
    E. All of the above
    Correct answer: A

Explanation

While all of the above answer choices may be effective for idiopathic intracranial hypertension (IIH), weight loss is considered to be the most effective and is even considered to be disease-modifying. Preceding a diagnosis of IIH is typically a 5–15% weight gain, and some studies suggest evidence of remission after 15% weight loss. Patients may benefit from weight loss programs or medications (such as glucagon-like peptide-1s [GLP-1s] or phentermine).

Acetazolamide is a carbonic anhydrase inhibitor, and while it is the mainstay of pharmaceutical treatment in IIH by directly reducing intracranial pressure (ICP), weight loss is still considered to be the *most effective* treatment.

Lumbar drains may be considered in severe cases but are invasive and do confer a greater risk of side effects and potential complications.

Optic nerve fenestration procedure may be considered in patients with significant or refractory papilledema who need time to lose weight but are at risk for imminent vision loss (the feared complication of IIH).

Other notable medications for IIH include topiramate, alternative carbonic anhydrase inhibitors, and/or furosemide. Other potential interventions for IIH include ventriculoperitoneal shunt (VPS), venous sinus stenting, and/or repetitive large-volume lumbar punctures.

References

Ahmad SR, Moss HE. Update on the Diagnosis and Treatment of Idiopathic Intracranial Hypertension. Semin Neurol. 2019;39(6):682–91. https://doi.org/10.1055/s-0039-1698744.

Mollan SP, Davies B, Silver NC, Shaw S, Mallucci CL, Wakerley BR, et al. Idiopathic intracranial hypertension: consensus guidelines on management. J Neurol Neurosurg Psychiatry. 2018;89(10):1088–100. https://doi.org/10.1136/jnnp-2017-317440.

30. A 22-year-old man with a history of anxiety, depression, and substance abuse presents to the emergency department with a headache that has gradually worsened since he awoke this morning and does not change with position. His vital signs are notable for tachycardia to the 130s, hypertension to 180s/120s. On exam, he is agitated and confused. You notice tongue fasciculations and general tremulousness. His CT scan of the head is normal. What is the best next step?
    A. Obtain LP
    B. Obtain MRI
    C. Initiate chlordiazepoxide protocol
    D. CT myelogram
    E. Rapidly lower blood pressure
    Correct answer: C

Explanation

This patient is suffering from withdrawal, likely from alcohol given the presence of agitation, tachycardia, hypertension, and tremulousness in the absence of other identifiable causes. In a recent animal model study, it was found that mast cell-specific receptor MrgprB2 plays a role in the development of alcohol-withdrawal-induced headache. In this study, spontaneous activation and hypersensitization of trigeminal ganglia neurons were shown. Chlordiazepoxide specifically is a long-acting benzodiazepine used for alcohol withdrawal. While chlordiazepoxide (and other benzodiazepines) do not necessarily improve the underlying headache, it is important to treat those in alcohol withdrawal to prevent worsening withdrawal symptoms, especially seizures.

Reference

Son H, Zhang Y, Shannonhouse J, Ishida H, Gomez R, Kim YS. Mast-cell-specific receptor mediates alcohol-withdrawal-associated headache in male mice. Neuron. 2024;112(1):113–23.e4. https://doi.org/10.1016/j.neuron.2023.09.039.

Linked questions: 31–32

31. A 13-year-old girl presents to the emergency department after getting hit in the head by another player during a soccer game. She did not lose consciousness, but she reports feeling dizzy, nauseous, and sensitive to light, with a severe right frontal headache. Her neurological exam is non-focal. What are best next steps?
    A. Admit patient to the hospital for close observation
    B. Obtain a non-contrast head CT for further evaluation
    C. Encourage resuming normal physical activity as soon as possible to aid in recovery
    D. Provide reassurance
    E. Encourage bed rest for at least 14 days following injury

    Correct answer: D

Explanation

This patient presents with a mild traumatic brain injury (mTBI) or concussion. No further imaging or workup is necessary as the mechanism of injury was overall mild, and there are no neurological deficits or clinical red flag symptoms. Brain imaging may be considered in patients with a severe injury mechanism, abnormal examination (Glascow Coma Scale <15 or focal neurologic deficits), and/or if symptoms are progressively worsening to evaluate for more severe neurologic injury, like intracranial hemorrhage or skull fracture.

After concussion, patients should be instructed to "relatively" rest for ~24–48 h following injury. There is no evidence to indicate that bed rest for 14 days would improve overall outcome. In fact, after ~24–48 h, patients should *slowly return* to their baseline activities with monitoring for worsening symptoms. Prolonged periods of rest are now associated with delayed recovery.

References

Guenette JP, Shenton ME, Koerte IK. Imaging of Concussion in Young Athletes. Neuroimaging Clin N Am. 2018;28(1):43–53. https://doi.org/10.1016/j.nic.2017.09.004.

Shaughnessy AF. Imaging Guidelines for Children With Mild Traumatic Brain Injury. Am Fam Physician. 2024;110(2):202–3.

Linked question

32. For the patient in the prior question, the patient's parents ask what medications can be used for quick improvement in her symptoms. Which of the following is your best response?
    A. There are unfortunately no medications for the pediatric population on treatment for this condition
    B. While medications can acutely help the disorder, they will make symptoms worse long-term and thus should be avoided in the acute setting at all costs
    C. The management of symptoms should be based on the primary headache disorder the patient's symptoms most closely resemble
    D. Preventive therapy should be implemented as soon as possible to improve overall outcomes
    E. None of the above

    Correct answer: C

Explanation

Management of Headache attributed to trauma or injury to the head and/or neck, as defined by the International Classification of Headache Disorders-3 (ICHD-3), is still being studied in the pediatric and general population. However, the general consensus reveals that posttraumatic headache should be treated as the primary headache it most closely resembles (in the case of this patient, that is migraine given the presence of nausea and photophobia).

Post-concussive syndrome and post-traumatic headache may improve with time and after 24–48-h period of relative rest. Preventive therapies may be considered, though it would be reasonable to wait ~4–6 weeks post-injury if symptoms are not improving or are occurring at least 1–2 times per week. Neutraceuticals such as magnesium, riboflavin, and melatonin may be effective for the pediatric population.

Acute symptomatic management may include over-the-counter anti-inflammatories (NSAIDs, acetaminophen), though it is important to counsel patients on avoiding medication overuse.

Activities should be limited in the first 24–48 h after injury, after which a gradual return to usual activities should be encouraged.

In some cases, non-pharmacological interventions like cognitive behavioral therapy (CBT) may be helpful on a case-by-case basis and pending access. Taken together, a multimodal approach encompassing relative rest, abortive therapies and, potentially, preventive, and behavioral therapies is best.

Reference

Patterson Gentile C, Rosenthal S, Blume H, Rastogi RG, McVige J, Bicknese A, et al. American Headache Society white paper on treatment of post-traumatic headache from concussion in youth. Headache. 2024;64(9):1148–62. https://doi.org/10.1111/head.14795.

Linked questions: 33–34

33. A 76-year-old man with a history of multiple myeloma, currently under treatment, presents for a third opinion after visiting several emergency departments with a chief complaint of headache. His headache is worse when lying down and better when sitting up. He also has blurry vision that has progressively worsened since the onset of these headaches several months ago. What is the best next step?
    A. Provide reassurance
    B. Consult oncology
    C. Obtain an MRI brain with and without contrast
    D. Consult ophthalmology
    E. Obtain a CT angiogram

Correct answer: C

Explanation

In a patient with malignancy and newer headaches, there are several key differential diagnoses that should be considered. The patient is receiving oncologic treatment (chemotherapy, immunotherapy, or radiation) so treatment complications should be considered (such as neurotoxicities, opportunistic infections, immune-mediated). Additionally, leptomeningeal spread of the malignancy is of concern. While oncology and ophthalmology consultations will be important, a contrasted MRI brain is the best next step in this case.

Linked question

34. MRI of the brain is shown above. What should you do next?

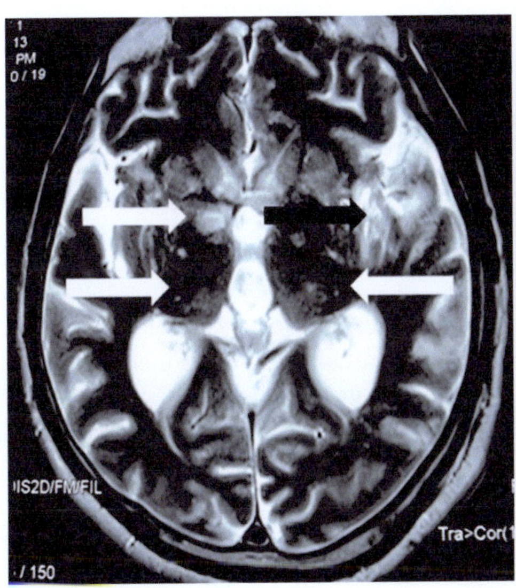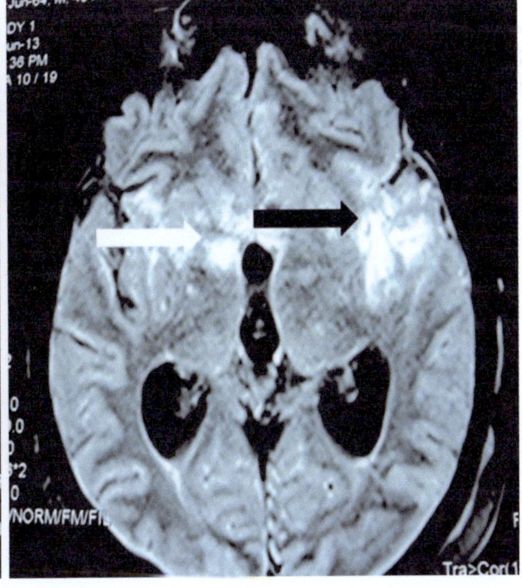

Axial MRI brain. (Source: Liyanage, D. S., Pathberiya, L. PS., Gooneratne, I. K., Caldera, M. HPC., Priyankara, WS. P., Gamage, R. CC-BY 2.0 (https://creativecommons.org/licenses/by/2.0/) via *BMC Research Notes*. Image has not been modified from source. Please see full attribution with citation below in references section for this question.)

A. Check HIV and CD4 count
B. Obtain a lumbar puncture with opening pressure
C. Start antimicrobial medications
D. Consult Ophthalmology
E. All of the above

Correct answer: E

Explanation

Brain MRI shows multiple nodular lesions in basal ganglia and thalamus. These nodules would be expected to enhance (not shown). These nodules are most likely cryptococcomas. In this immunocompromised cancer patient, HIV and a CD4 count should also be obtained since HIV can further increase a patient's risk of developing intracranial infection and impair the patient's ability to mount a response to treatment. A lumbar puncture (LP) should be pursued urgently to evaluate the cerebrospinal fluid (CSF) studies for specific infectious processes (e.g., cryptococcal antigen) and cytology, as well as to measure the opening pressure. Broad-spectrum antimicrobials should initially be started, including for cryptococcus. Ophthalmology should evaluate for papilledema and other potential ophthalmic involvement due to the pathologic, space-occupying process.

Important intracranial infections to remember in patients who are immunocompromised include cryptococcus, toxoplasmosis, streptococcus pneumoniae, herpes simplex virus (HSV), and cytomegalovirus (CMV).

Reference

Liyanage DS, Pathberiya LP, Gooneratne IK, Caldera MH, Perera PW, Gamage R. Cryptococcal meningitis presenting with bilateral complete ophthalmoplegia: a case report. BMC Res Notes. 2014;7:328. https://doi.org/10.1186/1756-0500-7-328.

Linked questions: 35–36

35. A 37-year-old patient presents with 6 months of stabbing pain in the ear and throat. The pain lasts anywhere from a few seconds to a couple of minutes and is often triggered by swallowing. What artery can cause these pathologic symptoms?
    A. Anterior inferior cerebellar artery (AICA)
    B. Posterior inferior cerebellar artery (PICA)
    C. Superior cerebellar artery
    D. Basilar artery
    E. None of the above

    Correct answer: B

Explanation

This patient is presenting with glossopharyngeal neuralgia. While this can sometimes be idiopathic, it is prudent to rule out a vascular cause. The posterior inferior cerebellar artery (PICA) is most commonly cited vessel in glossopharyngeal neuralgia. In severe cases, surgical decompression can be considered.

AICA can affect the facial nerve and potentially lead to hemifacial spasm.

The superior cerebellar artery (SCA) is often the culprit in trigeminal neuralgia, as it travels close to the trigeminal nerve's root entry zone.

Reference

Alafaci C, Granata F, Cutugno M, Marino D, Conti A, Tomasello F. Glossopharyngeal neuralgia caused by a complex neurovascular conflict: Case report and review of the literature. Surg Neurol Int. 2015;6:19. https://doi.org/10.4103/2152-7806.150810.

Linked question

36. For the patient in the prior question, an MRI of the brain is obtained and shows an abnormal upward looping of the posterior inferior cerebellar artery and enhancement of the glossopharyngeal nerve. What are best next steps?
    A. Neurointerventional consultation
    B. Trial of carbamazepine
    C. Trial of verapamil
    D. Dental referral
    E. A and B
    F. B and D

    Correct answer: E

Explanation

The imaging confirms neurovascular glossopharyngeal neuralgia. In such patients, structural intervention, typically by microvascular decompression (MVD), should be considered. Common vascular etiologies include a high-origin Posterior Inferior Cerebellar Artery (PICA), compression of the PICA on the supraolivary fossette, and an upward looping PICA

Carbamazepine is first-line pharmaceutical therapy for trigeminal neuralgia and glossopharyngeal neuralgia alike. Gabapentin may be the next line therapy to try in patients where carbamazepine is ineffective or contraindicated.

Verapamil is the first-line pharmaceutical therapy in cluster headache.

Dental referral would not be indicated in this patient.

References

Alafaci C, Granata F, Cutugno M, Marino D, Conti A, Tomasello F. Glossopharyngeal neuralgia caused by a complex neurovascular conflict: Case report and review of the literature. Surg Neurol Int. 2015;6:19. https://doi.org/10.4103/2152-7806.150810.

Han A, Montgomery C, Zamora A, Winder E, Kaye A, Carroll C, et al. Glossopharyngeal Neuralgia: Epidemiology, Risk factors, Pathophysiology, Differential diagnosis, and Treatment Options. Health Psychol Res. 2022;10(5):36042. https://doi.org/10.52965/001c.36042.

Linked questions: 37–38

37. A 29-year-old man presents with sudden onset left neck pain radiating into the left occipital region. His symptoms started suddenly while he was driving, although he is not sure if he made any triggering maneuvers. On exam, you notice right beating nystagmus on rightward gaze and left beating nystagmus on leftward gaze. He further notes that he has been intermittently dizzy, especially worse when turning his head, which has caused him to vomit once. What are best next steps?

    A. Perform an Epley maneuver
    B. Trial of meclizine
    C. Trial of sumatriptan
    D. Obtain vessel imaging
    E. A and B

    Correct answer: D

Explanation

In this patient with sudden onset left neck and radiating occipital pain and associated vertigo, vertebral artery dissection must first be evaluated for with vascular imaging. Red flag features include direction-changing nystagmus, provocation with head turning, associated emesis, or any other focal neurologic symptoms.

The Epley maneuver is designed to guide displaced crystals back toward the utricle in the treatment of benign paroxysmal positional vertigo (BPPV). First, performing the Dix–Hallpike maneuver, looking for torsional and upsetting ipsilateral nystagmus, can be diagnostic for BPPV. In this case where there is high suspicion for arterial dissection, such manual maneuvers should be avoided given the risk of potentially worsening the dissection.

Meclizine, a histamine H1 receptor antagonist, can be used as supportive treatment for the patient's symptoms only as a temporizing measure.

Triptans are used acutely in migraine headache management. Further, they are vasoconstrictive and should be avoided in patients with vascular issues, including acute arterial dissection.

Linked question

38. You obtain a CT angiogram for the patient in the prior question with *results* shown below. The patient reports worsening occipital headache pain. What are best next steps?

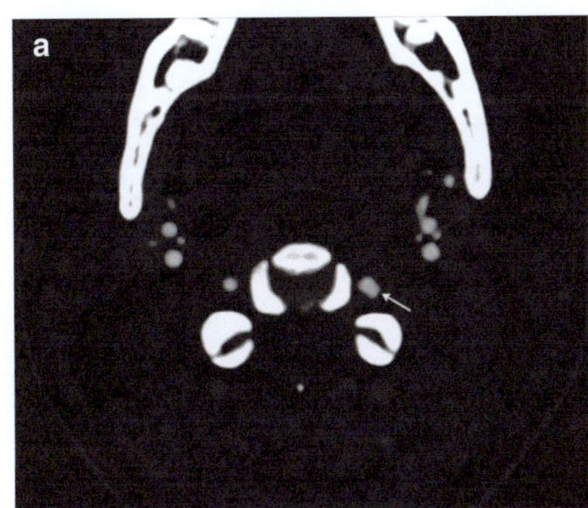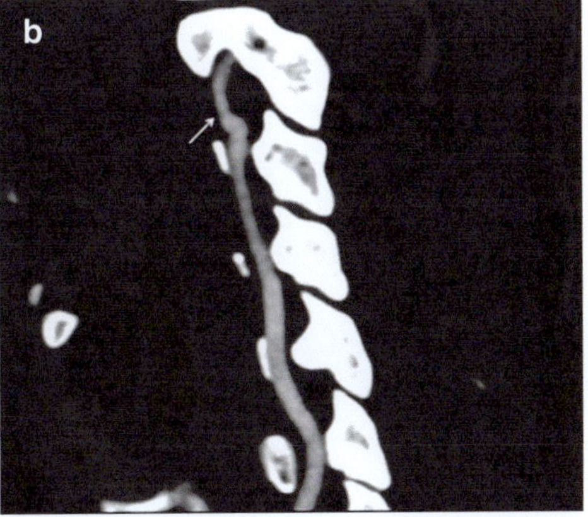

(**a**) Axial view and (**b**) sagittal view of CTA head and neck. (Source: Yvon, C., Adams, A., McLauchlan, D., Ramsden C. CC-BY 4.0 (https://creativecommons.org/licenses/by/4.0/) via Journal of *Medical Case Reports*. Image has not been modified from source. Please see full attribution with citation below in references section for this question.)

A. Provide reassurance
B. Obtain MRI brain without contrast
C. Discussion of antiplatelet versus anticoagulation therapy
D. Both B and C
E. None of the above

Correct answer: D

Explanation

CT angiogram of the head and neck confirms the suspicion of vertebral artery dissection. Potentially resultant strokes of the posterior circulation can be associated with severe headache. This combined with the patients' vertigo and direction-changing nystagmus warrants an MRI brain without contrast to evaluate the posterior fossa.

Typically, anti-platelet therapy is indicated for vertebral artery dissection. However, in some cases, anticoagulation may be preferred. Present research at the time of publication is mixed on the benefit of antiplatelet versus anticoagulation in cervical arterial dissection.

References

Yaghi S, Shu L, Mandel D, Leon Guerrero CR, Henninger N, Muppa J, et al. Antithrombotic Treatment for Stroke Prevention in Cervical Artery Dissection: The STOP-CAD Study. Stroke. 2024;55(4):908–18. https://doi.org/10.1161/strokeaha.123.045731.

Yvon C, Adams A, McLauchlan D, Ramsden C. Headache and transient visual loss as the only presenting symptoms of vertebral artery dissection: a case report. J Med Case Rep. 2016;10(1):105. https://doi.org/10.1186/s13256-016-0893-8.

Linked questions: 39–40

39. A 32-year-old woman with a history of episodic migraine and hypertension is 2 months postpartum and presents to the emergency room with a daily, dull headache that has been ongoing for 6 weeks. She has not had relief with acetaminophen or NSAIDs. What are best next steps?
    A. Trial rizatriptan
    B. Trial eletriptan
    C. Trial ubrogepant
    D. Obtain an MRI brain with and without contrast
    E. Provide reassurance

Correct answer: D

Explanation

Given this patient is postpartum, it is prudent to rule out secondary causes of headache. Important structural secondary headache considerations in the peripartum period include cerebral venous sinus thrombosis (CVST), intracranial hypotension (from recent epidural catheter placement or post-dural puncture headache [PDPH]), pituitary apoplexy, reversible cerebral vasoconstriction syndrome (RCVS), and posterior reversible encephalopathy syndrome (PRES). While migraine can also worsen peripartum, due to major changes in hormones during this time, secondary causes must be evaluated for prior to initiating treatment.

Linked question

40. For the patient in the prior question, MRI of the brain is obtained and shown below. What is the best next step?

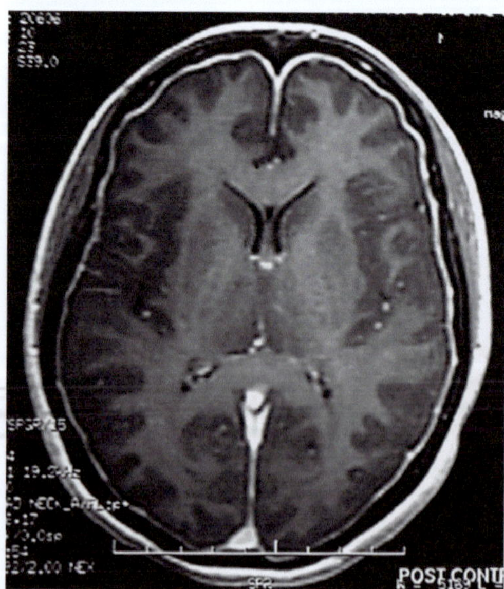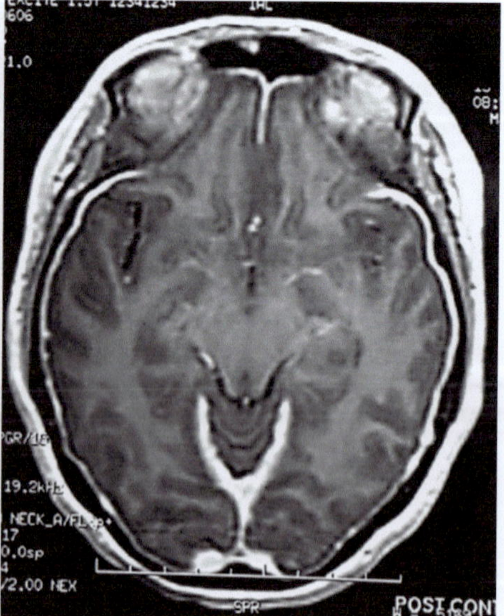

Axial MRI brain. (Source: Chang, T., Rodrigo, C., Samarakoon, L. CC-BY 4.0 (https://creativecommons.org/licenses/by/4.0/) via *BMC Research Notes*. Image has not been modified from source. Please see full attribution with citation below in references section for this question.)

A. Consult anesthesiology for consideration of blood patch
B. Lumbar puncture for further characterization of the findings
C. Encourage fluid intake and reassure the patient that the symptoms will resolve on their own
D. Consult neurosurgery for consideration of brain biopsy
E. None of the above

Correct answer: A

Explanation

MRI brain shows diffuse pachymeningeal enhancement consistent with intracranial hypotension, likely from recent epidural catheter placement resulting in post-dural puncture headache [PDPH]. Conservative management with caffeine, bed rest, and fluids is possible in the acute setting as some cerebrospinal fluid (CSF) leaks resolve on their own. However, in a patient with 2 months of symptoms, the leak is less likely to spontaneously resolve, and thus, an epidural blood patch (EBP) should be pursued. In a study conducted in 2021, conservative treatment was effective in 28% of patients, while EBP success ranged from 64% to 77%.

A lumbar puncture should be avoided, as this would further drop CSF pressure and could potentially worsen symptoms.

A brain biopsy is not indicated in this patient.

References

Chang T, Rodrigo C, Samarakoon L. Spontaneous intracranial hypotension presenting as thunderclap headache: a case report. BMC Res Notes. 2015;8:108. https://doi.org/10.1186/s13104-015-1068-1.

D'Antona L, Jaime Merchan MA, Vassiliou A, Watkins LD, Davagnanam I, Toma AK, et al. Clinical Presentation, Investigation Findings, and Treatment Outcomes of Spontaneous Intracranial Hypotension Syndrome: A Systematic Review and Meta-analysis. JAMA Neurol. 2021;78(3):329–37. https://doi.org/10.1001/jamaneurol.2020.4799.

Linked questions: 41–43

41. A 32-year-old woman is 28 weeks pregnant and comes into the emergency department for sudden onset, severe intractable headache. She tells you she has recently been feeling generalized weakness and craving salt. She is bradycardic, hypotensive, and hypoglycemic. What other finding is most likely evident?

A. Visual aura
B. Left inferior quadrantanopia
C. Bitemporal hemianopsia
D. Elevated cortisol
E. High TSH

Correct answer: C

Explanation

This patient is presenting with signs of adrenal insufficiency. Adrenal insufficiency is caused by failure of the pituitary gland to produce enough adrenocorticotropic hormone (ACTH) to stimulate the adrenal glands. In pregnancy, the pituitary gland enlarges under prolonged estrogen stimulation causing increased pressure in the sella turcica, potentially resulting in ischemia, thrombosis, swelling, and/or hemorrhage. The presence of acute-onset headache in this case suggests pituitary apoplexy, which would result in upward optic chiasm compression and a bitemporal hemianopia visual field deficit. Other symptoms of pituitary apoplexy may include ptosis, anisocoria, alteration of consciousness, and/or fever and, while it is rare to present with adrenal insufficiency, this is a serious complication that can result in headache.

Visual aura is a potential symptom of migraine headache. It is characterized by gradually progressive (5–60 min) positive visual phenomena in one side of the visual field, typically preceding headache onset.

Left inferior quadrantanopia would result from damage to the right parietal lobe or associated optic radiations.

Low cortisol is a result of adrenal insufficiency due to pituitary dysfunction.

Low TSH is often a result of pituitary dysfunction.

References

Grand'Maison S, Weber F, Bédard MJ, Mahone M, Godbout A. Pituitary apoplexy in pregnancy: A case series and literature review. Obstet Med. 2015;8(4):177–83. https://doi.org/10.1177/1753495x15598917.

Iglesias P. Pituitary Apoplexy: An Updated Review. J Clin Med. 2024;13(9). https://doi.org/10.3390/jcm13092508.

Linked question

42. For the patient in the prior question, MRI brain is shown *below*. What should the patient be monitored for?

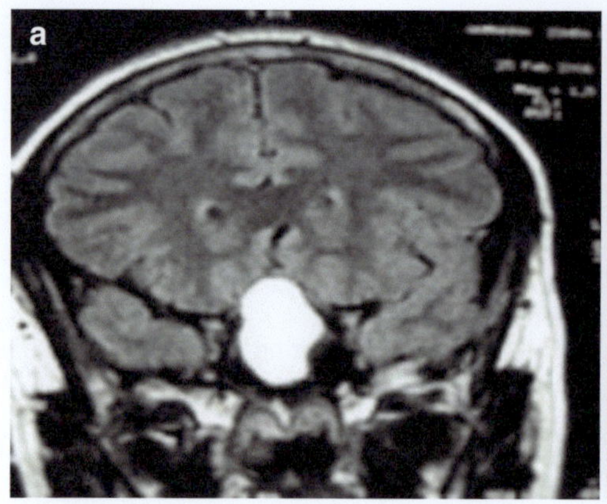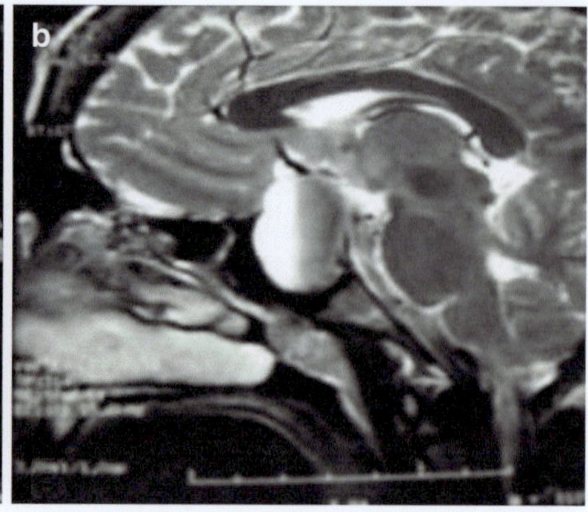

MIR brain, coronal (**a**), and sagittal (**b**) views. (Source: Chegour, H., Ansari, N. E. CC-BY 2.0 (https://creativecommons.org/licenses/by/2.0/) via *PanAfrican Medical Journal*. Image has been cropped from source. Please see full attribution with citation below in references section for this question.)

A. Hyponatremia
B. Hypothyroidism
C. Ophthalmoplegia
D. A and B
E. All of the above
Correct answer: E

Explanation

Pituitary apoplexy leads to hypopituitarism. This may result in hyponatremia (due to disruption of antidiuretic hormone [ADH]), hypothyroidism (due to disruption of thyroid stimulating hormone [TSH]), and hypocortisolism with resultant hypoglycemia and hyponatremia (due to disruption of adrenocorticotropic hormone [ACTH] and resultant cortisol production, respectively).

Ophthalmoplegia may also occur, due to compression by the apoplectic pituitary of cranial nerves III, IV, and VI passing through the cavernous sinus just lateral to the pituitary.

Reference

Chegour H, El Ansari N. Pituitary apoplexy during pregnancy. Pan Afr Med J. 2014;17:211. https://doi.org/10.11604/pamj.2014.17.211.4133.

Linked question

43. For the patient in the prior question, what is recommended for management of the above clinical scenario?
    A. Steroids
    B. Surgical consultation
    C. Pain management
    D. B and C
    E. All of the above
    Correct answer: E

Explanation

Pituitary apoplexy is considered a medical emergency. Surgery should be considered early in the disease course, and patients should be treated with IV glucocorticoids to treat adrenal insufficiency. In some cases, endogenous thyroxine must be used to treat hypothyroidism as well.

Given the acute and severe onset of headache, pain should be effectively managed as soon as possible as well.

Reference

Iglesias P. Pituitary Apoplexy: An Updated Review. J Clin Med. 2024;13(9). https://doi.org/10.3390/jcm13092508.

Linked questions: 44–45

44. A 68-year-old man presents to your clinic for the evaluation of a headache that started 3 weeks ago. He notes an episode of transient visual change in his left eye only, saying "things went black" for a few minutes. He otherwise describes having a reduced appetite. He notes he has recently visited several dentists for evaluation of pain with chewing. What is the most likely diagnosis based on this clinical scenario?
    A. Retinal migraine
    B. Migraine with visual aura
    C. Chronic migraine
    D. Giant cell arteritis
    E. Focal seizure
    Correct answer: D

Explanation

This elderly patient with transient *monocular* visual changes and jaw claudication (pain with chewing/motion) most likely has giant cell arteritis (GCA). GCA is an immune-mediated medium to large vessel vasculitis that can cause visual impairment (such as amaurosis fugax here), jaw claudication, constitutional symptoms, and local scalp tenderness. On exam, temporal artery tenderness or fullness may be, but is not always, observed.

Retinal migraine also causes monocular visual disturbances, but typically involves positive phenomena. While it is possible to have scotomas or transient blindness with retinal migraine, the other associated symptoms in this vignette make GCA the cannot miss diagnosis.

Similar to retinal migraine, migraine with visual aura and focal seizures affecting vision would typically involve positive phenomena. Although migraine could reduce appetite and cause pain involving the V3 region (the jaw), jaw *claudication* would not be likely. Further, it would be unusual for a migraine with visual aura or focal visual seizures to be monocular as described in this case.

Chronic migraine requires headache to be present for at least 15 days per month for at least 3 months.

References

Headache Classification Committee of the International Headache Society (IHS) The International Classification of Headache Disorders, 3rd edition. Cephalalgia. 2018;38(1):1–211. https://doi.org/10.1177/0333102417738202.

Lee AW, Chen C, Cugati S. Temporal arteritis. Neurol Clin Pract. 2014;4(2):106–13. https://doi.org/10.1212/CPJ.0b013e3182a9c62a.

Linked question

45. You inform the patient in the prior question of what you think the diagnosis could be. Which of the following is the best next step?
    A. Prescribe a preventive agent, as his headache is happening frequently enough
    B. Schedule a temporal artery biopsy
    C. Immediately obtain blood tests and prescribe prednisone
    D. Obtain an EEG
    E. All of the above
    Correct answer: C

Explanation

When there is a high clinical suspicion for giant cell arteritis (GCA) and potential visual compromise, prednisone should be prescribed right away. Further, blood tests, namely erythrocyte sedimentation rate (ESR) and C-reactive protein (CRP), should be sent to the lab as soon as possible.

A preventive agent is not indicated, as this is a secondary headache and should be managed by treating the underlying cause.

A temporal artery biopsy (TAB) is gold standard for diagnosing GCA. However, this patient has already had at least one episode of amaurosis fugax, and prednisone should not be delayed for other diagnostic tests or evaluations.

An EEG would be indicated if concern for epileptogenic etiology.

Linked questions: 46–47

46. A 24-year-old woman with a past medical history of systemic lupus erythematosus (SLE) presents to the emergency department for evaluation of headache. She notes that the headache is worse when lying down and better when sitting up, gradually started 2 weeks ago and has progressively worsened in severity. She does not usually get headaches. She denies any medication or supplement use aside from oral contraceptives. Which of the following tests (if any) should be obtained?
    A. No imaging, patient should be reassured and discharged with outpatient neurology follow-up
    B. Non-contrast head CT
    C. CT angiogram of neck
    D. MRI brain and MR venogram of brain
    E. Lumbar puncture
    Correct answer: D

Explanation

In this young woman with a new positional headache (suggestive of high intracranial pressure [ICP]), a history of a rheumatologic disease, and on an oral contraceptive, secondary headache should be suspected, namely cerebral venous sinus thrombosis (CVST).

For patients on estrogen therapy, specifically, presenting with a positional headache, the venous system should be further evaluated with brain MR venography (or CT venography). Also on the differential would be any space-occupying lesions, which would be best evaluated with brain MRI with and without contrast.

Non-contrast head CTs are best at evaluating bone and blood. Given you are more suspicious of a venous or parenchymal problem, this can be skipped. It is also good, if able, to avoid the unnecessary radiation that comes to CT scans.

Lumbar punctures (LPs) should not be pursued unless a space-occupying lesion is first ruled out, as there is a theoretical chance of brain herniation if performed prior to brain imaging.

Reference

van Crevel H, Hijdra A, de Gans J. Lumbar puncture and the risk of herniation: when should we first perform CT? J Neurol. 2002;249(2):129–37. https://doi.org/10.1007/pl00007855.

Linked question

47. For the patient in the prior question, imaging is obtained and shown below, what would you most likely see on ophthalmic evaluation?

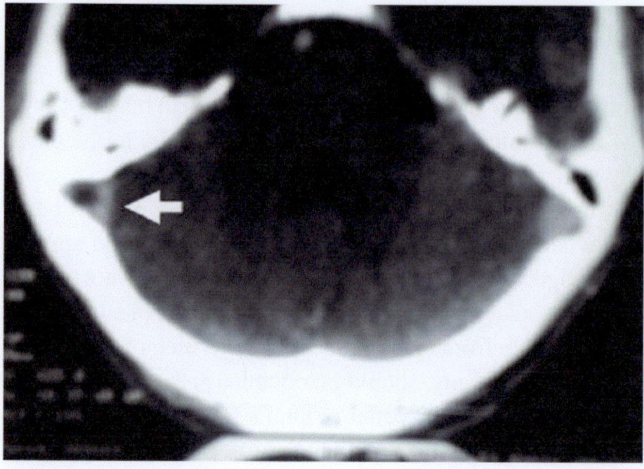

Axial CT. (Source: Souirti, Z., Messouak, O., Belahsen F. CC-BY 2.0 (https://creativecommons.org/licenses/by/2.0/) via PanAfrican Medical Journal. Image has not been modified from source. Please see full attribution with citation below in references section for this question.)

A. Relative afferent pupillary defect
B. Absence of venous pulsations
C. Cherry red spot
D. Altitudinal visual field defect
E. Enlarged cup to disc ratio
Correct answer: B

Explanation

The imaging shows a cerebral venous sinus thrombosis (CVST) in the right lateral sinus. In patients with CVST, you would expect to see one or more ophthalmic features of increased intracranial pressure (ICP), which may include hyperemia, blurring of optic disc margins (papilledema), absence of venous pulsations, venous dilation, and/or flame hemorrhages.

Relative afferent pupillary defect (RAPD) would be expected in optic neuritis.

Cherry-red spot can be seen in various genetic conditions, such as Tay–Sachs and Niemann Pick's disease, or in central retinal artery occlusion.

Enlarged cup-to-disc ratio can occur in conditions such as glaucoma or optic neuritis.

Reference

Souirti Z, Messouak O, Belahsen F. Cerebral venous thrombosis: a Moroccan retrospective study of 30 cases. Pan Afr Med J. 2014;17:281. https://doi.org/10.11604/pamj.2014.17.281.165.

Linked questions: 48–49

48. A 35-year-old male presents to your neurology clinic for evaluation. He notes an increase in his migraine frequency over the past 5 years. He also notes that his father had similar progression of his migraines and more recently has suffered from several strokes. You suspect a genetic etiology of the patient's symptoms. Which chromosome is most likely affected?
A. Chromosome 9
B. Chromosome 19
C. Chromosome 20
D. Chromosome 17
E. Chromosome 7
Correct answer: B

Explanation

The genetic syndrome described is most likely Cerebral Autosomal Dominant Arteriopathy with Subcortical Infarcts and Leukoencephalopathy (CADASIL). As the name implies, this is an autosomal dominant condition and is due to a mutation of the NOTCH3 gene on chromosome 19. The clinical presentation varies, but often starts as typical migraine headache in a patient's 30s. Later in life, it develops into recurrent strokes and dementia. A majority of patients with CADASIL and migraine do experience aura. The strokes are typically subcortical with classical lacunar syndromes.

Reference

Di Donato I, Bianchi S, De Stefano N, Dichgans M, Dotti MT, Duering M, et al. Cerebral Autosomal Dominant Arteriopathy with Subcortical Infarcts and Leukoencephalopathy (CADASIL) as a model of small vessel disease: update on clinical, diagnostic, and management aspects. BMC Med. 2017;15(1):41. https://doi.org/10.1186/s12916-017-0778-8.

Linked question

49. For the patient in the prior question, what MRI finding is most specific for this condition?
A. Cortical microbleeds
B. Hyperintensities in the anterior temporal lobes
C. Diffuse microvascular ischemic changes
D. Congenital narrowing of the cerebral aqueduct
E. Slit-like ventricles
Correct answer: B

Explanation

In CADASIL, patients are most likely to have anterior temporal lobe changes. This has been reported to have a high sensitivity and specificity (90%).

Cortical microbleeds may be seen in cerebral amyloid angiopathy (CAA). CAA can have variable presentations, including stroke-like episodes, headaches, a stepwise decline in cognition, and thus, it should be included in the differential diagnosis for this patient. However, the described progression from migraine at onset to later-stage disease symptoms in a first-degree relative makes CADASIL the most likely correct diagnosis in this instance. CAA can may also result in lobar hemorrhages. The diagnosis of CAA is primarily made by brain biopsy postmortem.

Diffuse microvascular ischemic changes may be present in CADASIL, but it is found in other conditions as well; hence, this finding is not specific to this condition.

Congenital narrowing of the cerebral aqueduct would result in an obstructive hydrocephalus, which is not the likely cause of this patient's clinical syndrome.

Slit-like ventricles may be present in conditions of cerebrospinal fluid (CSF) pressure dysregulation and is unlikely to be present in this patient.

Reference

Di Donato I, Bianchi S, De Stefano N, Dichgans M, Dotti MT, Duering M, et al. Cerebral Autosomal Dominant Arteriopathy with Subcortical Infarcts and Leukoencephalopathy (CADASIL) as a model of small vessel disease: update on clinical, diagnostic, and management aspects. BMC Med. 2017;15(1):41. https://doi.org/10.1186/s12916-017-0778-8.

50. A 24-year-old man presents to your clinic with episodic neck pain and headache. He was told by another neurologist that his symptoms are due to a Chiari malformation recently seen on neuroimaging. You have access to the images and confirm the cerebellar tonsils descend approximately 3 mm below the foramen magnum. On further history, he endorses accompanying sensitivity to light and sound but no nausea. Headaches last 5–6 h if untreated, but improve within 1 h following a combination of acetaminophen and ibuprofen. He thinks lack of sleep may be a trigger. Headaches are not positional, and he denies headache worsening with coughing or Valsalva maneuver. What is the best message to convey to this patient about what is causing his symptoms?
    A. You should see a surgeon to correct the Chiari malformation
    B. You should have a CT myelogram to evaluate for the presence of a CSF leak
    C. Your pain is likely caused by migraine, let's discuss various options for treatment
    D. The Chiari malformation is unlikely to be contributing to your headache
    E. Both C and D

Correct answer: E

Explanation

Chiari type I malformations may contribute to head and neck pain, but the severity typically depends on the severity of the malformation. Chiari malformations <5 mm below the foramen magnum are considered mild and are unlikely to be symptomatic. Headache attributed to Chiari malformation type I, as per the International Classification of Headache Disorders-3 (ICHD-3), would be precipitated by cough or Valsalva maneuver and/or associated with other symptoms and/or clinical signs of brainstem, cerebellar, lower cranial nerve, and/or cervical spinal cord dysfunction. Taken together, this patient likely has migraine given associated photophobia, phonophobia, and improvement in symptoms with over-the-counter medications.

Surgery would not be indicated for a mild, asymptomatic Chiari malformation.

Cerebrospinal fluid (CSF) leak should be on the differential when a "Chiari malformation" is called by radiology given it's potential to cause downward displacement of the cerebellar tonsils. Clinicians should ask about a positional nature (improvement with lying flat?) and about any triggering event(s) or trauma potentially associated with the headache onset.

Reference

Smith JH. Other Primary Headache Disorders. Continuum (Minneap Minn). 2021;27(3):652–64. https://doi.org/10.1212/con.0000000000000960.

Parmpreet Dhillon and Priya Purushothaman

Linked questions: 1–2

1. A 5-day-old born at 40 weeks of gestation with a normal head size after an uncomplicated birth presents with an episode of tonic stiffening of the right side. Several hours later, he has another seizure with tonic stiffening of the left side. Neurologic exam, Interictal EEG and MRI are unremarkable.

   Which of the following statements best describes the most likely prognosis for the child?
   A. Seizures often spontaneously resolve by age 6 months
   B. This patient has a diagnosis of hypoxic ischemic encephalopathy
   C. Seizures often require lifelong treatment
   D. Most patients with this syndrome have developmental delay
   Correct answer: A

Explanation

Onset of focal motor seizures between days 2 and 7 of age is typical in self-limited neonatal seizures, which previously used to be called "fifth day fits." Imaging and interictal EEG are expected to be normal—abnormal testing would suggest an alternative diagnosis. Despite frequent seizures, the neonate behaves normally between seizures, and seizures remit without impact on development.

Hypoxic Ischemic Encephalopathy (HIE) is the most common cause of neonatal seizures, but would likely have a history of a complicated birth, abnormal neurologic exam at birth, and abnormal MRI.

An abnormal interictal EEG, neurologic exam, or MRI may increase likelihood of refractory seizures and abnormal development.

P. Dhillon (✉) · P. Purushothaman
Division of Epilepsy, Department of Neurology, NYU Langone Health, New York, NY, USA
e-mail: Parmpreet.Dhillon@nyulangone.org; Priya.Purushothaman@nyulangone.org

Reference

International League Against Epilepsy (2024). SELF-LIMITED (FAMILIAL) NEONATAL EPILEPSY (SeLNE). https://www.epilepsydiagnosis.org/syndrome/self-limited-neonatal-overview.html. Accessed 30 Apr. 2025

Linked question

2. This patient's father reports that he also had a history of seizures as a neonate. What gene are you most likely to find a pathogenic mutation in?
   A. MECP2
   B. KCNQ2
   C. CHRNA4
   D. CDKL5
   Correct answer: B

Explanation

Self-limited neonatal seizures can be non-familial or familial. Pathogenic variants in KCNQ2 are the most common cause; pathogenic variants in KCNQ3 and in SCN2A are also reported. De novo variants of the same genes are responsible for the syndrome in neonates without family history.

Mutations in MECP2 lead to Rett Syndrome, a neurodevelopmental disorder primarily affecting girls, characterized by developmental regression, motor dysfunction, and autistic-like behavior.

Mutations in CHRNA4 can lead to autosomal dominant nocturnal frontal lobe epilepsy (ADNFLE), which is a genetic epilepsy syndrome characterized by seizures during sleep.

Mutations in the CDKL5 gene can lead to CDKL5 deficiency syndrome, a developmental and epileptic encephalopathy characterized by early-onset, often intractable, seizures, global developmental delay, and other neurological impairments.

Reference

International League Against Epilepsy (2024). SELF-LIMITED (FAMILIAL) NEONATAL EPILEPSY (SeLNE). https://www.epilepsydiagnosis.org/syndrome/self-limited-neonatal-genetics.html. Accessed 30 Apr. 2025.

3. A 1-day-old with microcephaly and hypotonia is noted to have episodes of stiffening. During video EEG, he is noted to have numerous tonic seizures. This is his background EEG:

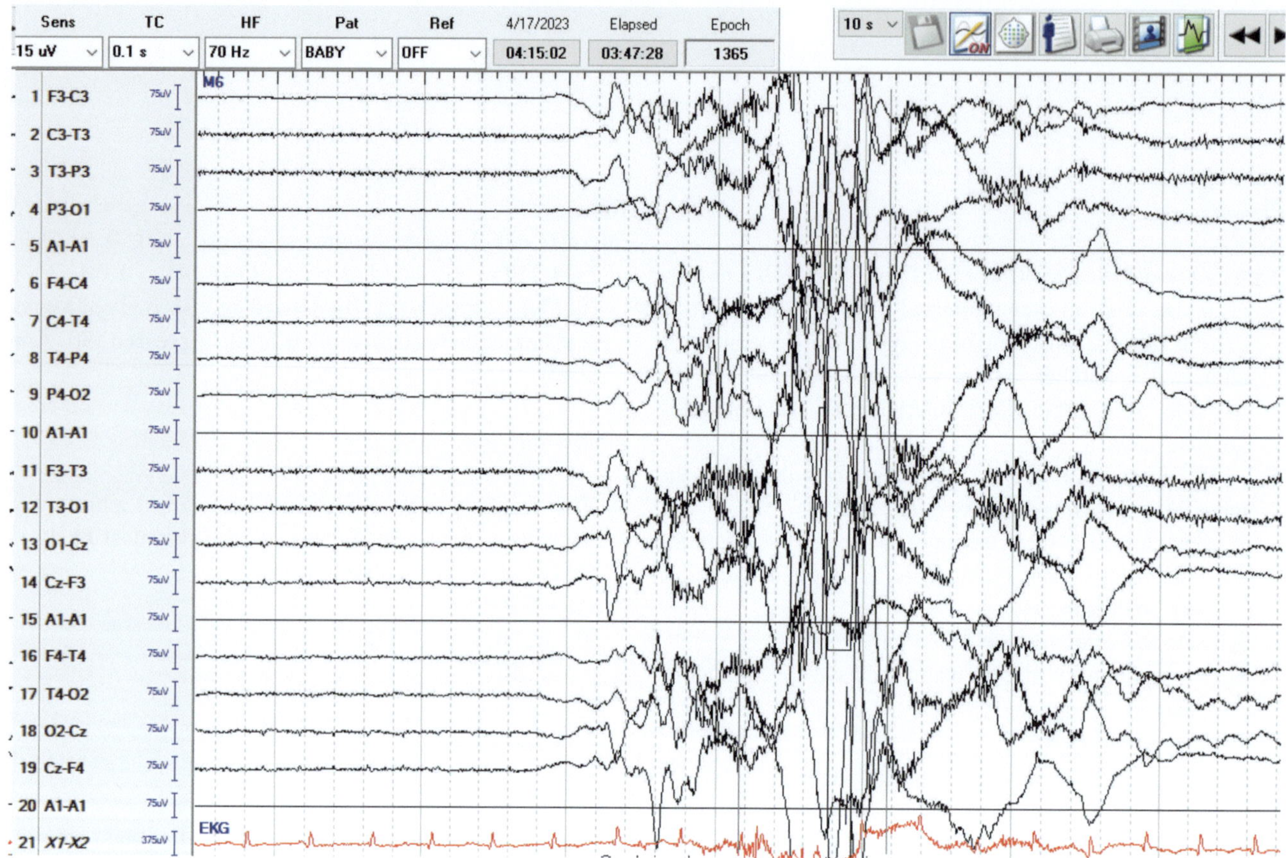

Background EEG of 1-day-old with hypotonia and tonic seizures. (Source: De-identified image courtesy of Dr. Parmpreet Dhillon, New York University Langone Health)

Which of the following is most likely true?
A. Patient is not at risk of developing other seizure types
B. Most patients with this syndrome will have normal developmental progress
C. Neuroimaging, metabolic, or genetic testing is likely to be positive
D. EEG will eventually normalize

Correct answer: C

Explanation

This EEG shows burst suppression.

Early infantile [developmental] epileptic encephalopathy (EIDEE) presents with medically refractory seizures in the early infantile period (0–3 months). Background EEG is notable for either burst-suppression or multifocal epileptiform discharges with diffuse slowing. Most children will have moderate to profound developmental impairment. A cause can be found in ~80% of cases. Seizures are usually medically intractable unless a treatable structural, genetic, or metabolic cause is found.

Previously known as separate entities, Early Myoclonic Encephalopathy (EME) and Early Infantile Epileptic

Encephalopathy (EIEE)/Ohtahara Syndrome are now both classified under Early Infantile Developmental and Epileptic Encephalopathy (EIDEE) in the 2021 International League against Epilepsy (ILAE) classification of epilepsy syndromes papers. EME may present with early myoclonus and later focal seizures and tonic spasms, and Ohtahara Syndrome may present with tonic spasms and later focal seizures and myoclonus.

References

International League Against Epilepsy (2024). Neonatal seizure. https://www.epilepsydiagnosis.org/seizure/neonatal-seizure-overview.html. Accessed 30 Apr. 2025.

International League Against Epilepsy (2024). Early-Infantile DEE. https://www.epilepsydiagnosis.org/syndrome/eme-overview.html. Accessed 30 Apr. 2025

Pressler RM, Cilio MR, Mizrahi EM, Moshé SL, Nunes ML, Plouin P, Vanhatalo S, Yozawitz E, de Vries LS, Puthenveettil Vinayan K, Triki CC, Wilmshurst JM, Yamamoto H, Zuberi SM. The ILAE classification of seizures and the epilepsies: Modification for seizures in the neonate. Position paper by the ILAE Task Force on Neonatal Seizures. Epilepsia. 2021 Mar;62(3):615–628. https://doi.org/10.1111/epi.16815. Epub 2021 Feb 1. PMID: 33522601.

4. What is the most common cause of neonatal seizures?
   A. Self-limited neonatal seizures
   B. Hypoxic-ischemic encephalopathy
   C. Early myoclonic encephalopathy
   D. Early epileptic encephalopathy/Ohtahara syndrome
   Correct answer: B

Explanation

Symptomatic neonatal seizures (or acute provoked seizures) provoked by an acute illness or brain insult are responsible for the majority of seizures in a neonate (~85%). Hypoxic-ischemic encephalopathy (HIE) may present as a newborn with signs of encephalopathy (low APGARs, decreased level of consciousness, decreased spontaneous activity, abnormal posture, tone, or reflexes), abnormal autonomic status, or abnormal blood gas analysis after a hypoxic-ischemic event occurring in the prenatal or intrapartum period.

Other neonatal epilepsy syndromes account for ~15% of neonatal seizures.

Reference

Gunasekaran V, Ighodaro ET, Govil-Dalela T. Neonatal Seizures and Neonatal Epilepsy. [Updated 2024 Nov 14]. In: StatPearls [Internet]. Treasure Island (FL): StatPearls Publishing; 2025 Jan-. Available from: https://www.ncbi.nlm.nih.gov/books/NBK609108/

5. A 6-month-old with Trisomy 21 presents with events characterized by a brief head drop and elevation of both arms occurring many times a day, clustered after awakening. These two images capture her background and the event of concern.

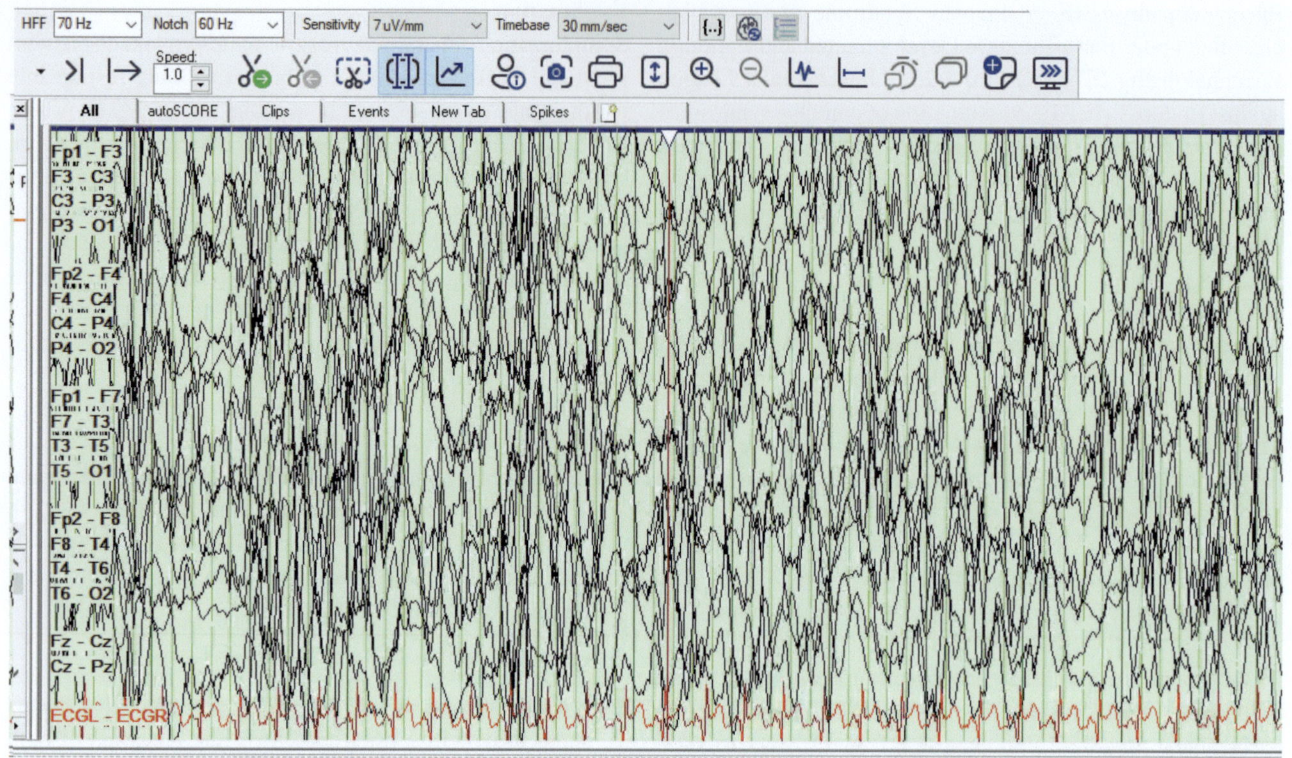

Background EEG. (Source: De-identified image courtesy of Dr. Parmpreet Dhillon, New York University Langone Health)

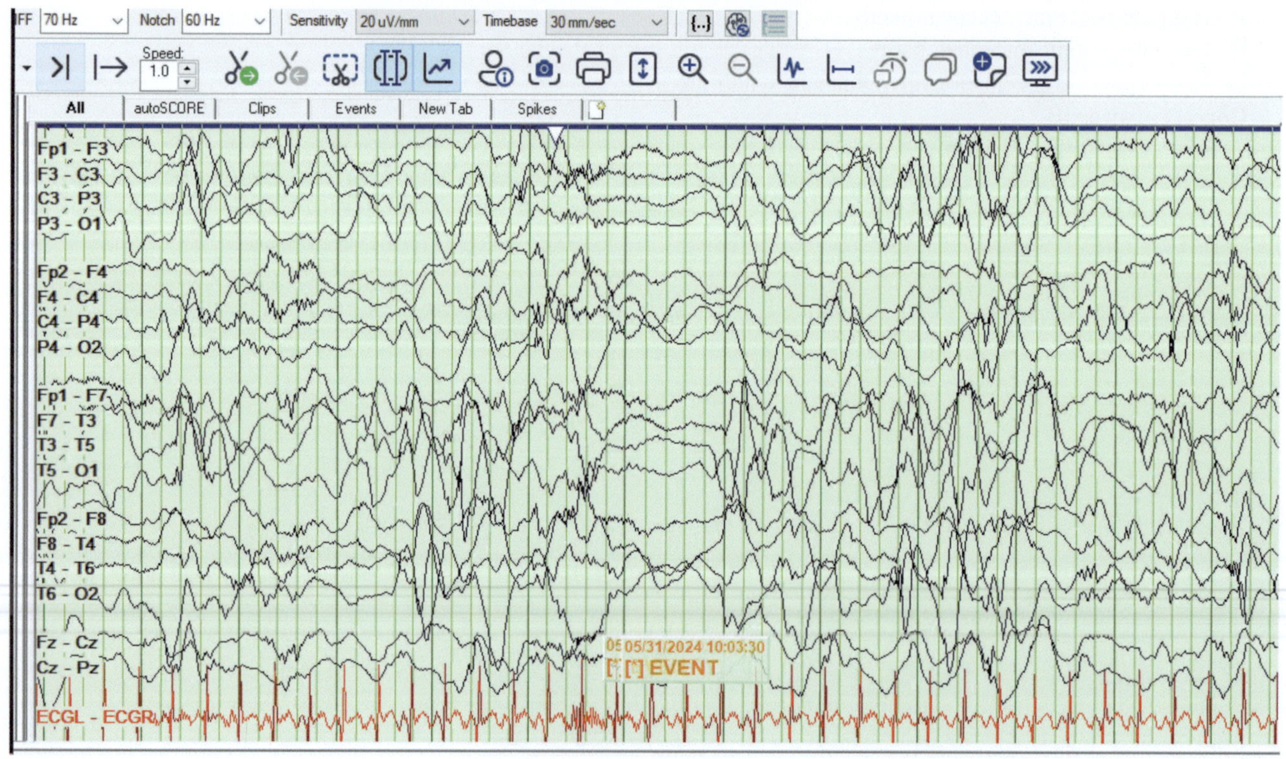

Event of concern. (Source: De-identified image courtesy of Dr. Parmpreet Dhillon, New York University Langone Health)

What is the best treatment for this patient's diagnosis?

A. Adrenocorticotropic hormone (ACTH)
B. Vigabatrin
C. Fosphenytoin
D. Phenobarbital
E. Carbamazepine
Correct answer: A

Explanation

The first image, which is at a sensitivity of 7 µV/mm, is notable for high-amplitude disorganized (no anterior-to-posterior gradient) slow waves with multifocal spikes (which may be better visualized in the second image), consistent with hypsarrhythmia. The second image, which is at a sensitivity of 20 µV/mm (decreasing the sensitivity from 7 to 20 makes the higher amplitude activity easier to see), is notable for a high-voltage slow wave, relative voltage attenuation, and overriding low-voltage fast activity at the time of the event, consistent with an epileptic spasm. EMG leads (in this case, EKG lead) can show a rhomboid shape during the spasm.

Epileptic spasms include a sudden flexion, extension, or mixed movement of proximal and truncal muscles lasting 1–2 s, typically occurring in a cluster on wakening. Infantile epileptic spasms syndrome is characterized by the onset of epileptic spasms in infancy (age 1–24 months). This syndrome includes West syndrome, where patients have a triad of epileptic spasms, hypsarrhythmia on EEG, and developmental plateauing or regression.

Steroids (primarily ACTH) are considered first-line therapy for infantile spasms in most children. In an infant with infantile spasms and tuberous sclerosis, vigabatrin is considered first-line treatment. Traditional antiseizure medications such as fosphenytoin, phenobarbital, and carbamazepine are not considered effective for epileptic spasms. Phenobarbital is considered the first line in the treatment of neonatal seizures.

References

International League Against Epilepsy (2024). Infantile Epileptic Spasms Syndrome. https://www.epilepsydiagnosis.org/syndrome/west-syndrome-overview.html. Accessed 30 Apr. 2025. https://www.ilae.org/files/ilae-Guideline/Summary-of-recommendations-for-infantile-seizures%2D%2D-Wilmshurst_et_al-2015-Epilepsia.pdf

Smith MS, Matthews R, Rajnik M, et al. Infantile Epileptic Spasms Syndrome (West Syndrome) [Updated 2024 Feb 1]. In: StatPearls [Internet]. Treasure Island (FL): StatPearls Publishing; 2025 Jan-. Available from: https://www.ncbi.nlm.nih.gov/books/NBK537251/

Taha M, Nordli DR 3rd, Kacker S, Oetomo A, Phitsanuwong C, Nordli DR Jr. Electroclinical features of myoclonic- tonic and spasm-tonic seizures in childhood. Epileptic Disord. 2024 Jun;26(3):369–374. https://doi.org/10.1002/epd2.20213. Epub 2024 Mar 27. PMID: 38536013.

Linked question: 6–7

6. A 6-month-old presents for evaluation after a prolonged seizure described as left arm and leg jerking that occurred in the setting of fever. She is discharged with a prescription for rectal diazepam as needed for future prolonged febrile seizures. A month later, she is noted to have frequent prolonged convulsions without fever. Her EEG shows generalized 2.5 Hz spike wave complexes. A year later, she is noted to have myoclonic seizures, developmental delay, and regression. Which of the following is the most likely diagnosis?
A. Childhood Absence Epilepsy
B. Early Myoclonic Encephalopathy
C. Epilepsy with Myoclonic and Atonic Seizures
D. Epilepsy of infancy with migrating focal seizures
E. Dravet Syndrome
Correct answer: E

Linked question

7. This 6-month-old from the prior question was found to have a loss of function mutation in SCN1A. Which of the following anti-seizure medications would be most appropriate to start?
A. Phenytoin
B. Valproic Acid
C. Ethosuximide
D. Lacosamide
E. Carbamazepine
Correct answer: B

Explanation

Onset of prolonged febrile hemi-convulsions in the first year of life, followed by drug-resistant afebrile seizures, other seizure types, and cognitive and behavioral impairments, is characteristic of Dravet Syndrome. The clinical diagnosis is supported by the presence of a loss-of-function mutation in the sodium channel gene SCN1A (found in over 80% of cases).

Anti-seizure medications that have sodium channel blocking properties, such as phenytoin, cenobamate, lacosamide, and carbamazepine, may aggravate seizures in this syndrome. The Dravet Foundation, based on an International Consensus Panel Study, recommends valproic acid as first-line treatment.

Childhood Absence Epilepsy (CAE) is characterized by frequent absence seizures between the age of 4 and 11 years old with EEG showing 3–4 Hz generalized spike wave discharges. Development is typically normal until seizure onset, but learning difficulties may appear. A majority of children outgrow this type of epilepsy. Ethosuximide is first-line treatment for absence seizures.

Early Myoclonic Encephalopathy (EME) is a type of Early Infantile Developmental and Epileptic encephalopathy (EIDEE) that typically presents in the neonatal or early infantile age with tonic, atonic, myoclonic seizures but may also have hemi-convulsions. EEG shows a burst-suppression pattern. Severe developmental delay and poor neurologic outcomes are typical.

Epilepsy with Myoclonic–Atonic seizures (previously known as Doose Syndrome) presents with predominantly myoclonic and atonic (though also generalized tonic–clonic) seizures in infancy to early childhood. EEG may be normal initially but may then show generalized spike and wave epileptiform discharges. Developmental delay may or may not be present. Two-thirds of patients outgrow this type of epilepsy.

Epilepsy of Infancy with Migrating Focal Seizures presents as frequent intractable multifocal seizures that can migrate from one cortical region to another in the same seizure. Characterized as a developmental and epileptic encephalopathy, infants may be normally developing until age 6 months, then may have developmental regression and microcephaly. Mutations in KCNT1 are the most common cause.

References

Dravet Foundation (2024). Diagnosis and Treatment. https://dravetfoundation.org/hcp-resources/diagnosis-and-treatment/. Accessed 30 Apr. 2025

Gogou M, Cross JH. Seizures and epilepsy in childhood. Continuum Lifelong Learning Neurol. 2022 Apr;28(2):428–456.

International League Against Epilepsy (2024). Dravet Syndrome. https://www.epilepsydiagnosis.org/syndrome/dravet-overview.html. Accessed 30 Apr. 2025

8. A 6-month-old developmentally normal child presents with frequent myoclonic jerks provoked by sudden noises. EEG shows 3 Hz polyspike and wave at the time of a myoclonic jerk that is triggered by photic stimulation. These events stop after 1 year, though he is noted to have developmental delay. What is his most likely diagnosis?
   A. Severe myoclonic epilepsy of infancy
   B. Benign myoclonus of infancy
   C. Myoclonic epilepsy of infancy
   D. Progressive myoclonic epilepsy
   Correct answer: C

Explanation

A myoclonic jerk occurring at the same time of a 3 Hz polyspike wave is consistent with myoclonic seizure. Frequent myoclonic seizures activated by photic stimulation, sudden noise, or touch that begin in infancy and self-remit within 6 months to 5 years of onset are typical in myoclonic epilepsy of infancy. Prior development is usually normal, and developmental outcome is normal in 60–85% of cases.

"Benign" myoclonus of infancy is characterized by episodes lasting 1–2 s with normal ictal and interictal EEG recordings. These occur in the first year of life and usually spontaneously resolve by age 2.

In Dravet Syndrome, previously known as severe myoclonic epilepsy of infancy, myoclonic seizures may be frequent; however, they typically occur in the second year of life, after a period of prolonged febrile seizures.

Progressive myoclonic epilepsies include Lafora body disease, Unverricht–Lundborg disease, mitochondrial encephalopathy with ragged-red fibers, type 3 neuronopathic Gaucher Disease, neuronal ceroid lipofuscinosis, and sialidosis. These epilepsies may present in late childhood or adolescence and are characterized by multiple seizures (myoclonic or tonic–clonic), progressive neurologic deterioration including ataxia, and/or dementia.

References

Balasundaram P, Anilkumar AC. Myoclonic Epilepsy of Infancy. [Updated 2025 Jan 22]. In: StatPearls [Internet]. Treasure Island (FL): StatPearls Publishing; 2025 Jan-. Available from: https://www.ncbi.nlm.nih.gov/books/NBK570566/

International League Against Epilepsy (2024). Epilepsy Imitators. https://www.epilepsydiagnosis.org/epilepsy-imitators.html#shud-attacks. Accessed 30 Apr. 2025

International League Against Epilepsy (2024). Myoclonic Epilepsy in Infancy. https://www.epilepsydiagnosis.org/syndrome/mei-overview.html. Accessed 30 Apr. 2025

9. A 5-year-old developmentally normal child has an episode of awakening from sleep, looks pale, vomits several times, and loses consciousness. This is followed by gaze deviation to the right and a bilateral tonic–clonic convulsion lasting for 30 min. Interictal EEG is notable for occipital spikes on a background with normal frequencies. Developmental progress is normal.
   Which of the following is the most likely diagnosis?
   A. Lennox–Gastaut Syndrome
   B. Self-limited epilepsy with autonomic seizures (Panayiotopoulos syndrome)
   C. Childhood epilepsy with centrotemporal spikes
   D. Childhood occipital visual epilepsy (Gastaut type)
   Correct answer: B

Explanation

Self-limited epilepsy with autonomic seizures (formerly known as Panayiotopoulos syndrome or early-onset benign occipital epilepsy) is characterized by the onset of focal autonomic seizures in early childhood that are often prolonged. The EEG commonly shows high-amplitude focal spikes typically activated by sleep, which may be focal or multifocal, particularly in the occipital region. Seizures are infrequent in most patients. Seizures are self-limiting with remission typically within a few years from onset.

Childhood occipital visual epilepsy, previously known as late-onset (benign) childhood occipital epilepsy or idiopathic childhood occipital epilepsy-Gastaut type, is characterized by focal sensory visual seizures in wakefulness. Seizures are brief but frequent, and they usually respond to anti-seizure medication and remit by puberty.

Lennox–Gastaut Syndrome is characterized by multiple seizure types (particularly tonic seizures) that are drug-resistant, cognitive, and behavioral impairments that may not be present at seizure onset, diffuse slow spike-wave, and generalized paroxysmal fast activity on EEG.

Self-limited epilepsy with centrotemporal spikes, previously known as benign childhood epilepsy with centrotemporal spikes or rolandic epilepsy, is characterized by hemifacial sensorimotor seizures that may evolve to focal to bilateral tonic–clonic seizures. This may occur in an otherwise normal child, and seizures often remit by puberty.

Reference

International League Against Epilepsy (2024). SELF-LIMITED EPILEPSY WITH AUTONOMIC SEIZURES (SeLEAS). https://www.epilepsydiagnosis.org/syndrome/panayiotopoulos-overview.html. Accessed 30 Apr. 2025

10. You see an 8-year-old who reports that once a month they have episodes where they see multicolored circles in their peripheral vision, which may increase in size and move, followed by deviation of the eyes or head, lasting for seconds to minutes. These episodes occur when they are awake only. They have seen ophthalmology, and their visual exam was normal. You perform an EEG, which shows occipital sharps.

    Which of the following is the most likely diagnosis?
    A. Migraine
    B. Self-limited epilepsy with autonomic seizures (Panayiotopoulos syndrome)
    C. Childhood epilepsy with centrotemporal spikes
    D. Childhood occipital visual epilepsy (Gastaut type)
    Correct answer: D

Explanation

Childhood occipital visual epilepsy, previously known as late-onset (benign) childhood occipital epilepsy or idiopathic childhood occipital epilepsy-Gastaut type, is characterized by focal sensory visual seizures in wakefulness. Elementary visual phenomena are typical, described as small multicolored circles seen in the peripheral vision, increasing in areas of the visual field involved and moving horizontally to the other side. This may be followed by gaze deviation or head version. Other occipital lobe seizure features may include blindness, complex visual hallucinations, and/or visual illusions. Seizures are brief but frequent, usually respond to anti-seizure medication and remit by puberty.

Self-limited epilepsy with autonomic seizures (formerly known as Panayiotopoulos syndrome or early-onset benign occipital epilepsy) is characterized by the onset in early childhood of focal autonomic seizures that are often prolonged. The EEG commonly shows high-amplitude focal spikes, typically activated by sleep, which may be focal or multifocal, particularly in the occipital region. Seizures are infrequent in most patients. Seizures are self-limiting with remission typically within a few years from onset.

Self-limited epilepsy with centrotemporal spikes, previously known as benign childhood epilepsy with centrotemporal spikes or benign Rolandic epilepsy, is characterized by hemifacial sensorimotor seizures that may evolve to focal to bilateral tonic–clonic seizures. This may occur in an otherwise normal child, and seizures often remit by puberty. As the name describes, EEG shows spikes in the centrotemporal head region. These spikes may be frequent and activate in drowsiness and sleep. They may be unilateral or bilateral and have a typical triphasic morphology with a transverse dipole (maximum negativity in centrotemporal electrodes C3/C4 and T3/T4 and maximum positivity frontally).

Visual symptoms in migraine auras tend to start more in the center of the visual field and move toward the periphery, whereas epileptic auras tend to start in the periphery. Progression to stereotyped gaze deviation and head version with EEG abnormalities are more characteristic of seizures than migraine.

Reference

International League Against Epilepsy (2024). Childhood Occipital Visual Epilepsy. https://www.epilepsydiagnosis.org/syndrome/late-childhood-occipital-overview.html. Accessed 30 Apr. 2025

11. A 2-year-old previously developmentally normal child presents with frequent seizures described as a brief jerk

and fall to the ground. His development is noted to stagnate. Three years later, he stops having seizures. Which of the following is the most likely diagnosis?

A. Lennox–Gastaut Syndrome
B. Dravet Syndrome
C. Ohtahara Syndrome
D. Doose Syndrome

Correct answer: D

Explanation

Epilepsy with Myoclonic–Atonic seizures (previously known as Doose syndrome) is a syndrome characterized by abrupt onset of multiple generalized seizure types, including myoclonic–atonic seizures in early childhood. Developmental stagnation or regression is typically seen during the phase of active seizures. Despite initially drug-resistant seizures, two-thirds of children can achieve epilepsy remission.

Lennox–Gastaut Syndrome is characterized by multiple seizure types (particularly tonic seizures) that are drug-resistant, cognitive, and behavioral impairments that may not be present at seizure onset, diffuse slow spike-wave, and generalized paroxysmal fast activity on EEG.

Ohtahara Syndrome (now classified under Early Infantile Developmental and Epileptic Encephalopathy/EIDEE) may present in early infancy (0–3 months) with tonic spasms, focal seizures, and myoclonus with a burst-suppression pattern on EEG.

Dravet syndrome is characterized by onset of prolonged febrile hemi-convulsions in the first year of life, followed by drug-resistant afebrile seizures, other seizure types, and cognitive and behavioral impairments.

Reference

International League Against Epilepsy (2024). Epilepsy Myoclonic Atonic Syndrome. https://www.epilepsydiagnosis.org/syndrome/epilepsy-myoclonic-atonic-overview.html. Accessed 30 Apr. 2025

12. A 4-year-old with global developmental delay and a history of refractory infantile spasms comes to your office with a new seizure type in sleep that seems consistent with tonic seizures. You perform an EEG, and his interictal EEG is noted below.

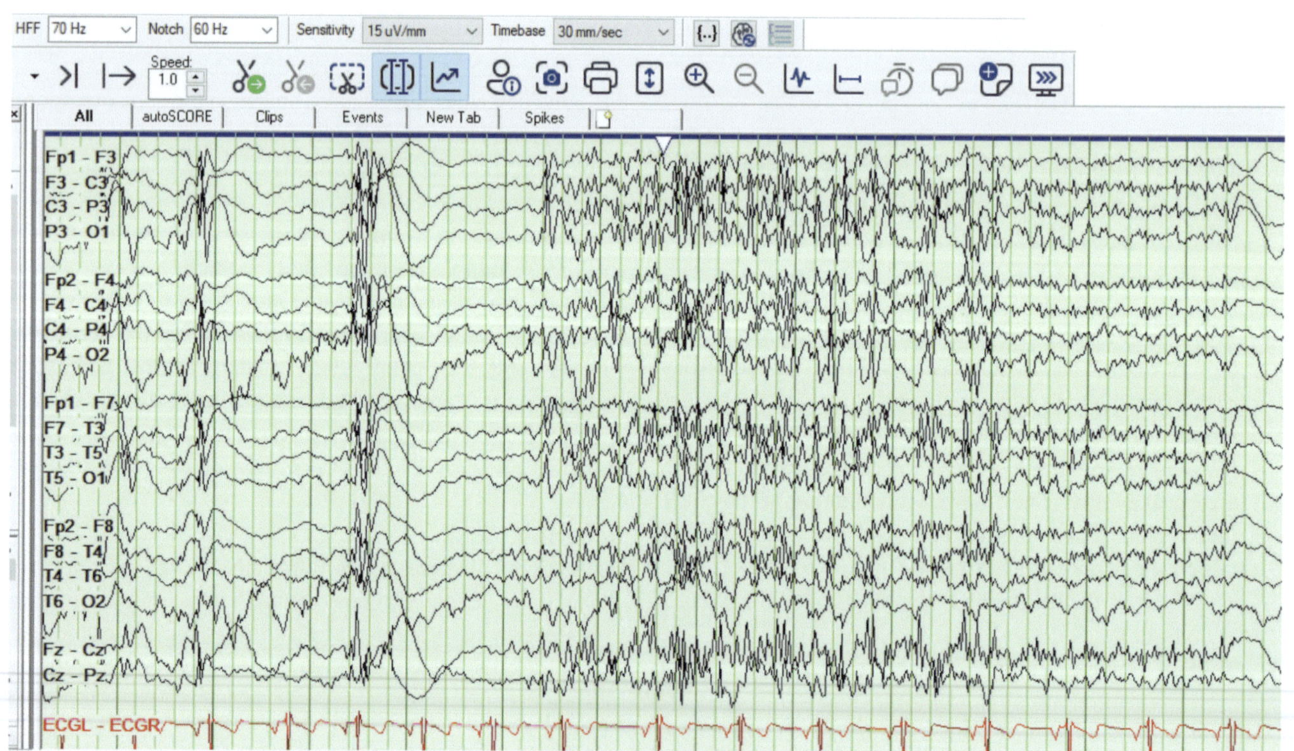

Interictal EEG for a 4 year old with global developmental delay, history of infantile spasms and a new seizure type in sleep. Source: De-identified image courtesy of Dr. Parmpreet Dhillon, New York University Langone Health

What is the most likely diagnosis?
A. Doose Syndrome
B. Panayiotopoulos syndrome
C. Childhood epilepsy with centrotemporal spikes
D. Childhood occipital visual epilepsy (Gastaut type)
E. Lennox–Gastaut Syndrome

Correct answer: E

Explanation

This EEG shows diffuse slow spike waves and paroxysmal fast activity.

Lennox–Gastaut syndrome is characterized by

1. multiple seizure types that are drug resistant (in particular tonic seizures in sleep)
2. cognitive and behavioral impairments (that may not be present at seizure onset) and
3. diffuse slow spike-wave and generalized paroxysmal fast activity on EEG

It is an epilepsy syndrome that can often evolve from a prior epilepsy syndrome/etiology and usually persists into adulthood. Peak age is 3–5 years. Most children have prior developmental impairment, and further stagnation or regression can occur when the syndrome emerges.

Epilepsy with Myoclonic–Atonic seizures (previously known as Doose syndrome) is a syndrome characterized by the usually abrupt onset of multiple generalized seizure types, including myoclonic–atonic seizures in early childhood. The background is normal at onset, and with increased seizure frequency, generalized slowing may be seen.

Self-limited epilepsy with autonomic seizures (formerly known as Panayiotopoulos syndrome or early-onset benign occipital epilepsy) is characterized by infrequent prolonged focal autonomic seizures in early childhood. The EEG commonly shows high-amplitude focal spikes typically activated by sleep, which may be focal or multifocal, particularly in the occipital region with an otherwise normal background.

Self-limited epilepsy with centrotemporal spikes, previously known as benign childhood epilepsy with centrotemporal spikes or Rolandic epilepsy, is characterized by hemifacial sensorimotor seizures that may evolve to focal to bilateral tonic–clonic seizures. EEG shows spikes in the centrotemporal head region with an otherwise normal background.

Childhood occipital visual epilepsy, previously known as late-onset (benign) childhood occipital epilepsy or idiopathic childhood occipital epilepsy-Gastaut type, is characterized by focal sensory visual seizures in wakefulness. EEG shows occipital sharps on an otherwise normal background in the majority of children.

Reference

International League Against Epilepsy (2024). Lennox-Gastaut Syndrome. https://www.epilepsydiagnosis.org/syndrome/lgs-overview.html. Accessed 30 Apr. 2025

Linked questions: 13–14

13. A 9-year-old developmentally normal child has a nocturnal seizure characterized by focal jerking of the left side of the face and hand, salivation, and inability to speak, followed by generalized tonic–clonic movements. The next year, he has a similar event involving the right side. Which of the following is most likely to be seen on EEG?
    A. Temporal spikes
    B. Central/temporal spikes
    C. Frontal spikes
    D. Generalized 3-Hz spike and wave discharges
    E. Generalized slow spike and wave discharges

Correct answer: B

Explanation

Self-limited epilepsy with centrotemporal spikes, previously known as benign childhood epilepsy with centrotemporal spikes or Rolandic epilepsy, is characterized by hemifacial sensorimotor seizures that may evolve to focal to bilateral tonic–clonic seizures. EEG shows spikes in the centrotemporal head region that may be unilateral or bilateral with an otherwise normal background.

Temporal-onset seizures typically consist of behavioral arrest, manual and oral automatisms, and variable degrees of loss of awareness and post-ictal confusion.

Frontal lobe seizures commonly occur from sleep and can appear bizarre with bilateral motor phenomena. They may include various different simple (clonic, tonic posturing, eye deviation) or more complex motor movements (such as cycling, rocking, and grimacing).

Absence seizures with generalized 3 Hz spike waves are typically very short periods of motor and behavior arrest, lasting seconds, without preceding aura or post-ictal confusion, and occur many times a day.

Generalized slow spike waves can be seen in Lennox–Gastaut syndrome, which is characterized by multiple seizure types including tonic seizures.

Linked question

14. You perform an EEG, which shows high-amplitude spikes over the centrotemporal head region that activate in sleep. Which of the following is the most likely true?
    A. Seizures will persist into adulthood
    B. Developmental delay will always be seen
    C. Seizures will self-remit during puberty

D. Scalp EEG would not capture seizures (there is a deep source in the frontal head region)

Correct answer: C

Explanation

In self-limited epilepsy with centrotemporal spikes, spikes are usually high-amplitude centrotemporal in location and activate in sleep. Seizures often remit by puberty. While behavioral or neuropsychological deficits may emerge, these often improve and do not always occur.

Developmental delay and seizures into adulthood would be more expected in Lennox–Gastaut Syndrome, which on EEG is characterized by diffuse slow spike wave and paroxysmal fast activity.

Ictal scalp EEG may show no changes if there is a deep source in the frontal head region, which can be seen in frontal lobe epilepsy.

Reference

Chowdhury FA, Silva R, Whatley B, Walker MC. Localisation in focal epilepsy: a practical guide. Pract Neurol. 2021 Dec;21(6):481-491. https://doi.org/10.1136/practneurol-2019-002341. Epub 2021 Aug 17. PMID: 34404748.

Linked question: 15–16

15. A 7-year-old girl is referred to you by her teacher for episodes of inattentiveness throughout the day. During these episodes, she appears to be daydreaming and does not respond to touch or direct questions from the teacher. She has never had a convulsion. She has a routine EEG done, which captures one of the episodes of inattentiveness.

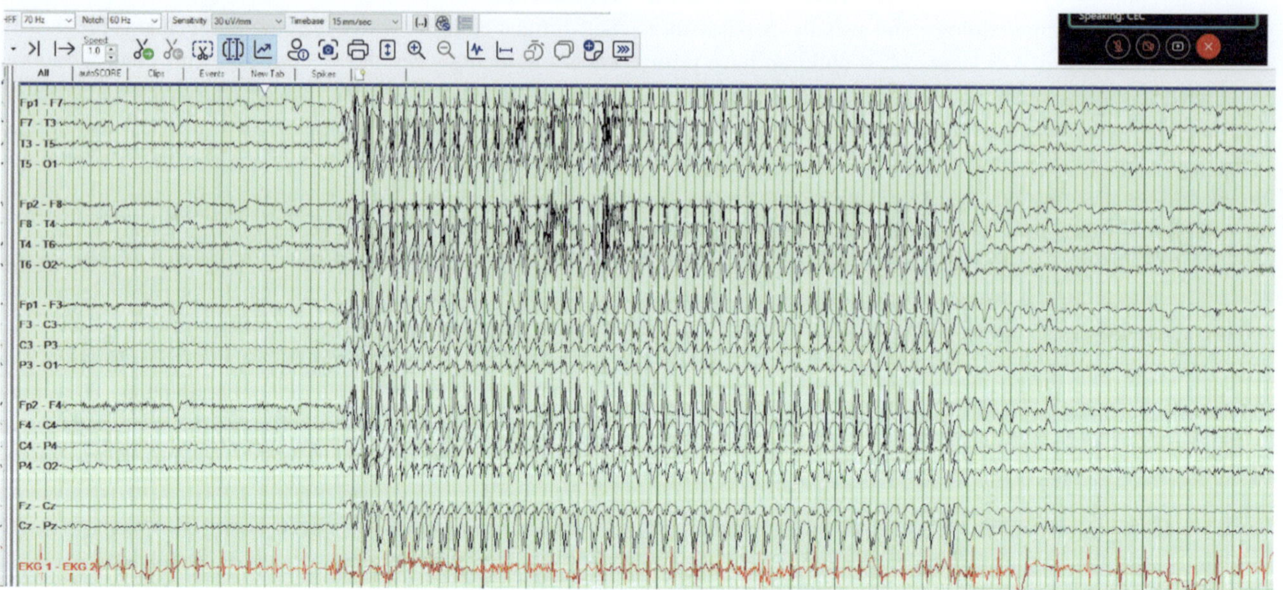

EEG capturing an event of inattentiveness. Source: De-identified image courtesy of Dr. Parmpreet Dhillon, New York University Langone Health

What is the best initial treatment for this patient?
A. Methylphenidate
B. Levetiracetam
C. Valproic Acid
D. Ethosuximide
Correct answer: D

Explanation

This EEG recording is seen at a time base of 15 mm/s, which is more condensed than the typical viewing speed of 30 mm/s, in order to capture the entire episode in one screenshot. This EEG is consistent with a clinical generalized absence seizure with behavioral arrest and altered awareness, associated with 2.5–4 Hz diffuse spike wave. Absence seizures can be provoked by hyperventilation and/or photic stimulation. Targeted treatment is with ethosuximide, which is thought to block T-type calcium channels.

Valproic acid is effective against absence seizures; however, it is known to have a higher rate of side effects. Lamotrigine is the third option for absence seizures, though thought to be less effective than Ethosuximide or Valproic Acid. Levetiracetam has not been shown to be as effective for absence seizures.

Reference

Kessler SK, McGinnis E. A Practical Guide to Treatment of Childhood Absence Epilepsy. Paediatr Drugs. 2019 Feb;21(1):15–24. https://doi.org/10.1007/s40272-019-00325-x. PMID: 30734897; PMCID: PMC6394437.

Linked question

16. The patient in the prior question starts Ethosuximide at a low but effective dose and does not have recurrent absence seizures. However, she returns a year later after having a generalized tonic–clonic seizure. What is your next step?
    A. Increase ethosuximide
    B. Switch to carbamazepine
    C. Add lamotrigine
    D. Tell patient and family that the original diagnosis is incorrect as convulsions never occur in childhood absence epilepsy
    Correct answer: C

Explanation

Ethosuximide is only effective against absence seizures, not generalized tonic–clonic seizures. Evidence for use of levetiracetam as the sole agent for absence seizures is not robust. Valproic acid or lamotrigine may be effective for both absence seizures and convulsions. Carbamazepine and other sodium channel blockers may worsen generalized seizures.

Convulsions are rare but may occur in childhood absence epilepsy.

Linked questions: 17–18

17. A 2-day-old neonate with an uncomplicated birth history is transferred from the nursery to the neonatal ICU for seizures. He is placed on EEG and continues to have frequent clinical and electrographic seizures, even after receiving high doses of phenobarbital, fosphenytoin, and levetiracetam. Serum and CSF glucose, MRI, and infection evaluation are normal.
    What is the best next intervention?
    A. ACTH
    B. Ketogenic diet
    C. Valproic acid
    D. IV pyridoxine
    Correct answer: D

Linked question

18. You trial IV pyridoxine, and the newborn stops having seizures. You perform genetic testing and are mostly likely to find a mutation in which gene?
    A. KCNQ2
    B. SCN1A
    C. ALDH7A1
    D. SCN2A
    Correct answer: C

Explanation

Common causes of neonatal seizures such as hypoxic-ischemic encephalopathy, stroke, hypoglycemia, and CNS infection are not present in this case. Treatable causes of neonatal refractory epilepsy should be considered next, including inborn errors of metabolism such as pyridoxine-dependent epilepsy (PDE). PDE is an autosomal recessive disorder in which a mutation in ALDH7A1 results in a deficiency of pyridoxine (vitamin B6) and accumulation of alpha-aminoadipic semialdehyde (alpha-AASA) and pipecolic acid. Newborns with this condition present in the first days of life with encephalopathy and refractory seizures (focal, generalized, tonic, infantile spasms) including status epilepticus. This condition typically responds rapidly to IV pyridoxine or pyridoxal phosphate (PLP). If response is inadequate, trials for other deficiencies with leucovorin (PNPO deficiency) and biotin (biotinidase deficiency) are attempted. Response to additional antiseizure medications is typically poor.

Valproic acid is considered first line for Dravet Syndrome but otherwise is generally avoided under the age of 2 as there is a higher risk of hepatotoxicity, especially if there is concern for a mitochondrial condition.

ACTH is first-line treatment for infantile epileptic spasms syndrome. Ketogenic diet is first-line treatment for GLUT1 and pyruvate dehydrogenase deficiency and generally non-medication second line for other causes of medically refractory epilepsy.

Reference

Kwon JM. Testing for inborn errors of metabolism. Continuum Lifelong Learning Neurol. 2018 Feb;24(1):37.

19. A 5-year-old boy presents with new onset convulsions, and his overnight EEG shows notable spike-wave activation in sleep. A few weeks later, his family reports that he has regressed. What type of regression would most likely lead to a diagnosis of Landau–Kleffner Syndrome?
    A. Cognitive
    B. Language
    C. Motor
    D. Behavioral
    Correct answer: B

Explanation

Spike-wave activation in sleep can be seen in self-limited epilepsy syndromes such as self-limited epilepsy with centrotemporal spikes. However, a regression within weeks of this EEG pattern in sleep raises suspicion for developmental and/or epileptic encephalopathy with spike-wave activation in sleep (DEE-SWAS, EE-SWAS). EE-SWAS is a spectrum of conditions with varied degrees of cognitive, language, behavioral, and motor regression associated with marked spike-wave activation in sleep. DEE-SWAS is used when there is preexisting neurodevelopmental impairment before the regression. Seizures and the EEG pattern of spike-wave activation in sleep typically improve around puberty.

Landau–Kleffner syndrome is a specific subtype of EE-SWAS, where regression affects mainly language, with an acquired epileptic aphasia; the aphasia can be expressive or receptive ("word deafness").

Reference

International League Against Epilepsy (2024). DEVELOPMENTAL AND/OR EPILEPTIC ENCEPHALOPATHY WITH SPIKE-WAVE ACTIVATION IN SLEEP (DEE-SWAS, EE-SWAS). https://www.epilepsydiagnosis.org/syndrome/ee-csws-overview.html Accessed 30 Apr. 2025

20. A 3-year-old previously healthy, developmentally normal child presents with prolonged focal status epilepticus in the setting of fever. After the seizure stops, she is noted to have persistent hemiparesis of the right side that does not resolve. Which of the following findings on MRI done immediately after the status epilepticus would be most consistent with a diagnosis of hemi-convulsion–hemiplegia–epilepsy syndrome?
    A. Ischemia in the distribution of the left middle cerebral artery
    B. Watershed infarcts over the entire left hemisphere
    C. Cytotoxic edema of the left hemisphere
    D. Normal MRI
    Correct answer: C

Explanation

Hemi-convulsion–hemiplegia–epilepsy syndrome is a rare epilepsy syndrome characterized by acute focal motor status epilepticus followed by hemiplegia in a young child. Acute imaging initially shows edema particularly of the subcortical white matter that later evolves to atrophy of one hemisphere. Later, children typically develop drug-resistant focal seizures.

References

International League Against Epilepsy (2024). HHE. https://www.epilepsydiagnosis.org/syndrome/hhe-overview.html. Accessed 30 Apr. 2025

Pfleger R, Acute phase of hemiconvulsion-hemiplegia epilepsy syndrome. Case study, Radiopaedia.org (Accessed on 30 Apr 2025) https://doi.org/10.53347/rID-29309

21. A 12-year-old presents with frequent events described as an arousal from sleep with tachycardia, vocalization, an expression of fear, with pedaling of the legs and rocking movements. Father reports that he has similar episodes. Which of the following can you see in autosomal dominant sleep-related hypermotor epilepsy?
    A. Normal EEG in wakefulness
    B. Normal EEG in sleep
    C. Frontal lobe epileptiform discharges in sleep
    D. All of the above
    Correct answer: D

Explanation

Sleep-related hypermotor (hyperkinetic) epilepsy (SHE) is a focal epilepsy syndrome with characteristic motor or hyperkinetic seizures. Etiology may be sporadic, but if familial is usually inherited in an autosomal dominant fashion, with a penetrance of approximately 70%.

Awake EEG is normal in most patients with no epileptiform abnormalities. 50% of patients may have epileptiform abnormalities over the frontal areas.

Reference

International League Against Epilepsy (2024). SLEEP-RELATED HYPERMOTOR (HYPERKINETIC) EPILEPSY (SHE). https://www.epilepsydiagnosis.org/syndrome/adnfle-eeg.html. Accessed 30 April 2025

22. A 14-year-old boy with no past medical history presents for evaluation of several months of staring episodes in school and at home, typically once a day. He has never had any jerking episodes nor any convulsive seizures. A routine EEG captures an episode of staring, see figure below. Parents ask about the natural history of the disorder. Which of the following is true?
    A. This is childhood absence epilepsy, and most outgrow the epilepsy in a few years
    B. This is juvenile absence epilepsy, and lifelong therapy may be required
    C. This is juvenile absence epilepsy, and most outgrow the epilepsy in a few years
    D. This is childhood absence epilepsy, and lifelong therapy may be required

Correct answer: B

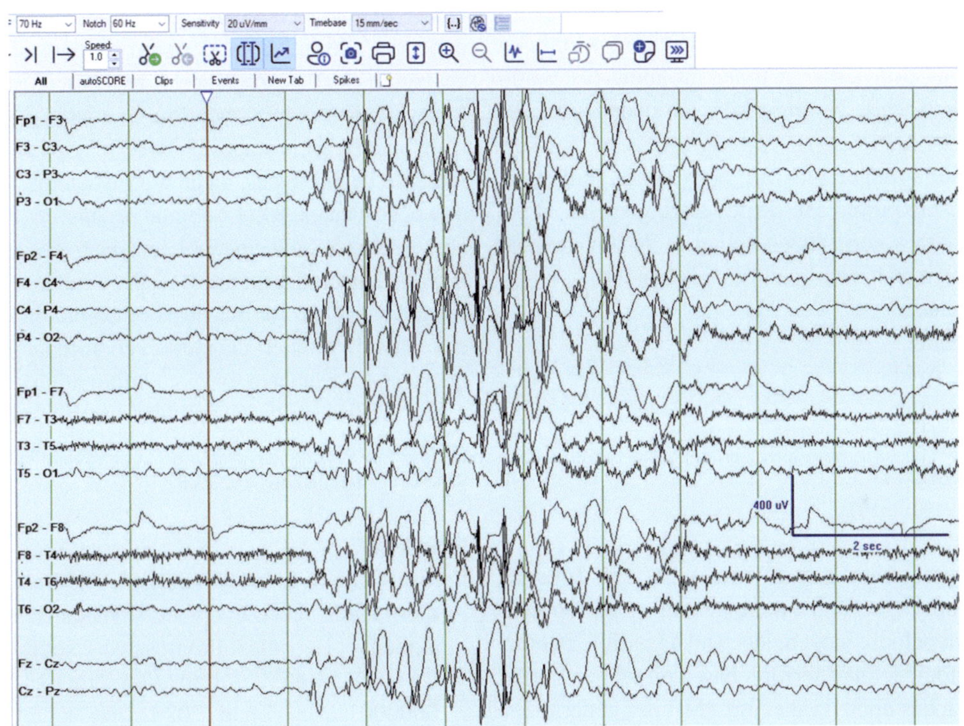

EEG, Sensitivity 20 μV/mm, Time base 15 mm/s. (Source: De-identified figure courtesy of Dr. Priya Purushothaman, New York University Langone Health)

Explanation

Based on the patient's age and seizure semiology, this is most consistent with juvenile absence epilepsy (JAE). The image shows EEG background with 3–4 Hz generalized spike-wave epileptiform discharges. While JAE can present during school-age years (6–9 years old) like childhood absence epilepsy (CAE), this patient's onset of seizures at 14 years old fits most with JAE. Further, CAE patients will have numerous seizures per day, whereas JAE patients may only have a few a day. CAE patients typically outgrow the epilepsy by teenage years, but patients with JAE often require treatment with anti-seizure medications for several decades, possibly lifetime.

Linked questions: 23–25

23. A healthy 15-year-old boy presents with 1 month of early morning arm jerks, at times dropping his toothbrush or comb while getting ready. On questioning, he shares that he also had an episode last year when he woke up with a tongue bite, full body aches, and drops of blood on his pillow. He denies staring spells. He is diagnosed with a generalized epilepsy. Which medication could worsen his early morning seizures?
    A. Levetiracetam
    B. Zonisamide
    C. Valproic Acid
    D. Carbamazepine
    E. Topiramate
    Correct answer: D

Explanation

This clinical presentation is most consistent with Juvenile Myoclonic Epilepsy (JME) given the patient's age, reported early morning myoclonic movements, and a possible nocturnal generalized tonic–clonic seizure, based on tongue bite in sleep and body aches upon awakening. JME is a generalized epilepsy, with seizures exacerbated by sodium channel blockers (e.g., carbamazepine, oxcarbazepine, and lacosamide), which are anti-seizure medications used in focal epilepsies. All other anti-seizure medication options listed are broad-spectrum and can help control generalized seizures.

Linked question

24. The previously mentioned 15-year-old boy is diagnosed with juvenile myoclonic epilepsy (JME). As the year goes on, he continues to have refractory myoclonic seizures and monthly generalized tonic–clonic seizures on therapeutic doses of valproic acid and zonisamide. He has progressive academic decline, worsening mood symptoms, ataxia and reports poor vision with blacking out episodes. What is the next best step in his clinical management?

    A. Provide reassurance to family that this is the expected natural history for JME
    B. Send genetic testing, including mitochondrial testing, and consider a skin biopsy
    C. Obtain a non-contrast CT brain
    D. Add phenytoin as the third anti-seizure medication
    Correct answer: B

Explanation

In most juvenile myoclonic epilepsy (JME) cases, seizures are well controlled on anti-seizure medications. Academic issues and mood disorders can be expected comorbidities in many pediatric epilepsy syndromes. However, this patient seems to have progressive symptoms with refractory seizures, ongoing cognitive decline as well as new systemic concerns with ataxia and vision changes. This should raise suspicion for a progressive myoclonic epilepsy (PME). Many PMEs are mitochondrial in etiology.

While the early stages of PME may present like JME with multiple seizure types, including myoclonic, tonic–clonic, and absence seizures, focal occipital seizures with transient blindness or visual hallucinations are relatively specific to Lafora disease, a neurodegenerative PME. Genetic testing is currently the gold standard for diagnosis of Lafora disease. Skin biopsy can provide further diagnostic confirmation. See following question–answer stem for more information on Lafora disease.

CT brain would not provide valuable information in this context. Phenytoin, which is a sodium channel blocker, can worsen generalized seizures.

Reference

Purushothaman P, McGinnis EM, Aldulescu M, Stack CV, Gertler TS. Pearls & Oy-sters: When Genetic Generalized Epilepsy Becomes Progressive. Neurology. 2021 Mar 2;96(9):454-457. https://doi.org/10.1212/WNL.00000 00000011293. Epub 2020 Dec 4. PMID: 33277415; PMCID: PMC8055328.

Linked question

25. As suspected, this patient's genetic result is consistent with a progressive myoclonic epilepsy (PME). For this specific PME, a skin biopsy is often completed as an ancillary study. Histopathology from a skin biopsy of his axilla (see image) shows scattered perinuclear, intracytoplasmic polyglucosan inclusions. Which gene is typically implicated in this disorder?
    A. EMP2A
    B. GABRA1
    C. STXBP1
    D. Lysine tRNA gene (MT-TK)
    E. DEPDC5
    Correct answer: A

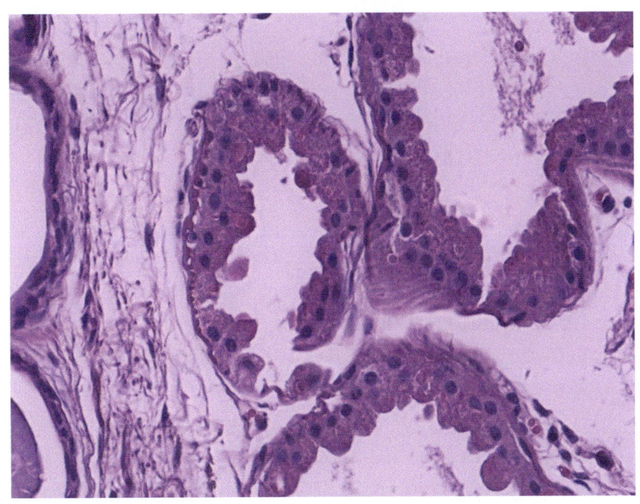

Histology of axillary skin biopsy. (Source: Zeka et al. via Journal of Medical Case Reports. 2022. CC-BY 4.0 (https://creativecommons.org/licenses/by/4.0/). Image has not been modified. Please see full attribution with citation below in references section for this question.)

Explanation

Histopathology image, pictured in the question, shows scattered perinuclear, intracytoplasmic inclusions in the secretory cells of apocrine sweat glands. These polyglucosan inclusions, known as Lafora bodies, are more readily apparent with periodic acid–Schiff stain.

To establish a diagnosis, genetic testing remains the gold standard, supported by ancillary skin biopsy. Lafora disease is an autosomal recessive disorder, clinically presenting as a progressive myoclonic epilepsy (PME), caused by biallelic loss of function variants in *EMP2A* or *NHLRC1*, which respectively encode laforin and malin. Physiologically, laforin (a phosphatase) and malin (an E3 ubiquitin-protein ligase) regulate glycogen chain formation; if absent, poorly branched and hyperphosphorylated glucose polymers aggregate in neurons, skin, liver, and skeletal muscle as insoluble polyglucosans, visualized as pathognomonic Lafora bodies on skin biopsy.

The GABRA1 gene encodes GABA-A receptor, and mutations of this gene are implicated in various non-progressive epilepsy syndromes, including juvenile myoclonic epilepsy, generalized epilepsy with febrile seizures plus (GEFS+) and Dravet syndrome. STXBP1 is the gene implicated in a severe developmental epileptic encephalopathy, often with seizure onset in early infancy. Lysine tRNA gene (MT-TK) is a mitochondrial gene implicated in Myoclonic Epilepsy with Ragged-Red Fibers (MERRF), though can also be seen in Leigh Syndrome. DEPDC5 is a mutation in the mTOR pathway associated with various epilepsy syndromes, including infantile spasms syndrome, familial focal epilepsy with variable foci (FFEVF), autoso-

mal dominant sleep-related hypermotor epilepsy (AD-SHE), and familial mesial temporal lobe epilepsies (FMTLE).

References

Baulac S, Baldassari S. DEPDC5-Related Epilepsy. 2016 Sep 29 [Updated 2023 Mar 9]. In: Adam MP, Feldman J, Mirzaa GM, et al., editors. GeneReviews® [Internet]. Seattle (WA): University of Washington, Seattle; 1993–2025.

Purushothaman P, McGinnis EM, Aldulescu M, Stack CV, Gertler TS. Pearls & Oy-sters: When Genetic Generalized Epilepsy Becomes Progressive. Neurology. 2021 Mar 2;96(9):454-457. https://doi.org/10.1212/WNL.0000000000011293. Epub 2020 Dec 4. PMID: 33277415; PMCID: PMC8055328.

Zeka N, Zogaj L, Gerguri A, et al. Lafora disease: a case report. J Med Case Rep. 2022;16(1):360. Published 2022 Oct 3. https://doi.org/10.1186/s13256-022-03537-x

26. A 15-year-old boy presents with episodic auditory hallucinations, at times with impaired awareness. Father and paternal grandmother share that they have also had similar auditory episodes, with father having a history of one focal to bilateral tonic–clonic seizure in adolescence. Routine EEG is normal. A prolonged overnight EEG shows rare left lateral temporal spikes. Which gene is implicated in this autosomal dominant epilepsy syndrome?
    A. LGI-1
    B. EPM2A
    C. SOX11
    D. SMN1
    Correct answer: A

Explanation

This clinical presentation is most consistent with autosomal dominant epilepsy with auditory features (ADEAF), which is a focal epilepsy syndrome characterized by auditory symptoms and/or receptive aphasia as the primary seizure semiologies. The auditory seizures may include simple sounds such as buzzing or ringing or be more complex, with specific voices. Age of onset ranges from adolescence to early adulthood. This epilepsy syndrome is usually well controlled with anti-seizure medications. Though identifying a genetic mutation is not required for the diagnosis, the most common gene identified in ADEAF is LGI-1. The LGI-1 gene encodes a protein involved in regulating the activity of voltage-gated potassium channels.

Mutations of the EPM2A gene are implicated in a progressive myoclonic epilepsy, specifically Lafora Disease. SOX11 mutations result in Coffin–Siris Syndrome, a rare congenital neurodevelopmental disorder with various dysmorphisms, intellectual disability and an unspecified epilepsy. SMN1 gene mutations lead to spinal muscular atrophy (SMA).

Reference

Michelucci R, Pasini E, Dazzo E. Autosomal Dominant Epilepsy with Auditory Features. 2007 Apr 20 [Updated 2024 May 9]. In: Adam MP, Feldman J, Mirzaa GM, et al., editors. GeneReviews® [Internet]. Seattle (WA): University of Washington, Seattle; 1993–2025.

27. A healthy, neuro-typical 7-year-old girl presents with 2 months of episodes of behavioral arrest, staring, and eyelid jerking. Father notes the episodes are increased when they are driving in the car on a sunny day. The patient shares that events can also occur in the shower when she is washing her face and forcefully closes her eyes. Sometimes she has eyelid twitching without behavioral arrest or altered awareness. EEG captures 4–6 Hz generalized poly-spike and wave epileptiform complexes, often following eye closure. Which of the following syndromes is the most likely diagnosis?
    A. Childhood Absence Epilepsy
    B. Lennox–Gastaut Syndrome
    C. Epilepsy with Eyelid Myoclonia (Jeavons Syndrome)
    D. Juvenile Absence Epilepsy
    Correct answer: C

Explanation

This clinical presentation is most consistent with epilepsy with eyelid myoclonia (E-EM), also known as Jeavons syndrome. E-EM is an idiopathic reflex epilepsy, typically provoked by light or photic stimulation at particular frequencies and may also be provoked with eye closure. Onset is in school-aged children (range 2–14 years old, peak 6–8 years), with a 2:1 female: male predominance. It is presumed to be genetic in etiology. Seizure types include eyelid myoclonia with or without absences, febrile seizures, and rarely other generalized seizures (GTC, typical absence alone, myoclonic). Electrographically, there are 3–6 Hz generalized spike-wave and/or polyspike-wave complexes interictally and may also be time-locked with seizures. Eye closure (fixation off sensitivity), photic stimulation, and hyperventilation can activate the EEG and elicit eyelid myoclonias. This is typically a life-long epilepsy; comorbidities include varying degrees of learning problems. Treatment options include valproate, lamotrigine, levetiracetam, and clobazam. Avoid sodium channel blocking agents. Anti-seizure medications can help control generalized tonic–clonic seizures and some absence seizures, though eyelid myoclonia can remain medically refractory. Consider specialized Zeiss (Z1) blue lenses to help with photosensitivity.

Reference

Smith KM, Wirrell EC, Andrade DM, et al. A comprehensive narrative review of epilepsy with eyelid myoclonia. *Epilepsy Res.* 2023;193:107147. https://doi.org/10.1016/j.eplepsyres.2023.107147

28. A full-term 9-month-old girl presents with several weeks of episodic, stereotyped crying and abnormal laughter. EEG captures and confirms the episodes as dacrystic and gelastic seizures. An MRI of the brain is most likely to show what finding?
    A. A focal cortical dysplasia in the right parietal lobe
    B. A Chiari I malformation
    C. An arteriovenous malformation in the left occipital lobe
    D. A hypothalamic hamartoma
    E. A normal MRI brain
    Correct answer: D

Explanation

In the clinical context of an infant with new-onset epilepsy, dacrystic and gelastic seizures are typically pathognomonic for a hypothalamic hamartoma (HH). HH is a rare, noncancerous lesion of the hypothalamus that occurs in 1 out of 200,000 children and teenagers worldwide (epilepsy foundation). Children with HH can present with precocious puberty, cognitive concerns, and various focal seizures, most notably dacrystic and gelastic seizures. Dacrystic seizures are focal seizures characterized by stereotyped crying without associated sadness or from a noxious trigger, and gelastic seizures are focal seizures with stereotyped uncontrolled, mirthless laughter. While the mechanism of pathophysiology of epilepsy in this context isn't well understood, it is thought to be a network disorder leading to a secondary epileptogenesis. Focal seizures can be refractory, often requiring multiple anti-seizure medications; ultimately, surgical resection and/or laser ablation of the lesion may be required.

The other focal lesions listed would not typically cause these rare focal seizure semiologies.

References

Hypothalamic Hamartoma—Epilepsy Foundation. https://www.epilepsy.com/causes/structural/hypothalamic-hamartoma

Scholly J, Bartolomei F. Gelastic seizures and the hypothalamic hamartoma syndrome: Epileptogenesis beyond the lesion? Handb Clin Neurol. 2021;182:143-154. https://doi.org/10.1016/B978-0-12-819973-2.00010-1. PMID: 34266589.

Linked questions: 29–30

29. A 7-year-old girl with history of speech delay presents with focal motor seizures of her right arm and right face with retained awareness. Exam is notable for right hemiparesis. The seizures become refractory to several anti-seizure medications and are now continuous. She is diagnosed with epilepsia partialis continua (EPC). Which of the following conditions is most strongly associated with EPC?
    A. Neurofibromatosis type 2
    B. Multiple Sclerosis
    C. Rasmussen's Encephalitis
    D. Amyotrophic Lateral Sclerosis
    Correct answer: C

Explanation

Epilepsia partialis continua (EPC) is a rare form of focal motor status epilepticus, typically without impaired awareness, leading to prolonged seizures involving small motor groups. EPC can last for hours, days, weeks, or even years. Of note, EPC may not always show an ictal correlate on scalp EEG. EPC may be caused by various etiologies, ranging from structural lesions to metabolic derangements. However, in this clinical context with the patient's right hemiparesis, Rasmussen's encephalitis is the likely cause. EPC is most closely associated with Rasmussen's encephalitis, which is a rare, progressive neuro-immunologic disorder, manifesting as inflammation of one hemisphere of the brain. See following question–answer stem for more information on Rasmussen's encephalitis.

Reference

Khan Z, Arya K, Bollu PC. Epilepsia Partialis Continua. [Updated 2023 Aug 28]. In: StatPearls [Internet]. Treasure Island (FL): StatPearls Publishing; 2025 Jan-.

Linked question

30. Which of the following is the most effective way to treat, and potentially cure, seizures associated with Rasmussen's encephalitis?
    A. Cerebral hemispherectomy
    B. High-dose ACTH injections
    C. Vagal nerve stimulator (VNS)
    D. Ketogenic diet
    Correct answer: A

Explanation

Rasmussen's encephalitis is a rare, progressive neuro-immunologic disorder, manifesting as inflammation of one hemisphere of the brain. In addition to medically refractory epilepsy, patients will have contralateral hemiparesis that can progress as well as cognitive decline. Neuroimaging typically shows progressive atrophy of one hemisphere. Beyond typical anti-seizure medications, immunomodulatory treatments may be trialed, including corticosteroids, intravenous immunoglobulins, plasmapheresis, and/or tacrolimus. However, the only definitive cure for Rasmussen's encephalitis is surgical treatment, specifically with a disconnection procedure such as (functional) hemispherectomy or hemispherotomy.

Reference

Varadkar S, Bien CG, Kruse CA, Jensen FE, Bauer J, Pardo CA, Vincent A, Mathern GW, Cross JH. Rasmussen's encephalitis: clinical features, pathobiology, and treatment advances. Lancet Neurol. 2014 Feb;13(2):195-205. https://doi.org/10.1016/S1474-4422(13)70260-6. PMID: 24457189; PMCID: PMC4005780.

31. A full-term 4-month-old female presents with seizure-like episodes. EEG background shows hypsarrhythmia and captures events of stiffening associated with a diffuse electro-decrement. Diagnostic evaluation raises concern for Aicardi Syndrome. What is the classic triad associated with Aicardi Syndrome?
    A. Focal seizures, hypomelanotic macules, dysmorphic facial features
    B. Infantile spasms, agenesis of the corpus callosum, chorioretinal lacunae
    C. Hemimegalencephaly, joint hypermobility, lens subluxation
    D. Generalized seizures, hypothalamic hamartoma, optic nerve hyperplasia
    Correct answer: B

Explanation

Aicardi Syndrome is a rare, neurodevelopmental disorder characterized by the classic triad of agenesis of the corpus callosum, distinct chorioretinal lacunae, and infantile spasms. This patient's EEG shows hypsarrhythmia and seizure-like episodes associated with an electrodecremental pattern, which are the hallmark features of infantile spasms syndrome.

Aicardi syndrome, an X-linked condition, predominantly affects girls, as it is lethal in boys. As more affected individuals have been identified, it is now understood that the syndrome can present without all three features of the classic triad. Other neurologic and systemic defects seen include various brain malformations (mostly polymicrogyria), optic nerve abnormalities, other seizure types, varying intellectual disability, and vertebral and rib abnormalities. Endocrinologic disorders may be present, with either precocious puberty or delayed puberty, given involvement of midline structures. Note: Aicardi syndrome is NOT related to Aicardi–Goutières syndrome, which is a distinct early-onset encephalopathy.

None of the other triad of symptoms are pathognomonic for a specific syndrome.

Reference

Sutton VR, Van den Veyver IB. Aicardi Syndrome. 2006 Jun 30 [Updated 2020 Nov 12]. In: Adam MP, Feldman J, Mirzaa GM, et al., editors. GeneReviews® [Internet]. Seattle (WA): University of Washington, Seattle; 1993–2025. Available from: https://www.ncbi.nlm.nih.gov/books/NBK1381/

32. Which of the following congenital malformations is not typically associated with seizures and/or epilepsy?
    A. Schizencephaly
    B. Lissencephaly
    C. Holoprosencephaly
    D. Chiari Type I malformation
    E. Periventricular heterotopia
    Correct answer: D

Explanation

All the listed cerebral malformations are associated with seizures and/or epilepsy except Chiari Type I Malformation (CM-I). In CM-I, the cerebellar tonsils are abnormally shaped and downwardly displaced below the level of the foramen magnum, typically ≥5 mm below the foramen magnum, though exact number may vary based on age (cerebellar tonsils have been shown to ascend with age) and other co-occurring symptoms. CM-I may be asymptomatic for several years, with the most common clinical features including headache, hydrocephalus, cerebellar dysfunction, and/or syringomyelia.

While an association between CM-I and epilepsy was clinically hypothesized, there is currently no supporting evidence in the literature.

Reference

Massimi L, Palombi D, Contaldo I, Veredice C, Chieffo DRP, Calandrelli R, Tamburrini G, Battaglia DI. Chiari 1 Malformation and Epilepsy in Children: A Missing Relationship. J Clin Med. 2022 Oct 20;11(20):6182. https://doi.org/10.3390/jcm11206182. PMID: 36294502; PMCID: PMC9604608.

33. A full-term male newborn is admitted to the NICU for poor feeding and hypotonia. His exam is notable for dysmorphic features (including high forehead, hypertelorism, and micrognathia), encephalopathy, severe hypotonia and hepatomegaly. On DOL 2, he develops focal–clonic seizures. During evaluation, plasma assay reveals elevations in multiple very long-chain fatty acids (VLCFA), concerning for Zellweger Syndrome. Which of the following can be seen on neuroimaging for Zellweger Syndrome?
    A. Lissencephaly
    B. Pachygyria
    C. Leukoencephalopathy with hypomyelination
    D. Polymicrogyria
    E. All the above
    Correct answer: E

Explanation

Zellweger Syndrome (ZS) is a rare, autosomal recessive peroxisomal disorder that manifests as various congenital anomalies involving the brain, liver, and kidneys; hence, it is also known as cerebrohepatorenal syndrome. ZS is often fatal in infancy, with the most common neurologic issues including profound hypotonia, seizures, encephalopathy, vision impairment, among other issues.

ZS results from a mutation in one of the PEX genes, which codes for a peroxisome assembly protein. Peroxisomes are organelles involved in various catalytic and anabolic cellular metabolism functions. When peroxisomes are dysfunctional, there can be an accumulation of very long-chain fatty acids (VLCFAs) in developing organs, among other complications. High intracellular VLCFAs are particularly harmful to the organizing brain. This leads to various neuronal migration defects of cortical neurons and other abnormalities, including lissencephaly, pachygyria, polymicrogyria, generalized or focal leukoencephalopathy, and brain atrophy.

Reference

Lee PR, Raymond GV. Child neurology: Zellweger syndrome. Neurology. 2013 May 14;80(20):e207-10. https://doi.org/10.1212/WNL.0b013e3182929f8e.

34. A full-term 2-month-old girl presents to your clinic for evaluation of right arm clonic movements. The patient and her family have recently immigrated to the USA from Burkina Faso. Parents share that she has a history of congenital cytomegalovirus (CMV). Which of the following structural abnormalities can be seen in a patient with congenital CMV?
    A. Microcephaly
    B. Polymicrogyria
    C. Peri-ventricular calcifications
    D. A and C only
    E. All the above
    Correct answer: E

Explanation

Congenital cytomegalovirus (CMV) is one of the most common congenital infections globally, with particularly high incidence in Sub-Saharan Africa, making it a major public health issue.

Depending on the gestational age of the fetus at the time of CMV infection, there can be a range of distinct neurologic issues. CMV has tropism for periventricular areas, but may also result in microcephaly, polymicrogyria, porencephaly, and ventricular dilatation. CMV is the leading cause of non-heritable sensorineural hearing loss (SNHL) and can also cause several long-term neurodevelopmental disabilities, including cerebral palsy, intellectual disability, vision impairment, and epilepsy. The most common clinical findings of CMV include neonatal jaundice, hepatosplenomegaly, petechiae, and small size for gestational age (SGA).

References

Payne H, Barnabas S. "Congenital cytomegalovirus in Sub-Saharan Africa-a narrative review with practice recommendations". Front Public Health. 2024 May 15;12:1359663. https://doi.org/10.3389/fpubh.2024.1359663. PMID: 38813410; PMCID: PMC11134569.

Teissier N, Fallet-Bianco C, Delezoide AL, Laquerrière A, Marcorelles P, Khung-Savatovsky S, Nardelli J, Cipriani S, Csaba Z, Picone O, Golden JA, Van Den Abbeele T, Gressens P, Adle-Biassette H. Cytomegalovirus-induced brain malformations in fetuses. J Neuropathol Exp Neurol. 2014 Feb;73(2):143–58. https://doi.org/10.1097/NEN.0000000000000038. PMID: 24423639.

35. Which of the following neurocutaneous syndromes is not associated with seizures or epilepsy?
    A. Sturge–Weber Syndrome
    B. Hypomelanosis of Ito
    C. Tuberous Sclerosis Complex
    D. Incontinentia Pigmenti
    E. All the above are associated with seizures and/or epilepsy

    Correct answer: E

Explanation

All the listed neurocutaneous syndromes are associated with seizures and/or epilepsy.

Sturge–Weber Syndrome, a rare congenital vascular disorder caused by somatic mosaic *GNAQ* pathogenic mutations, is associated with childhood-onset epilepsy in most patients. Their epilepsy may start with focal seizures, but generalized tonic–clonic seizures may also be seen. Hypomelanosis of Ito (HI) is a form of pigmentary mosaicism that has extracutaneous manifestations, typically neurologic, beyond the typical hypopigmentation of the skin (in whorls) along the Blaschko's lines. The most common neurologic features of HI include epilepsy and intellectual disability, though other issues like ataxia, attention-deficit hyperactivity disorder (ADHD), and autism spectrum disorder (ASD) can be seen. Tuberous Sclerosis Complex (TSC), an autosomal dominant neurocutaneous disorder, is the leading genetic cause of infantile spasms syndrome. TSC has variable phenotypic expression, resulting in a spectrum of neurologic issues ranging from intellectual disability, ADHD, ASD, focal epilepsy, and behavioral issues. Incontinentia Pigmenti, a rare X-linked dominant dermatologic disorder, can have systemic issues involving other neuroectodermal tissues such as teeth, hair, eyes, and the central nervous system (CNS). In the CNS, encephalopathy, cognitive impairment, and seizures can be seen.

References

Hübner S, Schwieger-Briel A, Technau-Hafsi K, Danescu S, Baican A, Theiler M, Weibel L, Has C. Phenotypic and genetic spectrum of incontinentia pigmenti - a large case series. J Dtsch Dermatol Ges. 2022 Jan;20(1):35–43. https://doi.org/10.1111/ddg.14638. Epub 2021 Dec 13. PMID: 34904373.

Northrup H, Aronow ME, Bebin EM, Bissler J, Darling TN, de Vries PJ, Frost MD, Fuchs Z, Gosnell ES, Gupta N, Jansen AC, Jóźwiak S, Kingswood JC, Knilans TK, McCormack FX, Pounders A, Roberds SL, Rodriguez-Buritica DF, Roth J, Sampson JR, Sparagana S, Thiele EA, Weiner HL, Wheless JW, Towbin AJ, Krueger DA; International Tuberous Sclerosis Complex Consensus Group. Updated International Tuberous Sclerosis Complex Diagnostic Criteria and Surveillance and Management Recommendations. Pediatr Neurol. 2021 Oct;123:50–66. https://doi.org/10.1016/j.pediatrneurol.2021.07.011. Epub 2021 Jul 24. PMID: 34399110.

Pavone P, Praticò AD, Ruggieri M, Falsaperla R. Hypomelanosis of Ito: a round on the frequency and type of epileptic complications. Neurol Sci. 2015 Jul;36(7):1173–80. https://doi.org/10.1007/s10072-014-2049-1. Epub 2015 Jan 14. PMID: 25586695.

Linked questions: 36–37

36. A full-term 5-month-old boy is diagnosed with infantile spasms syndrome and, during diagnostic evaluation, is found to have a mutation in the TSC1 gene. Which of the following is the next best step in management?
    A. Start high-dose ACTII
    B. Start the ketogenic diet
    C. Start vigabatrin
    D. Start everolimus

    Correct answer: C

Explanation

Tuberous Sclerosis Complex (TSC), an autosomal dominant neurocutaneous disorder, is the leading genetic cause of infantile spasms syndrome (ISS). Based on strong evidence for its efficacy in current literature, vigabatrin is the first-line treatment for ISS in the setting of TSC. If a therapeutic dosing of vigabatrin for at least 2 weeks has not resulted in clinical and EEG improvement, patients should then be initiated on ACTH and/or oral steroids, which is the first-line treatment for ISS in non-TSC cases. For more information on the side effect profile of vigabatrin, see the following question–answer stem.

Reference

Northrup H, Aronow ME, Bebin EM, Bissler J, Darling TN, de Vries PJ, Frost D, Fuchs Z, Gosnell ES, Gupta N, Jansen AC, Jóźwiak S, Kingswood JC, Knilans TK, McCormack FX, Pounders A, Roberds SL, Rodriguez-Buritica DF, Roth J, Sampson JR, Sparagana S, Thiele EA, Weiner HL, Wheless JW, Towbin AJ, Krueger DA; International Tuberous Sclerosis Complex Consensus Group. Updated International Tuberous Sclerosis Complex Diagnostic Criteria and Surveillance and Management Recommendations. Pediatr Neurol. 2021 Oct;123:50–66.   https://doi.org/10.1016/j.pediatrneurol.2021.07.011. Epub 2021 Jul 24. PMID: 34399110

Linked question

37. Which rare side effect of vigabatrin is potentially permanent?
    A. Retinal toxicity, specifically peripheral vision loss
    B. Valvular heart disease
    C. Vestibular dysfunction, specifically vertigo
    D. Pulmonary arterial hypertension
    Correct answer: A

Explanation

Vigabatrin is an anti-seizure medication (ASM) that works through irreversible inhibition of gamma-aminobutyric acid transaminase (GABA-T), leading to increased inhibitory gamma amino butyric acid (GABA) in the brain. The most common side effects include sedation and hypotonia, but vigabatrin carries an FDA black box warning for potential permanent retinal toxicity associated with peripheral vision loss. Though this risk may be related to the total cumulative dose, physicians monitoring children on vigabatrin should offer serial fundoscopic examinations to detect retinal changes early on.

The other listed symptoms are not typically associated with vigabatrin use.

Reference

Northrup H, Aronow ME, Bebin EM, Bissler J, Darling TN, de Vries PJ, Frost MD, Fuchs Z, Gosnell ES, Gupta N, Jansen AC, Jóźwiak S, Kingswood JC, Knilans TK, McCormack FX, Pounders A, Roberds SL, Rodriguez-Buritica DF, Roth J, Sampson JR, Sparagana S, Thiele EA, Weiner HL, Wheless JW, Towbin AJ, Krueger DA; International Tuberous Sclerosis Complex Consensus Group. Updated International Tuberous Sclerosis Complex Diagnostic Criteria and Surveillance and Management Recommendations. Pediatr Neurol. 2021 Oct;123:50–66.   https://doi.org/10.1016/j.pediatrneurol.2021.07.011. Epub 2021 Jul 24. PMID: 34399110.

38. A 14-year-old girl with cognitive impairment, frequent migraines, and hearing loss presents in non-convulsive status epilepticus. MRI shows a stroke-like lesion with hyperintensity over the left occipital region on T2-weighted FLAIR and DWI sequences, not confined to a vascular territory. Which of the following is true about the features of epilepsy associated with this disorder?
    A. Majority of patients have drug-refractory epilepsy
    B. Valproic acid is the first line anti-seizure medication
    C. Majority of patients initially present with non-epileptic functional seizures
    D. Seizures are rare with this disorder and only occur at late stage
    E. Seizures are typically unrelated to the stroke-like lesions
    Correct answer: A

Explanation

The patient described in this question stem has mitochondrial encephalomyopathy, lactic acidosis, and stroke-like episodes (MELAS), a rare mitochondrial disorder presenting with multi-organ involvement due to mitochondrial respiratory chain dysfunction. As the name implies, patients can have recurrent stroke-like events with ischemic changes seen on MRI in a non-vascular pattern, as well as migraines, hearing loss, diabetes mellitus, and drug-refractory epilepsy. Epilepsy is one of the most common clinical presentations of MELAS. The epilepsy and seizures are typically symptomatic from the stroke-like lesions. While non-epileptic functional seizures can co-occur in patients with epilepsy, epileptic seizures are predominant in MELAS. Valproic acid is contraindicated in most mitochondrial disorders as it can disrupt mitochondrial function, leading to hepatotoxicity and exacerbating symptoms of the underlying disorder.

References

Pia S, Lui F. Melas Syndrome. [Updated 2024 Jan 25]. In: StatPearls [Internet]. Treasure Island (FL): StatPearls Publishing; 2025 Jan-.

Yang X, Sun A, Ji K, Wang X, Yang X, Zhao X. Clinical features of epileptic seizures in patients with mitochondrial encephalomyopathy, lactic acidosis, and stroke-like episodes. Seizure. 2023 Mar;106:110-116. https://doi.org/10.1016/j.seizure.2023.02.014. Epub 2023 Feb 18. PMID: 36827862.

39. A 4-year-old boy with history of microcephaly, developmental delay, and ataxia develops new-onset epilepsy with two generalized tonic–clonic seizures, one provoked by fever. During his diagnostic evaluation, genetic testing reveals maternal deletion of chromosome 15q11.2-13.1, consistent with Angelman Syndrome (AS). What is the most typical finding seen on electroencephalogram (EEG) in patients with AS?
    A. 14-and-6 Hz positive spikes, typically unilateral
    B. High-amplitude rhythmic notched delta slowing, bifrontal maximal
    C. Normal EEG
    D. Wicket spikes, anterior or mid-temporal region
    Correct answer: B

Explanation

Angelman Syndrome (AS) is neurodevelopmental disorder caused by absence of the maternally inherited copy of the *UBE3A* gene (chromosome 15q11-q13). This gene is involved in genomic imprinting, with a functional maternal copy and an inactive or silenced paternal copy. Thus, deletion of the maternal copy of the *UBE3A* gene leads to AS phenotype, which can present as intellectual disability, microcephaly, gait ataxia, frequent laughter or smiling with an apparent happy demeanor, and seizures (febrile and nonfebrile). Patients with AS have characteristic electroencephalograms (EEGs) with large-amplitude slow (delta) waves. Intermittent spike and slow-wave discharges can be embedded in the delta activity, in which case they are described as a notched delta pattern. These EEG findings can be present even in the absence of seizures.

14-and-6 Hz positive spikes and wicket spikes are benign EEG variants seen typically during drowsiness and/or light sleep.

Reference

Dagli AI, Mathews J, Williams CA. Angelman Syndrome. 1998 Sep 15 [Updated 2021 Apr 22]. In: Adam MP, Feldman J, Mirzaa GM, et al., editors. GeneReviews® [Internet]. Seattle (WA): University of Washington, Seattle; 1993–2025.

Linked questions: 40–41

40. A full-term 30-month-old boy with history of microcephaly, hypotonia, and developmental delay presents for evaluation of staring spells and behavioral arrest, thought to be inattention. EEG captures these events and confirms atypical absence seizures with 2 Hz generalized spike-wave epileptiform discharges. During this admission, he develops a febrile illness with a 3 minute focal seizure that terminates without intervention. He is well-appearing. A lumbar puncture is obtained during evaluation and shows the following:

- Glucose: 10 (serum glucose 98)
- WBC: 1
- RBC: 1
- Protein: normal
- Meningitis-encephalitis viral panel: negative
- CSF bacterial and fungal cultures: negative

    Which of the following explains the CSF findings?
    A. CSF findings are consistent with a bacterial meningitis and requires meningitic-dosing antibiotic course
    B. CSF findings show low glucose, likely from a mutation in the KCNQ2 gene
    C. CSF findings are benign and do not require further workup
    D. CSF findings show low glucose, likely from a mutation in the SLC2A1 gene
    Correct answer: D

Explanation

The above clinical presentation of a patient with microcephaly, hypotonia, and developmental delay found to have hypoglycorrhachia (abnormally low glucose in the cerebrospinal fluid [CSF]) without an infectious cause raises concern for Glucose Transporter 1 Deficiency Syndrome (Glut1-DS), previously known as De Vivo Disease. Patients with Glut1-DS typically present with early-onset atypical absence seizures. Genetic testing will reveal a pathogenic mutation in the *SLC2A1* gene, which encodes for glucose transporter protein type 1 (Glut1), the primary protein that transports glucose across the blood–brain barrier. Thus, the classic CSF finding in these patients is hypoglycorrhachia.

Patients with bacterial meningitis would have a more prominent pleocytosis. *KCNQ2* gene mutations do not cause hypoglycorrhachia but rather are involved in various epilepsy syndromes, ranging from self-limited neonatal epilepsy to severe developmental and epileptic encephalopathies (DEEs)

Linked question

41. Outpatient genetic testing is completed for this patient and confirms *SLC2A1* gene variant and a diagnosis of GLUT1 deficiency syndrome. Which of the following is the next best step in management of his epilepsy?
    A. Start valproic acid
    B. Start the ketogenic diet
    C. Start lamotrigine
    D. Start high-dose oral prednisolone
    Correct answer: B

Explanation

Symptoms of Glucose Transporter 1 Deficiency Syndrome (Glut1-DS) are a result of an inability to appropriately transport glucose through the blood–brain barrier. Thus, by offering the brain a different energy substrate, the ketogenic diet, a strict high fat–low carbohydrate diet, circumvents the underlying metabolic defect as it allows for ketones to serve as the primary source of energy. While anti-seizure medications (ASMs) may be trialed, the ketogenic diet serves as a unique and effective treatment in Glut1-DS not only to treat seizures but also to slow or prevent neurodevelopmental deterioration.

Reference

Wang D, Sands T, Tang M, et al. Glucose Transporter Type 1 Deficiency Syndrome. 2002 Jul 30 [Updated 2025 Mar 6]. In: Adam MP, Feldman J, Mirzaa GM, et al., editors. GeneReviews® [Internet]. Seattle (WA): University of Washington, Seattle; 1993–2025. Available from: https://www.ncbi.nlm.nih.gov/books/NBK1430/

Kristen Yang, Doris Xia, and Sarah Levy

1. A 21-year-old female has tonic–clonic seizures that include early tonic extension of her left arm with her fist clenched while her right arm becomes flexed at the elbow. What area of the brain does the seizure involve to produce this finding?
   A. Right temporal lobe
   B. Left temporal lobe
   C. Left parietal lobe
   D. Left supplementary motor area
   E. Right supplementary motor area

   Correct answer: E

Explanation

The posturing described is consistent with the classic "figure-of-four sign," in which there is extension of the arm contralateral to the seizure focus and flexion of the arm ipsilateral to the seizure focus. This posturing is mostly seen in the tonic phase of a generalized tonic–clonic seizure and localizes to the supplementary motor area or premotor cortex of the frontal lobe. This finding is an important lateralizing sign, i.e., a semiologic finding that can be observed clinically and has shown a high likelihood of lateralizing the seizure onset. The fencing posture, which consists of elevation of the arm contralateral to the seizure focus, is another lateralizing sign.

Reference

Beniczky, Sándor, et al. "Seizure Semiology: ILAE Glossary of Terms and Their Significance." *Epileptic Disorders*, vol. 24, no. 3, 2022, pp. 447–95, https://doi.org/10.1684/epd.2022.1430.

K. Yang · D. Xia (✉) · S. Levy
Department of Neurology, New York University Langone Health, New York, NY, USA

NYU Langone and Bellevue Hospital, New York, NY, USA

New York University Langone Health, New York, NY, USA
e-mail: kristen.yang@nyulangone.org; doris.xia@nyulangone.org; sarah.levy@nyulangone.org

2. A 27-year-old male has seizures that begin with forced sustained posturing of his right arm followed by repetitive tapping and fumbling with his left arm. Where is the most likely origin of his seizures?
   A. Right temporal lobe
   B. Right frontal lobe
   C. Left frontal lobe.
   D. Left temporal lobe
   E. Left parietal lobe

   Correct answer: D

Explanation

The patient presents initially with unilateral dystonic hand posturing, which localizes to the temporal lobe. The seizure arises from the temporal lobe contralateral to the dystonic extremity. The tapping and fumbling described are consistent with hand automatisms, which localize to the ipsilateral temporal lobe when co-occurring with contralateral dystonic posturing.

References

Beniczky, Sándor, et al. "Seizure Semiology: ILAE Glossary of Terms and Their Significance." *Epileptic Disorders*, vol. 24, no. 3, 2022, pp. 447–95, https://doi.org/10.1684/epd.2022.1430.

Kotagal, P., Luders, H., Morris, H. H., Dinner, D. S., Wyllie, E., Godoy, J., & Rothner, A. D. (1989). Dystonic posturing in complex partial seizures of temporal lobe onset: a new lateralizing sign. *Neurology*, *39*(2), 196–196.

3. Which of the following findings would not be supportive of a diagnosis of Autosomal Dominant Epilepsy with Auditory Features (ADEAF)?
   A. Normal MRI brain imaging

B. Focal abnormalities on neurologic exam

C. Receptive aphasia that accompanies the seizures

D. Focal temporal epileptiform discharges

E. Normal developmental history

Correct answer: B

Explanation

The mandatory criteria for diagnosing ADEAF include focal sensory, auditory, or cognitive seizures with receptive aphasia and normal brain imaging. The auditory symptoms usually consist of humming or buzzing with accompanied sudden onset of inability to understand language. The onset is usually from 10 to 30 years old. The exclusion criteria consist of generalized onset seizures, generalized epileptiform discharges, severe intellectual disability, or focal findings on exam.

Reference

Michelucci R, Pasini E, Dazzo E. Autosomal Dominant Epilepsy with Auditory Features. 2007 Apr 20 [Updated 2024 May 9]. In: Adam MP, Feldman J, Mirzaa GM, et al., editors. GeneReviews® [Internet]. Seattle (WA): University of Washington, Seattle; 1993–2025. Available from: https://www.ncbi.nlm.nih.gov/books/NBK1537/

4. A 19-year-old girl presented to you for stereotyped night-time awakenings. Multiple habitual events were captured on video EEG, and she was diagnosed with frontal lobe epilepsy. Her grandmother experiences similar seizures. The patient also has two uncles with temporal lobe epilepsy; one has a focal cortical dysplasia, whereas her other uncle does not. She also has a cousin with autism but no seizures, and other family members are also unaffected. Her family is concerned about a genetic basis of her epilepsy. What syndrome might this be?

A. Juvenile myoclonic epilepsy

B. Temporal lobe epilepsy

C. Familial focal epilepsy with variable foci

D. Dravet Syndrome

E. Lennox–Gastaut Syndrome

Correct answer: C

Explanation

Familial focal epilepsy with variable foci (FFEVF) is an autosomal dominant epilepsy syndrome characterized by focal seizures that can originate from different cortical areas in different family members. It often presents with a wide range of focal seizure types, sometimes even in the same patient. Mutations in genes like DEPDC5, NPRL2, or NPRL3 are associated. The key features in this case are the variability in seizure focus and the family history of similar but non-identical epilepsy.

Juvenile myoclonic epilepsy (JME) is an idiopathic generalized epilepsy syndrome in which myoclonic seizures are the main seizure type, which often occur on awakening and involve brief sudden muscle jerks of the limbs or entire body. Patients can also have tonic–clonic and absence seizures. Age of onset is between 12 and 18 years old.

Dravet syndrome is a developmental and epileptic encephalopathy (DEE) that presents in the first year of life with prolonged, hemiclonic or generalized tonic–clonic seizures, frequently triggered by fever.

Lennox–Gastaut syndrome is a DEE with tonic seizures plus other seizure types, often atonic, myoclonic, and generalized tonic–clonic seizures.

Temporal lobe epilepsy is the most common type of focal epilepsy and consists of seizures, which originate from the temporal lobe.

References

Zhang, Y., Chen, J., Ren, J., Liu, W., Yang, T., & Zhou, D. (2019). Clinical features and treatment outcomes of Juvenile myoclonic epilepsy patients. *Epilepsia Open*, 4(2), 302–308.

Zuberi SM, Wirrell E, Yozawitz E, Wilmshurst JM, Specchio N, Riney K, et al. ILAE classification and definition of epilepsy syndromes with onset in neonates and infants: Position statement by the ILAE Task Force on Nosology and Definitions. *Epilepsia*. 2022; 63: 1349–1397.

5. A 28-year-old female presents with recurrent episodes of impaired consciousness with repetitive right-hand movements, which occurred only when she was at the opera and the lead actor sang a specific note. The patient attempted to trigger these episodes by playing the same opera music to herself at home, and she had a similar episode as above. What condition is this?

A. Reflex epilepsy

B. Juvenile myoclonic epilepsy

C. Familial focal epilepsy with variable foci

D. Autoimmune encephalitis

E. Non-epileptic attack

Correct answer: A

Explanation

Reflex epilepsy is defined by seizures that occur only when the patient is exposed to a specific stimulus, such as flashing lights, somatosensory stimuli, music, or even specific cognitive thought processes. Reflex seizures can be generalized or focal in nature.

Reference

Stern, John. "Musicogenic Epilepsy." *Handbook of Clinical Neurology*, vol. 129, Elsevier Health Sciences, 2015, pp. 469–77.

6. An 18-year-old boy was brought to the clinic by his parents due to progressive motor and cognitive difficulties over the past 3 years. He has developed involuntary jerking movements, especially affecting his arms and legs, which worsen with excitement or stress. He reports difficulty walking with frequent falls. He also reports waking up with blood on his pillow and finding that he had urinated in his sleep. On examination, the patient demonstrates dysarthria, ataxia, and brisk deep tendon reflexes. His uncle had similar symptoms but died before receiving a diagnosis. Which of the following is the most likely underlying genetic cause of this patient's condition?
   A. Autosomal dominant mutation in the HTT gene
   B. Autosomal recessive mutation in the CSTB gene
   C. X-linked mutation in the FMR1 gene
   D. Autosomal dominant mutation in the SNCA gene
   E. Autosomal recessive mutation in the PARK2 gene
   Correct answer: B

Explanation

This patient most likely has Unverricht–Lundborg Disease (ULD), a form of progressive myoclonic epilepsy. It typically presents with myoclonic seizures, ataxia, and cognitive decline. ULD is caused by mutations in the CSTB gene, which is inherited in an autosomal recessive manner. The disease commonly begins in childhood or adolescence and progresses over time, often with a family history of similar symptoms. The hallmark feature of ULD is myoclonus, especially triggered by stress or excitement.

The HTT gene is associated with Huntington's disease. A mutation in the FMR1 gene leads to Fragile X syndrome, which is the most common inherited cause of intellectual disability, especially in males. The SNCA gene mutation is associated with Parkinson's disease and other neurodegenerative diseases like multiple system atrophy (MSA). PARK2 gene mutations are associated with Parkinson's disease in younger patients (usually referred to as early-onset Parkinson's disease).

Reference

Crespel, Arielle, et al. "Unverricht-Lundborg Disease." *Epileptic Disorders*, vol. 18, no. s2, 2016, pp. S28–37, https://doi.org/10.1684/epd.2016.0841.

7. A 34-year-old woman presents to the neurology clinic with years of recurrent, brief episodes of altered consciousness, preceded by an aura of déjà vu, that then resolves. At times, these symptoms progress, and her family observes episodes of confusion and lip-smacking, often associated with automatisms such as repetitive hand movements. The episodes typically last for 1–2 min and have been occurring more frequently over the past 6 months. There is no significant family history of epilepsy. MRI of the brain shown below:

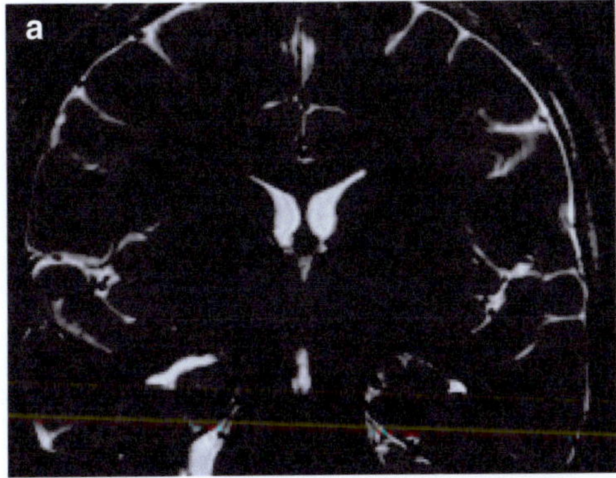
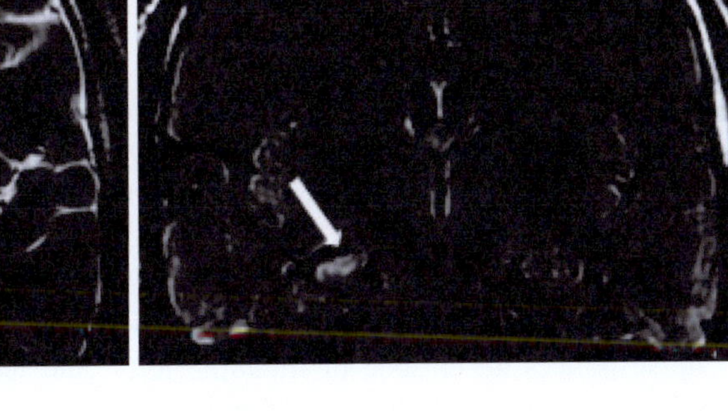

(**a**) Coronal T2 MRI and (**b**) Coronal FLAIR MRI. (Source: Abud LG, Thivard L, Abud TG, Nakiri GS, Dos Santos AC, Dormont D. CC-BY 4.0 (https://creativecommons.org/licenses/by/4.0/) via *Clinics (São Paulo, Brazil)*. Image has not been modified; Abud LG, Thivard L, Abud TG, Nakiri GS, Santos AC, Dormont D. Partial epilepsy: A pictorial review of 3 TESLA magnetic resonance imaging features. *Clinics (Sao Paulo)*. 2015;70(9):654–661. https://doi.org/10.6061/clinics/2015(09)10)

Which of the following is the most likely diagnosis?

- A. Focal seizures due to a cortical malformation
- B. Mesial temporal lobe epilepsy with hippocampal sclerosis
- C. Temporal lobe epilepsy without hippocampal sclerosis
- D. Frontal lobe epilepsy
- E. Juvenile myoclonic epilepsy

Correct answer: B

Explanation

This patient's presentation is consistent with mesial temporal lobe epilepsy (MTLE), which is often associated with hippocampal sclerosis and atrophy of the neighboring structures. The hallmark of MTLE is focal seizures originating from the temporal lobe, and semiology may include sensation of deja vu, epigastric rising, or fear, which may evolve into automatisms (e.g., lip-smacking, hand movements) and altered consciousness. The MRI findings of mesial temporal sclerosis are threefold: hippocampal atrophy, loss of internal architecture, and increased T2 signal. Hippocampal sclerosis may also develop as a sequelae of long-term uncontrolled seizures originating outside of the mesial temporal region.

References

Abud LG, Thivard L, Abud TG, Nakiri GS, Dos Santos AC, Dormont D. CC-BY 4.0 (https://creativecommons.org/licenses/by/4.0/) via *Clinics (São Paulo, Brazil)*. Image has not been modified.

Abud LG, Thivard L, Abud TG, Nakiri GS, Santos AC, Dormont D. Partial epilepsy: A pictorial review of 3 TESLA magnetic resonance imaging features. *Clinics (Sao Paulo)*. 2015;70(9):654–661. https://doi.org/10.6061/clinics/2015(09)10

Nayak CS, Bandyopadhyay S. Mesial Temporal Lobe Epilepsy. [Updated 2023 May 22]. In: StatPearls [Internet]. Treasure Island (FL): StatPearls Publishing; 2025 Jan-. Available from: https://www.ncbi.nlm.nih.gov/books/NBK554432/

8. A 68-year-old man is evaluated in clinic 3 months after an ischemic stroke affecting the right middle cerebral artery territory. He initially presented with left-sided face and arm weakness and neglect, which have partially improved. Two weeks after the stroke while undergoing rehabilitation, he develops intermittent periods of worsening deficits, and his nurse notices an episode of rhythmic left hand twitching lasting for 5 min, followed by fatigue. An EEG shows right frontotemporal sharp waves and frequent subclinical seizures. He has had no additional clinical seizures since that episode and is currently not on anti-seizure medication. Which of the following is the most appropriate next step in management?

- A. Initiate long-term antiseizure medication
- B. Recommend observation without treatment
- C. Repeat EEG in 3 months
- D. Start short-term antiseizure prophylaxis
- E. Refer for epilepsy surgery evaluation

Correct answer: A

Explanation

This patient had a late post-stroke seizure (occurring more than 1 week after stroke onset), which is a strong predictor of post-stroke epilepsy. The episode of left hand twitching was likely a seizure originating from his recent stroke, and the presence of subclinical seizures and epileptiform discharges further supports a diagnosis of epilepsy. Therefore, initiation of long-term antiseizure therapy is warranted.

Reference

Tanaka T, Ihara M, Fukuma K, et al. Pathophysiology, Diagnosis, Prognosis, and Prevention of Poststroke Epilepsy: Clinical and Research Implications. *Neurology*. 2024;102(11):e209450. https://doi.org/10.1212/WNL.0000000000209450

9. A 32-year-old woman presents with a 6-month history of focal-onset seizures characterized by right arm jerking and speech arrest lasting 1–2 min, followed by postictal confusion. Brain MRI reveals a left frontal lobe lesion with a "popcorn-like" appearance and a hemosiderin ring on susceptibility-weighted imaging. There is no evidence of surrounding edema or mass effect. EEG shows interictal sharp waves over the left frontotemporal region.

Which of the following is the most appropriate next step in management?

- A. Initiate antiseizure medication and monitor
- B. Immediate surgical resection of the lesion
- C. Brain biopsy to rule out neoplasm
- D. Whole-brain radiation therapy
- E. Genetic testing for CADASIL

Correct answer: A

Explanation

This patient's presentation meets criteria for focal epilepsy with suspected relation to the cerebral cavernous malformation (cavernoma), a vascular lesion that can irritate the cortex and lead to focal seizures. The characteristic MRI appearance (popcorn-like core with a hemosiderin ring) is typical of cavernomas. In a patient presenting with seizures and no acute hemorrhage or mass effect, the initial management is medical therapy with anti-seizure medication. Surgery is reserved for patients with medically refractory epilepsy or recurrent hemorrhage.

Reference

Rosenow, Felix, et al. "Cavernoma-related Epilepsy: Review and Recommendations for Management—Report of the Surgical Task Force of the ILAE Commission on Therapeutic Strategies." *Epilepsia (Copenhagen)*, vol. 54, no. 12, 2013, pp. 2025–35, https://doi.org/10.1111/epi.12402.

Linked questions: 10–11

10. A 22-year-old man is brought to the emergency department after a witnessed generalized tonic–clonic seizure. He has had a low-grade fever, headache, and confusion for the past 2 days. On examination, he is disoriented and cries out in pain when you try to move his neck. MRI brain shows hyperintensities in the right temporal lobe on T2-weighted and FLAIR sequences. Which of the following is the most likely cause of this patient's seizures?
    A. Neurocysticercosis
    B. Herpes simplex virus (HSV) encephalitis
    C. Bacterial meningitis
    D. HIV-associated progressive multifocal leukoencephalopathy (PML)
    E. Cryptococcal meningitis
    Correct answer: B

Explanation

This patient has clinical features (fever, altered mental status, seizure, temporal lobe involvement on MRI) that are classic for HSV encephalitis, which is the most common cause of focal encephalitis leading to seizures in adults. HSV has a predilection for the temporal lobes, often leading to early focal seizures.

Linked question

11. The patient from the prior question undergoes a lumbar puncture demonstrating pleocytosis and a positive HSV1 PCR. What is the most likely finding on EEG?
    A. Burst suppression
    B. Lateralized periodic discharges (LPDs)
    C. 3 Hz generalized spike and wave discharges
    D. Generalized discharges with triphasic morphology
    E. Delta brush
    Correct answer: B

Explanation

The patient presents with HSV encephalitis, which most commonly presents with lateralized periodic discharges (LPDs). LPDs may also be seen in other focal injuries to the brain including stroke or tumor.

Reference

Baykan B, Kinay D, Gökyigit A, Gürses C. Periodic lateralized epileptiform discharges: association with seizures. *Seizure*. 2000;9(6):402–406. https://doi.org/10.1053/seiz.2000.0435

12. A 19-year-old boy is evaluated for progressive difficulty in coordination and frequent myoclonic jerks. He began experiencing involuntary muscle twitches in his arms and legs at age 12, which have increased in frequency. Over the past year, he developed ataxia, hearing loss, and generalized tonic–clonic seizures. Neurologic exam shows dysarthria, gait instability, and multifocal myoclonus. EEG shows generalized spike-and-wave discharges. Muscle biopsy reveals ragged red fibers on modified Gomori trichrome staining. Serum lactate is elevated.
    Which of the following is the most likely diagnosis?
    A. Juvenile myoclonic epilepsy
    B. Friedreich ataxia
    C. Myoclonic epilepsy with ragged red fibers (MERRF)
    D. MELAS syndrome
    E. Lafora body disease
    Correct answer: C

Explanation

This patient has classic features of myoclonic epilepsy with ragged red fibers (MERRF), a mitochondrial disorder resulting from a mutation in the MT-TK gene (most commonly m.8344A > G) affecting mitochondrial tRNA for lysine. Key features include:

- Myoclonus (hallmark feature)
- Generalized epilepsy
- Cerebellar ataxia
- Sensorineural hearing loss
- Elevated lactate
- Ragged red fibers on muscle biopsy (abnormal mitochondria accumulating under the sarcolemma)

Reference

Velez-Bartolomei F, Lee C, Enns G. MERRF. In: Adam MP, Feldman J, Mirzaa GM, Pagon RA, Wallace SE, Amemiya A, eds. *GeneReviews®*. Seattle (WA): University of Washington, Seattle; June 3, 2003.

13. A 45-year-old man is brought to the emergency department after a witnessed generalized tonic–clonic seizure.

He is awake and alert upon arrival but appears tremulous and diaphoretic. He reports that he has been drinking "a fifth of vodka daily" for years and stopped abruptly 2 days ago. Vitals: HR 112, BP 148/92, Temp 37.5 °C. Neurologic exam is nonfocal. Labs show mild hypomagnesemia and hypokalemia. Head CT is normal. Which of the following is the most appropriate next step in his management?

A. Administer phenytoin for seizure prophylaxis
B. Begin alcohol withdrawal therapy and correct electrolytes
C. Order continuous EEG monitoring to rule out non-convulsive status
D. Initiate propofol for presumed refractory status epilepticus
E. Perform lumbar puncture to rule out meningitis

Correct answer: B

Explanation

This patient's seizure occurred within 48 h of alcohol cessation, with signs of autonomic hyperactivity (tachycardia, tremor, diaphoresis), consistent with alcohol withdrawal seizure. These seizures are typically generalized, occur early, and do not require anti-seizure medications, such as phenytoin, unless there is an underlying epilepsy.

Reference

Mauritz, M., Hirsch, L.J., Camfield, P., Chin, R., Nardone, R., Lattanzi, S. and Trinka, E. (2022), Acute symptomatic seizures: an educational, evidence-based review. Epileptic Disorders, 24: 26–49. https://doi.org/10.1684/epd.2021.1376

14. A 58-year-old woman is brought to the emergency room by her family for confusion and dizziness. They live out of state and are traveling on vacation. While waiting to be evaluated, the woman has a witnessed tonic–clonic seizure, which lasts 2 min. All of the following laboratory values could be implicated as cause for a possible acute symptomatic seizure EXCEPT:

A. Glucose of 500 mg/dL
B. Glucose of 65 mg/dL
C. Magnesium of 0.6 mg/dL
D. BUN of 105 mg/dL
E. Calcium 8 mg/dL

Correct answer: B

Explanation

All answers except for B are within the cutoff range of values for metabolic conditions, which may lead to acute symptomatic seizures in metabolic disorders as proposed by the International League against Epilepsy (ILAE). Serum glu-

cose <36 mg/dL or >450 mg/dL can be implicated as a cause for acute symptomatic seizures according to the ILAE. The other ranges implicated in acute symptomatic seizures include magnesium <0.8 mg/dL, BUN >100 mg/dL, and calcium <5 mg/dL.

Reference

Mauritz, M., Hirsch, L.J., Camfield, P., Chin, R., Nardone, R., Lattanzi, S. and Trinka, E. (2022), Acute symptomatic seizures: an educational, evidence-based review. Epileptic Disorders, 24: 26–49. https://doi.org/10.1684/epd.2021.1376

15. An 18-year-old healthy male collapses while standing during a 3-hour-long chorus performance. Witnesses report he turned pale and stiffened, followed by several seconds of rhythmic jerking movements of all limbs. The entire episode lasted about 30 seconds, and he regained consciousness within a minute. When asked about the episode, he recalls feeling lightheaded and sweaty right before passing out and remembers waking up to find everyone crowding over him, asking if he was alright. There was no tongue biting, incontinence, or postictal confusion. His physical exam and neurologic exam are normal. A 12-lead ECG shows sinus rhythm.

Which of the following is the most appropriate next step in evaluation?

A. Routine outpatient EEG
B. Start anti-seizure medications
C. Syncope workup
D. Brain MRI with and without contrast
E. Admit for video EEG monitoring

Correct answer: C

Explanation

This patient likely experienced convulsive syncope, a transient loss of consciousness due to cerebral hypoperfusion that can be accompanied by myoclonic or clonic posturing, often mistaken for a seizure. Key distinguishing features include:

- Preceding lightheadedness, pallor, and diaphoresis (vasovagal prodrome)
- Brief motor activity (<15–20 seconds)
- Rapid recovery with no postictal confusion
- No lateral tongue biting

Patients should undergo routine cardiac and neurological evaluations to confirm there is no underlying cardiac or neurological pathology contributing to the event, such as arrhythmia, hypertrophic cardiomyopathy, or carotid stenosis, for example.

Reference

Depositario-Cabacar, Dewi Frances T., et al. "Imitators of Epilepsy." *Epilepsy Board Review*, Springer New York, 2017, pp. 167–70, https://doi.org/10.1007/978-1-4939-6774-2_12.

16. A 35-year-old woman presents to the emergency room for recurrent episodes of confusion that progress to generalized shaking. The patient is placed on EEG, and two events are captured without EEG correlate. Which of the following characteristics would most strongly support non-epileptic events?
    A. Urinary incontinence
    B. Upward eye deviation
    C. Tongue biting
    D. Loss of consciousness
    E. Asynchronous limb movements
    Correct answer: E

Explanation

Asynchronous movements are a strong indicator for non-epileptic events. These movements are described as jerking or shaking movements that are non-rhythmic. Coordinated and rhythmic movements are more consistent with seizure activity. Upward eye deviation and tongue biting (typically midline rather than lateral) can be seen with non-epileptic events. Patients may be unresponsive during events as well as report loss of consciousness.

Reference

De Paola L, Terra VC, Silvado CE, et al. Improving first responders' psychogenic nonepileptic seizures diagnosis accuracy: Development and validation of a 6-item bedside diagnostic tool. *Epilepsy Behav*. 2016;54:40–46. https://doi.org/10.1016/j.yebeh.2015.10.025

17. A 24-year-old female is brought to the emergency room by her coworkers for a seizure. While examining her, she exhibits back and forth head shaking and pelvic thrusting, with non-rhythmic arm shaking that starts and stops repeatedly. Her eyes are closed throughout. She intermittently responds to your questions by nodding yes or shaking her head no. The ER physician informs you that she has received several rounds of benzodiazepines and a levetiracetam load, but her seizures have not stopped for 20 minutes. The plan is to intubate. What is the appropriate next step?
    A. Tell patient to stop
    B. Tell ED to intubate
    C. Trial Ativan
    D. Start video EEG monitoring, after reassuring ED and patient
    E. Trial Depakote
    Correct answer: D

Explanation

There are several features suggestive of non-epileptic seizures. These events are frequently unresponsive to benzodiazepines and are at risk of overtreatment due to misdiagnosis. Starting video EEG would allow confirmation of non-epileptic seizures by showing a lack of electrographic seizure correlate during the event. It is also important to keep in mind that a response to benzodiazepines is also not diagnostic of an epileptic seizure.

References

Mezouar N, Demeret S, Rotge JY, Dupont S, Navarro V. Psychogenic non-epileptic seizure-status in patients admitted to the intensive care unit. Eur J Neurol. 2021 Aug;28(8):2775–2779. https://doi.org/10.1111/ene.14941. Epub 2021 Jun 20. PMID: 34033167.

Viswanathan, N., & Benbadis, S. R. (2022). The diagnosis of functional seizures. *Pract. Neurol, 21*, 3.

18. A 21-year-old man reports recurrent episodes of transient left-sided weakness that develop slowly over 10–20 min and resolve within a few hours. These episodes are sometimes preceded by flashing lights in the right visual field and followed by severe, unilateral headaches with nausea. His father experienced similar episodes starting in adolescence. Neurological exam, EEG, and MRI are normal. Which is the most likely diagnosis?
    A. Transient ischemic attack
    B. Focal seizure
    C. Autosomal dominant disorder causing transient hemiparesis
    D. Conversion disorder
    E. Multiple sclerosis relapse
    Correct answer: C

Explanation

Hemiplegic migraine represents a rare subtype of migraine with aura in which the aura is unilateral motor weakness. The weakness as seen in this patient may also be accompanied by vision or sensory changes. Hemiplegic migraines may be inherited or occur sporadically. Given that this patient's father also had similar complaints, he most likely has Familial Hemiplegic Migraine (FHM), which is autosomal-dominantly inherited. Although seizures are not a criterion for diagnosis, there is a higher rate of seizures in FHM compared to sporadic hemiplegic migraines.

Reference

Kumar A, Samanta D, Emmady PD, et al. Hemiplegic Migraine. [Updated 2023 Jul 4]. In: StatPearls [Internet]. Treasure Island (FL): StatPearls Publishing; 2025 Jan. Available from: https://www.ncbi.nlm.nih.gov/books/NBK513302/

19. A 25-year-old woman with recurrent episodes of unilateral weakness and headache undergoes genetic testing. Which of the following genes is most commonly implicated in her condition?
    A. CACNA1A
    B. SCN1A
    C. PRRT2
    D. ATP7B
    E. SOD1
    Correct answer: A

Explanation

The syndrome described above is consistent with a hemiplegic migraine. CACNA1A-related Hemiplegic Migraine is a severe migraine attack consisting of migraines with associated unilateral weakness. CACNA1a is the most commonly associated mutation with familial hemiplegic migraines (FHM). SCN1A is associated with epilepsy including Dravet's syndrome. PRRT2 is associated with paroxysmal kinesigenic dyskinesia and FHM; however, it is the fourth most common gene associated with FHM. ATP7B is associated with Wilson's disease. SOD1 mutations are strongly linked with Amyotrophic Lateral Sclerosis.

Reference

Carrera, P., Stenirri, S., Ferrari, M., & Battistini, S. (2001). Familial hemiplegic migraine: a ion channel disorder. *Brain research bulletin*, *56*(3–4), 239–241. https://doi.org/10.1016/s0361-9230(01)00570-6

Yang K, Quiroz V, Ebrahimi-Fakhari D. PRRT2-Related Disorder. 2018 Jan 11 [Updated 2024 Jul 4]. In: Adam MP, Feldman J, Mirzaa GM, et al., editors. GeneReviews® [Internet]. Seattle (WA): University of Washington, Seattle; 1993–2025. Available from: https://www.ncbi.nlm.nih.gov/books/NBK475803/

Linked questions: 20–23

20. A 35-year-old man with a history of epilepsy. He feels his typical seizure aura and presents to the nearest emergency room. While in triage, he develops continuous tonic–clonic seizure activity, which persists for over 5 minutes. His anti-seizure medication regimen is unknown. His finger stick glucose is 89 mg/dL and vital signs are notable for tachycardia. The ER team applied supplemental oxygen, turned the patient onto his side, and suctioned oral secretions. Which of the following is the most appropriate next step in management?
    A. Administer IV lorazepam 4 mg
    B. Order an urgent MRI brain before treatment
    C. Start intravenous fosphenytoin
    D. Observe and wait for seizures to stop spontaneously
    E. Perform lumbar puncture to rule out meningitis
    Correct answer: A

Explanation

Benzodiazepines are the first line of treatment for convulsive status epilepticus after medical stabilization. Guidelines for the treatment of convulsive status epilepticus in adults and children lists Level A evidence for intramuscular midazolam, intravenous lorazepam, or intravenous diazepam. The recommended dosing for intravenous lorazepam is 0.1 mg/kg/dose, maximum dose 4 mg, which can be repeated once. A randomized trial investigating the treatment of benzodiazepine-refractory convulsive status epilepticus found that intravenous antiseizure fosphenytoin, levetiracetam, and valproic acid had no significant difference in rates of seizure cessation or safety. The patient in this question has not been treated with benzodiazepines yet, so intravenous fosphenytoin is not the appropriate next step. Neither additional diagnostic testing nor observation would be appropriate at this time.

Linked question

21. The patient from the prior question continues to seize and requires a second dose of lorazepam 4 mg before he stops convulsing. He remains unresponsive. His oxygen saturation is 70% despite supplemental oxygen, and he is unable to clear his oral secretions. Which of the following is the most appropriate next step in management?
    A. Administer additional IV lorazepam 4 mg
    B. Call the family to determine his home medication regimen
    C. Start EEG
    D. Intubation
    E. Perform a lumbar puncture to rule out meningitis
    Correct answer: D

Explanation

It is imperative to ensure that the patient's airway, breathing, and circulation are maintained. This patient is exhibiting signs of respiratory failure, which may be related to both convulsive seizures and the adverse effect of sedation from necessary pharmacologic interventions. However, it is important to note that uncontrolled convulsive status epilepticus is more likely than benzodiazepines to cause respiratory depression. Stabilizing the patient's airway and restoring ventilation through endotracheal intubation are the most appropriate next step in management.

Linked question

22. The patient is now intubated. Video EEG has been initiated. His wife reports that he is prescribed valproic acid, but he ran out of medication 3 days ago. This is what you see on the EEG:

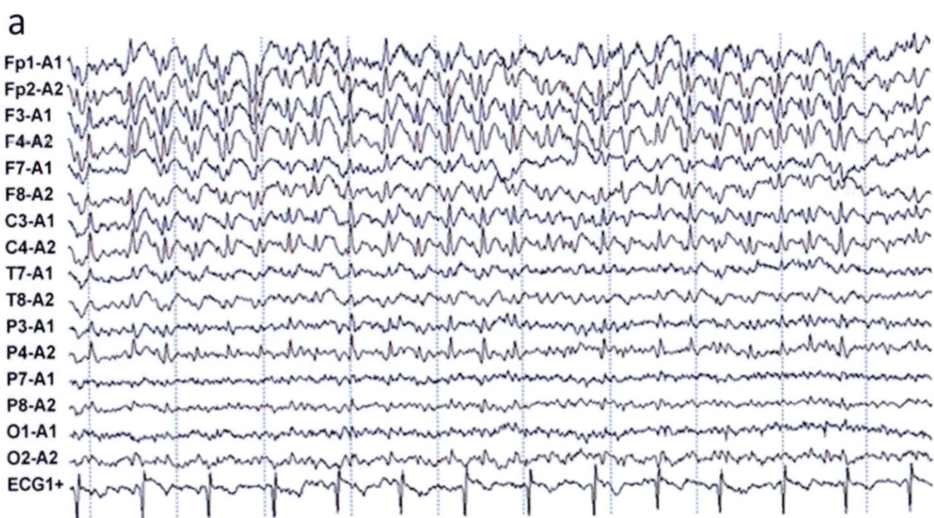

EEG. (Source: Wu et al. via Acta Epileptologica. CC-BY 4.0 (https://creativecommons.org/licenses/by/4.0/deed.en). Image has been cropped to include only panel A. Please see full attribution with citation below in references section for this question.

Which of the following is the **most appropriate next step in management**?
A. Extubate him
B. Load with IV pentobarbital
C. Load with IV valproic acid
D. MRI brain with and without contrast
E. Perform lumbar puncture to rule out meningitis
Correct answer: C

Explanation

The image shows 3 Hz spike and wave activity, which meets electrographic criteria for status epilepticus, which is now "nonconvulsive" as the patient's clinical movements have ceased. Sudden cessation of a patient's home antiseizure medication can cause breakthrough seizures and, in extreme cases, status epilepticus. The patient's home anti-seizure medication can be administered intravenously and loaded at a dose of 40 mg/kg in this setting. Pentobarbital would not be indicated at this time, as this medication is used for refractory or super refractory status epilepticus. Obtaining an MRI of the brain may be important if there are new focal examination findings, but treating the continued status epilepticus is the most appropriate next step at this time.

Linked question

23. The previous pattern on the patient's EEG resolved following administration of intravenous valproic acid. The EEG now revealed generalized slowing without epileptiform discharges. The patient was ordered for his home dose of medication. Twenty-four hours later, he was weaned off sedation and follows commands well enough to be extubated. You prepare to transfer him from the intensive care unit to the general neurology service. What is his diagnosis?
A. Acute symptomatic seizure
B. Epilepsia partialis continua
C. Convulsive status epilepticus followed by nonconvulsive status epilepticus
D. Meningitis
E. Refractory status epilepticus
Correct answer: C

Explanation

The patient presented in convulsive status epilepticus. EEG then revealed non-convulsive status epilepticus, which resolved after administration of the second anti-seizure medication. This case does not meet the criteria for refractory status epilepticus, which is defined by failure of two appropriately selected and dosed antiseizure medications to stop status epilepticus. An acute symptomatic seizure is defined as a "seizure occurring in close temporal relationship with an acute CNS insult," and since we know this patient has epilepsy, presented in status, and workup has revealed no other insult, this is not considered to be an acute symptomatic seizure. The patient's seizures consisted of loss of consciousness with whole body tonic–clonic movements, thus not characterized as epilepsia partialis continua. There was no evidence of meningitis.

References

Beuchat, Isabelle, et al. "Refractory Status Epilepticus: Risk Factors and Analysis of Intubation in the Multicenter SENSE Registry." *Neurology*, 2022, https://doi.org/10.1212/WNL.0000000000201099.

Glauser T, Shinnar S, Gloss D, et al. Evidence-Based Guideline: Treatment of Convulsive Status Epilepticus in Children and Adults: Report of the Guideline Committee of the American Epilepsy Society. Epilepsy Curr. 2016 Jan-Feb;16(1):48–61. https://doi.org/10.5698/1535-7597-16.1.48. PMID: 26900382; PMCID: PMC4749120.

Kapur J, Elm J, Chamberlain JM, et al. Randomized trial of three anticonvulsant medications for status epilepticus. N Engl J Med 2019;381(22): 2103–2113. https://doi.org/10.1056/NEJMoa1905795

Mauritz, Matthias, et al. "Acute Symptomatic Seizures: An Educational, Evidence-based Review." *Epileptic Disorders*, vol. 24, no. 1, 2022, pp. 26–49, https://doi.org/10.1684/epd.2021.1376.

Vossler, David G. "First Seizures, Acute Repetitive Seizures, and Status Epilepticus." *Continuum (Minneapolis, Minn.)*, vol. 31, no. 1, 2025, pp. 95–124, https://doi.org/10.1212/CON.0000000000001530.

Wu et al. via *Acta Epileptologica*. CC-BY 4.0 (https://creativecommons.org/licenses/by/4.0/deed.en). Image has been cropped to include only panel A. Wu, D., Liu, X., Yao, X. et al. Analysis of electroclinical features of nonconvulsive status epilepticus: a study of four cases. *Acta Epileptologica* 4, 4 (2022). https://doi.org/10.1186/s42494-021-00073-x

24. A 42-year-old woman with no significant medical history is brought to the ED with new-onset generalized convulsive status epilepticus. She received IV lorazepam 0.1 mg/kg twice, followed by a loading dose of fosphenytoin 20 mg PE/kg. She was intubated but continues to have tonic–clonic seizures, now ongoing for 40 minutes. Which of the following is the most appropriate next step in management?

A. Administer a different benzodiazepine as a single dose

B. Begin continuous infusion of midazolam with EEG monitoring

C. Perform urgent lumbar puncture to rule out viral encephalitis

D. Order emergent MRI brain before additional treatment

E. Attempt weaning of sedation after 30 min regardless of EEG findings

Correct answer: B

Explanation

This patient's condition meets the criteria for refractory status epilepticus, which is defined by failure to stop status epilepticus following a second antiseizure medication, such as intravenous fosphenytoin, valproic acid, levetiracetam, or phenobarbital if the first three options are not available. At this point in the status epilepticus algorithm, an appropriate next step is to initiate infusion of an anesthetic to treat seizures, which is commonly chosen by experts. Repeating a second non-anesthetizing medication is also an option. While many clinicians choose to administer an anesthetic infusion, there are no Class I randomized trials that determine this to be superior. Out of the choices provided above, B is the next best step.

References

Glauser T, Shinnar S, Gloss D, et al. Evidence-Based Guideline: Treatment of Convulsive Status Epilepticus in Children and Adults: Report of the Guideline Committee of the American Epilepsy Society. Epilepsy Curr. 2016 Jan-Feb;16(1):48–61. https://doi.org/10.5698/1535-7597-16.1.48. PMID: 26900382; PMCID: PMC4749120.

Vossler, David G. "First Seizures, Acute Repetitive Seizures, and Status Epilepticus." *Continuum (Minneapolis, Minn.)*, vol. 31, no. 1, 2025, pp. 95–124, https://doi.org/10.1212/CON.0000000000001530.

Linked questions: 25–26

25. A 30-year-old female with a history of a large right frontoparietal meningioma presents to the ED with a chief complaint of left hand twitching every few seconds for the last 3 hours. She is unable to suppress the twitching with her opposite hand. Her neurological exam reveals no other findings, and she is able to move her left hand despite the twitching. She has not had head imaging for several years. Which is the next best step in management?

    A. MRI brain with and without contrast

    B. Meningioma removal surgery

    C. IV steroids

D. Baclofen

E. Administer IV lorazepam 4 mg and intubate the patient

Correct answer: A

Explanation

The repetitive, non-suppressible left hand twitching is suspicious for focal motor seizures, which appear to meet criteria for epilepsia partialis continua (EPC), which is defined as focal motor seizures with preserved awareness lasting greater than 60 minutes or recurring with less than 10-second intervals. Obtaining updated imaging is the correct first step in this case. An MRI brain could reveal any changes to the meningioma, which may be responsible for the patient's acute symptoms, such as interval growth of the tumor or surrounding edema.

Steroids may be helpful to treat edema and thereby treat seizures; however, without imaging, it is unclear if edema is the cause of the patient's seizures. Baclofen is used to treat muscle spasms and stiffness, which is not the etiology of the patient's symptoms in this question. While some patients may benefit from benzodiazepines as a first-line treatment, it would be inappropriate to intubate for EPC. Surgery without repeat imaging would also be inappropriate.

Linked question

26. MRI brain of the patient in the prior question reveals that the patient's meningioma is larger than previously seen and now directly puts pressure on the hand knob of her motor cortex. Neurosurgery recommends resection, which has been scheduled in 2 weeks. Her CBC, BMP, LFT, and TFT labs are all normal. The left hand twitching is bothersome to the patient. Which is the next best step in management?

    A. Wait for resective surgery

    B. Lamotrigine

    C. IV steroids

    D. Baclofen

    E. IV levetiracetam load

Correct answer: E

Explanation

Guidelines recommended for loading doses of levetiracetam

An algorithm proposed in a recent systematic review for the management of epilepsia partialis continua (EPC) recommends loading doses of levetiracetam or phenytoin, though there is significant variability in pharmacological management in the literature. Oral anti-seizure medications, such as topiramate and carbamazepine, may control EPC in select patients; however, lamotrigine, due to the need for slow uptitration of dosing, would not provide timely seizure control.

Reference

Tan S, Ng JS, Devinuwara J, Ong ST, Virdi P, Goh R, El-Masri S, Kovoor J, Stretton B, Gupta A, Bellinge J, Zhang T, Gilbert T, Crawford G, Bergin P, Kimberly WT, Harroud A, Stacpoole S, Kiley M, Bacchi S. Management of epilepsia partialis continua: A systematic review. Seizure. 2025 Feb;125:79–83. https://doi.org/10.1016/j.seizure.2025.01.005. Epub 2025 Jan 4. PMID: 39813748.

27. A 28-year-old presents to the epilepsy clinic for follow-up and reports that she is interested in becoming pregnant within the next year. Which of the following anti-seizure medications has the highest risk of teratogenicity and should be avoided in this patient?
    A. Levetiracetam
    B. Lamotrigine
    C. Valproate
    D. Oxcarbazepine
    E. Gabapentin
    Correct answer: C

Explanation

Valproate use in pregnancy carries a higher risk of dose-related major congenital malformations than any other anti-seizure medication. The most commonly observed malformations included cardiac defects, hypospadias, and neural tube defects. It also carries an increased risk of reduced verbal IQ and autism.

Reference

Tomson, Torbjörn, et al. "Dose-Dependent Teratogenicity of Valproate in Mono- and Polytherapy: An Observational Study." *Neurology*, vol. 85, no. 10, 2015, pp. 866–72, https://doi.org/10.1212/WNL.0000000000001772.

28. A 56-year-old man presents to the emergency room for increased episodes of intermittent somnolence. He was recently started on a new anti-epileptic medication in addition to his phenobarbital. Which of the following anti-epileptic medications did he most likely start?
    A. Levetiracetam
    B. Valproate
    C. Lamotrigine
    D. Phenytoin
    E. Oxcarbazepine
    Correct answer: B

Explanation

Phenobarbital is metabolized by cytochrome P450 (CYP450). Valproate is a known CYP450 inhibitor, which will subsequently cause increased levels of phenobarbital. Phenobarbital toxicity presents as dizziness, increased tiredness, and respiratory depression.

Reference

Abou-Khalil, Bassel W. "Update on Antiseizure Medications 2025." *Continuum (Minneapolis, Minn.)*, vol. 31, no. 1, 2025, pp. 125–64, https://doi.org/10.1212/cont.0000000000001521.

29. Which of the following statements regarding sudden unexpected death in epilepsy (SUDEP) is incorrect?
    A. The highest rate of SUDEP occurs in epilepsy patients between the ages of 20 and 45
    B. There must be evidence of a recent seizure in order to support an SUDEP diagnosis
    C. An patient with epilepsy and intellectual disability has a higher rate of SUDEP
    D. SUDEP is a diagnosis of exclusion after other potential causes of death are ruled out
    E. SUDEP is more common among male epilepsy patients
    Correct answer: B

Explanation

SUDEP is a diagnosis of exclusion and is made when a patient with known epilepsy dies suddenly with no clear etiology. A diagnosis can be made with or without evidence of a preceding seizure. Other causes to rule out include trauma, drowning, and toxicological ingestions.

References

Keller AE, Ho J, Whitney R, Li SA, Williams AS, Pollanen MS, Donner EJ. Autopsy-reported cause of death in a population-based cohort of sudden unexpected death in epilepsy. Epilepsia. 2021 Feb;62(2):472–480. https://doi.org/10.1111/epi.16793. Epub 2021 Jan 5. PMID: 33400291.

Nashef, Lina, et al. "Unifying the Definitions of Sudden Unexpected Death in Epilepsy." *Epilepsia (Copenhagen)*, vol. 53, no. 2, 2012, pp. 227–33, https://doi.org/10.1111/j.1528-1167.2011.03358.x.

Thurman, David J., et al. "Sudden Unexpected Death in Epilepsy: Assessing the Public Health Burden." *Epilepsia (Copenhagen)*, vol. 55, no. 10, 2014, pp. 1479–85, https://doi.org/10.1111/epi.12666.

30. A 32-year-old man comes to the emergency room with a first-time tonic–clonic seizure. Basic blood work, including glucose, was within normal limits. Urinalysis and urine toxicology were negative. The seizure appears to be unprovoked. All of the following features would

encourage you to start this patient on an anti-seizure medication, EXCEPT:

A. Left frontal arteriovenous malformation found on MRI Brain
B. Seizure onset out of sleep
C. 4–5 Hz generalized spike and wave discharges on EEG
D. Past medical history of migraine
E. Right temporal encephalomalacia on CT Head

Correct answer: D

Explanation

All the features except for a history of migraine confer an increased risk of a second seizure within the first 2 years after the first seizure in an adult. According to guidelines published in 2016, the risk of seizure recurrence in the first 2 years is 21–54%. This value doubles if an adult has an epileptogenic brain lesion, evidence of a prior brain insult (E), nocturnal seizure (B), or an epileptiform EEG (C). The current definition of epilepsy from the International League Against Epilepsy (ILAE) includes: "(1) At least two unprovoked (or reflex) seizures occurring >24 hours apart; (2) one unprovoked (or reflex) seizure and a probability of further seizures similar to the general recurrence risk (at least 60%) after two unprovoked seizures, occurring over the next 10 years; (3) diagnosis of an epilepsy syndrome" (Fisher 2014).

References

Krumholz A, Wiebe S, Gronseth GS, et al. Evidence-based guideline: Management of an unprovoked first seizure in adults: Report of the Guideline Development Subcommittee of the American Academy of Neurology and the American Epilepsy Society. *Neurology*. 2015;84(16):1705–1713. https://doi.org/10.1212/WNL.0000000000001487

Fisher RS, Acevedo C, Arzimanoglou A, et al. A practical clinical definition of epilepsy. Epilepsia 2014;55:475–482.

Lawn ND, Pang EW, Lee J, Dunne JW. First seizure from sleep: clinical features and prognosis. Epilepsia 2023;64(10):2714–2724. https://doi.org/10.1111/epi.17712

Linked questions: 31–33

31. A 25-year-old woman with a history of depression presents to your office for follow-up of her epilepsy. Three months prior, she was admitted to the hospital following her second lifetime seizure. During admission, her habitual seizure, which consisted of the sensation of epigastric rising and behavioral cessation, was captured on video EEG with onset from the right temporal region. She was prescribed levetiracetam, which she has been taking twice a day as prescribed. Today, she reports worsening

irritability and hopelessness. Together, you and the patient decide to try a new antiseizure medication. Which medication might you recommend to your patient?

A. Valproic acid
B. Lamotrigine
C. Fenfluramine
D. Cannabidiol
E. Felbamate

Correct answer: B

Explanation

Lamotrigine is a widely used anti-seizure medication given its broad-spectrum efficacy, favorable safety profile, and potential mood benefits. Lamotrigine treats focal and generalized onset seizures. There is also low teratogenicity associated with Lamotrigine making it a preferred choice among those with childbearing potential. The main limitation is the need for a slow titration prior to reaching therapeutic levels due to dermatologic side effects. Lamotrigine acts by stabilizing voltage-dependent sodium channels, thus reducing excitability and release of excitatory neurotransmitters.

Linked question

32. For the patient in the prior question, you discuss the benefits of lamotrigine, including efficacy in focal onset epilepsy and potential for mood-stabilizing effects. The patient agrees to try it. What major risk must you counsel the patient about before beginning lamotrigine?

A. Gingival hyperplasia
B. Aplastic anemia
C. Prolongation of the PR interval
D. Stevens–Johnson Syndrome
E. Visual field constriction

Correct answer: D

Explanation

Stevens–Johnson syndrome is a potentially life-threatening skin rash that is associated with the use of lamotrigine. The highest risk is within 2–8 weeks of treatment initiation. Particular consideration is needed if a patient is also taking valproate as valproate will inhibit the metabolism of lamotrigine, thus causing increase in levels of lamotrigine and increase in the risk of toxicity. Gingival hyperplasia is a possible adverse effect of phenytoin. Aplastic anemia is a possible adverse effect of felbamate. Prolongation of the PR interval is a possible adverse effect of lacosamide. Visual field deficits have been seen with vigabatrin use.

Linked question

33. You successfully transitioned the patient in the prior question onto lamotrigine and off of levetiracetam. In

1 year, she updates you that she has become pregnant. What is your next step in management?

A. Instruct her to discontinue the medication immediately
B. Instruct her to halve the medication dosage
C. Obtain a drug level of the medication, as hormonal changes during pregnancy typically decrease concentration of lamotrigine in the blood
D. Obtain a drug level of the medication, as hormonal changes during pregnancy typically increase concentration of lamotrigine in the blood
E. Advise her to switch back to levetiracetam despite its negative effect on her mood

Correct answer: C

Explanation

During pregnancy, estrogen and progesterone induce hepatic glucuronidation, the main mechanism by which the body metabolizes lamotrigine. Women may experience an increase in lamotrigine clearance as early as 5 weeks of gestation with progressive rises in clearance into the third trimester. Given the significant risk for breakthrough seizures when levels drop, it is essential to monitor lamotrigine levels frequently throughout pregnancy.

References

Arfman IJ, Wammes-van der Heijden EA, Ter Horst PGJ, Lambrechts DA, Wegner I, Touw DJ. Therapeutic Drug Monitoring of Antiepileptic Drugs in Women with Epilepsy Before, During, and After Pregnancy. *Clin Pharmacokinet.* 2020;59(4):427–445. https://doi.org/10.1007/s40262-019-00845-2

Hilas, O., & Charneski, L. (2007). Lamotrigine-induced Stevens-Johnson syndrome. American journal of health-system pharmacy, 64(3), 273–275.

Kanner, Andres M., et al. "Practice Guideline Update Summary: Efficacy and Tolerability of the New Antiepileptic Drugs I: Treatment of New-Onset Epilepsy: Report of the Guideline Development, Dissemination, and Implementation Subcommittee of the American Academy of Neurology and the American Epilepsy Society." *Neurology*, vol. 91, no. 2, 2018, pp. 74–81, https://doi.org/10.1212/WNL.0000000000005755.

Karanam A, Pennell PB, French JA, et al. Lamotrigine clearance increases by 5 weeks gestational age: Relationship to estradiol concentrations and gestational age. *Ann Neurol.* 2018;84(4):556–563. https://doi.org/10.1002/ana.25321

Smith PEM. Initial Management of Seizure in Adults. *N Engl J Med.* 2021;385(3):251–263. https://doi.org/10.1056/NEJMcp2024526

34. Which of the following patients are possible candidates for evaluation for epilepsy surgery?

A. An adult with mesial temporal sclerosis who continues to have seizures after trying at least two appropriately selected and tolerated antiseizure medications
B. A child who is seizure-free on one anti-seizure medication but has a brain lesion in noneloquent cortex
C. A teenager currently on three anti-seizure medications with uncontrolled seizures, with no clear epileptogenic lesion on imaging, and whose genetic testing is in process
D. All of the above
E. A and B

Correct answer: D

Explanation

Referral for consideration of surgical therapy continues to be delayed. According to expert consensus, any patient who has drug-resistant epilepsy should be referred for epilepsy surgery evaluation. It is important to know the definition of drug-resistant epilepsy, which is defined by the International League Against Epilepsy as the failure to achieve sustained seizure freedom following adequate trials of two tolerated and appropriately prescribed antiseizure medications. The guidelines also recommend that a surgical referral be considered for any patient who may be seizure-free on 1–2 anti-seizure medications but has a brain lesion in a noneloquent cortex.

References

Jehi L, Jette N, Kwon CS, et al. Timing of referral to evaluate for epilepsy surgery: Expert Consensus Recommendations from the Surgical Therapies Commission of the International League Against Epilepsy. *Epilepsia.* 2022;63(10):2491–2506. https://doi.org/10.1111/epi.17350

Kwan P, Arzimanoglou A, Berg AT, et al. Definition of drug resistant epilepsy: consensus proposal by the ad hoc Task Force of the ILAE Commission on Therapeutic Strategies. *Epilepsia.* 2010;51(6):1069–1077. https://doi.org/10.1111/j.1528-1167.2009.02397.x

35. Which of the following statements regarding this EEG finding is incorrect?

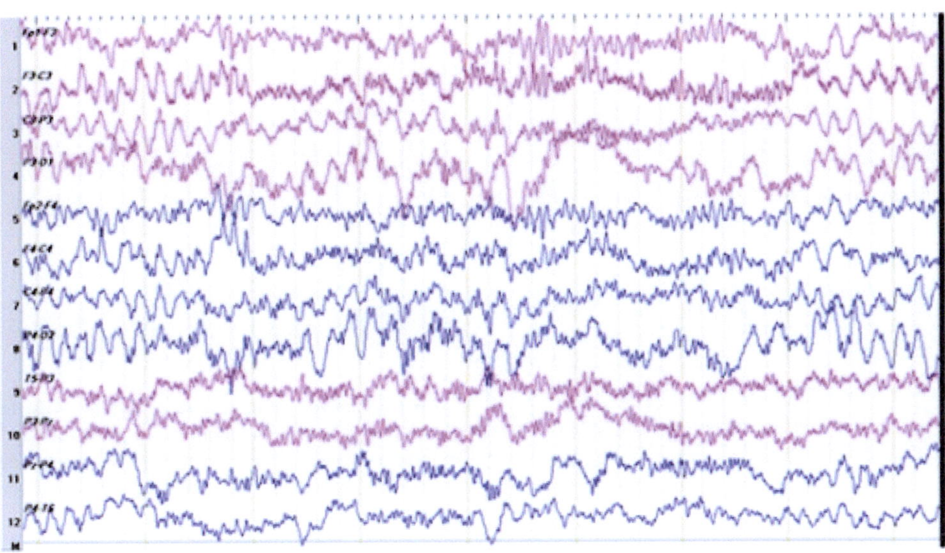

EEG during sleep. (Source: Ranasinghe et al. via *Journal of medical case reports (2015). CC-BY 4.0 (*https://creativecommons.org/licenses/by/4.0/). Image has not been modified. Please see full attribution with citation below in references section for this question.)

A. They do not correlate with cerebral development
B. They are observed primarily during stage 2 of NREM sleep
C. There is a strong association with memory consolidation
D. They are 11–16 Hz bursts that last 0.5–2 s
E. Variability in sleep is related to genetic factors

Correct answer: A

Explanation

This EEG depicts sleep spindles which are a hallmark of stage 2 non-rapid eye movement (NREM) sleep. They are characterized by 11–16 Hz bursts that last 0.5–2 s. There is a strong heritable component to sleep spindles and can reflect developmental or age-related changes.

References

Fernandez LMJ, Lüthi A. Sleep Spindles: Mechanisms and Functions. *Physiol Rev.* 2020;100(2):805–868. https://doi.org/10.1152/physrev.00042.2018

Lüthi A. Sleep Spindles: Where They Come From, What They Do. *Neuroscientist.* 2014;20(3):243–256. https://doi.org/10.1177/1073858413500854

Ranasinghe JC, Chandradasa D, Fernando S, Kodithuwakku U, Mandawala DE, Dissanayake VH. Angelman syndrome presenting with a rare seizure type in a patient with 15q11.2 deletion: a case report. *J Med Case Rep.* 2015;9:142. Published 2015 Jun 16. https://doi.org/10.1186/s13256-015-0622-8

36. A 23-year-old male presents with a history of multiple café-au-lait macules and axillary freckling. He mentions that his friends have started to tease him because he will suddenly stop responding and stare blankly with associated repetitive right hand movements. This is followed by immediate return to his normal activity. Which of the following statements is correct regarding his condition?

A. Patients with a specific NF1 mutation are at higher risk for developing epilepsy

B. The most common type of seizures in patients with NF1 are generalized tonic–clonic

C. NF1 patients with epilepsy have the same risk at developing developmental delays as those without epilepsy

D. Epilepsy in NF1 patients is most often associated with structural abnormalities including hamartomas, meningiomas, or vasculopathies

E. NF1 patients with epilepsy usually do not have any significant brain imaging findings

Correct answer: D

Explanation

The patient in the question stem has features of Neurofibromatosis type 1 (NF1), and the episode described is concerning for a focal impaired consciousness seizure. Focal onset seizures are more commonly seen in NF1 patients with epilepsy; however, generalized onset seizures may also occur. NF1 patients with epilepsy have a higher incidence of learning disorders compared to those without epilepsy. Additionally, there is no clear genotype–phenotype correlation linking a specific NF1 mutation to epilepsy risk. Most seizures in NF1 are a consequence of a structural brain abnormality such as gliomas, cortical malformations, or vascular malformations.

References

Bernardo P, Cinalli G, Santoro C. Epilepsy in NF1: a systematic review of the literature. *Childs Nerv Syst.* 2020;36(10):2333–2350. https://doi.org/10.1007/s00381-020-04710-7

Ostendorf AP, Gutmann DH, Weisenberg JL. Epilepsy in individuals with neurofibromatosis type 1. *Epilepsia.* 2013;54(10):1810–1814. https://doi.org/10.1111/epi.12348

37. A 34-year-old right-handed woman presents with a 10-year history of recurrent seizures characterized by sudden loss of awareness, unresponsiveness, and rhythmic movements of her left arm. She has tried multiple anti-seizure medications with no improvement in her seizure control. She undergoes a presurgical workup, and her MRI reveals a lesion at the right middle frontal gyrus with increased T2 signal and blurring of the gray and white junction. She undergoes surgical resection of the lesion, and the histopathology is shown below. Which of the following statements is most accurate regarding her diagnosis?

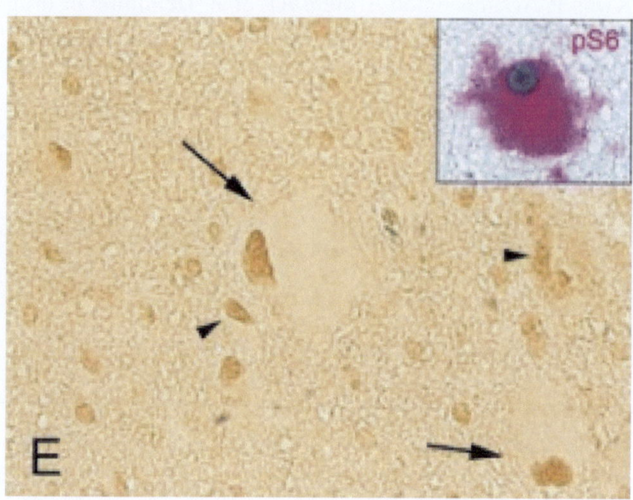

Histopathology of brain tissue. (Source: van Scheppingen et al. via Journal of Neuroinflammation. 2016. CC-BY 4.0 (https://creativecommons.org/licenses/by/4.0/). Image has been cropped to display only panel E. Please see full attribution with citation below in references section for this question.)

A. Focal cortical dysplasia (FCD) most often presents in adulthood

B. Abnormal MRI brain findings must be present to diagnose FCD

C. Surgical resection is rarely pursued in adults because seizures are usually well controlled with medications

D. The different types of FCD are characterized based on the size of the lesion

E. Balloon cells are a hallmark finding for FCD Type IIb

Correct answer: E

Explanation

Focal cortical dysplasia (FCD) is often associated with drug-resistant epilepsy. FCD is commonly diagnosed in childhood but can be found at any age. MRI of the brain can reveal a focal cortical dysplasia; however, up to 30% of FCDs may not appear on MRI. Surgical resection of the lesions can lead to improvement or resolution of seizures, though surgical outcomes depend on multiple factors. The ILAE developed a classification system of Types I, II, and III based on histologic findings. The hallmark feature of FCD Type IIb is balloon cells, which are pictured above.

References

Najm I, Lal D, Alonso Vanegas M, et al. The ILAE consensus classification of focal cortical dysplasia: An update proposed by an ad hoc task force of the ILAE diagnostic methods commission. *Epilepsia.* 2022;63(8):1899–1919. https://doi.org/10.1111/epi.17301

van Scheppingen J, Broekaart DW, Scholl T, et al. Dysregulation of the (immuno)proteasome pathway in malformations of cortical development. *J Neuroinflammation.* 2016;13(1):202. Published 2016 Aug 26. https://doi.org/10.1186/s12974-016-0662-z

38. A 37-year-old woman is waiting at a bus station when she has sudden head version followed by allover tonic and then clonic movements, falling to the ground. As the seizure does not stop after several minutes, her husband administers a medication intranasally, which aborts the seizure. Which rescue therapy did he most likely administer?
    A. Diazepam
    B. Midazolam
    C. Clonazepam
    D. Either A or B
    E. Either A or C

Correct answer: D

Explanation

The current FDA-approved intranasal rescue medications for adults are midazolam and diazepam. Recent studies have demonstrated safety and efficacy for both. Intranasal midazolam is approved for patients 12 years and older, and diazepam is approved for patients 6 years and older. The use of other benzodiazepines including intranasal formulations of lorazepam and clonazepam currently is not approved for seizure rescue therapy as their tolerability and pharmacokinetics remain under study.

References

Gidal B, Detyniecki K. Rescue therapies for seizure clusters: Pharmacology and target of treatments. *Epilepsia.* 2022;63 Suppl 1(Suppl 1):S34-S44. https://doi.org/10.1111/epi.17341

Li C, Benbadis SR. Use of new intranasal benzodiazepines at a typical adult epilepsy center. *Epilepsy Behav.* 2022;134:108867. https://doi.org/10.1016/j.yebeh.2022.108867

39. Which of the following statements best summarizes the use of a routine EEG in evaluating an adult following a first unprovoked lifetime seizure?
    A. A routine EEG should only be recommended if the neuroimaging is abnormal
    B. A routine EEG after a first lifetime seizure has high specificity and low sensitivity
    C. A routine EEG has greater diagnostic yield than an extended EEG study
    D. If the routine EEG is normal, a prolonged ambulatory EEG should not be pursued
    E. A routine EEG is not recommended after a first seizure because it rarely shows abnormalities and does not affect management

Correct answer: B

Explanation

Electroencephalogram (EEG) can help diagnose epilepsy following a seizure through the identification of interictal epileptic discharges. EEG is also necessary to classify abnormal events when seizures are in question. For a routine EEG, which is a study typically between 20 and 40 min, the specificity is high while the sensitivity is relatively low. EEG should still be pursued as part of the workup for a first lifetime seizure even when neuroimaging is normal as many patients with epilepsy do not have an identifiable epileptogenic lesion on CT scan or MRI. Prolonged EEG, such as ambulatory EEG, has a much greater diagnostic yield when compared to a routine EEG. Especially among higher-risk patients, a prolonged ambulatory EEG should be pursued if the initial routine EEG is non-diagnostic.

References

Baldin E, Hauser WA, Buchhalter JR, Hesdorffer DC, Ottman R. Yield of epileptiform electroencephalogram abnormalities in incident unprovoked seizures: a population-based study. *Epilepsia.* 2014;55(9):1389–1398. https://doi.org/10.1111/epi.12720

Burkholder DB, Britton JW, Rajasekaran V, et al. Routine vs extended outpatient EEG for the detection of interictal epileptiform discharges. *Neurology.* 2016;86(16):1524–1530. https://doi.org/10.1212/WNL.0000000000002592

Lena Bell and Dhristie Bhagat

1. What is the only triptan medication that is FDA-approved for children 6 years and older?
   A. Zolmitriptan
   B. Rizatriptan
   C. Almotriptan
   D. Sumatriptan/Naproxen
   Correct answer: B

Explanation

Rizatriptan is the only migraine treatment that that is FDA-approved for children 6 years and older. The other triptans listed are FDA-approved for patients 12 years and older.

Reference

Orr SL. Headache in Children and Adolescents. *Continuum (Minneap Minn)*. 2024;30(2):438–472. https://doi.org/10.1212/CON.0000000000001414.

2. A 7-year-old boy is brought to the neurologist due to concerns of inattention at school. Teachers report that he stares off at times and does not seem to respond for 30 s to 1 min. What is the most likely EEG finding in this patient?
   A. Generalized polyspike and wave discharges at a frequency of 3–6 Hz
   B. Slow (1.5–2.5 hz) spike and wave
   C. 3 Hz spike and wave
   D. Centrotemporal spikes
   Correct answer: C

L. Bell
Department of Neurology, NYU Langone Medical Center, New York, NY, USA
e-mail: lena.bell@nyulangone.org

D. Bhagat (✉)
Departments of Pediatrics, Ophthalmology and Neurology, Weill Cornell Medicine, NY Presbyterian Hospital, New York, NY, USA
e-mail: dhb2003@med.cornell.edu

Explanation

Patients with absence epilepsy have bilateral, symmetric 3 Hz spike-and-wave discharges during staring episodes. The EEG background is usually normal. Generalized polyspike and wave discharges at a frequency of 3–6 Hz are typical for Juvenile Myoclonic Epilepsy (JME). Slow spike-and-wave discharges (1.5–2.5 Hz) are the hallmark EEG finding in Lennox–Gastaut syndrome (LGS). Centrotemporal spikes are seen in patients with Benign Epilepsy with Centrotemporal Spikes (BECTS).

References

Pearl PL. Epilepsy Syndromes in Childhood. *Continuum (Minneap Minn)*. 2018;24(1, Child Neurology):186–209. https://doi.org/10.1212/CON.0000000000000056.

Sims KB, Peters JM, Musolino PL, et al. *Handbook of Pediatric Neurology, 1e*. Lippincott Williams & Wilkins, a Wolters Kluwer business; 2014. Accessed May 16, 2025. https://neurology.lwwhealthlibrary.com/book.aspx?bookid=2856§ionid=0.

3. An 8-month-old boy is brought to the pediatrician for evaluation of head nodding. A few times per day, his head seems to drop down for 1–2 s, and then he returns to his normal activities. The frequency has been increasing over the last few weeks, so he is referred to a neurologist. The neurologist notes no abnormalities on a thorough physical and neurologic exam, and episodes of concern are not witnessed. An EEG is obtained, which shows hypsarrhythmia. The neurologist is practicing in a resource-limited setting. What is the best first-line treatment for this condition?
   A. Vigabatrin
   B. Adrenocorticotropic hormone (ACTH)
   C. High-dose steroids (prednisolone)
   D. Levetiracetam
   E. Valproic Acid
   Correct answer: C

Explanation

The correct answer is C (high-dose steroids). The EEG shows hypsarrhythmia, the diagnostic interictal pattern seen in patients with infantile spasms. Treatment of infantile spasms includes prednisolone, ACTH, or vigabatrin. Vigabatrin has been shown to be particularly effective in children with tuberous sclerosis complex. There is no evidence to suggest that this patient has Tuberous Sclerosis (i.e., there is no mention of an "ash leaf spot" or hypomelanotic macule). In a resource-limited setting, prompt treatment initiation with prednisolone is the best option.

Reference

Pearl PL. Epilepsy Syndromes in Childhood. *Continuum (Minneap Minn)*. 2018;24(1, Child Neurology):186–209. https://doi.org/10.1212/CON.0000000000000568.

Linked questions: 4–5

4. A 15-year-old boy returns home from a party at 3 am and falls asleep. Later that morning, his parents hear a thud, run to his room to find him on the floor, jerking his arms and legs. The episode lasts 3 minutes. 911 is called, and he is admitted for EEG. What is this patient's EEG background most likely to show?
   A. 3 Hz Spike and Wave
   B. generalized 4–6 Hz spike- or polyspike-and-slow-wave activity
   C. occipital predominant multifocal spike and wave
   D. slow 1–2.5 Hz spike and wave
   Correct answer: B

Explanation

This patient most likely has Juvenile Myoclonic Epilepsy (JME). The EEG background in JME is characterized by: generalized 3–6 Hz spike- or polyspike-and-slow-wave activity. 3 Hz spike and wave is the EEG finding of absence seizures. Occipital predominant multifocal spike and wave is the hallmark EEG finding of Panayiotopoulos syndrome. Slow 1–2.5 Hz Spike-and-Wave EEG findings are characteristic of Lennox–Gaustaut Syndrome (LGS).

References

Pearl PL. Epilepsy Syndromes in Childhood. *Continuum (Minneap Minn)*. 2018;24(1, Child Neurology):186–209. https://doi.org/10.1212/CON.0000000000000568.

Sims KB, Peters JM, Musolino PL, et al. *Handbook of Pediatric Neurology, 1e*. Lippincott Williams & Wilkins, a Wolters Kluwer business; 2014. Accessed May 16, 2025. https://neurology.lwwhealthlibrary.com/book.aspx?bookid=2856§ionid=0.

Linked question

5. What is the best treatment for this condition described in the prior question?
   A. Phenytoin
   B. Carbamazepine
   C. High-dose steroids
   D. Valproic Acid
   Correct answer: D

Explanation

Valproic acid (VPA) is a good choice for this patient as it is very effective for treating seizures in patients with JME. It is important to note that VPA is a known teratogen and should be avoided in women of childbearing potential. Myoclonic seizures are WORSENED by sodium channel blockers like phenytoin and carbamazepine; thus, these should be avoided in this individual. High-dose steroids can be useful for other epilepsy syndromes like infantile spasms, Landau–Kleffner Syndrome, Electrical Status Epilepticus in Sleep (ESES), and autoimmune epilepsies, but there is limited evidence to support their role for treating JME.

References

Higdon LM. Autoimmune epilepsy. A newly recognized category of epilepsy caused by or associated with antibodies. Practical Neurology. 2025; May 15.

Pearl PL. Epilepsy Syndromes in Childhood. *Continuum (Minneap Minn)*. 2018;24(1, Child Neurology):186–209. https://doi.org/10.1212/CON.0000000000000568.

Sims KB, Peters JM, Musolino PL, et al. *Handbook of Pediatric Neurology, 1e*. Lippincott Williams & Wilkins, a Wolters Kluwer business; 2014. Accessed May 16, 2025. https://neurology.lwwhealthlibrary.com/book.aspx?bookid=2856§ionid=0.

Linked questions: 6–7

6. A 7-month-old boy, with normal development, presents with second seizure of life, characterized by shaking of left arm and left leg, after spending a warm summer day at the beach with his family. The seizure lasts 20 minutes and stops when lorazepam is administered by EMS. Two weeks prior, he had his first febrile seizure, characterized by generalized shaking of all his limbs, which stopped on its own after 2 minutes. What is the most likely genetic mutation in this patient?
   A. SCN2A
   B. SCN1A
   C. MECP2
   D. TSC2
   E. NF1
   Correct answer: B

Explanation

This patient most likely has Dravet Syndrome, a type of epilepsy syndrome that usually begins in the first year of life. It is characterized by prolonged febrile seizures (sometimes meeting criteria for status epilepticus), recurrent generalized and alternating unilateral tonic–clonic seizures. These patients are very sensitive to elevated temperatures, which can provoke additional seizures. Mutations of the SCN1A gene, a gene involved in the formation of sodium channels, are the cause of Dravet Syndrome in the vast majority of patients.

Mutations of SCN2A are associated with a variety of other epilepsy syndromes, but rarely associated with Dravet syndrome. Mutations of the MECP2 gene are the cause of Rett Syndrome. Mutations of the TSC2 gene are the cause of tuberous sclerosis complex. Mutations of the NF1 gene are the cause of neurofibromatosis type 1.

References

Pearl PL. Epilepsy Syndromes in Childhood. *Continuum (Minneap Minn)*. 2018;24(1, Child Neurology):186–209. https://doi.org/10.1212/CON.0000000000000568.

Sims KB, Peters JM, Musolino PL, et al. *Handbook of Pediatric Neurology, 1e*. Lippincott Williams & Wilkins, a Wolters Kluwer business; 2014. Accessed May 16, 2025. https://neurology.lwwhealthlibrary.com/book.aspx?bookid=2856§ionid=0.

Linked question

7. Which medication should be AVOIDED in this patient described in the prior question?
   A. Levetiracetam
   B. Phenytoin
   C. Clobazam
   D. Topiramate
   Correct answer: B

Explanation

Phenytoin, a sodium channel blocker, should be avoided in this patient with Dravet syndrome, as these agents can worsen seizures in these patients. The other agents listed have not been shown to worsen seizure frequency in Dravet Syndrome.

Reference

Pearl PL. Epilepsy Syndromes in Childhood. *Continuum (Minneap Minn)*. 2018;24(1, Child Neurology):186–209. https://doi.org/10.1212/CON.0000000000000568.

8. A 15-month-old girl with normal development, currently able to walk unassisted and able to say some words including "mama" and "dada", starts to have a developmental regression over the course of days. She stops speaking, develops an ataxic gait, diminished eye contact, and develops hand wringing movements and hand rubbing. What is the most likely mutation associated with this syndrome?
   A. MECP2
   B. SCN1A
   C. SCN2A
   D. CDKN1C
   Correct answer: A

Explanation

This patient likely has Rett Syndrome, which is characterized by developmental regression, gait abnormalities, and abnormal hand movements developing around 12–18 months. Mutation of the MECP2 gene is associated with Rett Syndrome. SCN1A is associated with Dravet syndrome, SCN2A is associated with various epilepsy syndromes, and mutations of the CDKN1C gene are associated with Beckwith–Wiedemann Syndrome, an overgrowth syndrome.

Reference

Sims KB, Peters JM, Musolino PL, et al. *Handbook of Pediatric Neurology, 1e*. Lippincott Williams & Wilkins, a Wolters Kluwer business; 2014. Accessed May 16, 2025. https://neurology.lwwhealthlibrary.com/book.aspx?bookid=2856§ionid=0.

9. The neurology team is consulted about a newborn baby who develops generalized, tonic–clonic seizures that eventually become well-controlled with phenobarbital. On exam, the patient has dysmorphic features including a long face, narrow forehead, almond-shaped eyes, and significant hypotonia. What is the most likely genetic abnormality in this patient?
   A. Partial/complete absence of maternal chromosome 15 (15q11-q13)
   B. Partial/complete absence of paternal chromosome 15 (15q11-q13)
   C. MECP2 gene mutation
   D. Trisomy 21
   E. FMR1 gene mutation
   Correct answer: B

Explanation

This patient likely has Prader–Willi syndrome, which is caused by partial/complete absence of paternal chromosome 15 (15q11-q13). These patients have certain characteristic physical features including long face, narrow forehead, almond-shaped eyes, and significant hypotonia on exam. A 2024 systematic review and meta-analysis found the prevalence of epilepsy in these patients to be approximately 11%.

Partial/complete absence of maternal chromosome 15 (15q11-q13) is associated with Angelman syndrome. MECP2 gene mutations are the primary cause of Rett Syndrome. Trisomy 21 is the cause of Down Syndrome. Fragile X syndrome is caused by a mutation in the FMR1 gene, which is located on the X chromosome.

References

Pascual-Morena C, Martínez-Vizcaíno V, Cavero-Redondo I, et al. Prevalence and genotypic associations of epilepsy in Prader-Willi Syndrome: A systematic review and meta-analysis. *Epilepsy Behav.* 2024;155:109803. https://doi.org/10.1016/j.yebeh.2024.109803.

Sims KB, Peters JM, Musolino PL, et al. *Handbook of Pediatric Neurology, 1e*. Lippincott Williams & Wilkins, a Wolters Kluwer business; 2014. Accessed May 16, 2025. https://neurology.lwwhealthlibrary.com/book.aspx?bookid=2856§ionid=0.

Linked questions: 10–14

10. A 12-year-old boy is noted to be falling asleep frequently in class. Mother notes that he falls asleep in the car abruptly on the way home from school. He becomes uncharacteristically irritable during soccer practice. Around this time, he also reports seeing shadows of monsters on the wall before he falls asleep. He also reports that he is unable to move his limbs upon waking up. This patient undergoes a polysomnogram. What will the results likely show?

    Mean sleep latency time of
    A. 11 minutes
    B. 9 minutes
    C. 6 minutes
    D. 15 minutes
    E. 32 minutes
    Correct answer: C

Explanation

This patient has clinical characteristics consistent with narcolepsy syndrome including excessive daytime sleepiness, hypnagogic (while going to sleep) hallucinations, and sleep paralysis. A sleep study (polysomnography) and daytime multiple sleep latency test (MSLT) are required to diagnose narcolepsy. Mean sleep latency (average time it takes for a person to fall asleep) of 8 min or fewer is consistent with a diagnosis of narcolepsy.

Reference

Maski K, Owens J. Pediatric Sleep Disorders. *Continuum (Minneap Minn)*. 2018;24(1, Child Neurology):210–227. https://doi.org/10.1212/CON.0000000000000566.

Linked question

11. What is the best treatment for this condition described in the prior question?
    A. Levetiracetam
    B. Serotonin–norepinephrine reuptake inhibitor
    C. Methylphenidate
    D. Selective serotonin reuptake inhibitor
    E. Tricyclic antidepressant
    Correct answer: C

Explanation

Stimulants like methylphenidate are the first-line pharmacologic treatment for pediatric narcolepsy. The other options listed are used to treat cataplexy, the sudden loss of muscle tone in response to an extreme emotion, which can be associated with narcolepsy, but there is no mention of cataplexy in this patient.

Reference

Maski K, Owens J. Pediatric Sleep Disorders. Continuum (Minneap Minn). 2018;24(1, Child Neurology):210–227. https://doi.org/10.1212/CON.0000000000000566.

Linked question

12. What would the CSF studies in this patient described in the prior question show?
    A. Low hypocretin
    B. High hypocretin
    C. Normal hypocretin
    D. Low leptin levels
    Correct answer: A

Explanation

Narcolepsy type 1 (the type of narcolepsy, which requires cataplexy for diagnosis, unlike Narcolepsy type 2, which is not associated with cataplexy) is caused by a loss of hypocretin-producing neurons in the hypothalamus, causing low CSF hypocretin levels. The relationship between CSF leptin levels and narcolepsy is less understood.

References

Maski K, Owens J. Pediatric Sleep Disorders. Continuum (Minneap Minn). 2018;24(1, Child Neurology):210–227. https://doi.org/10.1212/CON.0000000000000566.

Schuld A, Blum WF, Uhr M, et al. Reduced leptin levels in human narcolepsy. Neuroendocrinology. 2000;72(4): 195–198. https://doi.org/10.1159/000054587.

Siegel JM, Boehmer LN. Narcolepsy and the hypocretin system—where motion meets emotion. Nat Clin Pract Neurol. 2006;2(10):548–556. https://doi.org/10.1038/ncpneuro0300.

Linked question

13. The patient described in the prior question later develops episodes of falling to the ground when he is excited. Treatment for this condition includes:
    A. Selective serotonin reuptake inhibitor
    B. Serotonin–norepinephrine reuptake inhibitor
    C. Tricyclic antidepressant
    D. Sodium oxybate
    E. All the above
    Correct answer: E

Explanation

This patient likely has developed cataplexy. Treatment for cataplexy includes all of the above agents listed.

Reference

Maski K, Owens J. Pediatric Sleep Disorders. Continuum (Minneap Minn). 2018;24(1, Child Neurology):210–227. https://doi.org/10.1212/CON.0000000000000566.

Linked questions: 14–16

14. A 9-year-old girl presents with episodes of nighttime awakenings at which time she walks to her parents' room and is noted to have twitching of the left side of her face as well as drooling. This lasts approximately 1 minute. EEG is most likely to show:
    A. Hypsarrhythmia
    B. Electrical Status Epilepticus during Slow-Wave Sleep (ESES)
    C. Normal background, high-voltage sharp waves involving the centrotemporal regions
    D. Normal
    Correct answer: C

Explanation

The clinical description of these episodes is consistent with benign childhood epilepsy with centrotemporal spikes (BECTS), characterized by nocturnal episodes of seizures involving the unilateral face, characterized by twitching and drooling. Episodes are often preceded by unilateral facial paresthesia. Consciousness is usually preserved. Episodes typically last seconds to minutes. The EEG shows a normal background with sharp waves involving the centrotemporal region. Hypsarrhythmia is the EEG finding associated with infantile spasms.

Reference

Pearl PL. Epilepsy Syndromes in Childhood. *Continuum (Minneap Minn)*. 2018;24(1, Child Neurology):186–209. https://doi.org/10.1212/CON.0000000000000568.

Linked question

15. The MRI for this patient described in the prior question is most likely to show?
    A. Mesial temporal sclerosis
    B. Cortical malformation
    C. Normal
    D. Polymicrogyria
    Correct answer: C

Explanation

Most patients with BECTS have normal MRIs. The etiology is thought to be genetic, rather than structural.

Reference

Pearl PL. Epilepsy Syndromes in Childhood. *Continuum (Minneap Minn)*. 2018;24(1, Child Neurology):186–209. https://doi.org/10.1212/CON.0000000000000568.

Linked question

16. The patient described in the prior question has had a total of four lifetime episodes, though they are becoming less frequent. She has never had an episode during the day. All have been focal. What should the next step be?
    A. Start carbamazepine
    B. Start levetiracetam
    C. Watch and wait
    D. Start lamotrigine
    E. Start valproic acid
    Correct answer: C

Explanation

The prognosis of benign childhood epilepsy with centrotemporal spikes (BECTS) is excellent, with most patients achieving seizure freedom at approximately 15 years of age. The events are not interfering with patient's daily life and are becoming less frequent, and she has never had a generalized seizure; thus, it is appropriate to monitor clinically for now. All the other options listed would be appropriate considerations if the episodes become more frequent or generalize.

Reference

Pearl PL. Epilepsy Syndromes in Childhood. *Continuum (Minneap Minn)*. 2018;24(1, Child Neurology):186–209. https://doi.org/10.1212/CON.0000000000000568.

17. A 9-month-old ex-full term, developmentally appropriate infant is brought to the emergency department (ED) after episodes of generalized shaking. The first event occurred at 10 am and lasted 2 minutes, with return to baseline within 5 minutes. The second event occurred later that night at 10 pm, again lasting 2 minutes with prompt return to baseline, prompting the family to present immediately to the ED. Vitals reveal fever to 102°F, and the parent describes symptoms of cough and congestion for the past 2 days. What is the correct diagnosis?
    A. Simple febrile seizure
    B. Complex febrile seizure
    C. Dravet Syndrome
    D. Infantile Spasms
    E. Focal seizure
    Correct answer: B

Explanation

As the patient had two events in less than 24 hours, this is a complex febrile seizure. The typical age range for febrile seizures is 6 months to 5 years, and they require a fever within 24 hours before or after the seizure. Simple febrile seizures are generalized, last less than 15 minutes, and do not recur more than once in a 24-hour time period. They typically do not require further workup nor long-term anti-seizure medications.

Reference

Corsello A, Marangoni MB, Macchi M, Cozzi L, Agostoni C, Milani GP, et al. Febrile Seizures: A Systematic Review of Different Guidelines. Pediatr Neurol. 2024;155:141–8. https://doi.org/10.1016/j.pediatrneurol.2024.03.024.

18. A 5-month-old girl is referred to the neurology clinic for torticollis. On exam, you note an asymmetric very fine high-frequency, small-amplitude horizontal pendular nystagmus more in the right eye than the left eye. She also exhibits an intermittent head nod. She tracks consistently. She is otherwise developmentally appropriate, with no other medical history. What is the most likely diagnosis?
    A. Spasmus nutans
    B. Congenital myasthenic syndrome
    C. Congenital sensory nystagmus
    D. Ataxia telangiectasia
    E. Opsoclonus myoclonus syndrome
    Correct answer: A

Explanation

The classic triad of spasmus nutans is head bobbing, torticollis, and "shimmering" nystagmus that is often monocular or asymmetric. In a majority of cases, this is self-limited and resolves by 3 or 4 years of age, but rarely can be associated with intracranial lesions typically involving the optic chiasm.

Reference

Kiblinger GD, Wallace BS, Hines M, Siatkowski RM. Spasmus nutans-like nystagmus is often associated with underlying ocular, intracranial, or systemic abnormalities. J Neuroophthalmol. 2007;27(2):118–22. https://doi.org/10.1097/WNO.0b013e318067b59f.

19. A 3-month-old male infant is referred to pediatric neurology clinic after a prolonged stay in the neonatal intensive care unit due to recurrent apnea and poor feeding. He was born full-term after an uncomplicated pregnancy, but required respiratory support for several days after birth. On exam, the infant has diffuse hypotonia and subtle abnormal eye movements. His MRI brain is shown below. What is the most likely diagnosis?

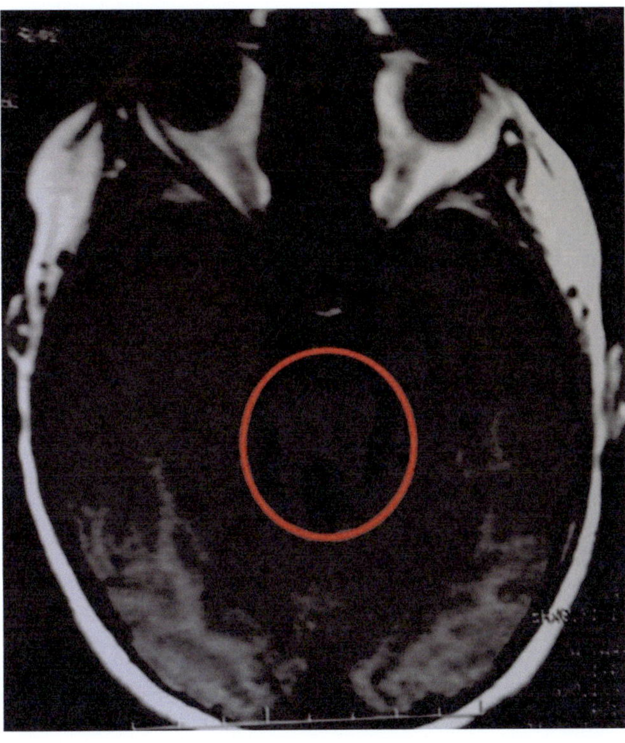

Axial MRI Brain. (Source: Roosing S, Hofree M, Kim S, et al. via Elife (2015). CC-BY 4.0 (https://creativecommons.org/licenses/by/4.0/). Image has been cropped. Please see full attribution with citation below in references section for this question)

A. Neonatal hypoxic-ischemic encephalopathy
B. Periventricular leukomalacia
C. Joubert Syndrome
D. Congenital myasthenic syndrome
E. Glycogen storage disease type II

Correct answer: C

Explanation

Joubert Syndrome often identified in the neonatal period presents with hypotonia, apnea or episodic hyperventilation, feeding difficulties, and oculomotor apraxia. The classic finding on MRI is the "molar tooth sign" due to cerebellar vermian hypoplasia.

References

Brancati F, Dallapiccola B, Valente EM. Joubert Syndrome and related disorders. Orphanet Journal of Rare Diseases. 2010;5:20.

Ghongade D, Moorthy S, Sreekumar KP, Prabhu NK. Neuroradiology. Indian J Radiol Imaging. 2008;18(1):96–98. https://doi.org/10.4103/0971-3026.38512.

Roosing S, Hofree M, Kim S, et al. Functional genome-wide siRNA screen identifies KIAA0586 as mutated in Joubert syndrome. Elife. 2015;4:e06602. Published 2015 May 30. https://doi.org/10.7554/eLife.06602.

20. A 4-month-old male infant ex-full-term born to a first-time mother with gestational diabetes but otherwise uncomplicated perinatal course, with a history of failure to thrive, is referred by his pediatrician for abnormal eye movements. Neurologic exam reveals nystagmus, and fundoscopic exam is concerning for bilateral optic nerve hypoplasia. Imaging reveals absence of the septum pellucidum. What is the best next step in management?
    A. Referral to pediatric endocrinology
    B. Referral to genetics
    C. Referral to pediatric ophthalmology
    D. Referral to occupational therapy
    E. Referral to nutrition

Correct answer: A

Explanation

Optic nerve hypoplasia with absence of a septum pellucidum is consistent with septo-optic dysplasia, more commonly seen in infants of first-time young mothers and those with gestational diabetes. This can be associated with other midline malformations and hypopituitarism. While referral to ophthalmology would be helpful in assessing visual function, and genetics would be helpful in testing for an underlying genetic mutation, endocrinology evaluation is most time-sensitive. Hypothyroidism is of particular concern, as this can lead to loss of IQ points monthly.

Reference

Gaitanis J, Tarui T. Nervous System Malformations. Continuum (Minneap Minn). 2018;24(1, Child Neurology):72–95. https://doi.org/10.1212/con.0000000000000561.

21. A 9-year-old girl presents to the emergency room with new morning headaches and vomiting. On exam, you note papilledema and a partial right cranial nerve 6 palsy, prompting imaging. An MRI brain reveals large heterogeneous enhancing cerebellar mass, with diffusion restriction. Which of the following features is most likely to be seen on pathology?
    A. Rosenthal fibers
    B. Homer-Wright rosettes
    C. True ependymal rosettes
    D. Pineocytomatous rosettes
    E. Plump keratin

Correct answer: B

Explanation

Medulloblastoma is a common pediatric infratentorial tumor, with heterogeneous enhancement and diffusion restriction on MRI. Pathology will reveal Homer-Wright rosettes. Pilocytic astrocytoma are also infratentorial; however, they do not classically diffusion restrict on imaging, and pathology would show Rosenthal fibers.

Reference

Wells EM, Packer RJ. Pediatric brain tumors. Continuum (Minneap Minn). 2015;21(2 Neuro-oncology):373–96. https://doi.org/10.1212/01.CON.0000464176.96311.d1.

22. A 7-month-old boy with macrocephaly and global developmental delay presents with refractory seizures and developmental regression. His neurologic exam is notable for diffuse spasticity in all four limbs. An MRI of the brain reveals symmetric T2 hyperintensity in the anterior white matter, involving the subcortical U-fibers. A mutation in which of the following genes is likely responsible for his presentation?
    A. GFAP
    B. ASPA
    C. ARSA
    D. PLP-1
    E. ABCD1
    Correct answer: A

Explanation

Infantile form Alexander disease typically presents before the age of 2, with megalencephaly, developmental delay or regression, refractory seizures, and spasticity. Imaging will reveal anterior white matter abnormalities involving the U-fibers, and pathology shows Rosenthal fibers within astrocytes—especially surrounding blood vessels. The underlying genetic mutation is within the GFAP gene.

Reference

Kuhn J, Cascella M. Alexander Disease. StatPearls. Treasure Island (FL): StatPearls Publishing Copyright © 2025, StatPearls Publishing LLC.; 2025.

23. A 7-month-old boy presents to the emergency department for increasing frequency of abnormal movements typically occurring upon falling asleep or waking up. Parents show you videos revealing stereotyped episodes of bilateral arm extension and neck flexion, clustering up to 15 times in a row. His past medical history and family history are unremarkable. Upon admission, video EEG shows a high-voltage, chaotic, disorganized background. The episodes of abnormal movements are also captured

on EEG—what is the most likely electrographic pattern correlate?
    A. 4–6 Hz generalized polyspike and wave
    B. Electrodecrement
    C. Delta brush
    D. 3 Hz generalized spike and wave
    E. Lateralized periodic discharges
    Correct answer: B

Explanation

This patient's presentation is consistent with infantile spasms, which typically present initially between 3 and 8 months of age. They are brief stereotyped movements that tend to cluster around waking and falling asleep, eventually leading to developmental regression if left untreated. The classic EEG background is hypsarrhythmia, high voltage, and disorganized, with generalized electrodecrement during spasms.

Reference

Hussain SA. Epileptic Encephalopathies. Continuum (Minneap Minn). 2018;24(1, Child Neurology):171–85. https://doi.org/10.1212/con.0000000000000558.

24. A 6-month-old boy presents with infantile spasms and recent developmental regression. Physical exam is notable for multiple hypopigmented macules visible under a Woods Lamp and hypotonia. An MRI brain is completed, revealing multiple subependymal nodules and cortical tubers. Which of the following screening tests is recommended?
    A. Hearing test
    B. Scoliosis screening
    C. Echocardiogram
    D. MRA
    E. Electromyography
    Correct answer: C

Explanation

This patient's hypopigmented skin findings, infantile spasms, and subependymal nodules and cortical tubers on imaging are consistent with tuberous sclerosis—a genetic multisystem syndrome arising from a mutation in the TSC1 or TSC2 gene. It is associated with cardiac rhabdomyomas, and thus, patients should have a screening echocardiogram especially if presenting under the age of 3. Other major features include angiofibromas, ungual fibromas, retinal hamartomas, subependymal giant cell astrocytomas, and angiomyolipomas.

Reference

Northrup H, Aronow ME, Bebin EM, Bissler J, Darling TN, de Vries PJ, et al. Updated International Tuberous Sclerosis Complex Diagnostic Criteria and Surveillance and Management Recommendations. Pediatr Neurol. 2021;123:50–66. https://doi.org/10.1016/j. pediatrneurol.2021.07.011.

25. A 6-year-old boy with a past medical history of ADHD and learning disability is referred for innumerable cafe au lait macules, the largest of which is 6 mm. His exam is notable for axillary freckling, and on chart review, his ophthalmologist noted Lisch nodules and choroidal abnormalities. Genetic testing would likely reveal a mutation on which chromosome?
    A. Chromosome 22
    B. Chromosome 17
    C. Chromosome 9
    D. Chromosome 15
    E. Chromosome 21
    Correct answer: B

Explanation
This patient meets the diagnostic criteria for neurofibromatosis type 1, caused by mutation in the NF1 gene on chromosome 17 encoding for neurofibromin. Familial cases are inherited in an autosomal dominant pattern, though approximately 50% of cases are sporadic.

Reference
Rosser T. Neurocutaneous Disorders. Continuum (Minneap Minn). 2018;24(1, Child Neurology):96–129. https://doi. org/10.1212/con.0000000000000562.

26. A 5-year-old girl who was previously healthy and developmentally appropriate presents with sudden speech regression. The family describes an increasing frequency of episodic behavioral arrest during which she is unresponsive, lasting less than 1 minute each time. Her neurologic exam is notable for difficulty following two-step commands, decreased vocabulary, and no other focal findings. An EEG reveals generalized spike-wave discharges. What is the most likely diagnosis?
    A. Autism Spectrum Disorder
    B. West Syndrome
    C. Rett Syndrome
    D. Stroke
    E. Landau–Kleffner Syndrome
    Correct Answer: E

Explanation
Landau–Kleffner Syndrome is a childhood-onset acquired epileptic aphasia, typically presenting between ages 3 and 8 years old with seizures and language regression. EEG characteristically demonstrates spike-wave discharges, and patients can have absence seizures or generalized tonic–clonic seizures more often during sleep.

Reference
Caraballo RH, Cejas N, Chamorro N, Kaltenmeier MC, Fortini S, Soprano AM. Landau-Kleffner syndrome: a study of 29 patients. Seizure. 2014;23(2):98–104. https:// doi.org/10.1016/j.seizure.2013.09.016.

27. A 3-year-old previously healthy girl presents with new speech regression. On exam, she has abnormal hand flapping and wringing movements near her face. Her parents note her first words were around 16 months—however, she has no verbal output during the appointment. What genetic mutation is the likely cause of her condition?
    A. SCN1A
    B. UBE3A
    C. GRIN2A
    D. MECP2
    E. SLC6A1
    Correct answer: D

Explanation
Rett Syndrome mostly affects females and presents with developmental regression, repetitive hand-wringing motions, cognitive impairments, and seizures. It is primarily caused by mutations in the MECP2 gene, encoding for the methyl-CpG-binding protein 2.

Reference
Ivy AS, Standridge SM. Rett Syndrome: A Timely Review From Recognition to Current Clinical Approaches and Clinical Study Updates. Semin Pediatr Neurol. 2021;37:100881. https://doi.org/10.1016/j. spen.2021.100881.

28. A 13-year-old boy with a past medical history of childhood-onset diabetes and scoliosis presents to your clinic with trouble walking. His exam reveals dysmetria on finger-to-nose testing, ataxic wide-based gait, decreased vibration and proprioception on sensory testing, and hyporeflexia. His eye movements are normal. Further workup reveals hypertrophic cardiomyopathy. A mutation in which gene is responsible for this patient's underlying condition?
    A. ATM
    B. PHYH
    C. CACNA1A
    D. FMR1
    E. FXN
    Correct answer: E

Explanation

This patient has Friedreich Ataxia, a hereditary ataxia caused by a trinucleotide expansion GAA in the FXN gene coding for frataxin, on chromosome 9q13. It typically presents with progressive ataxia, loss of reflexes, weakness, and posterior column spinal cord dysfunction. Age of onset is most often between 8 and 14 years old. It is associated with childhood onset diabetes, hypertrophic cardiomyopathy, and scoliosis.

Reference

Coarelli G, Wirth T, Tranchant C, Koenig M, Durr A, Anheim M. The inherited cerebellar ataxias: an update. J Neurol. 2023;270(1):208–22. https://doi.org/10.1007/s00415-022-11383-6.

29. A 6-month-old infant with a past medical history of jaundice is referred to your clinic for microcephaly and developmental delay. He was born full-term, but parents recall that he failed his newborn hearing screen; repeat testing was recommended but never scheduled. He has poor head control, inconsistent fix and follow on vision testing. His head circumference is at the 2nd percentile for his age. Blood work shows transaminitis. What is a likely characteristic finding on MRI brain for this patient?
    A. Periventricular calcifications
    B. Agenesis of the corpus callosum
    C. Basal ganglia calcifications
    D. Cortical atrophy
    E. Diffuse white matter abnormalities sparing the U-fibers

    Correct answer: A

Explanation

This presentation is consistent with congenital cytomegalovirus (CMV) infection. Clinical hallmarks can include microcephaly, sensorineural hearing loss, developmental delay, visual impairment with chorioretinitis, and hepatomegaly with transaminitis and jaundice. MRI can classically reveal periventricular calcifications, ventriculomegaly, and periventricular subependymal cysts in areas of focal necrosis.

Reference

Patel P. Congenital Infections of the Nervous System. Continuum (Minneap Minn). 2021;27(4):1105–26. https://doi.org/10.1212/con.0000000000000991.

30. An 8-year-old boy presents to your office for abnormal movements. For the past several months, multiple times per day, he has had a head jerk to the right. His mom notes for approximately 1 year prior to this, he used to blink repetitively throughout the day, although this has resolved. In the exam room, you note intermittent throat clearing from the patient with no other infectious symptoms. The patient describes these movements and sounds as voluntary, but something he has to do to feel more comfortable. His friends are beginning to notice, and rarely this will disrupt his classroom. What is the best first-line treatment for this?
    A. Cognitive behavioral therapy
    B. Clonidine
    C. Guanfacine
    D. Levetiracetam
    E. Oxcarbazepine

    Correct answer: A

Explanation

Motor and vocal tics for over a year are consistent with Tourette Syndrome. Most children will grow out of tics over time, and they do not need to be treated unless they are bothersome to the child. First-line treatment is cognitive behavioral therapy.

Reference

O'Malley JA. Diagnosing Common Movement Disorders in Children. Continuum (Minneap Minn). 2022;28(5):1476–519. https://doi.org/10.1212/con.0000000001187.

31. A 12-year-old boy with past medical history of short stature is referred by his pediatrician for generalized weakness. On exam, you note bilateral ptosis and restricted extra-ocular movements. An eventual muscle biopsy reveals ragged red fibers on trichrome stain. Which of the following screening tests should this patient receive?
    A. MRI brain with and without contrast
    B. MRA head and neck with and without contrast
    C. EEG
    D. ECG
    E. EMG

    Correct answer: D

Explanation

This patient has Kearns–Sayre syndrome, a mitochondrial disorder with onset before the age of 20 classically presenting with progressive external ophthalmoplegia. It is associated with short stature, cerebellar ataxia, pigmentary retinopathy, and complete heart block often requiring a pacemaker.

Reference

Shemesh A, Margolin E. Kearns-Sayre Syndrome. StatPearls. Treasure Island (FL): StatPearls Publishing Copyright © 2025, StatPearls Publishing LLC.; 2025.

Index